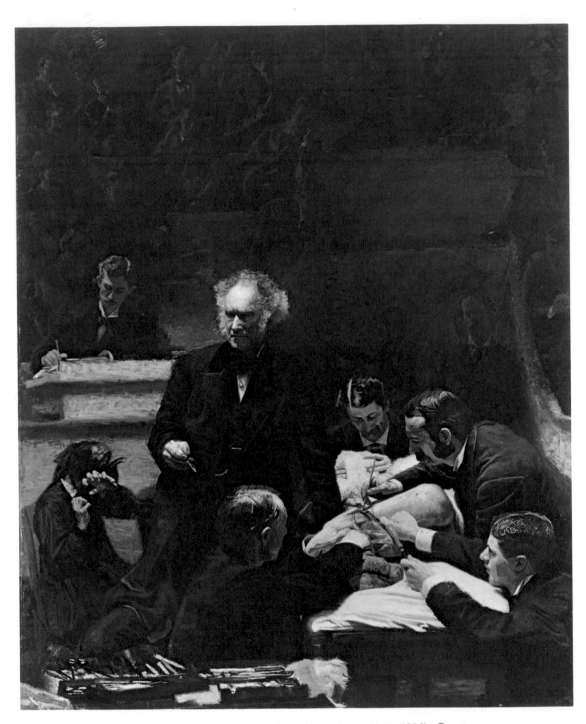

The Gross Clinic by Thomas Eakins (American, 1844–1916). Courtesy of Thomas Jefferson University, Philadelphia.

Two Centuries

of

American Medicine

1776
1976

JAMES BORDLEY, III, M.D.

Director Emeritus, Mary Imogene Bassett Hospital,
Cooperstown, New York; Clinical Professor of Medicine (Retired),
Columbia University College of Physicians and Surgeons;
Clinical Professor of Medicine, Albany Medical College

A. McGEHEE HARVEY, M.D.

Distinguished Service Professor of Medicine,
The Johns Hopkins University School of Medicine

W. B. SAUNDERS COMPANY · PHILADELPHIA · LONDON · TORONTO

W. B. Saunders Company: West Washington Square
Philadelphia, PA 19105

1 St. Anne's Road
Eastbourne, East Sussex BN21 3UN, England

1 Goldthorne Avenue
Toronto, Ontario M8Z 5T9, Canada

Library of Congress Cataloging in Publication Data

Bordley, James, 1900–

Two centuries of American medicine, 1776–1976.

Bibliography: p.

Includes index.

1. Medicine—United States—History.   I. Harvey, Abner
   McGehee, 1911–   joint author.   II. Title. [DNLM:
   1. History of medicine, Modern—United States WZ70
   AA1 B6t]

R151.B58   610'.973   75–19841

ISBN 0–7216–1873–1

Two Centuries of American Medicine   ISBN   0–7216–1873–1

Last digit is the print number: 9   8   7   6   5   4   3   2

DEDICATION

This book is dedicated to our wives
with gratitude for their patience
and never-failing support.

More than uncommonly incurious must be he who would not find delight in stemming the stream of ages; returning to times long past, and beholding the state of things and men.

(James Smithson: An examination of Egyptian colors. Annals of Philosophy 7:115, 1824)

Preface

To confine a comprehensive history of American medicine between the covers of a single volume would be an impossible task. Our purpose has been a more modest one: to relate in language that can be understood by the interested layman, as well as the physician, an account of the extraordinary advances in medical education and in the prevention and treatment of disease that have taken place during the two centuries of this nation's political independence (1776 to 1976). Most of the advances have occurred during the second of these centuries. In the first century of American history, the role of the physician was that of the Good Samaritan. His success depended upon his sympathy, his humanity, and his art. Lacking a scientific base, his therapy for the more serious maladies was founded upon false hypotheses and fanciful systems and was for the most part ineffective.

In the latter half of the nation's first century, scientific methods began to influence the development of medicine in Europe. Though the leading physicians in this country were familiar with what was happening abroad, medical education in the United States was then in such a deplorable state that the new developments had almost no effect upon the many young men who were entering practice each year. The one momentous American contribution to the advance was the introduction of surgical anesthesia.

In the 1870s, as the first century was giving way to the second, the seeds were sown for a forward movement. This was a period of fruitful transition for both medical education and medical science. The period also saw the introduction of technical developments that were to have a profound effect upon medical research and medical practice.

In the early years of the nation's second century, American medicine was engaged in improving its scientific base and in developing medical schools that could prepare and motivate those who were to build upon the new foundation. Laboratories for bacteriology, pathology, physiology, and pharmacology became essential features of medical schools. They were utilized for both teaching and research. Hospitals, which became the locus of clinical instruction in medicine and surgery, developed closer ties with those schools whose students they were serving, and the training of interns and residents became a responsibility of the medical school faculties. Many of the medical colleges of the earlier century, having neither the facilities nor the funds to keep pace with the new developments, gradually were forced out of existence.

The reorientation of medicine on a solid scientific base and the widely publicized discoveries of the specific causes of some of the most dreaded diseases aroused increasing public interest. After a century of decline in the eyes of the public, the medical profession within a few decades had become estimable and surprisingly productive. The future seemed so full of promise, as the twentieth century opened, that a succession of wealthy, public-spirited individuals began to contribute substantial sums of money for the support of medical education and medical research. In order to use these funds to the best advantage and to assimilate and apply the mass of new medical knowledge that was accumulating rapidly in this country and elsewhere, both medical practitioners and medical researchers had to become specialists in restricted fields. Otherwise they would have been submerged in the torrent of information. During the first century, the American practitioner had prided himself on being a jack-of-all-medical-trades, but by the middle of the second century he realized that for some of his sickest patients, precise diagnosis and adequate treatment could be accomplished only by specialists. The same was true of the research worker, who found it necessary to focus his attention on specialized scientific literature and to become expert in the use of special techniques.

After World War II, massive financial support for medical research came from the federal government. The atomic bomb had been developed by unlimited funding of nuclear research, and the belief became prevalent that in order to conquer the remaining great killer-diseases, such as cancer, cardiovascular disease, and kidney disease, it was necessary only to allocate huge sums to medical research. So much emphasis and so much money were devoted to research that medical education and medical care were relatively neglected at a time when both of these attributes of medicine were increasing almost prohibitively in cost. As a result of the concentration upon research, much new and valuable knowledge was acquired, and new forms of therapy were devised, but as the second century reached its end, the major killer-diseases were still unconquered. In the last decade of the nation's second century, the federal government shifted its principal emphasis, in the domain of medicine, from support of research to support of the planning and delivery of health services. A nagging residual question that can only be answered by future experience is whether medical care of the high quality made possible by a century of extraordinary progress in medical science can be delivered to the entire population at a level of funding, whether by taxation or insurance, that the public can afford and will tolerate.

The history of politics and government has been characterized by alternating periods of progression and retrogression; it undulates forward without, for any extended period, reaching higher ground; seeming never to learn from its failures nor to build upon its successes. The history of the United States has been no exception in this regard: our politico-governmental institutions are no better and perhaps are worse than they were when the Constitution was adopted in 1787. Science, on the other hand, moves forward by building on its successes; when it has reached higher ground, it maintains its height until new discoveries compel the next ascent. Since discoveries multiply and lead to other discoveries, science grows exponentially. This trend is clearly illustrated by the progress of medical science in the United States.

George Rosen* has observed that medical science in its historical development has advanced in a series of "explosion phenomena": after a

---

*Rosen, G.: Critical levels in historical process—a theoretical exploration dedicated to Henry Ernest Sigerist. J. Hist. Med. *13*:179, 1958.

period of relative quiescence, there is a gradual build-up to a critical level at which the explosion occurs. As examples, he cites: (1) The quiet build-up of bacteriology, which reached a critical level at about 1880, followed by the explosive discovery of the bacterial causes of many diseases within the span of little more than a decade. (2) The gradual growth of knowledge about nutrition, reaching a critical level at about 1910, followed by the explosive discovery of vitamins. In writing this history, we have dwelt upon these critical episodes in the progress of medicine. This was comparatively easy until about 1940, since the explosion phenomena followed one another with relatively little overlapping. But after World War II, a number of unusually violent explosions occurred almost simultaneously. For this reason, the treatment of medical research in Part III differs from that in Parts I and II: certain areas were selected for a more detailed account of the build-up to the critical level for each of several explosions. The chapters on Enzymes and Hormones, Medical Genetics, Immunology, Virology, and Cancer are of this type. As the story unfolds in each of these chapters, it becomes apparant that in spite of their disparate titles, it is not easy to tell where one begins and the other ends. Indeed, it was difficult for us to decide in which order the chapters should be presented; however they were arranged, the early chapters lacked information that came to light only in subsequent chapters. The theme which is common to all of them is molecular biology, which packs a detonating power whose full force is yet to be felt.

Throughout the book, but particularly in the sections describing the second century, space limitations forced us to make decisions, sometimes onerous ones, about what should be included and what should be left out. Our selection of material was guided by a desire to illustrate how the United States, in its two centuries of political independence, had progressed from a follower to a leader in medical education and medical research and to focus attention upon the principal events that were responsible for the change. We are aware that personal bias has influenced the selective process and that we unavoidably lay ourselves open to criticism for both misplaced emphasis and conspicuous omissions.

Our friend Owsei Temkin, who read part of the manuscript with the practiced eye of a professional medical historian, has pointed out that in our preoccupation with those developments that have led to improvements in the state of medicine, we have viewed medical history in the light of what we do now, emphasizing the extremes of what is far away from or what is near to our preferred way of doing things. As a result, we leave out of our account developments and personalities that the professional historian might consider important though they have not contributed to what we look upon as progress. We agree that this is fair criticism and that our readers should be forewarned of this aspect of our personal bias.

JAMES BORDLEY, III
A. McGEHEE HARVEY

April, 1976

Acknowledgments

John Romano furnished us with material helpful in the preparation of the chapter on psychiatry. Mrs. Monroe A. McIver loaned us some rare volumes relating to her ancestor, Dr. James Jackson, and the early years of the Massachusetts General Hospital.

Carol Bocchini of Baltimore, in addition to helping with the preparation of the manuscript, gave valuable assistance in carrying out research for portions of several chapters. We are also grateful to Patricia Fisher King of Baltimore and Amy Shapiro of the W. B. Saunders Company for their help in preparing and editing the mansucript.

The following offered helpful criticisms of portions of the manuscript: Paul Fenimore Cooper, Jr., John Eager Howard, John Imboden, Louis C. Jones, Boyd Lewis, Victor A. McKusick, Vernon Mountcastle, Daniel Nathans, Philip Norman, Albert Owens, Theodore Peters, Jr., Owsei Temkin.

We wish to thank the following for library assistance and the acquisition of photographs: Lucinda Keister of the National Library of Medicine; Ursula Poland, Librarian of the Albany Medical Center; and Ann L. Slocum, Medical Librarian of The Mary Imogene Bassett Hospital.

To John L. Dusseau and John J. Hanley of the W. B. Saunders Company we owe special thanks for their encouragement and advice.

Contents

xiii

PART THREE

Period of Explosive Growth–1946-1976

Because it deals with the vital interest of both indi-viduals and societies—with life and death, and with so much that matters in between—medicine has long had an unusually complex and intimate rela-tionship to social and cultural developments at large.... In other words, medical history involves social and economic as well as biologic content and presents one of the central themes in human ex-perience. After all, what is more basic in the life of any people than life itself?

Richard Harrison Shryock

PART ONE

The
First
Century–1776-1876

I

Introduction

I have lived myself to see the disciples of Hoffman, Boerhaave, Stahl, Cullen, Brown, succeed one another like the shifting figures of a magic lantern, & their fancies, like the dresses of the annual doll-babies from Paris, becoming, from their novelty, the vogue of the day, and yielding to the next novelty their ephemeral favor. The patient, treated on the fashionable theory, sometimes gets well in spite of the medicine.

(Thomas Jefferson to Dr. Caspar Wistar, 1807)

On March 4, 1797, George Washington turned over the reins of government to his successor, John Adams, and retired to his Virginia plantation, Mount Vernon. He was then 65 years old and still in such vigorous health that he resumed enthusiastically the strenuous life of a planter. "Agriculture," he said, "has ever been the most favourite amusement of my life . . . I begin my diurnal course with the sun; I mount my horse and ride round my farms until it is time to dress for dinner" (Blanton, 1933).

On December 12, 1799, according to his devoted secretary, Colonel Lear, Washington "rode abroad on his plantation from ten o'clock in the morning until three o'clock in the afternoon and the weather was very bad, rain, hail and snow falling alternately, with a cold wind." When he returned home, it was observed "that his neck appeared wet and that snow was hanging from his hair." On the morning of December 13, "he complained of a sore throat and remained indoors, but in the afternoon ventured out in the snow to mark some trees which he wished felled; upon his return it was noticed that he had developed a hoarseness, which increased in the evening, but he made light of it. He spent the evening reading the papers and when he met anything interesting, he read it as loud as his hoarseness would permit." Twenty-four hours later, Washington was dead.

The events that led up to his death were reported in the following let-

3

ter, which appeared in the local newspaper, the *Times* of Alexandria, Virginia, on December 19, 1799:

Messrs. J. and D. Westcott.

Presuming that some account of the late illness and death of General Washington will be generally interesting, and particularly so to the Professors and Practitioners of Medicine throughout America, we request you to publish the following statement.

Sometime in the night of Friday the 13th inst., having been exposed to rain on the preceding day, General Washington was attacked with an inflammatory affection of the upper part of the windpipe, called in technical language, cynanche trachealis. The disease commenced with a violent ague, accompanied with some pain in the upper and fore part of the throat, a sense of stricture in the same part, a cough, and a difficult rather than painful deglutition [swallowing], which were soon succeeded by fever and a quick and laborious respiration. The necessity of blood-letting suggesting itself to the General, he procured a bleeder in the neighborhood, who took from the arm, in the night, twelve or fourteen ounces of blood; he would not by any means be prevailed upon by the family to send for the attending physician till the following morning, who arrived at Mount Vernon at eleven o'clock on Saturday morning. Discovering the case to be highly alarming and foreseeing the fatal tendency of the disease, two consulting physicians were immediately sent for, who arrived, one at half past three and the other at four in the afternoon. In the interim were employed two copious bleedings; a blister was applied to the part affected, two moderate doses of calomel were given, and an injection was administered which operated on the lower intestines, but all without any perceptible advantage, the respiration becoming still more difficult and distressing. Upon the arrival of the first of the consulting physicians, it was agreed, as there were yet no signs of accumulation in the bronchial vessels of the lungs, to try the result of another bleeding, when about thirty-two ounces were drawn, without the smallest apparent alleviation of the disease. Vapors of vinegar and water were frequently inhaled, ten grains of calomel were given, succeeded by repeated doses of emetic tartar, amounting in all to five or six grains, with no other effect than a copious discharge from the bowels. The powers of life seemed now manifestly yielding to the force of the disorder. Blisters were applied to the extremities, together with a cataplasm of bran and vinegar to the throat. Speaking, which was painful from the beginning, now became almost impracticable, respiration grew more and more contracted and imperfect, till half after eleven o'clock on Saturday night, when, retaining the full possession of his intellect, he expired without struggle.

[Final two paragraphs of letter omitted.]

(Signed) James Craik, Attending Physician
Elisha C. Dick, Consulting Physician

The signature of Doctor Gustavus Brown of Port Tobacco, who attended as consulting physician, on account of the remoteness of his residence from the place, has not been procured to the foregoing.

Washington's last illness and its management serve to epitomize the state of medicine in the final quarter of the eighteenth century. Theories differed as to the nature of disease, but no major advances had been made beyond the ancient concepts of humoral pathology. Latin was still the official language of the European schools of medicine, and at the College of Philadelphia candidates for the medical degree were not given the option of writing their theses in English until 1789.

Diagnosis at that time depended largely on what one could see, hear, or feel in superficial observation of the patient. For example, *cynanche tra-chealis*, which was said to have caused Washington's death (the modern equivalent is laryngitis or croup, which in Washington's case may have been due to an acute streptococcal infection), was defined by Cullen in 1778 as "an inflammation of the glottis, larynx, or upper part of the trachea known by a peculiar croaking sound in the voice, by difficult respiration, with a sense of straightening about the larynx and by an attending pyrexia—and frequently produces such an obstruction of the air as suffocates and thereby proves suddenly fatal" (Lewis, 1932).

To make such a diagnosis one had only to stand by and watch the illness progress from hoarseness to suffocation. There is nothing to indicate that any of the attending physicians examined Washington beyond feeling his pulse and touching his skin in order to estimate the degree of fever. No mention is made of an examination of the throat or chest. All of the other observations could have been made from the foot of the bed. The failure to do more than this was not due to lack of training or competence on the part of the attending physicians, but rather it was due in part to the prevailing attitude toward disease and in part to the lack of adequate tools and techniques for diagnosis. Without having been taught the technique of percussion, and possessing neither thermometer, stethoscope, nor laryngeal mirror, one could not go far toward determining the cause of difficulty in breathing.

Though many of the physicians in Washington's day lacked adequate education and training, the three who attended him had received the best medical education that could be obtained in that era. Craik and Brown had studied at the renowned University of Edinburgh, and Dick was a graduate of the foremost American school, the Medical College of Philadelphia. If Benjamin Rush, America's most prominent physician of the 1790s, had been called in for consultation he would without question have approved both the diagnosis and the treatment.

During the first half of the nineteenth century, the medical profession in Europe, rising above the constraints imposed by fanciful theories, began to reassess its heritage and to combine the best of the past with the beginnings of a new clinical science. By closer and more critical observation of patients, by statistical analysis of the signs and symptoms of disease, and by correlation of clinical and autopsy findings, it became possible gradually to differentiate one disease from another. The first major advances were made in France and in the British Isles. Among the persons who played leading roles were Bichat, Corvisart, Laennec, Bretonneau, Bouillaud, and Louis in France; Addison, Bright, Hodgkin, and Parkinson in England; and Graves, Adams, Stokes, and Corrigan in Ireland. The names of many of these men have become attached to the diseases or manifestations of disease that they differentiated and characterized.

To appreciate the great progress that was made during the nation's first hundred years toward a better understanding of disease, one has only to read the series of lectures given to the medical students in Paris in the mid-1860s by the great French physician Armand Trousseau (*Lectures on Clinical Medicine*, 1868). His description of the clinical manifestations of such diseases as scarlet fever, diphtheria, rabies, typhoid fever, tetanus, the contagious diseases of childhood, and many others can scarcely be surpassed

5

today. Moreover, Trousseau manifested a freshness of outlook, an inquisitiveness, and a lack of dogmatism that were virtually unknown among the physicians of Rush's day. The extent to which some of the leaders of American medicine had moved in the same direction can be appreciated by reading the 1868 edition of Austin Flint's *Treatise on the Principles and Practice of Medicine*.

In addition to the advances in clinical medicine, there were revolutionary developments in the sciences basic to medicine (anatomy, physiology, biochemistry, pathology), particularly during the period 1840 to 1876. In Germany, Virchow and his colleagues had developed the science of cellular (microscopic) pathology and thereby had thrown much new light on the cellular abnormalities underlying disease. There had also been great progress in chemistry, particularly organic and physiological chemistry. Some crude, disease-related chemical analyses of blood and urine had been undertaken. Exciting discoveries in the field of experimental physiology were being made in France by Claude Bernard and his successor, Brown-Séquard, and by Johannes Müller, Helmholtz, and Karl Ludwig in Germany. Louis Pasteur in Paris and Robert Koch in Germany had created the science of bacteriology and had pointed the way for Joseph Lister's introduction of antiseptic surgery in Scotland. In 1876, as the first century of the American republic came to an end, Koch reported the isolation and cultivation of the anthrax bacillus, the first comprehensive identification of a bacterium causing a specific human disease.

Many of the advances in clinical medicine would not have been possible without the availability of new techniques such as percussion (tapping) of the chest and auscultation (listening through a stethoscope) and new diagnostic tools, including the clinical thermometer, the stethoscope, the ophthalmoscope, and the laryngeal mirror. Likewise, advances in cellular pathology would have been severely limited had not the microscope been improved by the development of achromatic lenses and compound objectives, which enhanced the resolving power and the practical utility of this instrument.

The better trained American physicians, particularly those who went abroad for all or part of their medical education, kept abreast of the new developments. However, the advances in the sciences basic to medicine had little impact upon medical practice or medical education in this country. American medical education was also deficient in clinical instruction. Students learned their medicine chiefly from books and lectures and had little or no experience at the bedside or in the autopsy room, though some had the privilege of visiting the patients cared for by their preceptor. Instruction of the type which could be obtained at the Hôpital de la Pitié and the Hôtel Dieu in Paris, Guy's Hospital in London, Meath Hospital in Dublin, and somewhat later in the great clinics of Germany and Austria, was nowhere available in the United States. It should be added, however, that though the average European physician was better educated, had a better understanding of scientific principles, and was more skilled in the differentiation of diseases, the therapy he offered was little better than that of his American counterpart, owing to the facts that the specific causes of disease had not been discovered and that specific therapeutic agents, with a few exceptions, were unknown.

The order in which we have chosen to present medical education and medical practice in the next two chapters may present problems for some readers. Education affects practice, and practice affects education; the two progress hand in hand and their histories are so intertwined that neither can be understood fully without knowledge of the other. The chapter on medical education, which we have given precedence, may therefore present some perplexities, but it is hoped that these will be resolved during the reading of the chapter on medical practice.

2

Medical Education

I believe we may safely affirm, that the inexperienced & presumptuous band of medical tyros let loose upon the world, destroys more of human life in one year, than all the Robinhoods, Cartouches, & Macheaths do in a century. It is in this part of medicine that I wish to see a reform, an abandonment of hypothesis for sober facts, the first degree of value set on clinical observation, and the lowest on visionary theories. I would wish the young practitioner, especially, to have deeply impressed on his mind, the real limits of his art, & that when the state of his patient gets beyond these, his office is to be a watchful, but quiet spectator of the operations of nature, giving them fair play. . . .

(Thomas Jefferson to Dr. Caspar Wistar, 1807)

HIGHER EDUCATION

Higher education in the United States during most of the nation's first century was dominated by theologians. College curricula were designed primarily to prepare students for the ministry. The faculties and governing boards of the best known institutions—Harvard, Yale, Princeton, Dartmouth, and Brown—were made up mostly of clergymen and were, with rare exceptions, narrowly sectarian. Even the University of Pennsylvania in the heart of Quaker territory, though it prided itself on being nonsectarian, had a strong religious tone; prior to the Revolution (when it was known as the College of Philadelphia) its chief executive and most of its faculty were clergymen, and one of its sponsors was the Archbishop of Canterbury. The College of William and Mary, in Virginia, had a more liberal tradition: Thomas Jefferson, when a student there, described his favorite teacher, a Scottish divine and mathematician, as "a man profound in most of the useful branches of science, with a happy talent of communication" (Garrett, 1971). This type of pedagogical emphasis on science was rare in the first century of American history. Andrew D. White, later to become the first president of Cornell University, said that when he was an undergraduate at Yale in the 1850s, the instruction in the best of the colleges was "narrow, their methods outworn, and the students, as a rule, confined to one simple,

9

single, cast-iron course, in which the great majority of them took no interest.

"Probably not one of us in the whole senior class [1853] had any idea of a chemical laboratory save as a sort of small kitchen back of a lecture desk, like that in which an assistant and a negro servant prepared oxygen, hydrogen and carbonic acid for the lectures of Professor Silliman. I was told that the new laboratory [just established at Yale] was intended for experiments, and my wonder was succeeded by disgust that any human being should give his time to pursuits so futile" (White, 1939).

At that time no institution in the United States deserved to be called a university. In 1780, by act of the Massachusetts legislature, *Harvard College* became *Harvard University,* surely a misnomer, since the "university" consisted of only a School of Arts with three professorial chairs—Divinity, Mathematics, and Oriental Languages (Harrington, 1905). At Harvard, as elsewhere, if science was taught it usually came under the title of *natural philosophy,* a descriptive science devoted largely to a study of the superficial characteristics and classification of plants and animals and far less weighty in the curriculum than *moral philosophy.*

The University of Michigan, which began to function at Ann Arbor in 1837, was the first American university to downgrade the classics and to assign a prominent position to its science courses. The first two appointees to its faculty were scientists.

EARLY MEDICAL SCHOOLS

None of the colleges in the colonies had a medical department prior to the 1760s. Young men who wished to become physicians either went to Europe for study or spent several years as apprentices to a practitioner who might, himself, have had no formal medical education. In many of the smaller communities there were no physicians of any type, and the practice of medicine was a part-time occupation for clergymen and some of the better educated farmers. It has been estimated that of the three to four thousand individuals practicing medicine in 1776, no more than 400 had received medical degrees (Davis, 1876). A large portion of these degrees had been conferred by the University of Edinburgh. Among 13 students receiving the M.D. degree at Edinburgh in 1765, five came from Scotland, five from the American colonies, two from England, and one from Ireland. Between 1765 and 1779, 112 Americans received M.D. degrees at that institution (Packard, 1931).

It is not surprising, therefore, that the University of Edinburgh provided the model for the only two medical schools to be established during the colonial period: the medical department of the College of Philadelphia in 1765 and the medical department of King's College in New York City in 1768. Only 51 medical degrees had been conferred by these two schools prior to 1776, when their operations were suspended because of the war.

In 1765, John Morgan (1735–1789), co-founder with William Shippen, Jr., of the Medical College of Philadelphia, wrote *A Discourse upon the Institution of Medical Schools in America.* He said that candidates for admission to the new college should have had (1) an apprenticeship, usually of at least

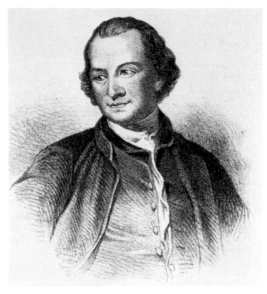

Figure 1. John Morgan, co-founder with William Shippen, Jr., of the Medical College of Philadelphia. (New York Academy of Medicine.)

three years, with a "reputable" physician; (2) education in the liberal arts, mathematics, and natural history; (3) a working knowledge of the Latin language and preferably also of French. The medical curriculum was to be a graded one, with subjects taught in the following order: anatomy, materia medica and botany, chemistry, physiology and pathology, and clinical medicine. Part of the clinical instruction was to be given by Dr. Thomas Bond at the Pennsylvania Hospital by means of lectures, demonstrations, and attendance upon patients. In emphasizing the importance of the hospital for clinical training, Morgan made a statement which was not to be heeded for another hundred years: "When two such important institutions as a medical college and a well regulated hospital contribute mutually to the advantage of each other, all ranks and conditions of people would no doubt most cheerfully unite in support of a common interest." Morgan's curriculum included neither surgery nor pharmacy, since he believed that the physician should not engage in the practice of either.

The school year for the College of Philadelphia was seven months in length (November to June). In the first year the preclinical subjects were taught and in the second year, clinical medicine, including experience at the Pennsylvania Hospital. At the end of the second year the student could take the examination for the degree of Bachelor of Medicine. He could not qualify for the degree of Doctor of Medicine until he had had three additional years of study and practice, had passed a stiffer examination, and had written, in Latin, a thesis which he had to defend before the faculty.

When the medical department of King's College was founded, there was no hospital in New York. In addressing the first class of medical graduates in 1769, Dr. Samuel Bard (1742–1821) lamented the fact that the city had no hospital and cited several reasons why a hospital should be built. "Another argument (and that by no means the least), for an Institution of this na-

11

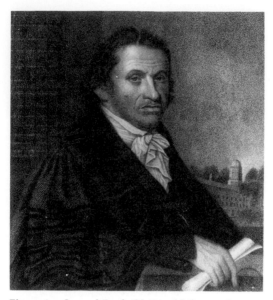

Figure 2. Samuel Bard. (National Library of
Medicine, Bethesda, Maryland.)

ture, is, that it affords the best and only means of properly instructing
Pupils in the Practice of Medicine." In this same address Bard warned the
young doctors of the need for continuing education: "Do not imagine, that
from this time your studies are to cease; so far from it, you are to be considered as but just entering upon them; and unless your whole Lives are one
continued series of Application ... in a Profession like this you have
embraced, where the Object is of so great Importance as the Life of a Man;
you are accountable even for the Errors of Ignorance, unless you have
embraced every Opportunity of obtaining Knowledge" (Bard, 1921).

Both of the prerevolutionary schools resumed operations after the war,
but their original names survived for only a few years. In 1791 the medical
department of the College of Philadelphia became the medical department
of the University of Pennsylvania (Wood, 1896), and in 1810 the medical
department of Columbia (formerly King's) College went out of existence
because it could not compete successfully with the College of Physicians
and Surgeons of New York, which had been established in 1807. (Years later
the College of Physicians and Surgeons became the medical department of
Columbia University.)

The Harvard Medical School was the third school to be established and
the first after the conclusion of the Revolutionary War. In 1781, at about the
time of the surrender of Cornwallis, the President and Fellows of Harvard
College requested Dr. John Warren (1753–1815) of Boston to prepare the
outlines of a plan for a "medical institution." Warren's background was
quite different from that of the founders of the schools in Philadelphia and
New York. He had never been abroad, had never attended a medical
college, and he possessed no medical degree. He had acquired his professional training by serving for a scant two years (from his 18th to his 20th
year) as an apprentice to an older brother who had a large practice in Boston. He had practiced independently in Salem, Massachusetts, for about

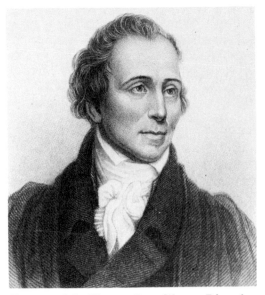

Figure 3. John Warren. (From Warren, Edward: The Life of John Warren, M.D. Boston, Noyes Homes and Company, 1874.)

two years when the Revolutionary War began. From 1775 to 1781 Warren served in the army as a hospital surgeon. There he won distinction both as a surgeon of unusual skill and as a teacher of anatomy. Though he lacked formal medical schooling, Warren had a broader educational background than most physicians of his day: at the age of 18 he had graduated from Harvard College, where he had proved himself to be a good classical scholar, "fluent in speaking the Latin language." His standing in the Boston community and his pious adherence to accepted religious doctrine were probably no less important than his reputation as a surgeon in leading the Harvard authorities to select him, at the age of 28, to prepare the plans for the Medical Institution. Warren's plans were accepted, and the formal opening of the school took place in 1783.

For the first 25 years of its existence, the school's faculty consisted of only three men: John Warren, Professor of Anatomy and Surgery; Benjamin Waterhouse, Professor of the Theory and Practice of Physic; and Aaron Dexter, Professor of Chemistry and Materia Medica. Waterhouse had received his medical education in Europe (in part at Edinburgh) and was considered to be the best trained physician in New England. Dexter, who had learned medicine as an apprentice to a Boston physician, did not possess a medical degree. These professorships were supported almost entirely by fees paid by students to purchase tickets for each professor's course of lectures. During the period 1783 to 1810 the total endowment available for medical school salaries was about $20,000, yielding an annual income of no more than $1000. Waterhouse, when he resigned in 1812, said that for a period of several years he had received no salary and at no time had it exceeded $400 (Cunningham, 1935).

When the Harvard Medical School opened there was no hospital in

13

Boston. Warren, who was well aware of the need for facilities for clinical instruction, tried unsuccessfully in 1784 to persuade the overseers of the Boston Almshouse to allow their institution to be used for this purpose. However, Waterhouse received permission in 1803 to take some of his students to see patients at the new Boston Marine Hospital. It was not until 1810 that permission was finally granted to make use of an eight-bed hospital ward at the Almshouse for clinical instruction in medicine and surgery. At the same time the Medical Institution moved from Cambridge to new quarters in Boston. Prior to that time the only medical instruction at Harvard consisted of lectures delivered in the college buildings at Cambridge. The facilities for clinical instruction remained quite inadequate until the opening of the Massachusetts General Hospital in 1821.

About a year after the Massachusetts General Hospital opened, James Jackson, who had succeeded Waterhouse as Hersey Professor of Physic, wrote a letter to the Harvard Corporation describing his teaching activities (Putnam, 1906):

> *I deliver one course of lectures annually to a class of medical pupils in Boston. . . . As, however, the term allotted for the course [three months] is not sufficiently long to discuss all the subjects, . . . I have, in addition, . . . commonly met my class two afternoons and always one afternoon in the week. One of these afternoons has been devoted to an extra lecture and the other to an examination of the pupils on the subject of the preceding week. . . .*

> *Since the Massachusetts Hospital has been opened I have taken the pupils there, sometimes one, sometimes two mornings in a week. . . . At the hospital I give a short clinical lecture after visiting the patients. . . . The time for the medical lectures is too short. I may add that the medical professors would be very happy to increase the length of this term. . . . The number of pupils attending the medical lectures has been gradually increasing within a few years from fifty to one hundred. Of these, generally four-fifths have attended my course; and . . . about one quarter have not paid for their tickets.*

The eager young men responsible for organizing the first three medical schools in the United States were fired with a zeal to improve medical education and medical practice in their native land. Most of them were, like Warren, under the age of 30, and none had attained his fortieth year. When Benjamin Rush joined the Philadelphia faculty in 1769 he was only 24 years old. At the opening of the medical department of King's College in 1768, Samuel Bard, Professor of the Practice of Physic and leader of the faculty, was just 25 years old.

The medical department of Dartmouth College was founded in 1797, and for the first decade of its existence Nathan Smith was its one-man faculty. As Oliver Wendell Holmes remarked, Smith occupied not just a chair but "a whole settee of professorships."

The medical school of Transylvania University at Lexington, Kentucky, founded in 1799, did not open until 1817. Twenty years after opening, this school, the first to be established west of the Allegheny Mountains, had a student body of more than 250, an outstanding faculty, probably the best medical library of the period, and the largest endowment of any medical school in the nation. Nevertheless by midcentury it was forced to close because it could not compete successfully with the schools in the more rapidly growing nearby cities, Cincinnati and Louisville.

The sixth medical school to be founded and the fifth to open was the University of Maryland. In about 1800, Dr. John B. Davidge, who had received his medical education in Europe, instituted at Baltimore a course of lectures on the principles and practice of midwifery. In the following two years the course was expanded to include lectures on anatomy and surgery. The lectures were delivered in Davidge's home and never were attended by more than a dozen students. Recognizing an increasing demand for medical instruction, Davidge erected an "anatomical hall," where he was joined by two other local practitioners, one of whom gave lectures on anatomy and physiology, the other, lectures on chemistry. The lectures on anatomy had scarcely commenced when an angry mob of citizens opposed to anatomical dissection attacked the new hall and demolished it. For the next several years Davidge and his associates gave their lectures and demonstrations at the county almshouse. In 1807 they applied to the Maryland legislature for permission to establish a medical college. A charter was granted, and the proprietors also were issued a license to raise funds by lottery for the construction of suitable buildings.

Though the new college bore the title *University of Maryland,* there was no university except for the medical component. Abraham Flexner said in 1910 that before the University of Maryland was founded, "a medical college had been a branch growing out of a living university trunk." This Maryland branch was not only the first to grow without a trunk but also the first to arise on an independent, proprietary basis, its proprietors being its faculty; and thus, said Flexner, "a harmful precedent was established" (Flexner, 1910). The precedent was followed by the flood of medical schools, large and small, urban and rural, which were founded during the remainder of the nation's first century.

Five medical schools were in operation in 1810. The number of students in attendance was approximately 650, of whom about 100 received medical degrees in that year. The pre-eminence of the University of Pennsylvania medical school at that time is shown by the fact that it was attended by 406 of the 650 students.

The population of the United States was then more than seven million. To serve this population there were only three public general hospitals: the Pennsylvania Hospital in Philadelphia, the New York Hospital in New York City, and the Charity Hospital in New Orleans. Though none of these hospitals was under the control of a medical school, all were used to a limited degree for clinical teaching.

Shortly after 1810 a unique type of medical school began to appear in the more remote areas of the country. These schools were established in rural villages, and their faculties were made up of two or three local practitioners. They were chartered by their respective states as independent educational institutions and were authorized to award the medical degree. The physical facilities of this type of school consisted of a room suitable for lectures, a small library containing books loaned by the local physicians, and perhaps one or two other rooms for anatomical and chemical demonstrations. Clinical instruction was by lecture and textbook, there being no provision for demonstration of patients or for observation of surgical operations or obstetrical procedures.

The first of the independent village schools was established in 1812 in

15

Fairfield, Herkimer County, New York. The official name of this school, *The College of Physicians and Surgeons of the Western District*, was so long that it was usually referred to as the *Fairfield School* or the *Herkimer School*. The second such school, the *Vermont Medical Academy*, was established in 1818 in the small, remote village of Castleton, Vermont. Its founders and faculty consisted of three local practitioners. The original agreement among the founders outlined their respective duties and responsibilities, specified how the students' fees were to be shared, and gave some indication of the facilities and plan of operation (Waite, 1935). The Fairfield school was in existence for 28 years and the Castleton school for 43 years.

In 1876 Dr. N. S. Davis gave an admirable though rather naïvely uncritical description of the development of medical education in the United States. The following paragraphs are taken from this account.

> *During the colonial period of our history, and for thirty or forty years subsequent to the achievement of our National Independence, it was the universal custom for young men who entered upon the study of medicine to become regularly apprenticed to some practitioner for a term of three or four years, during which time the preceptor was entitled to the student's services in preparing and dispensing medicines, extracting teeth, bleeding, and other minor surgical operations, and when more advanced in studies, in attending on the sick; and, in return, the preceptor became obligated to give the student detailed and thorough instruction in all the branches of medicine. Many of the more eminent practitioners often had several students in their offices at one time, constituting a small class who were drilled almost as regularly in their studies as they would be in a college. In some instances the term of apprenticeship was extended to six and even seven years, and was made to commence at the early age of fifteen or sixteen years. All these customs were brought by the emigrants from the parent country, and their perpetuation here was rendered more necessary by the sparseness of the population and the difficulty of access to medical schools.*

> *In the midst of such customs and at a period in the world's history when railroads, steamboats, and other means of speedy transit were unknown and when even post-coaches were rare, it was entirely reasonable that the first idea of the medical college should be to furnish the means for a rapid review of the several branches of medical science, aided by such experiments and appliances for illustration as could be commanded, and the whole concentrated into as small a part of the year as possible. The idea of the founders of medical schools in Great Britain and in this country was that the schools should **supplement** but **not supersede** the work of the preceptor and the medical apprentice. The study of anatomy by dissection, the illustration of chemistry by experiments, the clinical observation of disease at the bedside—all of these were capable of being carried on in the offices of preceptors to a very limited extent only. But by forming a college faculty of several preceptors, each eminently qualified in a particular department, and by having access to anatomical rooms, chemical laboratory, and hospitals for the sick, all the branches of medicine then recognized could be very well reviewed in the form of didactic instruction in five or six months of the year.*

The loss of physicians during the Revolutionary War, combined with the lack of new graduates during that period, created a serious shortage of practitioners to care for the growing population. As the settlers moved across the country, many physicians working in isolated communities had to practice surgery and midwifery and compound their own medicines. To meet these contingencies, the medical colleges began to lower their standards during the first decade of the nineteenth century. Students were admitted after only two years of apprenticeship and without specified educational prerequisites; the degree of Bachelor of Medicine was abolished, and the doctoral degree was awarded after only two years of attendance at school; the graduated curriculum was abandoned, the lectures of the second year being identical with those of the first; the school year was shortened from seven months to four months; and hospital experience was no longer required. All of these changes were well under way by 1810.

EXPANSION AND DETERIORATION, 1810–1840

In the years 1810 to 1840, while the population was increasing from 7 to 17 million, there was (as indicated earlier) a rapid increase in the number of medical schools. During that period 26 new schools were opened, many of them in small communities. In spite of the increase in the number of schools, the University of Pennsylvania attracted far more students than any other; there the average size of the class in the 1830s and 1840s was about 450, of whom well over 100 graduated annually.

The cost of medical education in the smaller schools rarely exceeded $100, but costs at the larger schools were somewhat higher. The cost at the University of Pennsylvania, for example, was reported in 1827 as follows: "Every medical student, upon entering the University, is obliged to pay five dollars as a matriculating fee. The price of admittance to the course of each profession [i.e., each professor's lecture course] is twenty dollars; and the aggregate cost of tuition for two years is two hundred and forty dollars. The expenses of graduation amount to forty dollars, of which each of the principal medical professors receives five, the provost three, the vice-provost two, and five dollars are paid to the secretary of the Board of Trustees, which, after defraying the cost of the diploma, is appropriated to the increase and preservation of the anatomical museum" (Wood, 1896). In other words, only the matriculating fee and the secretary's fee, a total of ten dollars, went to the medical school; all the rest went to the faculty. However, the faculty agreed to accept without fees six students each year, since "young men of high natural endowments, and strong inclination to the medical profession, are often deterred from entering into it by their inability to bear the necessary charges" (Wood, 1896).

In spite of the great increase in the number of medical colleges, there were many who entered the practice of medicine without formal schooling and after a pitifully skimpy apprenticeship. James Fenimore Cooper, in *The Pioneers* (1823), gave a somewhat overdrawn but apparently reliable account of the medical education of Elnathan Todd, whose real-life counterpart is said to have been the doctor in the rural village in which Cooper lived.

> *Elnathan, then about 15, was . . . dressed in a suit of homespun, dyed in the butternut bark; furnished with a* New Testament, *and a* Webster's Spelling Book, *and sent to school. [After he had attended school irregularly for two or three years, the schoolmaster and the boy's mother decided that he had] a natural love for doctoring.*
> *. . .*
>
> *[Therefore] the lad was removed to the house of the village doctor, a gentleman whose early career had not been unlike that of our hero, where he was to be seen, sometimes watering a horse, at others watering medicines . . .; then again he might*

17

be noticed lolling under an apple tree, with Ruddiman's Latin Grammar *in his hand, and a corner of Denman's* Midwifery *sticking out of a pocket....*

This kind of life continued for a twelvemonth, when he suddenly appeared at meeting in a long coat ... of black homespun....

[Three or four months later, he called, one evening] upon a young woman of his own class in life, ... and ... was called for the first time in his life, Doctor Todd, *by her prudent mother. The ice once broken in this manner, Elnathan was greeted from every mouth with his official appellation.*

Another year passed under the superintendence of the same master.... At the end of that period, Dr. Todd attained his legal majority. He then took a jaunt to Boston to purchase medicines, and, as some intimated, to walk the hospital; ... if true, he soon walked through it, for he returned within a fortnight....

The next Sunday he was married; and the following morning he entered a one-horse sleigh with his bride, having before him [a] box ... filled with home-made household linen, a paper-covered trunk, with a red umbrella lashed to it, a pair of quite new saddlebags, and a bandbox.

[After Elnathan had settled in his new home] ... time and practice did wonders for the physician. He was naturally humane, but possessed of no small share of moral courage.... In certain cutaneous disorders, very prevalent in new settlements, he was considered to be infallible; and there was no woman ... but would as soon think of becoming a mother without a husband, as without the assistance of Dr. Todd.

From time to time leaders of the profession, particularly those who had had experience in the medical schools and hospitals of Europe, complained about the gross inadequacies of the American system of medical education. As early as 1811 and again in 1813, Dr. Rush, who was nearing the end of his long term on the faculty, wrote to the trustees of the University of Pennsylvania urging that the entrance requirements be raised, that the length of the course be increased from two to three years, and that students be allotted time to receive bedside instruction. He asserted that under existing circumstances not more than one fourth of the graduates were qualified to practice medicine (Butterfield, 1951).

In New York the same Dr. Samuel Bard who had addressed the first graduates of King's College in 1769 told the graduating class of the College of Physicians and Surgeons in 1819 (Bard, 1921):

The great error in our system of education is, that we are too much in a hurry, and that our young men are ushered into the world, and commence the practice of their profession, at a period so early, and after a preparation so slight, that very few have acquired the prudence or the knowledge to govern their conduct ...: and hence arise the errors and failure of too many, and our general, and I am afraid I may say, too just, reputation for superficial attainments. Could we keep our youth at school until sixteen, at college until twenty and ... at the study of the professions, until twenty-four or twenty-five years of age, they would be more generally successful in life [and] we should have more respectability and eminence in our professional men.

The educational sequence which Bard considered so desirable, with preliminary schooling and four years of college preceding four or five years of professional training, was not to be realized until a century later.

Today we have grown accustomed to looking upon medical education as a period of graduate study undertaken only by those who have earned a bachelor's degree, but during the nation's first century the medical college was an undergraduate school of lower standing than the school of arts. The medical course was two years shorter than the arts course, and in the institutions which had both a school of arts and a school of medicine the educational requirements for admission to the latter were considerably less strict than those for admission to the former. The incongruity of this situation was apparent to Bard and to other leaders of the medical profession, but in spite of their repeated protests they seemed powerless to effect a change.

Among those protesting the inferior state of medical education was Daniel Drake (1785–1852), a peripatetic professor and author of an American medical classic, *The Diseases of the Interior Valley of North America.* He was one of the few physicians of his time to rise to distinction without benefit of a foreign education. In 1832 Drake wrote a brilliant little volume, *Practical Essays on Medical Education and the Medical Profession in the United States.* In it he attributes the deplorable state of medical education to the fact that each state "is ambitious to rival its neighbors in the number, if not the excellence of its institutions. But another cause is equally operative. This is the want of due care in the selection of Professors; by which the standard of professional excellence is depressed to a level that brings the office within the reach of unqualified aspirants; and offers to mediocrity of talents, a degree of encouragement which no age or nation ever before held out."

As Drake indicated, in most medical schools the teachers who held such titles as Professor of Anatomy, or Chemistry, or Physiology, or Pathology had no real claim to such titles. They were with rare exceptions general practitioners who engaged in teaching more or less as a spare-time occupation. The sciences basic to medicine were not looked upon as disciplines

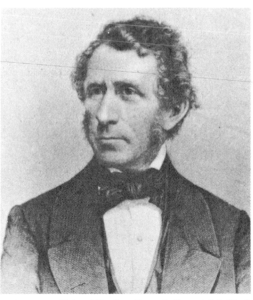

Figure 4. Daniel Drake. (From Jefferson Medical College Alumni Bulletin XXIV (3):6, Spring, 1975.)

19

worthy of independent study. Similarly, specialization in the clinical subjects was rare and almost never more than partial.

In 1838, Drake made the following recommendations to the *Medical Convention of Ohio:* that the medical school year be lengthened from four to five months; that the number of professorships be increased and that ampler provision be made for teaching the basic medical sciences; that the curriculum be reorganized so that the student could advance in gradual steps from the basic sciences to the practical clinical aspects of care of the sick; that there be stricter requirements for preliminary education; that no pupil be graduated before his twenty-first birthday and until at least four years after beginning the study of medicine. Drake urged that the various medical schools send representatives to a meeting at some central location to confer about these matters; "till when it would not be practicable, nor should it be expected that any single institution will attempt the reforms which are here proposed." Unfortunately, the proposed meeting of representatives was not held, and the reforms were not implemented.

In 1827 the Yale Medical School made an effort to establish higher standards for admission and graduation. Applicants for admission were required to demonstrate "a competent knowledge of the Latin language and some acquaintance with the principles of Natural Philosophy" as well as mastery of English studies. The medical course was increased in length to three years for college graduates and four years for others. Since none of Yale's competitors adopted these stiffer requirements, the New Haven institution experienced a serious reduction in the number of applicants for admission and in 1832 decided to abandon its experiment (Bell, 1960). Fourteen years later, the University of Pennsylvania increased the length of its annual medical school session from four to six months. No other medical college followed this lead, and after six years of steadily diminishing classes this experiment also was abandoned (Pepper, 1877).

EFFORTS TO EFFECT IMPROVEMENT, 1840–1870 Of the 26 states making up the Union in 1840, 16 had one or more medical schools. The number of students enrolled was approximately 2500, and the number receiving the M.D. degree that year was about 800 (Davis, 1877). During the years 1840 to 1870 many new medical schools were established. Most of them were small, badly planned, and poorly staffed and had a short life. The Civil War brought an end to some shaky ones. In spite of the discontinuance of many schools, the number in operation in 1870 was 80, of which 65 taught orthodox medicine, while 11 were homeopathic and 4 eclectic. The number graduating from the schools each year increased from about 800 in 1840 to more than 2500 in 1870 (Pepper, 1877). Almost all of the schools, even those with a university title, were still controlled and usually owned by practitioners who devoted part of their time to teaching in return for fees paid by students who bought tickets to their lectures. A notable exception to this arrangement was the medical school of the University of Michigan.

The Michigan medical school, founded in 1850, had several exceptional features. Ann Arbor was then a small village without hospital or other facil-

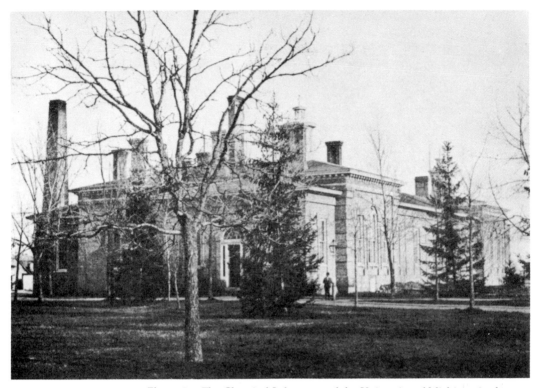

Figure 5. The Chemical Laboratory of the University of Michigan in the 1870s. The laboratory was a bud from the Medical School and was primarily for medical students. Michigan was the first university in this country to offer the facilities and require laboratory courses for students. (From Vaughan, Victor C.: A Doctor's Memories. Indianapolis, The Bobbs-Merrill Co., 1926.)

ities for clinical training. But unlike the village medical colleges previously mentioned, the Michigan school was not the casual child of the village doctors; rather it was born under the planned parenthood of the university. Science had acquired unusual prominence at Michigan. The first two men appointed to the faculty in the late 1830s were Asa Gray, the famous botanist, and Douglas Houghton, a chemist and geologist. The president of the university in the 1840s and 1850s was Henry Philip Tappan, who had received part of his education in Europe and who was a great admirer of the German educational system, in which the teaching of scientific subjects was assuming an increasingly important position. While Professor Silliman at Yale was struggling along with inadequate facilities for teaching chemistry, Michigan had established a separate chemical laboratory building where chemistry was taught as a science and not merely as a subject of practical utility (Vaughan, 1926).

In 1847, when the creation of a medical school at Michigan was first being considered, the Board of Regents appointed a committee to determine the expediency of such a step and to make recommendations for physical facilities, personnel, and other features. The chairman of the committee was not a local practitioner but a distinguished Detroit physician, well known for his broad interests in natural history. When on the recommendation of

21

this committee the medical school was opened in 1850, the university indicated its concern for the scientific aspect of medicine by transferring to the medical faculty Silas H. Douglas, the Professor of Chemistry who had organized the chemical laboratory in 1844.

According to Victor C. Vaughan, who was dean of the Michigan school from 1891 to 1921, the "Medical School was from its start a scientific, in contradistinction to a practical or clinical, institution. This was not altogether due to preference on the part of its founders and professors, but was a necessity. For twenty-five years it had no hospital—not a building which by any stretch of courtesy could be so denominated.... Indeed for many years the criticism of the School of most weight was that it had no hospital connection.

"Another argument against the school was that it is supported by the state. It was held that it is not a state function to provide a professional education." In this case, had it not been for state support, the medical school could scarcely have survived. The population of Ann Arbor was too sparse to permit the medical faculty to follow the example of other medical faculties and support itself by medical practice. The only way in which a qualified faculty of adequate size could be retained was by means of salaries paid by the state.

The lack of clinical facilities at Ann Arbor prior to the opening of the University Hospital in 1877 was partially overcome by the resourcefulness of Moses Gunn, Professor of Surgery on the founding faculty. According to Vaughan (1926), Gunn

> announced to the physicians of the state that the forenoons of Wednesday and Saturday would be devoted to consultations with them over their difficult cases.... There would be no charge to either the doctors or their patients so far as these consultations were conducted in the presence of the students. In this wise and mutually helpful way began that flow of the stream of the sick and injured citizens of Michigan to Ann Arbor.
>
> ...The doctors of the immediate vicinity did not bring their patients until the early morning of a clinic day. Those from greater distances lodged their patients in the hotel or some boarding house.... In some instances, probably in most, the professor had seen and examined the patient before he was brought before the class.... As a student I saw more than one surgical operation performed on a cadaver, or illustrated on a manikin, or figured in detail on charts, the day before I saw the operation on the patient.

Since there was no hospital, on clinic days "students carried patients on stretchers across the campus to the medical building, where the procedures ... were carried out"—presumably in one of the classrooms.

The medical school of the University of Michigan was in many respects a unique and pioneering institution. It exhibited some of the features of the university medical schools that would be developed in the years ahead. It was organized and strictly controlled by the university authorities. Its faculty, including its clinical professors, were on the payroll of the university and were not dependent upon income from practice or student fees. It thus avoided the commercial stigmata of other schools. It functioned as an integral part of a university that had a scientific rather than a theological tradi-

22

tion. Although the University of Pennsylvania established in 1874 the first full-fledged university hospital in the United States, the Michigan University authorities provided funds in 1869 to remodel a dwelling-house to serve as a temporary 20-bed hospital which was utilized for the clinical instruction of medical students. This was an inadequate, makeshift kind of hospital, but it was the first to be established under the full control of a university medical school. It functioned as a teaching hospital until the University of Michigan Hospital was opened in 1877.

Because of the inadequacies of the standard medical school programs, there were in some of the larger metropolitan centers opportunities for supplemental medical education. For example, in Boston for three decades prior to the Civil War there were several "private" medical schools. The most famous of these was the *Tremont Street School,* which was established in 1838. Its teachers, of whom there were four initially (including Jacob Bigelow and Oliver Wendell Holmes), were all members of the Harvard faculty. This school had two terms: a winter term (November through February) for which the tuition fee was $10, and a summer term (March through October) for a fee of $90. The winter session was designed to supplement the formal Harvard lectures that were delivered during the same four months. Classes were held only at night and consisted of discussions and quizzes on the subjects covered by the lectures of the day. Unique features of the summer session were its informality, its flexibility (students could take as many or as few subjects as they chose), its small classes, and the opportunity for close personal contact with a group of superior teachers. Led by their instructors, the students made rounds, observed methods of treatment, and watched surgical operations at the Massachusetts General Hospital, the Eye and Ear Infirmary, the Boston Dispensary, and the Children's Hospital.

The courses offered by the Tremont Street School covered a wide range and included subjects rarely or never included in a medical curriculum of that period. For example, Oliver Wendell Holmes, in addition to teaching auscultation and percussion, gave lectures and demonstrations in microscopical anatomy, using the most modern achromatic microscopes; and the great naturalist Louis Agassiz taught a course in embryology. There were also courses in comparative anatomy, surgical anatomy, chemistry, physiology, pathology, and a variety of clinical subjects including specialties such as dermatology, ophthalmology, and otology (Harrington, 1905).

During the period 1846 to 1851, when the average annual attendance at the Harvard Medical School was 133, an average of 44 students (about one third of the total student group) attended the Tremont Street School. In describing the relations between Harvard and the Tremont School the catalogue of the latter institution for the year 1856 stated: "The connection of the two schools affords an annual system of instruction which it is believed will be of the greatest value to students, and meet the demands of the Profession for the highest grade of medical instruction." The Tremont Street School did not award a degree.

Another private institution, the *Boylston Medical School,* was started in Boston in 1847 by six young physicians who planned to reform medical education. This school offered a three-year graded curriculum. The tuition fee was $100 per year. The financial arrangement differed from that of the typi-

23

cal proprietary school in that a single fee was paid to the school rather than multiple fees to individual professors. The Boylston School had a faculty of well-qualified teachers, almost all of whom were recent graduates of both Harvard College and Harvard Medical School. After operating with modest success for seven years without having authority to award medical degrees, the school petitioned the legislature in 1854 for power to grant the M.D. degree. The Harvard faculty, fearful of the competition which would be offered by a second fully chartered medical school in Boston, opposed the petition. In spite of this influential opposition, the petition was favored by the legislature. But Harvard won out in the end: it revised its course to meet some of the objections of the reformers, and it enlarged its faculty to make room for the leaders of the Boylston School. With the departure of its most active faculty members to accept jobs at Harvard, the Boylston School quietly passed out of existence (Harrington, 1905).

The changes in the Harvard medical curriculum that pleased the reformers took effect March 15, 1858, and were announced as follows in the catalogue for that year:

> *The Corporation of Harvard University, at the instance of the Medical Faculty, acting upon the experience of the Tremont Street School, which has extended over a quarter of a century, have decided to introduce a similar system of instruction into the Medical Department of the University.*
>
> *Accordingly, medical instruction will hereafter be given by the Faculty during the whole year with the exception only of appropriate vacations. The summer instruction which has hitherto been given by the Tremont Street School—an institution for private medical instruction—will for the future be given by the Medical Faculty of the College under the auspices of the University.*
>
> *By adopting this course—in reality extending medical instruction through the year, a part of which will be devoted to lectures, and a part to other modes of systematic study and training—the faculty believe that they are offering to medical students the best possible method of preparing themselves for the practice of medicine and surgery, and to the medical community the best assurance that Harvard University is using its utmost endeavors to elevate the character of the Medical Profession....*
>
> *During the winter session (November–February) lectures will be given as heretofore....*
>
> *During the summer term (March–October) instruction will be given by means of recitations, demonstrations, etc., in all the branches, ... except in Clinical Medicine and Clinical Surgery. Both the latter will be taught practically thro' the year at the Massachusetts General Hospital.*

The catalogue contained a recommendation by the faculty that the student devote three years to his medical studies and that he select his lectures and other courses so as to obtain a graduated program of study.

> *Students who want to go over the whole ground in a single year, and propose to follow the plan arranged for that purpose, will ...[find that] their opportunity for collateral reading and clinical observation will, of course, be more limited than if they remained in the school for a longer period....*
>
> *Terms for the Summer Session, $100.... For the Winter Session ... $80. Matriculation fee, $3, payable at once.*

Thus in 1858 Harvard not only offered but also strongly recommended a three-year course of graduated medical study, each year to consist of two terms running consecutively throughout the year. It should be noted, however, that the student was not required to pursue the recommended course. He could, if he chose, cover "the whole ground in a single year," or he could, alternatively, qualify for his medical diploma by attending only the four-month winter session of lectures for two years. Many students for economic or other reasons chose one of the shorter courses rather than the three-year program. Those who were able to take the full course recommended by the faculty obtained what was certainly a superior medical education for that period.

Regardless of the course chosen by the student, the decision as to whether he should receive his M.D. degree was determined by an oral examination. This was conducted in a large room in which the professors of the nine principal subjects were seated at intervals. The student circulated from one professor to the next and was quizzed at each station along the way. Every ten minutes a bell sounded and the candidate moved along to the next station. In this manner the students were examined by nine professors for ten minutes each. When all of the students had been examined, each professor was given a piece of cardboard, white on one side and with a large black spot on the other. As the dean called out the name of each candidate the nine examiners simultaneously thrust forward their cards so that the dean could see one or the other side. If he saw no more than four black spots the student was awarded his degree. Thus a candidate might be quite ignorant of the four most important branches of medicine and still receive a degree which entitled him to engage in practice (Harrington, 1905; James, 1930).

At about the same time that the reformers of the Boylston School were initiating the movement that eventually frightened Harvard into revising its curriculum, Nathan Smith Davis became the spokesman of another movement to reform medical education. In 1843 Davis, then only 26 years old, was practicing medicine in Binghamton, New York, and was elected a delegate to the State Medical Society. At several meetings of the Society he urged that a strong stand be taken regarding educational standards. Since the Society was unwilling to act alone in this matter, Davis decided to try to initiate action at a national level. He persuaded the State Society to sponsor a meeting in New York City to which medical societies and medical colleges throughout the country were invited to send representatives. At this meeting, which was held in 1846, the attendance was discouragingly small: only 119 delegates were present and half of these were from New York state. Approximately two thirds of the medical colleges sent no representatives. Nevertheless, the discussions of medical education and medical licensure that took place at the meeting aroused enough interest to justify the scheduling of a second meeting for the following year. The meeting in 1847 was better attended, consisting of 239 delegates from 22 of the 29 states then in the Union. The principal result of this session was the founding of the *American Medical Association,* which held its first convention the following year. As it turned out, many years would pass before the new Association would give effective support to Davis's objectives. During the first 30 or 40 years of its existence, the Association's attitude toward education was more

25

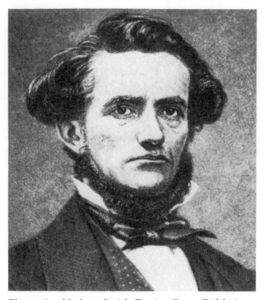

Figure 6. Nathan Smith Davis. (From Fishbein, Morris: A History of the American Medical Association, 1847–1947. Philadelphia, W. B. Saunders Co., 1947.)

that of a debating society than of a crusading legion. At the Association's meetings strong voices urged change, but equally strong voices argued for the maintenance of the status quo.

Opposition to raising the standards came chiefly from physicians who had a vested interest in the proprietary system under which American medical education was organized. The physician-proprietors of the colleges were afraid that upgrading of the admission requirements or the curriculum would put their schools out of business. It was, as President Eliot of Harvard remarked some years later, "in the pecuniary interest of the teachers composing a medical faculty to have as many pupils as possible, and grant as many degrees as possible, their receipts being proportionate to the number of fees paid for attendance at lectures and for graduation."

Davis did not give up his campaign for educational improvements with the founding of the American Medical Association. In 1849 he moved to Chicago to join the faculty of Rush Medical College. Several years later he resigned his Rush professorship because he could not persuade the dean to adopt educational reforms (Bell, 1973). Finally in 1859 Davis organized the Chicago Medical College (soon thereafter to become the Medical Department of Northwestern University) "for the express purpose of testing the practicability of establishing a school with a thoroughly graded and consecutive system of instruction" (Davis, 1876). The length of the medical course was increased from the customary two years with terms of four months each to three years of six months each. Students were required to receive clinical instruction at a hospital and to perform practical work in the chemical and microscopic (histological) laboratories. Although this college offered a new and well-planned course of study it is noteworthy that the faculty was of the traditionally proprietary type. It is also noteworthy that the

26

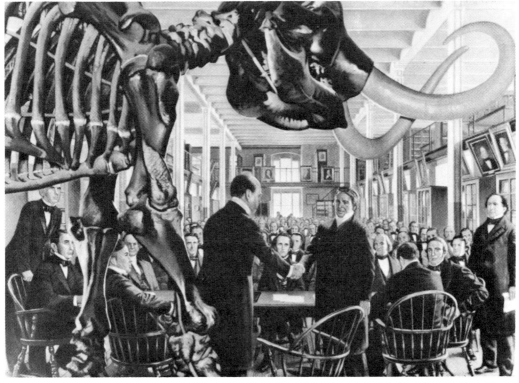

Figure 7. Founding of the American Medical Association. (From Great Moments in Medicine, Parke, Davis and Company. Detroit, Northwood Institute Press, 1966. Stories by George A. Bender. Courtesy of Parke, Davis and Company © 1961.)

college did not succeed in leading other schools to follow its example. However, in reporting in 1876 on the progress of his educational venture, Davis said, "The very satisfactory success of this institution during the past fifteen years, and its present prosperity certainly demonstrate the practicability of the scheme."

The other medical schools, with a few exceptions, disregarded the example set by Davis. Throughout the 1870s and beyond, they continued to offer a curriculum consisting of didactic lectures and demonstrations only, with minimal or no provision for bedside instruction. The lectures in the clinical subjects such as medicine, surgery, and obstetrics were presented simultaneously with the lectures in the preclinical subjects, such as anatomy, chemistry, and physiology, without any attempt to provide a graduated course of study. Although a student might attend medical school for two or three years, he heard substantially the same lectures during his second or third year as he heard during his first year.

The state of medical education in 1869, when he became president of Harvard University, was described by Charles W. Eliot as follows (Sabin, 1934):

There were no requirements for admission to our medical schools. To secure admission a young man had nothing to do but to register his name and pay a fee.... In consequence hundreds of young men joined the medical schools who could barely

27

read and write.... The total period of required attendance for the degree of Doctor of Medicine did not exceed, in the best schools, three winter terms of four months each. The main means of instruction were lectures, surgical exhibitions in large rooms appropriately called theatres, rude dissecting rooms with scanty supervision, and clinical visits in large groups.... A majority of young medical practitioners were, therefore, uncultivated men with scanty knowledge of medicine and surgery who had had opportunity for but a small amount of observation by the bedside and but little experience in hospitals.

On another occasion President Eliot said, "It seems almost incredible that the grossly inadequate training ... should be the recognized preparation of aspirants to a profession which was called learned, and which pre-eminently demands a mind well stored and a judgment well trained,... a profession in which ignorance is criminality, and skill a benefaction,...."

Eliot objected to the practice of awarding the M.D. degree to Harvard students who had passed only five out of nine 10-minute oral examinations. When he suggested to Dr. Henry J. Bigelow (then leader of the medical faculty) that it might be preferable to give written rather than oral examinations, Dr. Bigelow replied that "the students should not be expected to pass written examinations since half of them could hardly write" (Morison, 1965).

In support of Eliot's remarks about the "learned" medical profession it may be said that of 12,400 graduates of Harvard, Yale, Princeton, Dartmouth, Brown, Union, Amherst, and Hamilton, in the years 1800 to 1845, 25 per cent became clergymen, whereas only 7 per cent became physicians (Hudson, 1966). Viewed from another angle, in 1850–51 the proportion of students entering Yale's professional schools with bachelor's degrees was as follows: divinity school, 80 per cent; law school, 65 per cent; medical school, 26 per cent (Bell, 1960).

Whereas Eliot was inclined to place the blame for the low standards of medical education on the proprietary system, Davis (1876) believed "that our system,... with all its defects, had developed in strict consonance with the spirit of a free and enlightened people." He attributed the deterioration of educational standards to "the general acceptance of the [medical] college diploma as full admission into the profession, thereby uniting in the hands of the same men the business of teaching and the power of licensing." He believed this situation to be

wholly responsible for the fact that, while we have sixty-three [orthodox] medical colleges today [1876], one-third of them are so located that they can afford their students no advantages for clinical instruction worthy of mention; and all, except three or four, still attempt to crowd instruction ... [into] annual college terms of from sixteen to twenty weeks, and exact only two such strictly repetitional courses for graduation.... During the century under consideration [1776–1876], the system of private medical pupilage has undergone a complete change. At the beginning ... the private study, under a master, was a protracted and serious work, and the resort to the college was simply to review and more fully illustrate that work. But steadily, as medical colleges increased in number, as populations became more dense, and as steamboats and railroads increased a thousand-fold the facilities for travel, the work of private pupilage relaxed.... The relations of student and preceptor have become merely nominal,... consisting of little more than the registry of the student's name in the doctor's office, permission to read the books of his library or not as he chooses, and the giving of a certificate of time of study....[Hence the] collegiate studies [have now] become the student's chief reliance for the acquisition of medical knowledge [while the colleges have forsaken] their only appropriate function as institutions for imparting medical instruction and advancing medical science [and have been] hampered and perverted from their natural course by assuming the office of licensing institutions.

Davis urged that the colleges assume full responsibility for teaching and that full responsibility for granting licenses be taken over by government. However, he cautioned that "to invoke the patronage of either National or State governments, in this country, in the regulation and support of medical schools, is simply equivalent to asking that the lobbies of every legislative body in the country shall be annually filled with the log-rolling satellites of every 'pathy' and 'ism' of the day, [and] that the professorships of our colleges shall be transformed into political sinecures...."

Except for Davis's experiment in Chicago, little was done to alter the course of medical education until the 1870s, when real changes began to take shape, largely through the influence of educators who were not members of the medical profession. During the 1850s and 1860s a number of young American scholars spent long periods of study at European universities, particularly in Germany. Among the members of this group were a few who eventually became university presidents (in the years indicated), including Charles W. Eliot, Harvard University, 1869; James B. Angell, University of Michigan, 1871; and Daniel C. Gilman, Johns Hopkins University, 1875. These men recognized the inadequacies of American medical colleges, and with European models in mind they were able to devise ways to achieve improvements. Furthermore, they were not bound by loyalty to the medical profession, and they had the courage to insist on higher standards of medical education within their own institutions in spite of the loud protests of the physician-proprietor faction. The good work of these good men had just gotten under way when the first century of American medicine ended.

3

Medical Practice

*. . . if the appearance of doing something be necessary to keep alive the hope &
spirits of the patient, it should be of the most innocent character. One of the most
successful physicians I have ever known, has assured me, that he used more
bread pills, drops of colored water, & powders of hickory ashes, than of all other
medicines put together. It was certainly a pious fraud.*

(Thomas Jefferson, 1807)

DISEASES AND EPIDEMICS
The medical problems with which physicians were faced in the first century were very different from those of the present day. Infectious diseases were paramount. The death rate among children was appalling. To be convinced of this, one has only to walk through a cemetery of the mid-nineteenth century and note the graves of those who died before reaching their tenth year. Diarrheal diseases, diphtheria, measles, and scarlet fever accounted for many of the deaths. Tuberculosis was widespread and was responsible for invalidism and many deaths in early adult life. People of all ages succumbed in the great epidemics of yellow fever and cholera. In the yellow fever epidemic of 1793 it was estimated that some 8000 inhabitants of Philadelphia, which then had a population of about 45,000 contracted the disease, and there were over 4000 deaths. The dead included 10 physicians and many medical students who had assisted in caring for the ill.

The great epidemics of our first century were, to the people of those days, as mysterious as they were terrifying. They came stealthily, spread relentlessly, and killed without respect for age or rank. It must have been obvious to intelligent people that the doctors knew neither how to prevent disease nor how to cure it. The best medical advice was to flee the affected area with all possible haste, and this practice was followed by most of those possessing the means to do so. The sense of helplessness was of course due to ignorance about the cause of the disease and about how it was spread; the terror of confronting a remorseless, invisible enemy. We know today that yellow fever is caused by a specific virus, that it is transmitted from

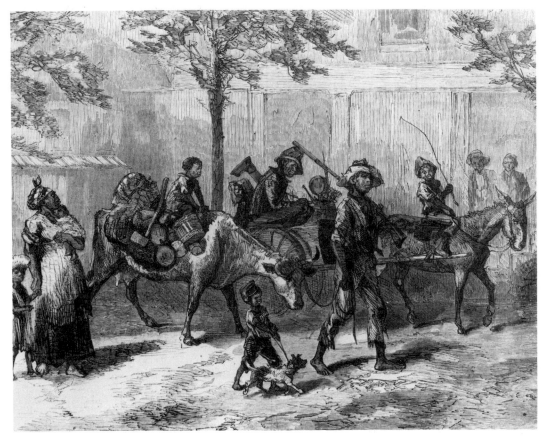

Figure 8. En route for Kansas: poor Negroes fleeing from the yellow fever in Memphis. (National Library of Medicine, Bethesda, Maryland.)

person to person only by the bites of particular varieties of mosquitoes, and that once it has been introduced into a community its spread can be halted only by getting rid of the mosquito (which in those days was accomplished without human intervention by the onset of cold weather) or by a campaign of preventive vaccination. The following description of an epidemic of yellow fever shows what happened when actions were governed by blind fear rather than by knowledge (quoted material from Tucker, 1968).

New York City experienced seven serious epidemics of yellow fever between 1791 and 1822, the episode in the latter year being somewhat more severe than its predecessors. The population of the city was then concentrated behind the busy waterfront at the southern tip of Manhattan. The 1822 epidemic started in early July, when two young girls living in the grimiest section of the waterfront contracted the disease. Deaths from yellow fever began to be reported on August 1. By November 2, when the epidemic was nearing its end, 1236 deaths had been recorded. As the death list mounted, the city was seized first by alarm and then by panic. Quicklime and coal were burned in the gutters to purify the "contaminated air." Residents were ordered to leave the most severely affected areas, and further intercourse with these areas was prevented by sealing them off with high wooden fences. The newspapers were filled with advertisements for quack remedies and preventives. People ventured out of their houses only on the most urgent business. "If they were unhappy enough to meet a friend on the way neither shook hands, but, exchanging a few words at a distance, each sought, bowing and scraping, to get to the windward of the other as they passed."

Throughout August people gradually deserted lower Manhattan by crossing the water to Brooklyn or New Jersey or by traveling by carriage and cart to upper Manhattan. One resident wrote at the time that the yellow fever "has utterly desolated the lower portions of the city. Thousands have left, and other thousands, panic-stricken, are daily leaving. Stores and dwellings are closed and deserted. The custom house, post office, all the banks, insurance offices, and other public places of business have been removed to the upper part of Broadway and to Greenwich Village. . . .

By September 1, in the "once bustling lower city . . . the only noise to break the stillness was the rumbling of hearses and the footsteps of nurses and physicians."

A Scottish businessman who landed in New York at the height of the epidemic found that "the whole of the business part of the city" had been "removed out to the fields which skirt the suburbs." There "an immense variety of wooden buildings, such as may be seen at Glasgow during the Fair" had been constructed and "the business transacted here during two months was prodigious; some of these buildings were fitted up as hotels, where 200 to 300 people were boarded, but the accommodations for beds, etc. . . . were none of the best. For such accommodation, however, people were very happy to pay an extravagant price; and in many instances . . . respectable persons were obliged for nights to bivouac in the fields. . . . In this irregular and temporary city in the field, you might find in one group, banking houses, insurance offices, coffee houses, auctioneers' sales rooms, dry goods, hardware and grocery stores, milliners' shops, barbers' shops and last though not least a suitable proportion of grog and soda-water shops."

In 1832, 1849, 1866, and 1873, cholera epidemics took a heavy toll in the cities of the Atlantic and Gulf coasts and spread up the Mississippi Valley into the Middle West. On July 29, 1832, while the epidemic of that year was still raging, it was announced that in New York City there had been 3506 cases of cholera with 1435 deaths (Smith, 1941). In that same year in New Orleans (population, 50,000), there were said to have been 6000 cholera deaths (Mason, 1932). In the epidemic of 1849, the death toll in New York between May and August exceeded 5000 (Rosenberg, 1971). During this same summer, while a Mississippi River boat was traveling from New Orleans to Louisville, 50 of its passengers died of cholera (Smith, 1941).

Though it did not occur in such dramatic, widely publicized epidemics, diphtheria was a constant threat and was responsible for the death of many children even in remote rural areas. Hertzler (1938), recalling his childhood experiences in rural Kansas during the 1870s, tells of a neighboring family in which eight out of nine children died of diphtheria within a period of 10 days.

Although vaccination against smallpox was introduced in the United States about 1800, this disease continued to be a major problem. Epidemic typhus appeared sporadically, and there were large outbreaks in 1846 and 1847 traceable to Irish immigrants. Typhoid fever, which was first clearly

33

distinguished from typhus by two Americans, Gerhard in 1837 and Bartlett in 1842, was an ever present threat, and large outbreaks with high mortality occurred from time to time. Syphilis was not uncommon, but the mortality from this disease is obscure, since the more serious late manifestations were not then recognized. Streptococcal infections in the form of erysipelas, scarlet fever, and childbed fever were common. Though nothing is known about the incidence of streptococcal and pneumococcal infections of the respiratory tract, it may be presumed that it was high. It seems probable that George Washington's final illness was due to a streptococcal infection. Malaria was prevalent in the southern states and frequently had serious consequences in spite of the availability of quinine.

Since the causes of infectious diseases were not known and since it was difficult to distinguish one from another, particularly in the early stages of the illness, all of these diseases were treated in a more or less similar manner. There is little doubt that in many cases the treatment did more harm than good.

BENJAMIN RUSH AND HIS THERAPY

American medical practice in the late eighteenth and early nineteenth centuries was dominated by the precepts and teachings of Benjamin Rush. Rush graduated from the medical department of Edinburgh University in 1768. After serving as the first Professor of Chemistry at the Medical College of Philadelphia, he was elected to the chair of the Theory and Practice of Physic in 1789, and when the college was merged into the University of Pennsylvania in 1791, he became Professor of the Institutes of Medicine (i.e., physiology and pathology) and of Clinical Medicine. From 1783 to 1813 he was physician to the Pennsylvania Hospital.

Rush was active in politics, an ardent patriot, and a signer of the Declaration of Independence. His energy both in public affairs and in the pursuit of his profession seemed boundless. Among his many contributions to the medical literature, perhaps the most original and enduring were his descriptions of cholera infantum (diarrheal disease of infants) and dengue fever and his account of the great Philadelphia epidemic of yellow fever in 1793. His monograph on insanity was ahead of his time. Garrison (1917), the medical historian, characterized Rush as "a man of highly original mind, well read, well trained in his profession, an attractive, straightforward teacher . . . sometimes wrong-headed as well as strong-headed." The last of these traits was at no time more evident than when Rush was defending his fanciful theory of disease and the system of therapy based upon this mistaken concept.

Rush believed and taught that disease, particularly disease manifested by fever, was due to the accumulation of a bodily poison that exerted its harmful effect by causing a nervous constriction of the small blood vessels. His therapy was designed to rid the body of the poison and to bring about a relaxation of the nervous excitement. Elimination was promoted by bleeding, by administering drugs to induce vomiting, purging, sweating, and salivation, and by drawing the poison to the surface by cupping (applying suction cups) and blistering the skin. Calomel was sometimes given in such

34

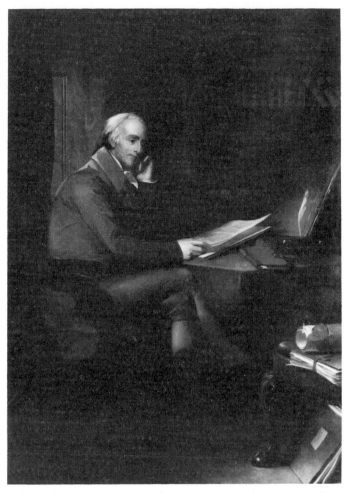

Figure 9.   Benjamin Rush. (Courtesy of Pennsylvania Hospital.)

large doses that it caused the hair and the teeth to fall out. His treatment for yellow fever consisted of daily bleedings of 12 ounces or more of blood and daily purging with a mixture of calomel and jalap, until the patient either recovered or died. About half of his yellow-fever patients were in the latter category. One of his patients was bled 22 times in 10 days, losing a total of 176 ounces of blood—an average of more than a pint a day. Rush cautioned his students that in bloodletting nothing could be worse than timidity, saying that it was frequently desirable to bleed a patient to the point of unconsciousness. Even in his obstetrical practice Rush bled his patients, 30 ounces at the beginning of labor, and at the same time administered purgatives (Rucker, 1941).

Some of Rush's contemporaries did not agree with his system of medicine and believed that his bleeding and purging were excessive. But he was such a renowned patriot, such a forceful and energetic person, such a prolific writer, and he had such a large following among those who had attended his lectures at the medical college and elsewhere that his influence was widespread and long-lasting.

In 1876 Yandell commented on Rush's writings: "He was more generally read and followed not only than any other medical writer of this country, but than all other writers in medicine put together. . . . His writings form, as a whole, a body of philosophical medicine — defective indeed, in many points — but exhibiting a breadth of view, an originality of thought and conception, an accuracy and extent of observation, and a terseness, vivacity, and clearness of style, that compare well with the best medical work of the period."

We wonder today how people had the fortitude to call a doctor, knowing that they would have to submit to the harsh treatment employed by Rush and his many followers. They did so because of the high mortality rate of the diseases then prevalent, because the practices were advocated by Rush, and because it was commonly believed that without medical intervention the natural outcome of disease was death. As Oliver Wendell Holmes said some years later, Rush spoke "habitually of nature as an intruder in the sick room" (Lloyd, 1930). Rush's methods continued to be practiced, with some modifications, for several decades after his death. The erosion of his system, which came about slowly, was attributable to several factors:

(1) Young physicians who had gone overseas to study in Paris under Louis, in London under Addison and Bright, and in Dublin under Graves and Stokes had learned to distrust dogmatism and had brought back fresh ideas about how one disease could be distinguished from another by utilizing new techniques and new tools. For a small and select group of physicians, the spirit of critical inquiry was replacing blind reliance on authority.

(2) It began to be realized that at least some diseases are self-limited and will run their course and subside without benefit of a physician. In his discourse *On Self-limited Diseases* (1835), Jacob Bigelow (1787–1879) of Boston was the first to make a clear and convincing statement on this subject. Oliver Wendell Holmes said that Bigelow's discourse did "more than any other work or essay in our language to rescue the practice of medicine from the slavery to the drugging system which was a part of the inheritance of the profession." Bigelow's thesis actually had been foreshadowed by Nathan Smith (1762–1829) of New Haven, who wrote in his discussion of the treatment of typhoid fever (*A Practical Essay on Typhous Fever, 1824*), "I have never been satisfied that I have cut short a single case; [the disease] has a natural termination like other diseases that arise from specific causes." This brief statement, which embodies both the concept of self-limited disease and the belief that diseases have specific causes, was wholly incompatible with the teachings of Rush.

(3) Public antagonism toward the harsh therapy of the Rush school made many people reject orthodox physicians and turn to quacks and cultists who employed gentler remedies. This competition from irregular practitioners forced the profession to examine more critically the rationale of its therapeutic measures.

Among the more articulate public antagonists was William Cobbett, an English writer and politician who came to the United States in 1792 and remained long enough to make life miserable for America's leading physician. Cobbett was a master satirist whose articles were read with relish by many prominent citizens in New York and Philadelphia. His antagonism

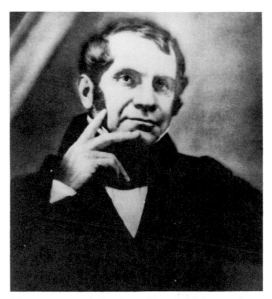

Figure 10.   Jacob Bigelow. (National Library of Medicine, Bethesda, Maryland.)

toward Rush initially was politically motivated, and he seized upon Rush's reputation as a champion of bleeding and purging to discredit him in the eyes of the public. He made a study of the mortality in the great Philadelphia epidemic of yellow fever (1793) and strove to create the impression, probably not far from the truth, that many of Rush's patients had died not of yellow fever but of exsanguination. He suggested that Rush had an irrational and unquenchable passion for extracting human blood.

After weeks of persecution by Cobbett's pen, Rush sought revenge by suing his detractor for libel. The case was tried before what Cobbett described as a packed bench and packed jury. The verdict was in favor of Rush, who was awarded $5000 for damages. Cobbett recorded with ill-concealed glee that on the very day in 1799 on which the verdict was rendered, George Washington expired at Mount Vernon "in precise conformity to the practice of Rush."

Rush's victory in court failed to silence Cobbett. Instead, it attracted more readers to the campaign against bleeding and purging and encouraged Cobbett to publish a new periodical, *Rush-Light,* which continued to disparage Rush's therapeutic methods. After the fifth number of *Rush-Light* had been published, Cobbett, to avoid a second trial for libel, boarded ship in June, 1800, and set sail for his native shore. At about the same time, Rush, badly shaken emotionally and professionally, withdrew from practice and spent the remaining 13 years of his life serving as treasurer of the United States mint, writing his memoirs, delivering medical lectures at a somewhat slower pace, and turning his attention to the problems of insanity (DeJong, 1940). In the ensuing years bloodletting was gradually discredited as an indiscriminate therapeutic procedure. Medical textbooks recommended it with diminishing enthusiasm. But it still had its champions: Henry I. Bowditch, a highly respected Massachusetts physician, pub-

37

lished a paper in 1872 entitled *Venesection* [i.e., bloodletting], *its abuse formerly — its neglect at the present day*.

PRACTITIONERS, GOOD AND BAD

The intellectual caliber and cultural background of the practitioners of the first century covered a broad spectrum. At one end were the country doctors, many of whom did not have even a high school education and some of whom could barely read and write. They had learned their medicine from a preceptor whose teaching might or might not have been supplemented by a brief sojourn at a pitifully inadequate medical college. The interests of this class of physician were severely limited and strictly practical. They were incapable of utilizing or even understanding the new scientific developments. To them medicine was neither a science nor an art but rather a respectable occupation in which one's professional ministrations were guided by a sort of cookbook regimen.

At the other end of the spectrum, in the larger population centers was a relatively small number of physicians, well educated, articulate, learned in the science of their day, and with a keen awareness of the significance and utility of the new developments. The majority of this class of practitioner had spent from one to four years in the great medical teaching centers overseas. Oliver Wendell Holmes was an outstanding example of the physicians of this type.

Holmes was born in 1809 and grew up in Cambridge, Massachusetts, which was then little more than a country village where scholarly attainments outshone every sort of worldly success (Spiller et al., 1974). He attended Phillips Academy and then Harvard College, from which he grad-

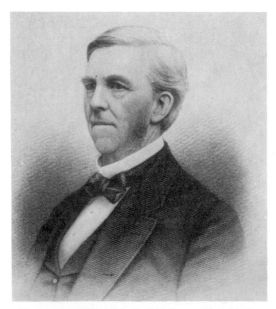

Figure 11. Oliver Wendell Holmes. (New York Academy of Medicine.)

uated in 1829. After spending a year "yawning over law books" he decided that he would rather be a physician than a lawyer and began his medical apprenticeship. In 1833 he went to Europe, where he remained for two and a half years, most of the time in Paris studying medicine under Louis and the other great French masters. When he returned to the United States he took his M.D. degree at Harvard and then began the practice of medicine.

In the period 1829 to 1836 Holmes had won attention as a poet and essayist. His poem "Old Ironsides" had become popular throughout the nation. In the eyes of the people who lived around him he was a literary man, and many of them refused to take him seriously as a physician. As a result, Holmes never had a very extensive practice. This was of no great concern to him, for his real interest was in the scientific side of medicine and medical education. He was an excellent lecturer and a lucid and effective writer on medical as well as literary topics. In the years 1838 to 1840 he spent three months each fall as Professor of Anatomy at Dartmouth. Thereafter, his pedagogical activities were confined to Harvard, where he was dean from 1847 to 1853 and Professor of Anatomy from 1847 to 1882. In 1843 he read before the Boston Society for Medical Improvement the first of his famous papers *On The Contagiousness of Puerpural Fever*. As a hobby Homes studied optics: he experimented with microscopes and cameras and invented a hand stereoscope. Throughout his long life (which ended in 1894) he kept up his literary activities. When the *Atlantic Monthly* was founded in 1857 he gave it its name and was one of its regular contributors. It was in this magazine that he published some of his best poetry and most of the essays of his popular *Breakfast Table* series. In spite of his literary fame, Holmes always considered medicine to be the center and focus of his career. His public addresses and widely read articles in support of orthodox medicine did much to clarify the reasons for the profession's opposition to homeopathy and other cults.

There were others with intellectual endowments and broad interests similar to those of Holmes. Most of these men were located in Boston, New York, or Philadelphia, with a few in the smaller cities and towns and a rare two or three in the rural areas. Among these were those who tried to keep American medicine abreast of the advances that were being made in Europe, who sponsored or edited a few first-class medical journals, and who tried, for a long time without success, to raise the standards of medical education and to establish qualifications and examinations for medical licensure.

A significant fact is that none of these men was a full-time specialist in any field of clinical medicine or surgery. John Morgan's pronouncement in 1765 that medicine did not embrace surgery or pharmacy might have been workable in Britain, but it was out of the question in the United States because of the sparseness and wide dissemination of the population. In most communities the lone medical practitioner could not escape being a surgeon and obstetrician, and he had to stock his own drugs and prepare his own medicines. The typical American practitioner became a jack-of-all-medical-trades. Not only did he undertake every type of clinical work but also in most medical colleges it was he who taught the preclinical (basic medical) sciences.

Beginning in the mid-nineteenth century, a gradually increasing number of physicians in the larger cities became known as having a special interest and competence in dealing with diseases affecting certain anatomical areas such as the throat and larynx, the eyes, the skin, or the female genital tract. Professional societies and journals specializing in these subjects began to appear. However, with rare exceptions, physicians did not become full-time practitioners of any clinical specialty; they devoted at least part of their time to general practice. Such was still the case in 1876 when Samuel D. Gross of Philadelphia, who was one of the most eminent professors of surgery, wrote his review of the progress of surgery in the United States during the previous century:

> *Although this paper is designed to record the achievements of American surgeons, there are, strange to say, as a separate and distinct class, no such persons among us. It is safe to affirm that there is not a medical man on this continent who devotes himself exclusively to the practice of surgery. On the other hand, there are few physicians, even in our larger cities, who do not treat the more common surgical diseases and injuries, such as fractures, dislocations, and wounds, or who do not even occasionally perform the more common surgical operations. In short, American men are general practitioners, ready for the most part, if well educated, to meet any and every emergency, whether in medicine, surgery, or midwifery. Of late, the specialists have seriously encroached upon the province of the general practitioner, and, while they are undoubtedly doing much good, it is questionable whether the arrangement is not also productive of much harm. The soundest, and therefore, the safest, practitioner is, by all odds, the general practitioner. . . .*

In the foregoing address, Gross unwittingly exposed the fact that the nonspecializing professors of surgery of whom he was so proud had failed to grasp the significance of the most important surgical development of their day. In speaking of the antiseptic surgical technique that Lister had introduced 11 years previously and which was already being employed with success by some of the leading surgeons of Europe, Gross said, "Little, if any faith is placed by any enlightened surgeon on this side of the Atlantic in the so-called carbolic acid treatment of Professor Lister." At about the same time, on the Pacific side of the nation, R. Beverly Cole, a general practitioner but also Professor of Diseases of Women and Children and Dean of the Medical School of the University of California, not only was pooh-poohing Lister's antisepsis but also was denying the contagiousness of childbed fever in spite of the fact that its contagiousness had been convincingly demonstrated by Holmes and Semmelweis (Gardner, 1940).

The following is a description of surgery in the Middle West in the 1870s and 1880s (Hertzler, 1938):

> *Operations in rural districts, even for the simplest of lesions, were practically unknown. In those days all wounds suppurated. It was the common practice for the surgeons in that day to operate garbed in the Prince Albert coat then regarded as the only fitting garment for the professional man. The cuff was turned up by the more fastidious. In the first operation I witnessed the surgeon threaded the needles with silk and then stuck them in the lapel of his coat so as to have them readily accessible when needed. He held the knife in his teeth when not in actual use.*
>
> *. . . Injuries which today seem comparatively trivial were treated by amputation. . . . The experience was that if amputation was not done death from infection would*

most likely follow, an end not obviated, however, in many cases by amputation, because the wound made by the amputation often became infected and killed the patient. The vessels were tied by silk threads cut long so they could be pulled out after the end of the vessel sloughed off; that is, if the patient did not die of secondary hemorrhage. . . .

When removal of a lesion required an abdominal incision, death from peritonitis almost invariably followed.

Mark Twain, with his talent for voicing the latent frustrations of the common man and with his typical humorous exaggeration, gave this description in his autobiography of the physicians of the days of his youth, about 1850 (Bragman, 1925):

They not only attended an entire family for twenty-five dollars a year, but furnished the medicines themselves. . . . Castor oil was the principal beverage. The dose was half a dipperful, with a dipperful of New Orleans molasses added to help it down and make it taste good, which it never did. The next standby was calomel; the next, rhubarb; and the next, jalap. Then they bled the patient and put mustard plasters on him. It was a dreadful system, and yet the death rate was not heavy. The calomel was nearly sure to salivate the patient and cost him some teeth. . . . Doctors were not called in cases of ordinary illnesses; the family grandmother attended to those. Every woman was a doctor, and gathered her own medicines in the woods, and knew how to compound doses that would stir the vitals of a cast-iron dog. And then there was the 'Indian doctor,' a grave savage, remnant of his tribe, deeply read in the mysteries of nature, and the secret properties of herbs; and most backwoodsmen had high faith in his powers and could tell of wonderful cures achieved by him.

This mock sufferance of the ministrations of the family doctor, the grandmother, and the Indian "doctor" was later replaced in Twain's writings by a sense of bitterness and intolerance. His personal frustrations as a patient led him to conclude that the medical profession was not only ineffective but also bigoted and pompous (Bragman, 1925):

The doctor's insane system has not only been permitted to continue its follies for ages, but has been protected by the State and made a close monopoly — an infamous thing, a crime against a free man's right to choose his own assassin. . . .

Fifteen years ago I had a deep reverence for the physician and the surgeon . . . now I have neither reverence nor respect for the physician's trade, and scarcely any for the surgeon's. I am convinced that of all quackeries, the physician's is the grotesquest and the silliest. And they know they are shams and humbugs.

CULTS AND QUACKS
As was mentioned previously, some people in the early nineteenth century, in order to escape the more violent forms of therapy practiced at that time, turned to quacks and cultists. Other factors contributing to the acceptability of these irregular practitioners include the following: (1) The relative scarcity of orthodox physicians led residents of many newly settled areas to welcome anyone who claimed to be a practitioner of the healing arts. (2) The best educated and most competent physicians were usually

41

located in the more thickly populated communities, whereas many of those who practiced elsewhere were so indifferently trained that there was little to distinguish them from the cultists. (3) Though orthodox physicians were usually more competent in the field of diagnosis, the medicines available to them were, with rare exceptions, no more effective than the quack's herbs. (4) Neither an M.D. diploma nor a license was required for the practice of medicine. Some states had licensing laws, but these were not enforced. Since quacks and cultists usually assumed the title of "Doctor," and since the law made no distinction between the quack and the possessor of the M.D. degree, the unsophisticated layman had little to guide him in the choice of practitioners.

The quacks practiced independently and usually moved along from one community to another with such rapidity that their mistakes and inadequacies rarely overtook them. The cultists, on the other hand, were composed of better organized, more stable groups, each basing its practice on its own peculiar system of medicine.

A cult known as the *Thomsonians* acquired many followers and for a time was considered a serious threat to orthodox medicine. The founder of this cult, Samuel Thomson, was born on a New England farm in 1769 and had no formal education (Ball, 1925). As a boy he became interested in the wild plants on the family farm and learned something about their physiological and toxic effects by experimenting on himself and his friends. Since no physician lived nearby, his family and neighbors allowed him to prescribe herbal remedies for their ills. In time he became an itinerant herbalist, and in the first decade of the nineteenth century, in order to provide a basis for his ministrations he concocted his own medical system. He proclaimed that disease was due to an excess of "cold" in the body. Accordingly, his therapy consisted of hot baths and the administration of herbs to eliminate or neutralize the cold. Thomson was evidently a convincing salesman: among the endorsements which he obtained for his system was one from Benjamin Waterhouse, the Professor of Medicine at Harvard. In 1813 he persuaded the United States Patent Office to issue a patent for his system and thereafter sold the rights to employ his methods. About 1830 Thomson's followers established several schools, which were known as botanico-medical colleges.

In the 1850s Thomsonianism began to lose its momentum, and by 1860 all but one of its colleges had ceased operation. What was left of the Thomsonians joined forces with the rising *Eclectic* cult. The latter sect had a better system of education and attempted to combine the teachings of Thomson with what were considered to be the best features of orthodox medicine. By 1876 there were four colleges of eclectic medicine and surgery, whose graduates enjoyed their greatest vogue during the nation's second century.

Other cults whose popularity depended in part upon their advocacy of gentler methods of treatment included the following:

(1) The *Grahamites,* a cult founded in the 1830s by Sylvester Graham (1794–1851) of Pennsylvania, held that many forms of illness were initiated or aggravated by calomel and the other "poisonous drugs" then in common use. The Grahamites taught that the maintenance of good health depended upon the observance of hygienic measures, the avoidance of alcoholic

drinks, a diet of "natural" vegetable foods, and the use of whole-wheat flour (which became known as "Graham flour") rather than refined flour in preparing the daily bread. The Graham cracker has been the most enduring product of this cult.

(2) The cult of *hydropathy* was imported into the United States from Germany in the 1840s. The hydropaths advocated the avoidance of drugs and the use of various types of waters not only internally but also externally in the form of therapeutic baths. They also stressed exercise, good hygiene, and a diet of "natural" foods similar to that of the Grahamites.

(3) The cult of *osteopathy* began to take shape in the mind of Andrew T. Still (1828–1917) in the 1860s. His experience as a soldier in the Civil War, the death of three of his children in an epidemic of meningitis in 1864, and the obvious inability of the medical profession to deal effectively with epidemics of yellow fever, cholera, typhoid fever, and other diseases convinced Still that the strong drugs employed by orthodox physicians were not only useless but also harmful and frequently lethal. Still's observations led him to devise his own fanciful theory of the causes of illness. In 1874 he announced a new system of therapy in which spinal manipulation and body massage were substituted for drugs.

(4) *Christian science* was a cult whose therapy, based solely on religious faith, was gentler than that of all the others. Its foundation was laid in 1875 by Mary Baker Eddy's *Science and Health*.

Of greater importance than the foregoing sects during the second half of the first century was the cult of *homeopathy* (Kaufman, 1971). The educational standards of this cult were high, much higher than those of the Thomsonians, the Grahamites, and the hydropaths, and higher than those of many orthodox schools. Initially, homeopathy did not arouse the antagonism of the established profession, because its founder had begun his career as an orthodox physician and because its adherents included graduates from the regular medical colleges. Like Thomsonianism it attracted many of its patients by offering simple and mild methods of therapy.

Samuel C. Hahnemann (1755–1843), the founder of homeopathy, lived in Germany and received his medical degree in 1779 from the University of Erlangen. He was more a philosopher and theorist than a practicing physician. In an experiment conducted on himself he found that when he took relatively large doses of quinine he developed fever, a rapid pulse, and other symptoms of the type exhibited by patients suffering from malaria. Since malaria could be cured by the administration of quinine, Hahnemann theorized that the key to therapy was to administer a medicine that when given to a healthy person would produce symptoms similar to those of the disease to be treated. Further experimentation convinced Hahnemann of the correctness of this hypothesis and led him to announce the first law of homeopathy: *similia similibus curantur* (likes are cured by likes).

Hahnemann also believed that his experiments proved that large doses of medicine served to aggravate illness and that small doses supported the "vital spirit" of the body in its effort to overcome disease. This led to the second principle of homeopathy, *the law of infinitesimals*. Hahnemann considered a drug dose of no more than 1/500,000 or 1/1,000,000 of a grain to be a "high potency" dose. But he warned that such minute amounts would not be effective unless prepared by the physician himself in a ritual in which the vial containing the medicine was struck against a leather pad in a prescribed manner. Only thus, he claimed, could the latent state in the medicine be "excited and enabled to act spiritually upon the vital forces." In the years ahead this mystical component of Hahnemann's teachings was to raise questions about his credibility. Another of his teachings which led not only to doubt but also to ridicule was his claim that chronic diseases such as dermatitis, asthma, deafness, and insanity were the result of medicines administered by orthodox physicians to cure "the itch."

The first homeopathic practitioner to cross the Atlantic was Hans B. Gram, who settled in New York in 1825. Until 1840 homeopathy spread slowly and was treated with tolerance and respect by the established profession. In 1830 a review of Hahnemann's works appeared in the *American Journal of the Medicial Sciences.* Though critical of some of his tenets, it treated him as a sincere physician and declared that homeopathy might furnish "a means, among others of alleviating human suffering." In 1832 Hahnemann was elected an honorary member of the *Medical Society of the County of New York.* In a paper read before the *New York State Medical Society* in 1838, it was noted that homeopathic therapy was mild, pleasant, and harmless, and it was proposed that a hospital open its wards for an experiment in which one group of patients would be treated by homeopaths and another group by orthodox methods, in order to discover the relative merits of the two systems. Further evidence of respect was manifested by a number of physicians, trained in orthodox schools, who joined the ranks of the homeopaths, believing that they could still practice orthodox medicine while substituting Hahnemann's *materia medica* for the bleeding, purging, blistering, and other severe therapies which they had previously employed.

As the popularity of homeopathy increased and as more physicians forsook the orthodox fold to embrace the principles of Hahnemann, tolerance and respect gave way to bitterness and ridicule. The medical journals expressed surprise that such an "absurd" system should have attracted so large a following. The physicians who had transferred their allegiance to the new sect were characterized as dishonest and unprincipled; before long they would regret having "trimmed their sails to catch the popular breeze." The formidable Dr. Oliver Wendell Holmes, in two lectures delivered in 1842, argued that homeopathy had no rational basis; that *similia similibus curantur* and its other laws were no more than delusions; and that it was, in fact, a dangerous form of quackery. To explain the homeopaths' claims of therapeutic success, Holmes made a statement which would have shocked and outraged the profession of Rush's day; 90 per cent of the cases commonly seen by a physician, he asserted, "would recover, sooner or later, with more or less difficulty, provided nothing were done to interfere seriously with the efforts of nature." The clear implication of Holmes's argument was that although homeopathy was quackery, in 9 out of 10 cases its infinitesimal doses of medicine interfered less with the healing powers of nature than did the harsher measures of the orthodox practitioner; it was in the treatment of the 10 per cent of serious illnesses that the true physician excelled.

The comments on Holmes's lectures in some of the lay press indicated that the public, at least a significant part of it, could not care less about the accusation of quackery so long as homeopathy provided a way to escape "the nauseous drugs, the offensive draughts . . . and all the painful and debilitating expedients of our present system."

In the eyes of the established profession, homeopathy posed a far greater threat than the other cults. Unlike the Thomsonians, many homeopaths were educated and respected members of their communities. Their medical journals carried sophisticated articles, which in addition to promoting their own system, exposed the weakness of what they called "allopathic" (orthodox) medicine. In the 1830s and 1840s homeopathic practitioners still held membership in the regular medical societies; it was not easy to exclude them, since many homeopaths were graduates of orthodox medical colleges. Nevertheless, during the 1840s and 1850s one medical society after another adopted rules to exclude homeopaths regardless of their educational background or standing in the community. At the same time many societies mounted campaigns to convince the public of the "dangers" of the homeopathic system.

There were several indications that the public was not in sympathy with this campaign and that many people considered it to be a bigoted and self-serving effort on the part of the orthodox profession: (1) Articles in some of the lay press voiced this point of view. (2) State legislators, under pressure to adopt and enforce stricter licensing laws, refused to take any action that would exclude from practice homeopaths or other cultists on whom so many citizens depended for their medical care. (3) The Michigan state legislature, after a running battle with the state board of regents, finally succeeded, in 1875, in forcing the University of Michigan to appoint to its faculty two homeopathic professors and to grant a doctorate to homeopathic graduates. Although the university then appeared to have two medical schools, this was not strictly the case. The homeopathic students attended the regular medical school lectures in the basic medical sciences and some clinical subjects, but they learned how to dose their patients from the professors of homeopathy.

EVIDENCE OF ENLIGHTENMENT   In the early 1840s the leaders of orthodox medicine began to realize that the public was not going to reject homeopathy simply because it was accused of being irrational and absurd. The doctors knew that their own educational system was faulty and that many of their medical colleges were turning out graduates who deserved little more professional respect than the quacks. They foresaw that the best way to reestablish the reputation of the profession and to regain the support and goodwill of the public was to raise their own educational standards. As previously noted, it was chiefly with this goal in view that the American Medical Association was organized in 1847.

Educational improvements were slow in coming, but even before significant advances were made there were indications that the public image of orthodox medicine vis-à-vis the cultists was destined to improve. Fortunately, the Rush system had been abandoned, for this system was no less fanciful, no less absurd, and no more defensible than that of the homeopaths. While homeopathy remained committed to rigid laws and doctrines,

45

orthodox medicine was no longer tied to dogmas that would impede its future growth. The medical textbooks of the 1870s clearly demonstrate that during the preceding 50 years there had been vast improvements in diagnostic methods and in the differentiation of diseases. The established profession had every reason to be proud of its accomplishments, though it was difficult to convince the public that there was any value in advances that did not lead directly to more effective methods of treatment. Auspiciously, on the far side of the Atlantic the foundations were being laid for a true science of medicine. These developments would transform American medicine as the second century progressed and would lead to rational methods of prevention and treatment which the public could applaud.

4

Public Hygiene
and Preventive
Medicine

The same measures which are needed to protect a city against occasional epidemics of cholera are needed at all times to protect it against other infectious diseases, such as typhoid fever, which, although they do not come with the terrible impetuosity of cholera, steadily do their deadly work, and in the course of time destroy among us far more lives than cholera.

(William Henry Welch, in arguing for
permanent public health laboratories)

Little progress was made in the United States during its first century in the fields of hygiene and preventive medicine. This was due in part to the lack of knowledge regarding the agents which cause disease and in part to the lack of involvement of government in health matters. In view of the Tenth Amendment to the Constitution, since no powers in health matters were specifically delegated to the federal government, the health of the people was considered to be a responsibility of the states. The Marine Hospital Service was created by an Act of Congress in 1798. However, this service was concerned not with public hygiene or prevention of disease but rather with the operation of hospitals for the care of disabled merchant seamen.

Of the 38 states that made up the Union in 1876, twelve had state boards of health. The first of these to be established was that of Louisiana in 1855 and the second that of Massachusetts, in 1869. None of these state boards had become really effective by 1876. In 16 states there were laws requiring registration of births, deaths, and marriages, but according to Bowditch (1876) the laws were either defective or poorly enforced in all except two states; and even in these there was doubt as to the reliability of the statistics. Information obtained by Bowditch in 1875–76 from 143 towns throughout the United States indicated that only 49 made any effort to assure the purity of their water supply. "That is to say, nearly two-thirds of the people of this Union are living in a senseless disregard as to whether they are drinking pure water or water which, though sparkling and tasting

47

pleasant, may be loaded with every species of filth!" Bowditch added that in "not a few cities which take water from rivers," including Philadelphia, Pennsylvania, and Albany, New York, the municipal sewers emptied into the river at a point above that from which the water supply was drawn.

As has already been mentioned, some of the states adopted but did not enforce licensing laws to protect the people from unqualified medical practitioners. Some states also adopted quarantine laws, which were designed to prevent the entry of epidemic diseases from foreign lands. In this endeavor a few states were more energetic and successful than others, but since there were no effective barriers between states, the result for the nation as a whole was no better than that of the most neglectful state. A physician in Boston in the mid-nineteenth century declared "that he could keep Boston free of smallpox if he could prevent the citizens from meeting immigrants from Maine, who flocked, most of them unvaccinated adults, into the city limits" (Bowditch, 1876).

A change in professional and public attitudes toward contagion and sanitation resulted from the cholera epidemics that ravaged the country between 1832 and 1873. For centuries it had been known that the commoner childhood diseases such as chickenpox, measles, and mumps were passed from one individual to another by close personal contact; that they were, in other words, contagious. However, it was not understood how some of the great epidemic diseases of high mortality (yellow fever, typhus, cholera, malaria) were propagated. For example, it seemed clear that yellow fever and malaria were not passed from person to person by close contact. Rush taught that yellow fever was not contagious. He believed that the great Philadelphia epidemic of 1793 began in the waterfront area not because people ill of the disease had been brought into port by ships from the West Indies (as was unquestionably the case) but because a damaged cargo of coffee had been dumped in the dock area and had decomposed, giving rise to "noxious effluvia." He emphasized his disbelief in the contagion theory by saying "I rested myself on the bedside of my patients, and I drank milk or ate fruit in their sick rooms."

Rush was, of course, both right and wrong: yellow fever is not spread by personal contact, but neither is it caused by bad air. This puzzle was not solved until a century later, when the mosquito was revealed to be the missing link in the transmission of yellow fever.

Cholera, unlike yellow fever, was a new disease to America. Its spread to all parts of the world from its usual confines in India has been attributed to the more numerous and more rapid means of travel that became available in the early decades of the nineteenth century. At the time, little was known about how the disease traveled except that it appeared to be transported by its victims. An epidemic which started in India in 1826 crept overland across Persia, Russia, and Europe and then made its way by ship across the Atlantic, reaching Canada and the United States in 1832. A similar worldwide spread from the Indian focus brought cholera to the United States in 1849 and 1866. In the period of 34 years between the epidemics of 1832 and 1866, as has been so well described and documented in Rosenberg's *The Cholera Years* (1962), there was a radical change in the attitude toward methods of dealing with cholera.

The most devastating effects of cholera always fell upon the poor, who lived in cheap, crowded, slovenly neighborhoods. In Richmond, Virginia, in 1832, nine tenths of those who died of cholera were buried in the poorhouse graveyard, and in New York City, of 100 cholera deaths on a single day in July, 95 were buried in the Potter's Field. The slums were invariably harder hit than the better sections of a city. In the 1830s and 1840s the slums of American cities were at their worst: crowded tumble-down housing, stinking outdoor privies, tainted drinking water, "swill" milk, pigs rooting through the piles of garbage in the streets. The slums were also the habitat of prostitutes, drunkards, criminals, and other social outcasts. In 1832 it was generally believed that moral dereliction rather than sanitary deficiency attracted cholera to the slums. The sermons delivered from many pulpits proclaimed that the cholera epidemic was a manifestation of the Will of God. God's wrath had fallen upon the moral delinquents in order that their fate might serve as a lesson to society to mend its evil ways. It seemed not only useless but also impious to try to thwart the Divine Will. The obvious inability of the medical profession either to prevent or to cure cholera encouraged the belief that one's best hope of survival lay in prayer, strict observance of the Ten Commandments, and penance for one's sins.

By the time the epidemic of 1866 came along, new facts had come to light concerning the propagation of cholera. In the 1850s, John Snow (1813–1858), an English physician, had shown that the disease was spread in London by contaminated drinking water. In the same period there were strong indications that it was the sanitary rather than the moral transgressions of the slums that determined their vulnerability to cholera. Hopefully, the prevention of spread within a city was not beyond the power of ordinary men; it might not even need the leadership of a doctor or a priest. It did not require the expertise of either of these professions to arrange for a water supply that was not contaminated by sewage and to attend to the enforcement of general sanitary measures. Most of the larger cities prior to 1866 had created boards of health, made up largely of "ordinary men," to cope with these matters. As a result, in the cities which had made the greatest progress in correcting their hygienic deficiencies, the epidemic of 1866 ran a shorter course than its predecessors and was less disruptive of urban life.

The experience with cholera made it clearer than ever before that local government had an important role to play in guarding the health of the public. It had also demonstrated with equal clarity, as Bowditch pointed out in 1876, that the spread of epidemics from state to state could not be checked by the states' acting independently. As a result of the lessons taught by cholera, Bowditch proposed that the responsibility for public hygiene and preventive medicine be assigned to a "National Health Council composed of representatives from each state, and a Secretary of Health, the peer of other Secretaries in the National Cabinet." He also proposed that there be "a National System for the registration of all Births, Marriages and Deaths." As a general title for the measures which he advocated, Bowditch employed the expression "State Preventive Medicine." When he used this term he had in mind certain developments in Britain and in Germany (Bowditch, 1876).

In Germany, Max von Pettenkofer (1818–1901), who had begun his professional career as a chemist in the 1840s, had become increasingly interested in the problems of sanitation and had carried out a number of experiments in the field of hygiene. He was responsible for the development of departments of hygiene in three universities, and in 1865 he became the first Professor of Hygiene in Germany. Pettenkofer's concept of public hygiene was as advanced as it was inclusive. He considered its realm of concern to embrace the atmosphere, clothing, housing, ventilation, heating, lighting, soil conditions, drinking water, foods (including milk, meat, and vegetables), sewerage and disposal of human feces, burial regulations, the hazards of trades and factories, regulations for the handling of poisonous substances, and registration of births, deaths, and causes of death. He persuaded the city of Munich, which then had a population of 170,000, to adopt a number of hygienic measures for improvement of housing, water supply, sewage disposal, and other influential factors in sanitation. An impressive argument in favor of these measures was the economic one. Pettenkofer maintained that if Munich, where the death rate was then more than 40 per 1000 population per year, could succeed in bringing its sanitation up to the standard already achieved in London, where by 1856 the death rate had been reduced to 22 per 1000 per year, the saving to the city and its citizens would amount to 25 million *gulden* annually. By 1876 Munich still had far to go to achieve this objective, but it was on its way to becoming one of the world's showplaces of urban sanitation and beauty. In that year Pettenkofer opened in Munich the world's first Hygienic Institute (Hume, 1925).

While in Germany the activities in the field of public hygiene were being carried out at the municipal level, those in Great Britain had come to involve the entire nation. The industrial revolution had changed the inhabitants of Britain from rural to urban dwellers. The cities, notably London, were teeming with ill-housed and ill-clad poor people and were filthy and disease-ridden. John Snow had shown how cholera was spread in London.

In 1873 another English physician, William Budd (1811–1880), had published his treatise *Typhoid Fever: Its Nature, Mode of Spreading, and Prevention,* which provided strong evidence that typhoid fever was spread by the excreta of patients having the disease, either by contamination of drinking water, by personal contact, or by other means. The work of Snow and Budd pointed to practical ways to prevent the spread of some of the most dreaded epidemic diseases; but it was apparent that the measures needed to achieve this end would require action by government at some level. Fortunately, another series of events was preparing the way for action of this type.

The leader of a movement to correct the evils of the crowded cities, Edwin Chadwick (1800–1890), was not a physician but a government official and a disciple of Jeremy Bentham (1748–1832), proponent of the social philosophy "the greatest happiness of the greatest number." After publishing, in the 1830s and 1840s, a series of reports on the deplorable hygienic conditions of the cities, Chadwick succeeded in making the government realize its responsibility for the health of the nation. His reports emphasizing "the national prevalence of sanitary neglect" were publicly printed and widely read. The attitude of a top-flight politician who had been won over to the cause of public hygiene was voiced by Benjamin Disraeli in 1872 when in speaking of sanitation he said: "Gentlemen, it is impossible to overrate the importance of the subject. After all, the first consideration of a Minister should be the health of the people" (Rolleston, 1934).

In the United States the members of the medical profession, with rare exceptions, did not encourage the involvement of government in health matters, though the precedent for such involvement existed. Benjamin Franklin recalled, in 1786, that when he was a boy living in Boston, a complaint had come "from North Carolina, against New England Rum, that it poison'd their People, Giving them the Dry Bellyache, with a Loss of the Use of their Limbs. The Distilleries being examin'd on the Occasion, it was found that several of them used leaden Stillheads and Worms [coils], and the Physicians were of Opinion, that the Mischief was occasioned by that Use of Lead. The Legislature of the Massachusetts thereupon pass'd an Act, prohibiting under severe Penalties the Use of such Stillheads and Worms thereafter." The Act to which Franklin referred was passed in 1723 by the legislature of "His Majesty's Province of Massachusetts-Bay in New-England" (Malloch, 1931). This law, which was strictly enforced, apparently put an end to lead poisoning by New England rum.

Such an excursion by government into the area of preventive medicine was rare in North America until well into the nineteenth century. In 1876, Bowditch said, "The medical profession as a body has heretofore taken very little interest in the ideas underlying preventive medicine, and hygiene, private or public." He pointed out that "the first and strongest efforts in behalf of State Preventive Medicine" had been exerted by the laity rather than the profession. The efforts to which Bowditch referred were initiated by Lemuel Shattuck of Boston, a student of social problems who in 1850 presented to the Massachusetts Legislature "a most exhaustive State Paper entitled 'Report of the Sanitary Commission of Massachusetts.'" This report "laid down all the principal ideas and modes of action" for government participation in the fields of hygiene and preventive medicine. In spite of this, the report was virtually ignored until 1869, when a "State Board of Health of laymen and physicians, exactly as Mr. Shattuck recommended, was established by Massachusetts. Dr. Derby, its first secretary, looked to this [Shattuck's] admirable document as its inspiration and support" (Bowditch, 1876).

In the 1870s the movement that had been initiated by Shattuck gathered strength. Additional states established boards of health. In 1872, the *American Public Health Association* was founded and began to play an active role in the promotion of public hygiene and preventive medicine. Still, in 1876, Bowditch declared regretfully that "a large majority of the States and Territories of this Union are not yet sufficiently enlightened to appreciate the duty devolving on them to be careful of the health of their people."

An Act of Congress in 1875 provided that a surgeon-general of the Marine Hospital Service should be appointed by the President, with the consent of the Senate. Three years later Congress gave broad powers to the Service to cooperate with state and local health authorities in the control of epidemic diseases such as yellow fever and cholera. Thus, as the second century began, the Marine Hospital Service was on its way toward becoming the United States Public Health Service.

51

5
Hospitals

About the end of the year 1750, some persons, who had frequent opportunities of observing the distress of such distempered Poor as from Time to Time came to Philadelphia, *for the Advice and Assistance of the Physicians and Surgeons of that City. . . . and considering moreover, that even the poor inhabitants of this city, though they had homes, yet were therein but badly accommodated in Sickness. . . . and several of the Inhabitants of the Province, who unhappily became disordered in their Senses, wandered about, to the Terror of their Neighbors, there being no Place (except the House of Correction) in which they might be confined. . . . did charitably consult together, and confer with their friends and acquaintances, on the best means of relieving the distressed. . . . and an Infirmary, or Hospital, in the manner of several lately established in* Great Britain, *being proposed, was so generally approved, that there was reason to expect a considerable subscription from the Inhabitants of this City, towards the support of such a Hospital. . . .*

(Benjamin Franklin, 1754)

Although the Hôtel Dieu was established in Quebec in 1646, the first hospital to be founded in the British colonies of North America appears to have been "St. Philip's Hospital in Charlestown in Carolina." This institution, which was built in 1736 to serve the paupers of St. Philip's parish, was not a hospital in the modern sense. It was characterized as a "good, substantial, and convenient Hospital, Workhouse, and House of Correction." In line with its multiple functions the warden was authorized "to take, besides his salary, fees and profits from the inmates or their labour, and to use 'fetters or shackles' or 'moderate whipping' on the inmates, or to 'abridge them of their food' if the necessity arose" (Waring, 1932). Apart from its functions as a workhouse and house of correction the "hospital" did, indeed, care for the indigent sick of the parish, and to supervise this service a physician was employed at a regular annual salary. In 1740 his salary was £ 150 per year, but this was gradually increased to £ 1000 per year by the time of the Revolutionary War. Shortly after the War, the hospital passed out of existence.

53

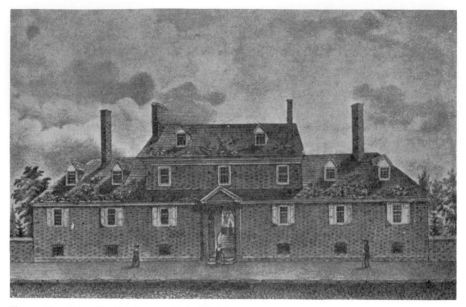

Figure 12. Friend's Almshouse, Philadelphia.

St. Philip's Hospital seems to us today to have been a strange sort of hospital, but it was not at all strange for its time. Early eighteenth-century hospitals served only the poverty-stricken members of the community, and they housed not only the sick but also the aged, the halt, the blind, and the feeble-minded. They also provided a home for paupers who had no home of their own. It was not unusual for the hospital to be combined with the workhouse. In the mid-eighteenth century a number of new hospitals were established in England and Scotland. These institutions adhered to the tradition of caring only for the poor, but they turned their attention increasingly to the provision of medical and surgical care, to the gradual exclusion of the workhouse functions.

The only permanent public general hospital to be established during the colonial period in the territory that was to become the United States was the *Pennsylvania Hospital.* The movement to build this hospital was started in 1750 by Dr. Thomas Bond, aided by his friend Benjamin Franklin. Shortly after the hospital opened in 1751, Franklin described its intended functions as follows:

(1) To provide suitable lodgings and other conveniences for "such distempered Poor as from Time to Time came to *Philadelphia,* for the Advice and Assistance of the Physicians and Surgeons of that City . . . providing good and careful Nurses, and other Attendants for want whereof many must suffer greatly. . . ."

(2) To provide housing for the medical care of the "poor Inhabitants of this City" who, though they might have homes of their own, "yet were therein but badly accommodated in Sickness, and could not be so well and so easily taken Care of in their separate Habitations, as they might be in one convenient House, under one Inspection and in the Hands of skillful Practitioners."

(3) To afford a haven for "several of the Inhabitants of the Province,

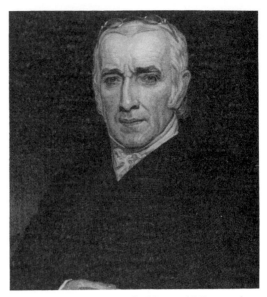

Figure 13. Thomas Bond. (National Library of Medicine, Bethesda, Maryland.)

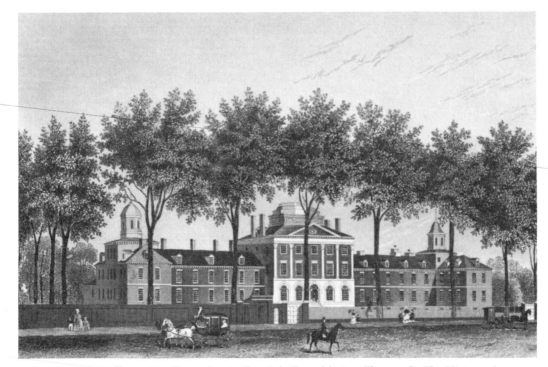

Figure 14. Pennsylvania Hospital. (From Morton, Thomas G.: The History of the Pennsylvania Hospital, 1751–1895. Philadelphia, Times Printing House, 1897.)

who unhappily became disordered in their Senses, wandered about, to the Terror of their Neighbors, there being no Place (except the House of Correction) in which they might be confined, and subjected to proper Management for their Recovery. . . ."

(4) To establish a hospital "in the Manner of several lately established in *Great Britain* . . ." (Cohen, 1954). Here, then, was a hospital without workhouse connotations which was to provide housing and medical, surgical, and nursing care for the poor people of Philadelphia and the surrounding country.

One function of the hospital not mentioned by Franklin became apparent a few years later, when "the Attending Physicians brought with them their office students, or apprentices, to follow the practice of the house, to apply dressings and render other assistance." Still later "an actual indenture was drawn up, by which the friends of the apprentice regularly bound him to serve the hospital for a period of five years, and the Managers on their part agreeing to instruct him in the art of medicine, etc. On leaving the hospital service, the young man had a suit of 'cloathes' and an engrossed certificate, if he completed his engagement satisfactorily. Beside the apprentices there were occasionally other resident pupils. . . . After the establishment of the Medical Department of the University of Pennsylvania, the apprentices attended lectures while serving the hospital." In 1824 a rule was adopted by the hospital "requiring Residents to be graduates in medicine previous to entering upon their duties in the Hospital" (Morton, 1897).

In 1766, Dr. Thomas Bond announced to the medical students of the College of Philadelphia that he would offer at the Pennsylvania Hospital a course in which he would "give you the best information in my power of the nature and treatment of chronical diseases, and of the proper management of ulcers, wounds and fractures. I shall show you all the operations of surgery, and endeavour . . . to introduce you to a familiar acquaintance with the acute diseases of your own country, in order to which, I shall put up a complete Meteorological Apparatus, and endeavour to inform you of all the known properties of the atmosphere which surrounds us, and the effects its frequent variations produce on animal bodies . . ." (Morton, 1897). Dr. Bond thus announced the first in-hospital instruction for medical students.

Although the *New York Hospital* obtained a Royal Charter in 1771, it did not function during the colonial period. Its original buildings were destroyed by fire as they were nearing completion in 1775, and new buildings were under construction when British troops occupied New York City. These buildings served as soldiers' barracks during the war and were not utilized as a hospital until 1791. In 1794 a distinguished Frenchman visiting New York gave this account of the new hospital (Roberts and Roberts, 1947):

This one does not belong to the city, having been built and maintained by private subscriptions. The subscribers, among whom are many Quakers, appoint two directors from their number. As a rule this hospital has fifty or sixty patients of both sexes. The sexes are separated. The death rate is one in twenty. The building is made up of a ground floor and an upper story. Each patient has a wooden bed, a mattress and sheets. Negroes are put in wards by themselves. Patients pay two dollars a week if they are able to do so. Four physicians give their services each quarter. A surgeon is attached to the hospital. In all it has twenty-four employees. The annual expense of the hospital is reckoned to be between two and three thousand dollars. The kitchens and the laundry are down in the cellars. There are four small rooms for lunatics, only one of which is occupied. There is a yard where patients are allowed to walk, and plans call for planting trees in it. A vegetable garden takes up part of the grounds, and some flowers are grown in it.

There has been some criticism of this hospital, and if it had any foundation, it would be truly serious. This is the charge that it refuses to accept sick persons if they have no money, particularly those afflicted with chronic diseases. It is further charged that such unfortunates go to the City Hospital [i.e., City Almshouse] and die there.

The third public general hospital to operate in the United States was the *Charity Hospital of New Orleans.* Actually this hospital antedates the New York Hospital, but New Orleans did not become United States territory until Louisiana was purchased in 1803.

In addition to the three general hospitals that were in existence in 1810, temporary hospitals had been established from time to time to perform special functions. A famous hospital of this type was the *Bush Hill Hospital,* which served Philadelphia so well during the great yellow fever epidemic of 1793 (Lane, 1936). "Fever hospitals" such as Bush Hill were usually supported by public funds and served the poor people of the community. They ceased operation as soon as the epidemic subsided. There were also the crude Army hospitals of the Revolutionary War and the Marine hospitals, which were established under the sponsorship of the federal government. After 1810 there was a gradual increase in the number of urban hospitals for the care of the sick poor.

The first major hospital to be organized after 1810, the *Massachusetts General Hospital,* from an early date exhibited features which were not to be adopted by most other hospitals until many years later: (1) special provisions for training both undergraduate and graduate medical students; (2) emergency services at all hours, day and night, provided by physicians always available at the hospital; (3) an outpatient department with hours designated for different types of specialty services; (4) admission of paying patients as well as those of the pauper class; (5) the maintenance of detailed case-records.

The founding of the Massachusetts General Hospital was chiefly due to the efforts of two young doctors, James Jackson, who had just been appointed Professor of Clinical Medicine at Harvard, and J. C. Warren, Assistant Professor of Surgery. Both of these men had had experience in the best-known teaching hospitals of London. It was they who had persuaded the Harvard authorities to allow the medical school to be moved from Cambridge to Boston; and it was they who had persuaded the overseers of the Boston Almshouse to allow the small ward of that institution to be used for the clinical instruction of medical students. They were well aware of the shortcomings of the Almshouse and were anxious to organize a hospital that would provide educational opportunities similar to those of the London hospitals with which they were familiar. In 1810 they inaugurated a campaign to persuade wealthy Bostonians to contribute funds for the construction and support of such a hospital. A statement of the type reiterated during the campaign was the following: "A hospital is an institution abso-

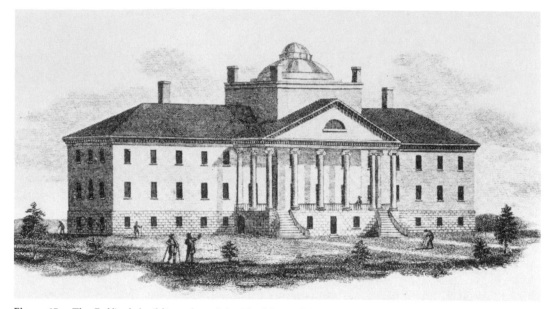

Figure 15. The Bulfinch building, the original building of the Massachusetts General Hospital. (From Myers, T. G.: History of the Massachusetts General Hospital. Boston, Griffiths-Stillings Press, 1929.)

lutely essential for a medical school, and one which would afford relief and comfort to thousands of the sick and miserable. On what other object can the superfluities of the rich be so well bestowed?''

Although the corporation of the proposed hospital held its first meeting in 1811, the War of 1812 and other unforeseen problems delayed construction. It was 1821 before the hospital was opened to receive patients. The original hospital building had an unusual appearance owing to its disproportionately large dome, a new feature designed to provide lighting for the surgical amphitheater on the top floor. The building contained beds for 93 patients. That the public did not know how to make use of their new institution is indicated by the fact that for three weeks after the hospital opened, only one patient applied for admission and at the end of the first year the patient census was only 12.

In 1822 the Trustees made a public statement describing the facilities and services offered by the hospital (Myers, 1929):

In the center are the rooms for the superintendent, the apothecary, attendants, and the kitchen. In the upper part of the center is also the operating theater. The wings are divided into apartments for patients; those of the males being distinct from the females. The staircases and entries are of stone. The apartments are supplied with heat by [wooden] pipes from a furnace in the cellar. They are also supplied with water, by pipes running by the side of the air flues, in order to prevent freezing in winter. The hospital is under the immediate care of the superintendent and it is visited and examined by a committee of the trustees every Thursday. . . . The physician and surgeon, independent of their regular duties in the hospital, will give advice to outpatients, to whom medicines will also be distributed gratuitously. The physician, Dr. Jackson, attends for this purpose, at the hospital, on Thursdays, at 12:00, and the surgeon, Dr. Warren, at the same hour on Tuesdays and Fridays. On

58

the latter day persons affected with disorders of the eyes will particularly receive medical advice.

The situation of the Hospital . . . allows it to be approached by water, by all the New England States which border upon the ocean.

The hospital offers peculiar advantages to those who require surgical operations. . . . There is a room expressly prepared for this purpose, with a light adapted to it, and in case of accident or emergency, there are instruments, dressings, medicines and skillful attendants, all within call and reach of the operator, and also in case of pain or accident following an operation there is always a physician in the place ready to administer relief both day and night. . . . The trustees consider this the most favorable arrangement in the hospital, and one upon which great value deserves to be placed.

Though the trustees have appropriated six beds to poor patients, they possess at this time no funds to provide for that expense, but they have thought proper to do it in a just expectation that the hospital would be remunerated by the generosity of the public.

The statement that there was "always a physician in the place" referred to the *Resident Physician* (who was also superintendent of the hospital) and his assistant, the *Apothecary,* both of whom had living accommodations in the hospital. The Resident Physician, whose appointment was a permanent one, was a man of experience, able to supervise the medical and surgical care of the patients with the advice and assistance of the *Visiting Physician,* Dr. Jackson, and *Visiting Surgeon,* Dr. J. C. Warren. The Apothecary was a recent medical school graduate of limited experience. His appointment was for one year only, and his duties corresponded in many respects to those of a twentieth century intern. He assisted the Resident Physician in the day-to-day care of patients, and he was the "clinical clerk." It was due to his efforts that "the earlier volumes of case-records stand as models of their kind, for completeness, accuracy and neatness" (Putnam, 1906). The Visiting Physician and the Visiting Surgeon made regular teaching rounds to the patients of their respective services (see Jackson's letter, p. 14), and the Visiting Surgeon also performed the more difficult operations. It was J. C. Warren who performed the first operation using ether anesthesia in 1846. Since then the hospital dome, which still exists, has been known as the *Ether Dome.*

In 1828 the Apothecary was replaced by two young medical graduates, each appointed for one year, one entitled *House Physician,* the other, *House Surgeon.* In the late 1840s the number of men appointed to these positions began to increase, and at the same time it was decided to choose the appointees from among medical students. The title was then changed to *House Pupil.* In 1850 five House Pupils were appointed. In 1860 they were given permission to sleep and take their breakfasts in the hospital, and in 1861 they were provided full board. A floor plan of the hospital in 1872 shows that House Pupils had the following accommodations: a bedroom large enough for six beds, a bathroom (one of the only two in the entire hospital), and a separate dining room. In addition there was a small lecture hall across the corridor from the bedroom. In 1873, on the recommendation of President Eliot of Harvard, the hospital began to select its House Pupils on the basis of competitive examinations open to students of all medical schools who had completed the third year of their medical studies. Since the length of the medical course at most schools was then no more than two years, only Harvard students and a few others were eligible for the examinations, but the number of others would increase as additional schools adopted the three-year curriculum. In 1875 there were seven House Pupils, four surgical and three medical.

St. Vincent's Hospital, in New York City, which was built in 1850, was the first hospital in the United States to include in its architectural plan a group of rooms for private patients (Freidson, 1963). Although the Massachusetts General Hospital accepted paying patients prior to this date, it is not known just when it began to set aside rooms specially furnished and decorated for private patients. In 1864 the hospital had "seven private rooms of different sizes and grades situated in different parts of the institution, not in a separate building. . . . Some of these rooms were fitted up very luxuriantly, and very little about them suggested a 'sick room.' The heavy damask lambrequins surrounded by gilt cornices, and the lace draperies and soft carpet dispelled all thoughts of a patient's room" (Myers, 1929).

The Massachusetts General Hospital was in many respects a pioneering institution. That it was by no means typical of contemporary hospitals may be gathered from W. Gill Wylie's *Boylston Prize-Essay* (Harvard University) for 1876. This essay provides an excellent description of hospitals in the latter part of the nation's first century. The following passages are quoted from Wylie's account.

> *More than five years ago, while a surgeon on the Resident House-Staff of Bellevue Hospital, a large pauper-hospital of this city [New York], I had an excellent opportunity for seeing the bad effects of poor nursing and defective construction on the welfare of patients. At that time, with rare exceptions, the nurses were ignorant and in some cases worthless characters, who accepted the almost impossible task of attending to and nursing from twenty to thirty patients each. There were no night-nurses; the night-watchmen—three in number to a hospital of eight hundred beds—were expected to give assistance to patients requiring attention during the night. The hospital building, originally an old prison and almshouse erected sixty years ago, had been added to, and was now a massive stone structure, with three stories and a basement. The wards were only separated from each other by the intervening partitions inclosing the water-closets and bath-rooms, which were without ventilation, except as they opened into the wards. In some instances there were only six windows to wards of twenty beds.*

> *The sanitary condition of the hospital was shocking. . . . I saw . . . patients die from septic diseases contracted in the wards after the slightest surgical operations or injuries. From forty to sixty percent of all amputations of limbs proved fatal; and I saw a strong, healthy man die from pyaemia [popularly known as "blood poisoning"] following an amputation of a great-toe.*

In the year 1871, 7514 patients were treated in the wards of Bellevue Hospital; of these, 1102 died, 36 of pyemia and 33 of puerperal peritonitis (childbed fever) among 376 women delivered. The overall death rate was 14.7 per cent, and the maternal death rate from puerperal sepsis was 8.7 per cent. Between 1871 and 1876, through the efforts of several public-spirited individuals and organizations, a great improvement took place at Bellevue,

60

and Wylie says, "Since the introduction of trained nurses, the removal of lying-in patients, the reduction in the number of beds from eight to six hundred, and the use of Lister's antiseptic dressings, the condition of the hospital has been very much improved." In fact, during this five-year period Bellevue had become one of the country's most progressive public hospitals. It had taken steps to reduce overcrowding; it was one of the first American hospitals to adopt Lister's methods; it had decided that the risk of puerperal sepsis was too high to warrant having a maternity service in a general hospital; and it had established the first American *Training-School for Nurses.*

Wylie points out that hospital construction prior to 1850 had been designed to conserve expense by providing spaces into which as many patients as possible might be crowded. In the late eighteenth century the renowned old Hôtel Dieu of Paris, an immense structure, housed more than 5000 patients. One of its typical barnlike wards contained two to three hundred double-beds, each occupied by two to six patients. It is not surprising that under these conditions infections spread like fire. The death rate in this hospital was appalling. "During the prevalence of the plague as many as sixty-eight thousand died within the hospital in one year" (Wylie, 1877).

It gradually became apparent to discerning physicians and surgeons that the high mortality rate in the large urban hospitals was related to overcrowding. In 1869, J. Y. Simpson, the Scottish gynecologist, gathered statistics showing that of 2089 amputations performed in urban hospital practice, 855 patients (41 per cent) died; while of 2098 amputations performed in country practice (principally operations in the home) only 226 patients (11 per cent) died. On the basis of this study Simpson urged that the large hospitals be replaced by small cottage hospitals of cheap construction so that it would be feasible to set them on fire or to tear them down every few years if the rate of septic (infectious) complications seemed to warrant it (Ashhurst, 1927). Semmelweis had shown two decades previously that the rate of such complications could be greatly reduced by less drastic measures. In his maternity ward in Vienna he had reduced the mortality due to puerperal sepsis from 12 per cent to 1.3 per cent simply by insisting that everyone, before examining his patients, must wash his hands thoroughly in a solution of chloride of lime.

In 1860, when Joseph Lister moved from Edinburgh to Glasgow, the Glasgow Infirmary was notorious for its "unhealthiness." In the overcrowded surgical wards there was a frightful death rate from wound infections, pyemia, erysipelas, and gangrene. It was in order to prevent these fatal complications that Lister began, in 1865, to experiment with antiseptic dressings. Within a few years the incidence of sepsis had been markedly reduced. Lister himself believed that an important preliminary to his success was his refusal to permit overcrowding on his wards (Ashhurst, 1927):

. . . *the managing body, . . . anxious to provide hospital accommodation for the increasing population of Glasgow, for which the Infirmary was by no means adequate, were disposed to introduce additional beds beyond those contemplated in the original construction. It is, I believe, fairly attributable to the firmness of my resistance in this matter that, though my patients suffered . . . in a way that was sickening and often heart-rending, so as to make me sometimes feel it a questionable privilege to be connected with the institution, yet none of my wards ever assumed the frightful condition which sometimes showed itself in other parts of the building, making it necessary to shut them up entirely for a time.*

61

The larger urban hospitals in the United States were also beset by a high rate of infections and needed to close down a ward from time to time to permit "cleansing and purification." William Gibson, Chief of Surgery at the Philadelphia General Hospital in the mid-nineteenth century, announced to his students each year at about Christmas time: "This is the season of the year when erysipelas prevails in the wards; we will do no more operations until the first of March!" (Ashhurst, 1927).

In spite of Lister's work and the progress of bacteriology in Europe, the "germ theory" of infections had not been accepted in the United States by 1876. The high incidence of infections in hospitals was still considered to be due to "bad air" in a crowded space. These were the factors that determined the architectural plan of hospitals, as Wylie pointed out in 1876:

> *More than a hundred years ago it was clearly shown that a large number of sick people should never be assembled under the same roof, as it is impossible to supply each patient with the requisite amount of fresh air on account of the large quantities of poisonous gas thrown off from the lungs and emanating from the bodies, the wounds and excretions of the patients, and continually infecting the air; that in a large building the foul air of one part could not be prevented from permeating the whole structure—in this way one infectious case being liable to infect all the inmates.*

These principles did not significantly influence the design of hospitals until after 1850, when recognition of them was forced to the fore by tragic experiences in two wars. Florence Nightingale's observations during the Crimean War (1854–55) led to the publication in 1859 of her *Notes on Hospitals,* in which she advocated that hospitals should consist of small, pavilion-type wards joined by open-air corridors. The experience during the American Civil War confirmed the soundness of Miss Nightingale's recommendations and, according to Wylie, formed the basis for the establishment of the following principles for the construction of hospitals:

> *1. That the hospital should be placed on a large area of ground, so that the pavilions can be widely separated from the administrative buildings and from each other.*
>
> *2. That the wards should be only one story in height, and be ventilated by openings along the ridge of the roof.*
>
> *3. That the ward-pavilions should be put up not to remain for generations to come, but only so long as they are free from infection; and that when once they are infected, they should be destroyed, and replaced with entirely new structures.*

The first civilian hospital to be constructed according to plans developed during the Civil War was built in Germany. This was a one-story ward-pavilion hospital constructed in Leipzig in 1867–68. "During twelve months, Prof. Thiersch, who has charge of the surgical clinic, performed 266 serious surgical operations, and did not lose a single case from pyemia; while prior to the construction of the new pavilions, in the old stone hospital . . . he lost forty to fifty amputations from this cause annually" (Wylie, 1877).

In 1873, two small (45 by 55 feet), free-standing, one-story wards were built at the Massachusetts General Hospital. "These were the first wards of

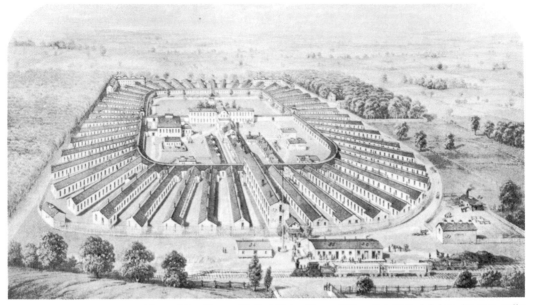

Figure 16. Mower United States General Hospital, Philadelphia. An unusually large Civil War hospital.

the pavilion type to be built in this part of the world. They were modeled somewhat upon the plan of army field-hospitals, with such modifications as climate and greater permanency required. Particular attention was paid to heating and ventilation. . . . It was not expected that they would be used for longer than six or seven years, as by that time they would have become 'hospitalized' and useless, and it would be necessary to tear them down. Therefore, temporary materials were used in their construction" (Myers, 1927). One of these buildings was designed as an open ward of 20 beds; the other was divided into eight rooms for paying patients — the hospital's first private ward. The charge for private patients in this building was $35 per week. Though built for a life of only six or seven years, the two pavilions were still in use at the end of the nineteenth century.

Wylie emphasized that the pavilion type of construction was preferable not only for control of infections but also for keeping down building costs: "The New York Hospital now being completed is a building of seven stories, to contain a hundred and fifty beds. The contract for the building alone is $432,000" ($2836 per bed). The contract for building a one-story pavilion at the Presbyterian Hospital of Philadelphia for 28 beds was $12,000, or a cost of $428 for each bed." The heating apparatus and furnishings made the total $15,000, or only $535 for each bed." The money appropriated by the Massachusetts General Hospital for the two small pavilions mentioned above was only $15,000.

There was a great flurry of hospital construction in the United States after the Civil War. In New York City alone, between the close of the war and 1876, six new hospitals were built, "the smallest of these, with the ground it stands on, costing about half a million dollars." It is remarkable that only one of the six hospitals, and this one only in part, utilized the plan of hospital construction advocated by Miss Nightingale and adopted by the United States Army. This was owing to the fact that the pavilion type of construction requires a larger plot of ground than was usually available within the confines of a city. That the pavilion plan was considered by the experts to be preferable when ample space was available was proved by the plans submitted for the Johns Hopkins Hospital in 1875.

Though we cannot deal adequately with the development of hospitals for the mentally ill, it is noteworthy that during the early years of the nineteenth century a movement was started which revolutionized the institutional care of the insane. Prior to 1815 the mentally ill were cared for largely in an appendage to the local almshouse. In describing the care of the insane at that time, the Reverend John S. Bartlett, who served as chaplain of the Boston Almshouse from 1807 to 1810, wrote, "There were generally from 10 to 20 in the house, and although the care was taken of them which the circumstances of the house would afford, yet there was no proper place for their confinement and rest; a 20-foot building, with several cells opening into a long entry, in each of which cells was a board cabin or berth, with loose straw, a pail for necessary purposes, was their only accommodation. The violent were confined in strait jackets, and the filth and wretchedness of the place were dreadful. At that time there were no places of refuge for the insane in Massachusetts except in a few private houses in the country, owned and managed by Doctors. . . . The mode of managing the insane then was most cruel, and unfavorable to recovery. Whipping, etc., was often resorted to . . ." (Myers, 1929).

The preceding description of the situation in 1810 was written by Bartlett in 1839. During that interval a great change had taken place in the care of the insane. For centuries, mentally deranged people had been subjected to the most cruel forms of institutional management: confined in cells lacking even the most primitive comfort; restrained by strait jackets, handcuffs, and leg irons; and abandoned by family and friends, they were without hope of recovery. However, reform in the care of the insane was begun in England in 1792 by William Tuke, and in 1794 he founded the Quaker Retreat in York. Similar reforms were initiated in France in 1795 under the leadership of Philippe Pinel. These two men and their followers brought about a gradual change in the attitude toward insanity. Small mental institutions were established in which a more humane, sympathetic type of treatment was provided, frequently with gratifying results: recovery and a return to a useful life. In the United States one of the first to appreciate the advantages of more humane treatment was Benjamin Rush. In the year before his death he set forth his liberal views on this subject in his treatise *Medical Inquiries and Observations upon the Diseases of the Mind,* the first general treatise on psychiatry written in America. Deutsch (1937) says that in writing this book Rush "fully earned the title by which he was known to later generations—'the father of American Psychiatry.'"

Rush had had a long experience with mental disease as Physician to the Pennsylvania Hospital. One of Franklin's original arguments for the establishment of this hospital was that it would be used for "the cure and treatment of lunaticks" in order that "they may be restored to reason and become useful members of the community." From its very beginning a large segment of the hospital had been devoted to the care of the insane, but the methods employed were little better than those described by the Reverend Mr. Bartlett. Rush began to agitate for the employment of more humane management as early as 1789, before the work of Tuke and Pinel, but his most advanced thinking on this subject was expressed in a long letter addressed to the Managers of the Pennsylvania Hospital, dated September 24, 1810. In spite of its length, this letter was so advanced in providing insight into the problems of the institutional management of mental patients that it is quoted here in full (Butterfield, 1951):

Gentlemen,

When our late illustrious fellow citizen Dr. Franklin walked out from his house to lay the foundation stone of the Pennsylvania Hospital, he was accompanied by the late Dr. Bond and the managers and physicians of the Hospital. On their way Dr. Bond lamented that the Hospital would allure strangers from all the then provinces in America. "Then," said Dr. Franklin, "our institution will be more useful than we intended it to be." This answer has been verified in a remarkable manner, and particularly in the relief our Hospital has afforded to persons deprived of their reason from nearly all the states in the Union. As great improvements have taken place in the treatment of persons in that melancholy situation within the last thirty years, I beg leave to lay an account of them before you as far as I have been able to obtain them from the histories of asylums for mad people in foreign countries, as well as from my own experience during five and twenty years' attendance upon that class of patients in the Pennsylvania Hospital. By adopting them, we may extend the usefulness and reputation of the Hospital, and thus contribute to add to the high character our city has long sustained for wise and benevolent institutions. The improvements which I wish respectfully to submit to your consideration are as follow:

1. That small and solitary buildings be erected at a convenient distance from the west wing of the Hospital for the reception of patients in the high and distracted state of madness, in order to prevent the injuries done by their noises to persons in the recent or convalescent state of that disease, and to patients in other diseases by depriving them of sleep or by inducing distress from sympathy with their sufferings.

2. That separate floors be appropriated for each of the sexes.

3. That certain kinds of labor, exercise, and amusements be contrived for them which shall act at the same time upon their bodies and minds. The advantages of labor have been evinced in foreign hospitals, as well as our own, in a greater number of recoveries taking place among that class of people who are employed in the ordinary work of the Hospital than in persons elevated by their rank in life above the obligations or necessity of labor. Exercise and amusements should be the substitutes for labor in such persons. The amusements should be swinging, seesaw, riding a hobby horse or in what are called flying coaches, playing at chess and checkers, listening to the music of a flute or violin, and in making short excursions into the city or country. Perhaps kinds of labor might be discovered for every class of mad people of such a nature as to afford a small addition to the funds of the Hospital.

4. That an intelligent man and woman be employed to attend the different sexes whose business shall be to direct and share in their amusements and to divert their minds by conversation, reading, and obliging them to read and write upon subjects suggested from time to time by the attending physicians. While we admit madness to be seated in the mind, by a strange obliquity of conduct we attempt to cure it only by corporeal remedies. The disease affects both the body and mind, and can be cured only by remedies applied to each of them.

5. That no visitor be permitted to converse with or even to see the mad people (the

65

managers and officers of the Hospital excepted) without an order from the attending physician, unless he depute that power to one of the resident apothecaries. Many evils arise from an indiscriminate intercourse of mad people with visitors, whether members of their own families or strangers. They often complain to them of the managers, officers, and physicians of the Hospital, and at times in so rational a manner as to induce a belief that their tales of injustice and oppression are true. Madness, moreover, which might have been concealed in individuals and in families is thereby made public. Nor is this all. The anticipation of being exposed as a spectacle to idle and sometimes to impertinent visitors is the chief reason why our hospital is often the last instead of the first retreat of persons affected by madness. "I would rather die," said a young gentlemen of respectable connections in our city a few years ago who felt the premonitory signs of that disease, "than to be gazed at and pitied in the cell of a hospital." To prevent this poignant evil, he discharged a musket ball through his head a few days afterwards.

6. That a number of feather beds and hair mattresses, with an armchair, be provided for the use of the cells of all those persons who pay a liberal price for their board and whose grade of madness is such as not to endanger any injury being done to those articles.

7. That each of the cells be provided with a close-stool with a pan half filled with water in order to absorb the fetor from their evacuations. The inventor of this delicate and healthy contrivance (Dr. Clark of New-Castle in England) deserves more from humanity and science than if he had discovered a new planet. Figure to yourselves, gentlemen, the sufferings of persons in a small room from inhaling the fetor of their stools for hours after they have discharged them into a chamber pot! Contrast the difference of this situation with that in which those persons passed days and nights of sickness and confinement in their own houses! But other and greater evils have followed the use of chamber pots in the cells of our Hospital. A Mr. Searle of Salem in Massachusetts lost his life in the year 1794 in consequence of the mortification of a wound upon his buttock brought on by one of them breaking under him, and there is good reason to believe that the malignant fever of which George Campbell died in the month of August last was induced by his being constantly exposed to the exhalations from the feces of mad people in emptying their chamber pots and cleaning their cells.

I am aware that it will be impracticable to carry into effect all the matters suggested in this letter in the present state of the funds of our Hospital, but the comfort of the mad people and the reputation of the institution are inseparably connected with the immediate adoption of some of them. There is a great pleasure in combatting with success a violent bodily disease, but what is this pleasure compared with that of restoring a fellow creature from the anguish and folly of madness and of reviving in him the knowledge of himself, his family, his friends, and his God! But where this cannot be done, how delightful the consideration of suspending by our humanity their mental and bodily misery! Degraded as they are by their disease, a sense of corporeal pleasure, of joy, of gratitude, of neglect, and of injuries is seldom totally obliterated from their minds.

I shall conclude this letter by an appeal to several members of your board to vouch for my having more than once suggested most of the above means for the recovery and comfort of the deranged persons under your care long before it pleased God to interest me in their adoption by rendering one of my family an object of them.

I am, gentlemen, with great respect and esteem, your sincere friend and servant, Benjn:Rush.

Rush's recommendations received serious consideration by the managers, and the less costly ones were adopted. However, his principal objec-

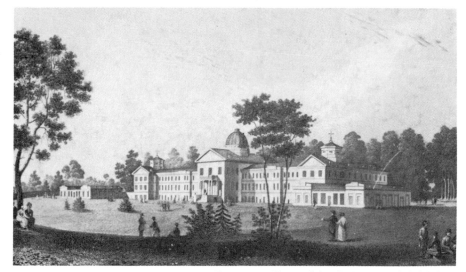

Figure 17. Hospital for the Insane, Philadelphia.

tives were not attained until 28 years after his death when, in 1841, a new, separate hospital specially designed for the care of the mentally ill and constructed at a cost of $265,000 was opened on a 100-acre estate in the country (now West Philadelphia).

In addition to the Pennsylvania Hospital, only two institutions were significantly involved, prior to 1815, in the care of mental patients: the Insane Hospital at Williamsburg, Virginia, established in 1768, and the Friends' Asylum at Frankford, Pennsylvania, opened in 1817.

In the light of the success of humane care in France and England, small mental institutions began to appear in a number of communities along the Atlantic seaboard in the 1820s and 1830s. These institutions employed what became known as "moral treatment," which was "an enlightened, kindly, and personal approach to patient care." As a result of "moral treatment" many patients who formerly would have been incarcerated for life were returned to their homes either well or much improved (Greenblatt, 1975).

The period of "moral treatment" did not extend far beyond the 1850s. Though some of the private institutions, such as the McLean Asylum and the Pennsylvania Hospital, succeeded in maintaining a humane, open, and individualized type of therapy, the state and municipal institutions which provided most of the care for mentally deranged patients were overwhelmed by the rapid increase in the population and the flood of immigrants. These institutions grew larger and larger, but they had neither the funds nor the staff to manage their patients properly. The result was "the isolation, overcrowding, neglect, and dehumanizing of the mentally ill throughout the country" (Greenblatt, 1975).

In 1873, there were in the United States 149 hospitals with 35,453 beds. Approximately one third of these hospitals were for the mentally ill (Rosen in Freidson, 1963). It seems probable, therefore, that there were no more than about 25,000 general hospital beds to serve a population of 40 million. Today a population of that size would require about 200,000 general hospital beds.

67

6

Medical Licensure
and
Medical Literature

MEDICAL
LICENSURE
In England there had been at least nominal regulation of the practice of medicine for more than two centuries. Henry VIII had decreed that no person should practice medicine without first being examined by a committee of physicians or by the bishop of his diocese. In 1518 a Royal Charter was granted to the College of Physicians of London empowering it to examine and license candidates for the practice of medicine. In the eighteenth century, though the College still had its licensing powers, many of those who practiced did so without a license. The American colonists who traveled to the mother country in the eighteenth century to obtain their medical education seem to have shown little interest in seeking the credentials of the Royal College, being content to return home with a medical degree or some other evidence of having acquired medical training. John Morgan, cofounder of the Medical College of Philadelphia, was one of the few exceptions to this generalization: in 1764 he became both a Licentiate of the Royal College of Physicians of London and a Fellow of the Royal Society (Morton, 1897).

Most physicians in the colonies had not had a formal medical education, and their only license to practice consisted of a certificate of competence signed by the preceptor under whom they had served an apprenticeship. Such certificates were not required for practice, and there was no serious effort to protect the public from medical impostors until 1772, when the province of New Jersey adopted a law requiring physicians to pass an examination for licensure, to be conducted by two judges of the Supreme Court.

After the Revolutionary War, state medical societies were organized, at first in the New England states, which were granted charters giving them power to examine and certify the competence of candidates for the practice of medicine and surgery. Membership in these societies was equivalent to a license to practice.

In 1783, when the newly founded Harvard Medical School announced that it intended to certify its graduates as qualified to practice medicine, its

69

authority to do so was challenged by the Massachusetts Medical Society. The Society claimed that the legislature had granted it a "positive and explicit right" to examine and license candidates for the practice of medicine and surgery. After prolonged controversy, it was finally agreed between the two parties that the university had the right to confer medical degrees but that only the Medical Society had the right to license practitioners.

As new states were added to the Union some of them enacted laws either granting to medical colleges the authority to license their graduates or authorizing medical societies to examine and license those who sought the right to practice. These laws were never very effective in eliminating poorly qualified practitioners. Even in Philadelphia, which was reputed to possess the elite among medical practitioners, in 1800 two thirds of the physicians and surgeons listed in the city directory were neither members of the local medical society nor graduates of any medical school (Bell, 1970). With the expansion of the nation and the clamor for more physicians to care for the people in the newly settled areas, the state laws seemed so unrealistic that no effort was made to enforce them.

The deterioration in the quality of medical care during the first three decades of the nineteenth century led many of the states to withdraw the licensing privilege from medical societies and to create boards of medical examiners appointed by the state governors. For the most part these boards accepted diplomas from "recognized" medical colleges as grounds for licensing without an examination. All other candidates had to be examined. Since this mechanism made it possible for sectarian practitioners to obtain a license which would put them on an equal footing with regular physicians, the orthodox profession opposed the examining boards. In the spirit of Jacksonian democracy prevalent during that period, many laymen also objected to the boards, claiming that they placed a legal barrier in the way of a free choice of physicians. The examining boards, therefore, lacked the professional and public support which were needed to make them effective. In the decade or two prior to the Civil War most states repealed their licensing laws, and the field of medical practice was again thrown open to any and all who cared to call themselves doctors.

After the Civil War, the rapid advances in medical science and the reluctance of the medical colleges to give up their established pattern of operation induced the leaders of the profession and many informed citizens to agitate anew for state licensing laws. It was held that such laws were necessary not only to protect the public but also to force the medical colleges to modernize their curricula and upgrade their standards. One of the strong arguments in favor of establishing state boards of medical examiners was that the medical degree had become accepted as a license to practice and that the proprietors of many medical schools, because of their pecuniary interest in graduating as many students as possible, had failed to withhold the degree from those who were not qualified to practice. This criticism was directed not only at the orthodox schools but also at the homeopathic, eclectic, and other sectarian schools whose diplomas and certificates had theretofore been accepted as a warranty of medical competence.

As the nation's first century neared its end, several states enacted licensing laws creating boards of medical examiners, including Texas in

70

1873, Kentucky and New York in 1874, New Hampshire in 1875, and Vermont and California in 1876. This started a movement which would continue, with public support, for two decades, at the end of which all states would have licensing laws.

MEDICAL   When the first century opened there were no reg-
LITERATURE   ular medical publications of any type. According
                      to Billings (1876), up to the commencement of the
Revolutionary War the body of American medical literature consisted of one
medical book, three reprints, and about 20 pamphlets. The one book, which
was written by John Jones (1729–1791), the first Professor of Surgery at
King's College, New York, appeared in 1775 under the title "Plain, Precise,
Practical Remarks on the Treatment of Wounds and Fractures." Billings
(1876) states that it was a mere compilation of the published work of several
European surgeons and contained only a single original observation.

The first original medical journal of the United States was the *Medical
Repository*, a quarterly edited in New York by three physicians (Elihu H.
Smith, Samuel L. Mitchell, and Edward Miller), which appeared in 1797 and
continued in existence until 1824. The *Repository* contained a great variety
of literary material, including some poetry, but little of lasting value to medicine except for Physick's report of his autopsies on cases of yellow fever
and the papers of Stearns and Prescott on the use of ergot in obstetrical
practice.

For seven years the *Repository* was the country's only medical periodical. After that medical journals began to appear in increasing numbers,
most of them short-lived and containing little of value. The journals found
it difficult to make ends meet, even though they sold for what was considered a high price: subscription rates ran from $1.50 to $5.00 per year. To
help cover the rather high publication costs most journals also carried advertisements. In 1838, the *American Journal of the Medical Sciences* charged
$6.00 per page to advertisers (Shafer, 1935). In 1843 one of the better jour-
nals announced that it would accept advertisements from publishers, book-
sellers, druggists, instrument makers, importers, medical schools, hospitals,
and societies, and all other medical notices. In 1848 the Committee on Medical
Literature of the American Medical Association reported "the advertising
portion of the journals seems to be considered by some editors as beyond
the jurisdiction of medical ethics. It is to this opinion, or more probably to
mere inadvertence, that the physician owes the privilege of reading before
he opens one of the prominent journals, the notice of one Dr. Beech's Medical Works, for which he has received numerous gold medals from the
various crowned heads of Europe, and diplomas from the most learned
colleges in the old world."

Two medical journals which began publication in the early part of the
nineteenth century were of a quality far above that of most of their competitors, and both of these journals are being published today according to the
same high standards: (1) the *New England Journal of Medicine and Surgery*
made its appearance in 1812; in 1828 it merged with the *Boston Medical In-
telligencer* and adopted the new name the *Boston Medical and Surgical Jour-*

nal; it is now the *New England Journal of Medicine.* (2) The *Philadelphia Journal of Medical and Physical Sciences* made its appearance in 1820; in 1828 it merged with the *Philadelphia Monthly Journal of Medicine and Surgery* and adopted the name which it still bears, the *American Journal of the Medical Sciences.*

In addition to the journals, a number of textbooks and treatises were published during the nation's first century. Many of these were reprints or translations of the works of foreign authors. But there were also a number of textbooks of American origin. A few of these were excellent for their time, and some of them won a reputation in foreign countries.

A standard reference book valued by all physicians and pharmacists, *The United States Pharmacopeia,* was proposed by the Massachusetts Medical Society in 1808, and the first issue appeared in 1820. Following its initial publication, revised editions have been issued at intervals of ten years.

In addition to the journals, treatises, textbooks, and odd pamphlets, the medical literature also contained the *Transactions* of many state and local medical societies. Most of the state societies published their Transactions in volumes of greater or lesser bulk.

The rate of growth of the periodical literature is indicated by the following statistics: In 1848 the Committee on Medical Literature reported to the American Medical Association that the number of journals being published in the United States was about 20; in 1876 Yandell reported that, since 1797, 195 journals had been started and that about 50 were still being published in the year of his report. This was evidently an underestimate, for in 1881 Billings informed the International Medical Congress in London that in reviewing the publications for that year for the *Index Medicus* he had found that 655 volumes of journals and transactions had been published in that year, of which 156 had been produced in the United States. The corresponding numbers for other countries were as follows: Germany, 129; France, 122; Great Britain, 54; Italy, 65; and Spain, 24.

Organizations that were soon to swell the volume of medical literature were the national specialist societies which were founded during the last quarter of the nation's first century: American Pharmaceutical Association, 1852; American Ophthalmological Society, 1864; American Otological Society, 1868; Association of Medical Superintendents of American Institutions for the Insane, 1870; American Public Health Association, 1872; American Neurological Association, 1875; American Gynecological Society, 1876; American Dermatological Association, 1876; American Laryngological Association, 1878; American Surgical Association, 1879.

7

Cost of Medical Care

Thomas Dimsdale, an English physician whose treatise entitled *Thoughts on General and Partial Inoculation* (for smallpox) was published in 1776, journeyed to Russia to inoculate Catherine the Great and her son Grand Duke Paul. For this trip he received from Her Majesty a fee for service of £10,000 plus £2000 to cover travel expenses, plus a pension of £500 per year for life (Bishop, 1932). This was exceptional remuneration for service to exceptional people, but there were other London practitioners of that period who had annual incomes of £10,000 to £20,000, a vast sum for the time (Shryock, 1930).

In America fees were far more modest, even when the most prominent physicians rendered services to the most exceptional people. When George Washington was at the height of his fame and a person of considerable wealth he paid a total of £482 for medical services during the entire period 1772 to 1792, or roughly £24 per year for care of himself, his family, and some 200 slaves. It is of interest that before the Revolutionary War, Washington paid a physician a fixed annual fee of £15 to render these same services (Blanton, 1933). This clearly indicates that the payment of an annual inclusive fee for the care of a relatively large group of people was acceptable practice long before the advent of the twentieth century.

It was, of course, in the interest of plantation owners to obtain medical care for their slaves. Washington's letters and account books show that he spared no pains and no funds to accomplish this. His accounts make several references to payments to Negro "doctors." Blanton says that "their fees were small and they were probably called in to treat only minor complaints."

In 1855, George Jones, a Florida plantation owner, received bills from two physicians for the care of his slaves. The first was a bill for $43 for "Attendance on Lucy in difficult labor." The second was a bill for $143 for services and medicine provided throughout the year 1855. In many parts of the country it was customary in the mid-nineteenth century for physicians to submit bills at the end of the year for all services rendered during that year. In some areas if the annual bill was not paid by the end of January, the doctor charged interest for any unpaid portion of the account (Rosen, 1946).

That the doctor's bills (then as now) were frequently the last to be paid

73

was indicated by Benjamin Rush. In a list of various phobias he includes the "Doctor-phobia," which he says, half-humorously, "might be supposed to be caused by the terror of a long bill, but that excites terror in few minds, for who ever thinks of paying a doctor's bill while he can use his money to advantage in another way" (Deutsch, 1937).

Samuel D. Gross, who has been mentioned several times in foregoing sections, graduated from Jefferson Medical College in 1828. During the year 1828–29 he attempted to carry on a general practice in Philadelphia, but his income was so small (about $300 for the year) that he moved to Easton, Pennsylvania, in 1830. In his autobiography he notes that "as the charges were very low I made little beyond my expenses." He was paid fifty cents for a house call in town and one to two dollars, depending on distance, for out-of-town calls, including a small charge for medicine, which it was the custom for the physician himself to prepare. Gross adds, "These charges were beyond doubt very contemptible; but then it is to be borne in mind that rent, provisions, and clothing were very much lower than they are now [1880s]. A chicken, for example, could be bought at six to ten cents, and the best quality of beef at about eight to nine cents." When Gross moved again, this time to Cincinnati in 1833, he had less than $250 to carry wih him. In Cincinnati "the charges were also miserably low." The fee for a house call was one dollar. In his first year in practice there his income was about $1400.

In the period 1815–1876 most medical societies published a document which was known as either a Fee Bill, a Fee Table, or a Table of Charges. These documents were intended to guide the members of the society as to the proper fee to submit for each service rendered. In 1825 the New England Journal of Medicine and Surgery (XIV, pp. 50–51) stated that "the ultimate object of a fee table . . . has been to produce uniformity and as nearly as possible, to adapt professional charges to the present state of communities and times. It has one other object. The law nowhere settles the precise value of professional opinion or advice. A fee table settles this, and equally lessens the chances of embarrassment or imposition" (Rosen, 1946).

In general the fees shown in the fee tables were intended to serve only as a guide to minimum charges. However, this was not always the case. For example, when the fee bill of the Union Medical Society of Knightstown, Indiana, was adopted in 1862 it was *"Resolved,* that this fee bill is as binding on the members of the society as their by-laws or constitutions; and that any one violating the same may be arraigned and tried, as for any other violation of the laws of the society" (Rosen, 1946).

A pathetic little note was attached by the secretary of the New Castle (Indiana) Medical Society to the fee bill adopted by his society in 1862: "The above fee bill looks small when compared to other fee bills I have noticed, and yet we have trouble to get that much. There are always quacks putting themselves forward and doing what they do for half price, and some men think more of the almighty dollar than their family's lives, and it seems as though we are blest with a goodly number of that class here" (Rosen, 1946). The charges in the New Castle fee bill were indeed small: seventy-five cents for a house call *and medicines* during the day; one dollar for the same at night. It is worth noting that the difficulty in collecting such small fees in this rural area was attributed to competition from quacks.

The fee tables of the societies located in cities such as Philadelphia, New York, and Boston displayed charges several times higher than those of the rural societies. The following tabulation shows selected items from the fee bills of the College of Physicians of Philadelphia (1843) and of the Medical Society of Washington County, New York (1837) (derived from material in Rosen, 1946):

	Urban Philadelphia	Rural N.Y. State
Visit to doctor's office for verbal advice	$1.00–10.00	$0.50
Charge for written advice	5.00–20.00	?
Ordinary house call	1.00–2.00	0.50
Extra for travel over 1 mi./per mi.	1.00	0.50
Night house call	5.00–10.00	0.75
Vaccination	5.00	1.00
Maternity—natural labor	10.00–30.00	4.00
Reductions of fractures	5.00–10.00	2.00–10.00
Removal of stones—urinary bladder	100.00–200.00	50.00
Hernia—reduction by operation	25.00–100.00	20.00
Passing urethral catheter	1.00–10.00	1.00–2.00

About 20 years later there was the same sort of difference between urban and rural fee bills. The following items were selected from the table of the Medico-Chirurgical Society of the City of New York (1860) and that of the Union Medical Society of Knightstown, Indiana (1862) (Rosen, 1946):

	Urban N.Y.	Rural Indiana
Visit to doctor's office for verbal advice	$1.00–2.00	$0.50
Charge for written advice	5.00–15.00	?
Ordinary house call	1.50–3.00	0.75–1.00
Extra for travel over 1 to 1.5 mi./per mi.	0.50–1.00	0.75–1.00
Night house call	5.00–10.00	1.10–1.50
Vaccination	1.50–3.00	0.50
Catheterization—urethral	3.00–10.00	?
Maternity—natural labor	10.00–50.00	5.00
Reduction of fractures	10.00–50.00	5.00–30.00
Removal of stones from bladder	100.00–500.00	?
Hernia—reduction by operation	50.00–500.00	50.00
Operation for cataract	100.00–500.00	40.00–75.00
Excision of tonsils	25.00–50.00	5.00

It may be noted in the fee bills that the charge for written advice was relatively high, almost as high as the charge for maternity care. This was doubtless attributable to the amount of time that the physician had to devote to composing a long letter of advice including elaborate prescriptions. Such letters were usually written in longhand by the physician himself, and the amount of time devoted to such activity, unless checked by a formidable fee, might have become intolerable. Benjamin Rush wrote in 1798: "So much of my time has lately been taken up in answering letters for advice for which I have received no compensation, and for which I am obliged to pay the postage, that I have been compelled to resolve to reply to no letter for advice which is not accompanied with a fee, unless it comes from persons who acknowledge themselves to be poor" (Butterfield, 1951).

Reviewing a number of fee bills for the period 1815–1875, one finds that the recommended charges are generally within the limits of the foregoing tabulations. They are almost always higher in the city than in the country, and the charges for ordinary items such as office visits and house calls show little tendency to rise during the six decades. However, after the introduction of anesthesia, the tables show an increasing number of surgical procedures for which fees of $100 to $500 are listed.

The cost of medical care in the first century of the republic was almost always limited to the doctor's fee and a small charge for medicines. Even the latter might be provided without charge as part of the doctor's service. With a few exceptions, only the indigent went to a hospital prior to 1850, when St. Vincent's Hospital in New York City offered private accommodations for paying patients (Friedson, 1963). Even as late as the 1870s almost all patients who were above the poverty level were cared for in their homes, where doctors did not hesitate to perform complicated surgical operations and difficult obstetrical procedures. Hence, patients had no hospital bill and, of course, no bills for x-rays, laboratory tests, expensive medicines, and the many other items which make up the cost of medical care today.

8

Research

Without theory, practice is but the routine born of habit. Theory alone can bring
forth and develop the spirit of invention. It is to you specially that it will belong
not to share the opinion of those narrow minds who disdain everything in science
which has no immediate application. You know Franklin's charming saying?
He was witnessing the first demonstration of a purely scientific discovery, and
the people round him said: "But what is the use of it?" Franklin answered them:
"What is the use of a new-born child?"

(Louis Pasteur)

There was no systematic research and very little research of any type
during the first century of American medicine. The American contributions
to medical progress that are cited at the end of this chapter were concerned
for the most part with the natural history of diseases or with improvements
in surgical methods. In only a few instances were experiments involved.

In the early part of the nation's first century, when physicians in Europe
were concentrating their research efforts on trying to correlate post-mortem
findings with the manifestations of disease observed in the patient before
death, Americans rarely undertook this type of study. A variety of factors
contributed to this posture: (1) There was a strong popular aversion to autopsies and human dissection. So strong was the feeling that mobs of riot-
ing citizens occasionally attacked those who were suspected of conducting
anatomical studies. (2) The education of physicians came from a combination
of on-the-job training under a preceptor and didactic lectures. All emphasis
was on private practice, and there was neither stimulation nor time for original studies. Fame and emoluments went to the physician who had a large
and fashionable practice. Time devoted to research could only impede
one's climb to the social eminence which was honored by both profession
and public. (3) The widely accepted theories of Benjamin Rush stultified
research. Since the great Dr. Rush affirmed that all illness was due to a
single cause, why be inquisitive, why perform an autopsy? (4) The utilitarian spirit of the American public at that time was not conducive to research.
During the period of ascendancy of clinical research in France (1820–

1860) a few young Americans (Holmes, Gerhard, and others) returned from Paris intellectually invigorated and filled with the spirit of inquiry. They were also filled with the spirit of iconoclasm and therapeutic nihilism. If all the medicines in America were thrown into the Atlantic Ocean, said Oliver Wendell Holmes, "it would be so much better for mankind and so much worse for the fishes." This type of negativism came from the most highly qualified members of the profession at a time when American medical education was at its worst and when public confidence in the orthodox physician was at a low ebb. The honesty and forthrightness of the nihilists, although in a sense admirable, served further to tarnish the image of orthodox medicine and to diminish the likelihood of public support for medical research.

In 1840 Samuel D. Gross of Louisville, Kentucky, undertook an experimental study on wounds of the intestines. Seventy dogs were utilized in these experiments, the first to be reported in this country in which a large number of experimental animals were involved. This study was not supported by any medical school, or the government, or by philanthropy. Gross had to provide and feed his own dogs and to employ a man to look after them. Since his income was then less than $1000 per year, the cost of the experiments imposed an almost intolerable financial burden (Gibbon, 1926).

During the period of low public confidence, the American Medical Association tried unsuccessfully to secure the adoption of two measures which would have provided building blocks for medical research. First, in 1855 the Association appealed to state legislatures to require registration of vital statistics. Not only was this effort unsuccessful but also it was ridiculed in some legislative chambers as "a trick of the doctors." Secondly, in 1872 the Association urged the adoption of a standard and uniform nomenclature of diseases, which would be utilized by physicians throughout the country. The recommended system was adopted by the Marine Hospital Service but went no further. Shryock (1947) states, "The only medical problems that appealed to legislators in the 1870's were the old ones of quarantines and sanitary science."

Though the federal government was not to provide medical research funds for another three or four decades, several departments of the government were taking steps in the 1860s and 1870s which would contribute to the development of medical science. The inefficient and disorganized state of the Army Medical Corps in the early months of the Civil War led to public demand for improvement. As a result, in 1861, the United States Sanitary Commission was created. The commission brought about the appointment of Dr. William A. Hammond as Surgeon-General of the Army. Hammond was a well-qualified physician, and he proved himself to be a competent and imaginative administrator. Among his accomplishments was the inauguration, in 1862, of the Army Medical Museum. After the war, this museum became the locus of some of the earliest planned medical research to be carried out in the United States.

In 1865, Dr. J. J. Woodward, working at the museum, was the first in the United States to report the use of aniline dyes for histopathological studies (microscopic studies of diseased tissues), and he did pioneering work in photomicrography (photographs taken through a microscope). It was also shortly after the Civil War that Congress permitted the Department of Agriculture to devote some of its funds to studies of the health of farm animals. The excellent research on infectious diseases which was carried out under the auspices of this Department was just getting under way at the end of the first century of American medicine. The Army also made a major contribution to future research when it diverted $80,000 in unused hospital funds, left over from the Civil War, for the improvement of the Surgeon-General's library. John Shaw Billings, who was in charge of the library at that time, utilized these funds and others subsequently appropriated not only to improve but also to greatly expand the library's collections and to devise ways to make the collections more accessible and more useful to medical scientists. In 1876 Billings published a "Specimen Fasciculus" of an index catalogue of authors and subjects. This specimen was the forerunner of the great *Index Catalogue of the Surgeon-General's Library*, of which the first volume would appear four years later.

Throughout the nation's first century medical research as such received neither encouragement nor financial support from the medical schools. But as the century was drawing to a close the university schools were beginning to move in a direction which would soon lead them to combine research with their educational activities. In 1871 the first physiological laboratory in the United States was established at Harvard, with young Henry P. Bowditch in charge. Bowditch had just returned from Europe, where he had demonstrated his ability in neurophysiological research. At Yale in 1874, Russell H. Chittenden was appointed Director of the first American laboratory of physiological chemistry, but before the laboratory was actually opened Chittenden went to Europe and spent several years working with leaders in the field.

Two British scientists, the physicist John Tyndall and the naturalist and physician Thomas H. Huxley, who made lecture tours of the United States in the 1870s, did much to arouse American colleges and universities to their opportunities and obligations in scientific research. In 1873 Tyndall observed astutely that the American people showed a "widespread public preference for sensational discovery, even if based on little or no evidence." That observation seems as valid today as it was a century ago.

Notwithstanding a lack of direct emphasis on medical research, Americans made a number of discoveries and innovations. The following brief paragraphs cite some of the more significant American contributions to medical progress during the nation's first century.

The most momentous contribution was the introduction of surgical anesthesia. In 1844, *Horace Wells,* a dentist of Hartford, Connecticut, began cautiously to utilize nitrous oxide ("laughing gas") to induce transitory sleep during dental extractions. In 1845 he made a rather unconvincing public demonstration of his method at the Massachusetts General Hospital. At the same hospital in 1846, another dentist, *William T. G. Morton* of Boston, who had experimented with ether for dental extractions, administered this volatile agent for a surgical operation performed by John C. Warren. Within a few months of this highly successful and thoroughly convincing demonstration, Morton's method was being used throughout the Western world to make possible surgical and obstetrical procedures which previously could not have been undertaken (Bigelow, 1876; Osler, 1917; Ball, 1925; Roth, 1932).

Benjamin Franklin (1706–1790), though not a physician, contributed significantly to medical resources by inventing the bifocal lens. Franklin, who had

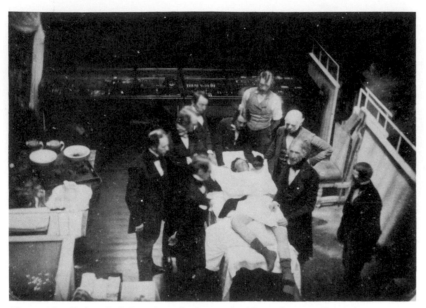

Figure 18. Early administration of ether at the Massachusetts General Hospital. (New York Academy of Medicine.)

first exhibited his genius for scientific experimentation when as a young man he flew a homemade kite in a thunderstorm, demonstrated his concern for the infirmities of age when, as an old man, he invented what he called double spectacles. (Single spectacles had been in use for many centuries.) In 1784, in a letter to a friend, he wrote, "I cannot distinguish a letter even of large print, but am happy in the invention of double spectacles, which, serving for distant objects as well as near ones, make my eyes as useful to me as ever they were."

In May, 1785, Franklin wrote from France, where he was representing the new United States government, that he "formerly had two pairs of spectacles, which I shifted occasionally, as in travelling I sometimes read and often want to regard the prospects. Finding this change troublesome, and not always sufficiently ready, I had the glasses cut out and half of each kind associated in the same circle, the least convex, for distant objects, the upper half, and the most convex, for reading, the lower half: by this means, as I wear my glasses constantly, I have only to move my eyes up or down, as I want to see distinctly far or near, the proper glasses being always ready. This I find more particularly convenient since my being in France; the glasses that serve me best at table to see what I eat, being the best to see the faces of those on the other side of the table who speak to me, and when one's ears are not well accustomed to the sound of a language, a sight of the movement in the features of him that speaks helps to explain; so that I understand French better by the help of my spectacles."

Philip Syng Physick (1768–1837) of Philadelphia has been called "the father of American surgery." He spent four years abroad, where he was a favorite of the celebrated John Hunter. His growing reputation as a surgeon led to his appointment to the chair of surgery at the University of Pennsylvania in 1805. Physick devised new surgical operations and made many contributions toward improvements in surgical technique, including the introduction of absorbable sutures made of various animal tissues. "Physick has left no works to commemorate his fame or to record his vast experience, a few short papers in

80

the medical press of the day comprising the whole of his contributions to the surgical literature of the country" (Gross, 1876).

Benjamin Waterhouse, the first Professor of Medicine at Harvard, introduced vaccination against smallpox into the United States in 1800. To prove its value to a skeptical community, he designed a controlled clinical experiment, which was carried out on an island near Boston. Nineteen vaccinated children and two unvaccinated children were exposed to smallpox under identical conditions. The unvaccinated children contracted the disease while the vaccinated children all remained well (Christian, 1933; Ann. Med. Hist., 1927).

John C. Otto of Philadelphia, in 1803, wrote the first account of hemophilia, in which he described an investigation of a family of "bleeders" (Otto, 1803).

In 1807 *John Stearns* of Saratoga County, New York, was the first to publish an account of the physiological effects of ergot, in which he reported both its ability to stimulate and strengthen uterine contractions and its power to constrict small blood vessels. He explained how ergot could be utilized to speed up childbirth and to control postpartum hemorrhage. His observations were soon confirmed by others and within a short time ergot was recognized as the most valuable oxytocic (i.e., promoting rapid labor) drug available to obstetricians (Thomas, 1876).

Daniel Drake, in 1840, was the first to write a clinical description of "milk sickness." During the first half of the eighteenth century this disease caused many deaths and much serious illness among the frontiersmen of the Middle West and actually delayed the settlement of that area. Nancy Hanks Lincoln, mother of Abraham Lincoln, died in Indiana in 1818, and the cause is said to have been milk sickness. The cause of this disease was discovered not by physicians but by an Ohio farmer, who in some remarkably well-controlled homespun experiments on farm animals, proved that the human illness was the result of drinking milk which came from cows that had fed on the white snakeroot (Woglom, 1949).

Ephraim McDowell (1771–1830), a frontier physician in Danville, Kentucky, was the first in the world to succeed in removing a diseased ovary, which contained a tumor weighing 22 pounds (1809). Before his death he had performed thirteen such operations with eight recoveries, a remarkable achievement in the early days of the nineteenth century. His operations were performed on an ordinary household table without benefit of anesthesia (Gray, 1968).

In 1811 *Elisha North* of New London, Connecticut, wrote *A Treatise on a Malignant Epidemic, Commonly Called Spotted Fever.* This work, based on personal observations of more than 200 patients in a single epidemic, gave the first adequate description of cerebrospinal fever (meningitis). North was among the first to emphasize the importance of a clinical thermometer for the study of fevers (Pleadwell, 1924).

In the 1820s and 1830s *William Beaumont,* a U.S. Army Surgeon, carried out a long series of carefully planned experiments on a man who had a permanent opening into his stomach resulting from an abdominal wound received in 1822. These classic experiments provided the first clear insight into the nature of gastric digestion (Miller, 1929 and 1933).

In 1831 chloroform was discovered by *Samuel Guthrie,* a chemist of Sachett's Harbor, New York. For a number of years this substance was looked upon as a chemical curiosity with a pleasant odor and an ability to intoxicate. It was not until 1847 that its anesthetic qualities were recognized and put to use by James Y. Simpson, Professor of Obstetrics at Edinburgh. For the next 40 to 50 years,

81

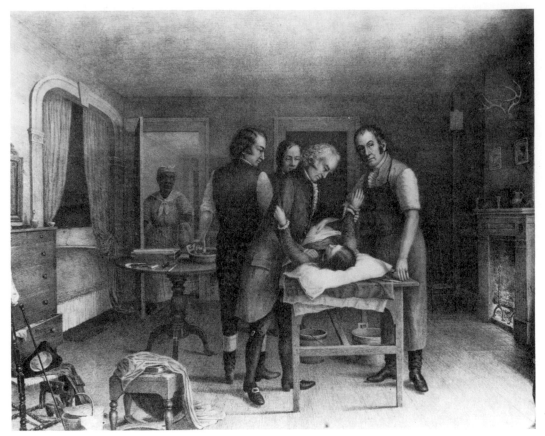

Figure 19. The first ovariotomy, performed by Ephraim McDowell; the patient, Jane T. Crawford. (National Library of Medicine, Bethesda, Maryland.)

in Europe, chloroform surpassed ether in popularity as an anesthetic agent (Clarke, 1876).

In 1837 *W. W. Gerhard* of Philadelphia was the first to make a clear differentiation between typhus fever and typhoid fever. Gerhard was also the first to point out that meningitis may result from the development of tubercles in the meninges (Gerhard, 1837; Clarke, 1876).

In 1843 *Oliver Wendell Holmes* of Boston wrote an important paper *On the Contagiousness of Puerpural Fever*. In 1847 *Samuel Kneeland, Jr.,* of New York directed attention to the connection between puerpural fever and epidemic erysipelas (Clarke, 1876).

In 1850 *Henry I. Bowditch* of Boston introduced thoracentesis for drawing off accumulations of fluid in the chest. His apparatus consisted of a sharply pointed needle-like punch, some tubing, and a suction pump designed by Dr. Morrill Wyman. This procedure at first met with strong opposition and criticism from prominent physicians on both sides of the Atlantic, but its utility and safety were finally acknowledged. By 1875 Bowditch had performed thoracentesis successfully 325 times on 204 patients (Clarke, 1876; Atwater, 1972).

C. W. Pennock of Philadelphia in 1839 contributed to diagnostic implementation by devising a flexible-tube stethoscope to replace the stiff and awkward wooden implement first employed by Laennec (Clarke, 1876).

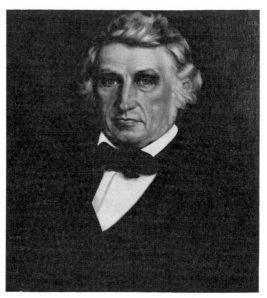

Figure 20. William Beaumont. (National Library of Medicine, Bethesda, Maryland.)

Although Benjamin Rush had encountered and described dengue fever in 1778, the first comprehensive description of an epidemic of this disease appeared in 1850 in a paper written by *S. H. Dickson* of South Carolina (Clarke, 1876).

William W. Reid of Rochester, New York, in a series of observations, dissections, and experiments reported in 1851 and 1855, laid down the principles for the reduction of dislocations by simple manipulation. His methods were

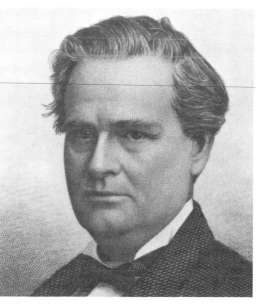

Figure 21. J. Marion Sims. (National Library of Medicine, Bethesda, Maryland.)

quickly accepted and won for him an international reputation. "Like Byron, he woke up one morning and found himself famous. . . ." (Gross, 1876).

J. Marion Sims (1813–1883) devised new implements, including the duck bill speculum, and new procedures, including the lateral position (Sims position) for examining and treating the female genital tract. In 1852 he won worldwide attention by reporting the first successful closure of an opening that allowed urine to flow from the bladder into the vagina. In 1853 he moved from Alabama to New York City and became the first surgeon in the United States to practice as a specialist in diseases of women. Sims's treatise, *Clinical Notes on Uterine Surgery* (1866), was translated into several languages and was widely read in Europe, where Sims was considered to be America's most original and gifted surgeon (Thomas, 1876).

In 1872 *Morrill Wyman* of Cambridge, Massachusetts, published a small volume entitled *Autumnal Catarrh,* which gives a description of what we now call hay fever. He differentiated it from the common type of catarrh (common cold), described its seasonal incidence, and listed many areas in the United States, chiefly in mountainous terrain, where those afflicted could obtain relief from their symptoms (Clarke, 1876).

In 1875, *William Pepper* of Philadelphia gave the first description of the abnormalities in the bone marrow that are characteristic of pernicious anemia.

Samuel D. Gross (1805–1884) was America's leading general surgeon of the mid-nineteenth century. His *Elements of Pathological Anatomy* (1839) was the first exhaustive study of this subject to be published in the English language. His *Practical Treatise on Foreign Bodies in the Air Passages* (1854) was the first work of its kind in any language. He was the first to carry out well-planned, large-scale surgical studies utilizing experimental animals. His well-illustrated two-volume *System of Surgery* went through seven editions btween 1859 and 1882. Gross served successively as Professor of Pathology and Anatomy in the Medical Department of Cincinnati College (1835–1840); Professor of Surgery at the University of Louisville, Kentucky (1840–1856); and Professor of Surgery at Jefferson Medical College, Philadelphia (1856–1884). His stature in the eyes of contemporaries overseas is evidenced by the fact that he received honorary degrees from Oxford University in 1872, Cambridge University in 1880, and the University of Edinburgh in 1884 (Gibbon, 1926).

Austin Flint, Sr., did much to improve and systematize methods of physical diagnosis and gained recognition abroad as an authority on the diagnosis of diseases of the heart and lungs. His textbook, *A Treatise on the Principles and Practice of Medicine; Designed for the Use of Practitioners and Students of Medicine,* went through six editions between 1866 and 1886. It was widely used both in the United States and in Europe and unquestionably had a favorable influence upon the development of medicine in this country.

The American discoveries and innovations cited above, though impressive individually, contributed to the progress of medicine largely in a peripheral sense. They were haphazard, not part of a broad plan, and they did not result in the creation of a foundation upon which a scientific structure could be erected. This was in sharp contrast with the consistent and progressive development of clinical diagnosis and physiology in France and of cellular pathology, biochemistry, and physiology in Germany. The Europeans were creating a firm base for modern medical science, while the American contributions (anesthesia excepted) did no more than fill in, largely by chance, a few gaps in the rising structure.

9

The Transition Period–The 1870s

*I . . . hope & believe that it is from this side of the Atlantic that Europe, which
has taught us so many other things, will at length be led into sound principles in
this branch of science, the most important of all other, being that to which we
commit the care of health & life.*

(Thomas Jefferson, 1807)

**THE NATIONAL
SCENE**
In 1876 the population of the United States was
approaching 45 million. Of this total, only about
12 million lived in the cities; the remainder lived
on farms or in rural villages. Some of them could remember the mist and
smoke over Baltimore harbor in 1814 through which Francis Scott Key had
dimly seen the nation's flag. Since then the number of stars that spangled
the banner had more than doubled. Colorado was admitted to the Union as
the thirty-eighth state in 1876. Though the country had just been spanned
by a transcontinental railroad, much of the land was still wild and un-
settled.

The anguish of the Civil War was a vivid memory to all who had
passed their teens. In the southern states the war's desolation and the abolition of slavery had wrecked the economy. In Washington the reins of government were held by military heroes, the greatest of whom, Ulysses S.
Grant, had occupied the White House for two presidential terms—eight
years of political scandal and corruption. The nation was in the depths of a
depression that had begun with the Panic of 1873: businesses were failing;
unscrupulous stock manipulators were gaining control of the country's largest industry, the railroads; newly organized labor groups were threatening
to go on strike; and the farmers were complaining about poor pay for their
crops and about monetary policies that undercut the value of their hard-
earned dollars. In reaction to the unrest and hard times there had been a
sharp decline in immigration, from over 400,000 in 1873 to less than 150,000
in 1876. Thus, industry was deprived of its principal source of cheap
labor—newly arrived immigrants.

85

The politico-economic policy of the party in power was in tune with Herbert Spencer's *laissez-faire* philosophy; the less government interfered with industry, the better.

The typical farmhouse — the place where most Americans lived — was of wooden frame construction and had no indoor plumbing. A pump in the yard supplied water, and there was an outdoor privy. The proximity of the privy to the pump was a not uncommon cause of illness. Heat in winter came from wood-burning stoves, and lighting was by kerosene lamps. Horses did the heavy farm work and transported the farmer to the nearby village, where he sold his produce and bought the things he needed. In the village there were a school, two or three churches, several general stores, one or two lawyers, and a doctor who in spite of his limited education had to serve as physician, surgeon, obstetrician, dentist, pharmacist, and veterinarian.

The homes of the city dwellers varied from the palatial establishments of the wealthy to the shabby, crowded, disease-ridden slums of the poor. The overcrowding in the slum neighborhoods of the port cities was aggravated by the flow of immigrants, who tended to remain in the city where they had disembarked.

The cities had grown by spreading horizontally. Vertical growth was limited to buildings that were no more than eight or nine stories in height, and there were very few of these. The skyscraper, a peculiarly American contribution to urban architecture, would have to await the development of steel-frame construction and the electrically powered elevator. A third requisite, central heating, had just become available: in 1874 William Baldwin devised the first efficient steam radiator.

By 1876 all of the larger cities possessed municipal "waterworks," in some instances bringing in pure water from distant reservoirs, but more frequently sucking up, from a river which flowed through or near the city, water which was of poor quality and often grossly contaminated. Piped systems for disposal of sewage, if available, were usually inadequate and poorly planned. Too frequently, even in major cities such as Philadelphia and Albany, sewage was deposited in the river or lake from which the water supply was drawn, without regard for the proximity of the two systems. Many of the poorer residents had no way to dispose of their trash and sewage except by throwing them into the streets. In the slums a single outdoor privy frequently served several families. Bathing was performed in a seldom-used portable tin tub. In 1876 the most luxurious homes still did not have bathrooms as we know them today. However, hotels were advertising bedrooms that contained wash basins with hot and cold running water. The modern type water closet began to be installed in the homes of the wealthy in the 1880s and 1890s.

In the field of literature the authors of the period of romanticism were giving way to a new generation of realists. Among the more prominent of this new group were Mark Twain, William Dean Howells, and Bret Harte. Mark Twain in his *Innocents Abroad* (1869) did much to debunk the misty romance of foreign lands and to arouse pride in the United States. Twain's most widely read book, *The Adventures of Tom Sawyer*, appeared in 1876.

The principal topic of conversation among scientists was Charles Darwin's most recent book, *The Descent of Man* (1871). A majority of biologists seemed, with varying reservations, to have accepted Darwin's radical theories. However, these theories did not so quickly prevail in the halls of religion. The preachers and congregations of those Protestant sects that demanded a literal interpretation of the Bible proclaimed without reservation that the true story of the descent of man was contained in the Book of Genesis. They had difficulty only in deciding whether Darwin was a deluded dreamer or an agent of the Devil.

TOWARD BETTER NUTRITION   Farmers' children could drink wholesome, fresh milk, but in the cities the children, particularly the children of poor families, had very little milk. What they had was of poor quality; it was frequently diluted with water and was handled in such a manner as to guarantee heavy contamination. There can be little doubt that part of the high mortality rate in city-dwelling infants and children was attributable to contaminated milk. A major improvement in urban milk supplies occurred in 1856, when Gail Borden, who had devised a process for condensing milk, established a plant in Litchfield, Connecticut, for the purpose of supplying New York City with large quantities of condensed milk made from fresh farm milk collected under specified conditions of cleanliness. The condensed product was delivered in sealed containers to New York and Brooklyn for twenty-five cents a quart. Since each quart could be diluted five to seven times to produce the equivalent of fresh milk, the cost of the final product was about four cents per quart. Infants in the city could then be fed a nourishing milk formula at low cost and without the usual contaminants. In 1875 the Borden Company began also to deliver in the city fresh whole milk that had been collected on farms under special sanitary supervision. This product was carted from door to door in large cans from which it was ladled into receptacles provided by the customer. Delivery in individual milk bottles did not begin until a decade later.

The household icebox, which could be used to prevent milk and other perishable foods from spoiling, came into use at about the time of the Civil War. At first the icebox was dependent upon natural ice; but even in the colder parts of the country the natural ice supply could not be relied upon during the summer months. In 1876 Carl von Linde, in Germany, invented the ammonia-compression ice-making machine. Shortly thereafter commercial ice plants were being built in the United States, and ice could be delivered the year round.

Of even greater importance than refrigeration for improvement in the American diet was the flowering of the canning industry. The preservation of food by heating in sealed glass containers began about 1800. Tin-plated cans replaced glass jars on a small scale in England about 1812. Commercial canning in the United States began with the canning of oysters in Baltimore in 1826. Other seafoods, fruits, berries, vegetables, and meats were added to the list of canned goods within the next several decades.

Canned foods in the early years were in limited supply and were too expensive for wide distribution. Two problems interfered with quantity production: (1) The processing time was too long. It took six hours to cook and sterilize the contents of the cans when they were immersed in ordinary

87

boiling water (212° F). (2) The cans were made individually by hand, a process which severely limited the number produced. The first of these problems was solved in 1861, when a Baltimore canner added calcium chloride to the water in which the cans were immersed, raising its boiling point to 240° Fahrenheit and reducing the processing time to about 30 to 45 minutes. A solution to the second problem began to emerge in the 1870s, when the first steps were taken to mechanize the manufacture of cans. It was after these improvements had been introduced that canned foods began to be sold in quantity (Keuchel, 1972; Boorstin, 1973).

The greater availability of meat also had a marked effect upon the diet of city dwellers. After the Civil War, Texas was glutted with millions of longhorn cattle, which could be bought for two or three dollars a head. At the same time cattle were selling in the Eastern markets for ten to twenty times this amount. In order to take advantage of the huge profits promised by this price differential, the long cattle drives were organized. It was during this period that the cowboy came into prominence. The long drives reached their height in the 1870s. In the peak year, 1871, some 600,000 head of cattle were driven north to the railheads in Missouri, Kansas, Nebraska, Wyoming, and Montana. During the drives, precautions had to be taken against Indian raids upon the moving herds. The Indians were then waging the last of their battles to retain possession of their hunting grounds, and in 1876 Colonel Custer made his famous "last stand." When barbed wire became available commercially, in 1874, it was used extensively to fence the farms of the Plains. This development, together with the extension of the rail lines into the cattle country, put an end to the long drives.

The cattle that had reached the rail lines were transported to the Middle West, chiefly Chicago, where they were slaughtered. Most of the meat was then shipped to the Eastern cities. At first the shipments could be made only during cold weather, but in the late 1870s young G.F. Swift of Chicago utilized the recently invented railway refrigerator car to ship fresh-dressed beef to the Eastern seaboard the year round.

Navel orange trees were first planted in Southern California in 1873. This initiated the great citrus fruit industry which in time would supply in abundance an almost indispensable component of the American diet.

DISCOVERY AND INVENTION

Several momentous developments in the field of technology occurred in the 1870s. In 1876 Alexander Graham Bell transmitted the first understood *telephone* message. In the same year the *internal combustion engine,* which was to have such a powerful effect upon life in America, was invented in Germany. In 1873 the first commercially successful *typewriter* was designed and manufactured by Alexander Sholes, a Milwaukee printer. At about the same time James Ritty of Dayton, Ohio, was trying to think up ways to keep his clerks from pilfering money from the cash drawer of his cafe-saloon. He devised, and in 1879 patented, the first *cash register,* soon to become an indispensable feature of stores and other commercial establishments. Prior to the 1870s *photography* was left to professionals. Few amateurs were capable of coping with the paraphernalia and tribulations of the wet-plate tech-

88

nique which was then employed. In 1877 George Eastman, a clerk in a Rochester bank, bought his first camera. Two years later he invented and patented a machine for dry-coating photographic plates and was on his way to making photography a popular and affordable hobby for amateurs.

Those who attended the Philadelphia Centennial Exposition of 1876 had an opportunity to see an English invention, a new form of lighting produced by electric arc lights burning brightly in the open air. Thomas A. Edison, who opened his laboratory in Menlo Park, New Jersey, in the centennial year, knew about the arc light but considered it impractical because in burning the arc was self-destructive, and the intensity of the light could not be controlled. In 1878 Edison began to work intensively on the development of a new type of *electric light* that would not have the faults of the arc light and would be safe enough and cheap enough for use in the home. By the fall of 1879 not only had he applied for a patent on his incandescent light bulb but also he had devised a power plant and wiring circuits to create a system that could be used to light thousands of homes.

Petroleum, which had been "discovered" in Pennsylvania, had a remarkable relationship with medical history. The American Indian, before the arrival of the white man, had used crude "rock oil" as a medicine, and by the nineteenth century the white man had added this substance to his *materia medica*. Petroleum, labeled *American Oil,* was first offered for sale not in barrels but in small bottles at the apothecary's counter. It was promoted as a cure for any and all human ills, and many thousands of bottles were sold.

In 1854 the Pennsylvania Rock Oil Company was organized to obtain and exploit this popular medicine. The company bought land near Titusville, Pennsylvania, where seepage of rock oil into ponds and streams had long been observed. Samples of the oil were sent to Professor Benjamin Silliman, Jr., at Yale. He was asked to analyze the oil and to determine whether it might have some commercial application in addition to its use as a medicine. In 1855 Silliman reported that it was an excellent lubricant and that a distillate of the oil burned with a bright, steady, nonsmoky flame. It was evident that the oil might serve as a substitute for the inadequate tallow candle and the expensive whale oil, which were then the principal sources of household illumination. The problem of how to obtain the oil in quantity was not solved until Edwin L. Drake, an employee of the Pennsylvania Rock Oil Company, conceived the notion that one might drill for oil just as one drilled for water. Drake hired a professional well-driller and in August, 1859, struck oil less than 70 feet below the surface. Within a few years wells in western Pennsylvania and in neighboring Ohio were producing crude oil by the thousands of barrels, and refineries had been devised for distilling kerosene from the crude material.

In 1876 two men who were to have a profound effect upon the development of medical science could have been seen walking about the oil fields of Pennsylvania and Ohio. Neither was a physician. One was a Russian scientist, Dmitri Ivanovich Mendeleev, who had been involved in the opening of the oil fields in the Caucasus (Jaffe, 1931). In 1876 he had been sent to the United States by the czar's government to learn about American methods of production and refining. Seven years before setting out on this trip, Mendeleev had discovered the periodic arrangement of the chemical elements. His *periodic table* brought order out of relative chaos in the science of chemistry and provided a major step toward the recognition and understanding of the radioactive elements and isotopes which were to be so useful to medicine.

The second man walking the oil fields was John D. Rockefeller, who had been born in New York state, the son of a peddler of patent medicines. In 1862, at the age of 25, Rockefeller used funds acquired in business operations to purchase a part interest in a small oil refinery in Cleveland. Within a few years he had bought out his partners and was the sole owner of the refinery. In 1870 he incorporated the Standard Oil Company of Ohio, and by 1876 he was busy absorbing his competitors or squeezing them out of business, in order to amass the great fortune much of which would eventually be used for the advancement of medical education and medical science.

Not all of the inventions of the 1870s were to affect health favorably. Cigarettes, introduced from Europe in the 1850s, were initially made by tedious "roll-your-own" methods. Their popularity was limited until about 1875, when a machine was invented to manufacture them in quantity. Three-quarters of a century would pass before the ill effects of the manufactured product would become apparent.

THE MEDICAL SCENE

While medical science and clinical diagnosis had made significant progress during the first century, few improvements were perceptible to the average layman other than the following: (1) the abandonment of the harsher methods of treatment that had been employed regularly in the early years of the century; and (2) the use of anesthesia for surgical operations. Though the layman might not be aware of it, anesthesia and better control of infections had made operative surgery not only less painful but also less hazardous, and the better American surgeons were widely acknowledged to be among the best in the world. In other branches of medicine improvement was less apparent. Epidemics still raged (an epidemic of cholera in 1873 and an epidemic of yellow fever in 1878). The same old diseases—typhoid fever, diphtheria, malaria, tuberculosis, diarrheal diseases of children, etc.—took the same heavy toll. In treating these diseases most doctors admitted, at least to themselves, that they were powerless, and the public suspected that this was the case. Yet in spite of their lack of confidence in doctors as a group, many people admired and trusted their physicians and sometimes idolized them. At the same time they knew others whom they considered to be ill educated and untrustworthy. Unhappily, the ill-educated segment of the profession was still on the increase.

Under the leadership of Nathan Smith Davis in Chicago and President Eliot at Harvard, the standards of medical education were definitely rising, but the upward movement was limited to a few schools—those bold enough to run the risk of adopting a graded three-year curriculum. In this movement the schools of Northwestern and Harvard universities were joined in the 1870s by the schools of Syracuse, Pennsylvania, and Michigan universities. There was also a small increase in the proportion of college

90

graduates applying for admission to these schools, though the educational *requirements* for admission were virtually nonexistent.

While these few schools were raising their standards, other developments were having an adverse effect. In the ten years 1867 to 1876 more new medical schools were founded than in any previous decade: 21 of the orthodox variety and 5 homeopathic. Most of these schools were of the poorest quality, thus serving to depress the average level of competence of medical school graduates.

To provide a closer look at the medical scene in the 70s we shall quote the observations of several men who lived in that period and knew it thoroughly. Commenting on the educational background of medical students, the British naturalist Thomas H. Huxley had this to say in Baltimore in 1876:

> At present, young men come to the medical schools without a conception of even the elements of physical science; they learn, for the first time, that there are such sciences as physics, chemistry and physiology.... Much of the first session is wasted in learning how to learn, ... and in awakening their dormant and wholly untrained powers of observation and of manipulation. It is difficult to over-estimate the magnitude of the obstacles thrown in the way of scientific training by the existing system of school education. Not only are men trained in mere book-work, ignorant of what observation means, but the habit of learning from books begets a disgust of observation. The book-learned student will rather trust to what he sees in a book than to the witness of his own eyes.

William H. Welch, who received his A.B. degree from Yale in 1870, was one of the small group of students who graduated from college before entering medical school. As an undergraduate Welch excelled in the classics and for more than a year after graduation he tried to obtain an appointment as a Professor of Classical Languages. Failing in this, medicine was his second choice, and he entered The College of Physicians and Surgeons, New York, in 1872. Unlike most of his contemporaries, Welch spent three rather than two years in medical school. He was mature enough and wise enough to plan his own graded course of study. Furthermore, his studies extended beyond the limits of the usual winter session of lectures and even beyond the limits of his own medical school. He spent much time at the excellent library of the New York Hospital, took a course at the University Medical College, and attended a summer session at Bellevue Hospital Medical College.

In 1907 Welch briefly described his memories of his school days, which were perhaps somewhat colored by nostalgic loyalty to his alma mater (Welch, 1908):

> One can decry the system of those days — the inadequate preliminary requirements, the short courses, the faulty arrangement of the curriculum, the dominance of the didactic lecture, the meager appliances for demonstrative and practical instruction — but the results were better than the system.... Our teachers were men of fine character, devoted to the duties of their chairs, they inspired us with enthusiasm, interest in our studies and hard work, and they imparted to us sound traditions of our profession; nor did they send us forth so utterly ignorant and unfitted for professional work as those born of the present, greatly improved methods of training ... are sometimes wont to suppose.

91

Commenting on the foregoing statement, Abraham Flexner (1910) said that it was not applicable to more than about a half-dozen medical schools of that period.

Another person who observed that the results were sometimes better than the system was President Eliot. After damning the system and deploring the ignorance and uncouthness of its products, Eliot felt constrained to add, "It speaks volumes for the educating force of medical practice that out of such raw material there could be produced, in the course of years, so fair a proportion of skillful, humane, and successful practitioners." Eliot, situated as he was in Boston and having contacts not only with the Harvard faculty but also with other leading medical educators, probably saw more of the "fair proportion" than did the rest of his fellow countrymen.

In the farm country of the middle states the picture was far less favorable. Hertzler, who spent his childhood in Kansas in the 1870s, gives the following account of what he observed in his early years:

> Most of the doctors had never attended a medical school. Most of them had "read medicine" with some active doctor but many just bought a book....We had one doctor in our town who had been to medical school—that is, to Keokuk Medical College—spending there two years of five months each....
>
> Many of the doctors of that day had drug stores [and they] examined patients as they were seated beside the counter in view of other customers, and loafers. That is to say, the patients' tongues were looked at, and the more thorough, if they had a watch, counted their pulses; then medicines were handed out from the stock on the shelves.
>
> It was generally believed by the laity in our community that...two-thirds of the doctors went to hell. The third saved were homeopaths with beards. Most of the doctors of that day were addicted to liquor, smoked pipes and did not go to church. ...My father believed...that approximately all doctors were parasites of society. He cannot be blamed for his uncomplimentary opinion of doctors because the small fortune he spent for alleged medical skill for members of his family netted just about nothing.

Hertzler may have been drawing a caricature of the rural physicians of his childhood, but his picture is based on authentic observations: many doctors were poorly educated, their habits were not always the best, their examination of patients was cursory, they dispensed medicines promiscuously, their therapy was for the most part ineffective, and, at least in some parts of the country, they were regarded as parasites on society, and regular practitioners were considered less admirable than homeopaths.

In 1877, William Pepper, Professor of Clinical Medicine at the University of Pennsylvania, delivered an address entitled *Higher Medical Education, the True Interest of the Public and the Profession*. Pepper shared the concerns about American medical education previously expressed by Drake, Davis, Eliot, and others; but he was particularly troubled by the degradation of the profession resulting from "the enormous overproduction of medical men."

> The Civil War, which broke out in 1861, soon attained such gigantic proportions that, both at the north and south, a large increase in the number of medical men was necessary to supply the demands of the army and navy. Following the termination of the war in 1865, came a period of inflated prosperity, when the development of

our country progressed at an incredible rate. The tide of immigration was setting like a mighty flood towards our shores; our railroad system was stretching its iron threads in every direction, weaving its wonderful network at the rate of 5000 miles a year; every day witnessed the establishment of new centers of mining and manufacturing industry, or the opening of new fields of agricultural wealth throughout the land; villages and even towns sprang into existence as though at the touch of a magician's wand. Side by side with this marvelous expansion came an equally rapid growth in the numbers of the medical profession. There was already enough, and more than enough, of unemployed medical talent in the cities and large towns that should have been drawn upon to supply the new demand, but none the less briskly went on the work of multiplying medical schools and of glutting the market with hastily manufactured doctors.

In 1873, overproduction and excessive development had reached a point of such extreme tension that it needed but a slight jar to dash to pieces the fictitious prosperity of the country. The crash came, and our overgrown industries were prostrated amidst the ruins of princely fortunes. Since then scarcely any branch of business has offered sufficient chances of profit to tempt new capital to seek investment in it. [As a result of this more young men have been diverted toward a medical career.] The returns of the Commissioner of Education for 1875 show that at the annual commencements of the 65 regular medical schools in that year there were 2597 graduates. . . . [In addition there were 391 graduates of the eclectic and homeopathic colleges.] It is within safe limits to estimate the number of practitioners of medicine who were qualified in 1875 at somewhat over 3000. . . . [In addition to the locally trained physicians, the census of 1870 showed that foreign-born and foreign-educated physicians had entered the country between 1860 and 1870 at an annual rate of 289.] Further, it is well known that it is an almost universal custom in America for druggists to prescribe over their counter, and thus to conduct a medical practice often of very considerable size. According to the census report of 1870 there were 17,369 druggists and traders in medicine.

Pepper contends that the ranks of the medical profession "have been fearfully overstocked by the reckless selfishness of the medical schools; . . . there are but few classes of the community of which a larger proportion are not earning a living than of the medical profession." As evidence of overcrowding in the profession Pepper cites the proportion of physicians to population in various countries: 1 to 600 in the United States, 1 to 1672 in Great Britain, 1 to 1814 in France, 1 to 2500 in Austria, 1 to 3000 in Germany, 1 to 3500 in Italy, and 1 to 7500 in Sweden.

"It is known to all men," says Pepper, "that for years the representative medical associations have loudly denounced the system of education in our medical schools; that for years the leading members of the profession have acknowledged its defects and urged immediate reform; that for years the pages of the most influential medical journals have overflowed with eloquent appeals and unanswerable arguments in favor of an elevated standard of education." In spite of all these efforts nothing had been done to correct the situation and now "medical diplomas and degrees conferred by 'bogus' universities, can be openly bought for 50, 30 even 20 dollars, without attendance on a single lecture or without the pretense of the slightest medical knowledge. . . . scarce a month passes without the exposure, in some of the leading foreign papers, of cases of horrible malpractice by ignorant quacks holding a 'bogus' American diploma. . . .

"The unscrupulous and unprincipled adventurer, the imposter and the quack, the men who have failed to pass the foreign examination boards, all of these flock to the United States as to a field where, without restriction, they may assume the title of physician and practice on an equality with the regular profession" (Pepper, 1877).

In concluding his address Pepper made recommendations for the improvement of medical education and announced that the University of Pennsylvania was instituting a new three-year graded curriculum which embodied all of his recommendations except for an examination prior to matriculation; "it was not thought feasible to insist upon this immediately, but all are agreed that it must be instituted as soon as possible."

In 1878, John Shaw Billings, who was then involved in the preparation of plans for the Johns Hopkins Hospital and Medical School, contributed *A Review on Higher Medical Education*, from which the following excerpts are taken:

The condition of medical education in this country may be briefly summed up as follows: —

There are now 65 medical schools in the United States, besides those devoted to homeopathy, eclectic and botanic systems, etc. During the winter of 1876–7, these 65 schools had 7141 students, of whom 2313 graduated as doctors of medicine in the spring of 1877. There were employed in these schools 515 professors, and 279 other teachers with various titles.

In five of these schools there is a graded course of three years, and in two a preliminary examination is required, although of a low grade. Of the remaining schools about 15 are doing fairly good work, work as good as there is a demand for, and are prepared to improve as rapidly as public opinion and financial necessities will permit.

The rest of the schools are doing poor work, and will probably continue to do it. Many of them owe their existence to the desire of two or three gentlemen to advertise themselves without coming under the ban of the Code of Ethics. What an individual may not do is yet permissible to a corporation. The profit from such schools does not come from the fees of the students, but from the advertisement, and from the consultation cases which the graduates bring to the professors. . . .

The amount of general education and time of study required by our medical schools are about the same as, or perhaps a little less than, those required for veterinary medicine abroad.

. . . The various attempts which our physicians have made to produce a change for the better have not as yet produced any striking results, but the attention of the non-medical public, which is after all the party most immediately interested, and is probably the only source from which effectual reform can be expected, has been to some extent aroused, so that it is probable that in the course of time our legislators will provide some means by which the public can distinguish the properly trained physician. . . .

Let us turn now to the remedies proposed for the condition of things in the United States. As far as protection to the public from incompetent practitioners is concerned, the majority of the medical profession are probably of the opinion that the government should interfere in some way, but in what way is by no means generally agreed upon. . . .

Dr. Pepper thinks that each State should prescribe the number of years to be devoted to medical studies before graduation, and should create a State board of ex-

aminers, who alone should have the right to confer licenses to practise within the limits of the State. This would probably be an effectual remedy, provided that public sentiment would permit the infliction of penalties upon those who practised in violation of the law. Such a public sentiment does not exist at the present time, and we do not believe that it will exist for a long time to come.

. . . The experience of Harvard and of the University of Pennsylvania show that extending the course of study to three years will be a financial success. Far more important, however, than lengthening the curriculum, is the establishing [of] a satisfactory preliminary examination. It is at the very beginning that incompetent men should be rejected, and this for their own sake.

No such examination has yet been tried in this country, nor can it probably be maintained by an institution which is not so endowed as to be comparatively independent of the students' fees. . . .

Thus far we have been considering the subject of medical education from the point of view from which the majority of authors and essayists view it, namely, as designed to produce medical practitioners, — as fitting men for the art or handicraft of medicine. This is the article for which the demand is evident, and the supply corresponds. . . .

What is the prospect in this country for the production of men qualified to teach medicine and the cognate sciences, and to carry on original research? We think it probable that this also we may hope to see accomplished. A new university is just now taking shape in Baltimore which has, to a great extent, the means to undertake this special work, and the authorities of which are now considering this problem of medical education with reference to the mode in which they should organize their medical department. Let us hope that their decision will be a wise one, and that a sufficient number of young men may be found in this country to appreciate the opportunity which will thus be afforded them.

Finally, a view of the American medical scene in the 70s is presented by an account which appeared in the *Lancet* (London) in 1874. An English surgeon, Sir John Eric Erichsen, who visited the United States in that year, felt that he should report his observations "because I believe that too little is known of American surgery in this country." The medical profession "appears to me to occupy in America . . . a far higher social status than it does in this country. The reason for this seems tolerably obvious. In the absence of an exalted hierarchy in an established church and of great dignitaries of the law, these professions do not offer sufficient inducement for men of the highest intellectual calibre to enter them. Medicine therefore stands prominent as probably the best-educated, certainly the most scientific, and consequently . . . the most respected, of the professions. . . .

"Surgery in the United States certainly stands at a very high level of excellence. The hospital surgeons throughout the country have struck me as being alike practical, progressive, and learned in a very high degree. In practical skill and aptitude for mechanical appliances of all kinds, they are certainly excelled by no class of practitioners in any country."

Erichsen's evaluation of those who practiced surgery in the United States may have been tempered by "the warm and hospitable and hearty welcome that was given to me wherever I went, east or west, north or south, from New York to Chicago, from Boston through Philadelphia and Baltimore to Washington." Nevertheless, his praise seems genuine, and in

95

the cities which he specifically mentions, he doubtless saw the best that American surgery had to offer.

Erichsen's comments on American medical education are also of interest:

> . . . the course of education required is generally shorter than with us, and no preliminary examination in the way of matriculation is required. . . . This undoubtedly is a great evil. . . . The chief difference [between English and American schools] that I have observed is in the method of communicating clinical instruction. The medical schools in the principal cities of the States, especially New York and Philadelphia, are so enormous that the classes would be too large to be conducted through the wards of a hospital. Classes numbering from 600 to 800 are not uncommon. At Professor Pancoast's introductory lecture at Jefferson College, Philadelphia, there were probably 600 students present; and at my last visit to the clinical theatre at Bellevue Hospital, New York, it was estimated that a thousand students were present. It therefore becomes necessary to bring the patient to the students, rather than, as with us, the pupils to the patient. This is done by raising him off the framework of his bed on a small platform running on wheels, and thus carrying him . . . into the clinical theatre. . . .

Shifting from medical education to hospitals, Erichsen writes,

> The Hospitals of the United States are, as with us, supported by voluntary contributions or by endowments from wealthy benefactors. . . . these institutions are numerous and well-organized. America has two sets of hospitals, the old and the new. Like England in some of its larger towns, it is still embarrassed by the hospitals erected in pre-sanitary days, . . . in which septic diseases are readily generated and become largely destructive to the patients. These institutions are, however, undergoing a process of conversion which will speedily do away with many of the evils inseparably connected with such buildings.

> . . . antiseptics are not so much needed in the American hospitals as in ours. The object of antiseptics is to prevent contamination of a wound by septic impurities from without. These sources of contamination do not exist in such hospitals as those I have been describing to the same extent as they do in less perfectly constructed and less hygienically conducted establishments. . . . In America it is attempted to accomplish by improved construction of hospitals, and by close attention to hygienic requirements, those great results which we are here driven to attain by "antiseptic" methods of treatment. . . . [In England], under the present system we begin at the wrong end. . . . we allow the septic poison to be generated, and then, before it can be implanted on the wound, seek to destroy it by the employment of chemical agents.

It would appear that Erichsen's American experience had impressed him with the value of what would be called today an "aseptic" environment. Another decade or two would elapse before Lister's cumbersome antiseptic procedures would be superseded in operating rooms by the aseptic technic which prevails today. Asepsis, with its sterilization of surgical dressings and surgeon's gowns, its boiling of instruments, its use of sterile rubber gloves, and other measures, is nothing more than an enhanced and formalized version of the "close attention to hygienic requirements" which Erichsen observed in American hospitals.

These hospitals, as Erichsen noted, were supported by contributions and endowments provided by the public. Community responsibility for and generosity toward hospitals had been a tradition since the founding of the Pennsylvania Hospital in colonial days. Medical schools, on the other hand, did not enjoy this type of public support. Throughout the first century, medical schools were considered to be and indeed were self-sustaining commercial enterprises. In the eyes of the public they neither needed nor deserved the generous financial backing accorded hospitals. In consequence, few medical schools had endowments or sources of income other than student fees. In 1870, the endowment funds of Harvard Medical School, perhaps as plentiful as any, yielded an income of some $2000 per year—scarcely enough to pay for the care and upkeep of the building.

THE PHYSICIAN'S MEDICINES   Even the most erudite and experienced physician had few effective medicines at his command. Some of those which were effective were unknown to the poorly educated practitioner; others he knew not how to use. The short list of effective therapeutic agents in the 1870s included the anesthetics (ether, chloroform, and nitrous oxide); opium and its alkaloids (morphine was first used extensively during the Civil War to ease the pain of the wounded); digitalis, which was used chiefly for cardiac edema; ergot, to stimulate uterine contractions and to control postpartum hemorrhage; mercury in the form of an inunction for syphilis and in the form of calomel to purge and salivate; various cathartics of botanical origin; iron, usually in the form of Blaud's pills for anemia; quinine for malaria; amyl nitrite, which was first recommended for the relief of angina pectoris by Sir Thomas Lauder Brunton in 1867 but was still not well known in 1876; sulfur ointment for the itch (scabies); green vegetables or citrus fruit for the prevention or treatment of scurvy. These various medicines were administered either by mouth, by rectum, by inhalation, or by application to the skin. The hypodermic syringe had been introduced by the French surgeon Pravaz in 1851. He employed it to inject "chloride of iron" into vascular tumors to coagulate their contents. Although it was subsequently used for other restricted purposes, the danger of infection limited its use until the physician had learned how to prevent infections by the preparation of sterile solutions.

LOOKING AHEAD   No one could have prophesied in 1876 that the next century would be, beyond measure, a century of fantastic medical progress and that American medicine would contribute mightily to the advance. We can see, in retrospect, that the principal elements initiating and helping to sustain the forward movement were then already discernible:

(1) Prominent educators had recognized the deplorable state of medical education and were beginning to do something about it. Their efforts would soon be strengthened by the benefactions of several wealthy philanthropists and by the return to American medical schools of young men who were then being trained in the foremost laboratories of Europe. Represent-

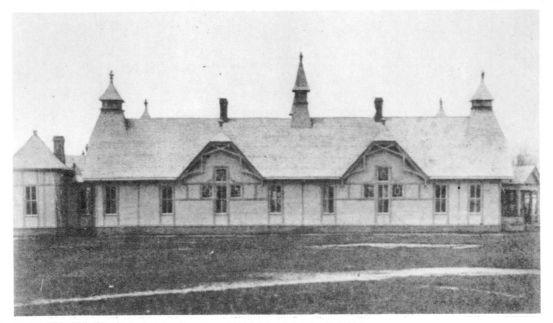

Figure 22. Pavilion Hospital, University of Michigan School of Medicine, 1875. This wooden building, accommodating about 150 patients, with operating theatre, was planned under the supervision of E. S. Dunster, Professor of Obstetrics and Gynecology, and was of the type employed in the latter part of the Civil War. (From Vaughan, Victor C.: A Doctor's Memories. Indianapolis, The Bobbs-Merrill Co., 1926.)

atives of 22 medical schools met in 1876 to form a *Provisional Association of American Medical Colleges,* which would, in time, play a leading role in raising the standards of medical education.

(2) A start had been made in providing facilities and personnel for basic medical research. The first university-based medical research laboratories had been founded: the laboratory of physiology under Henry P. Bowditch at Harvard (1871) and the laboratory of physiological chemistry under Russell H. Chittenden at Yale (1874).

(3) Drinking water contaminated by human excreta had been implicated in the spread of at least two epidemic diseases, cholera and typhoid fever. The knowledge that certain diseases were potentially preventable gave impetus to the formation of state and municipal boards of health and to the appointment of public health officers. The American Public Health Association was founded in 1876, and in 1879 Congress established the National Board of Health.

(4) Hospitals were beginning to assume a new role in the provision of health services and in the clinical instruction of medical students. Hospital architects were paying more attention to functional design and to the need to prevent the spread of intramural infections. That the hospital was no longer to be merely a haven for sick paupers was indicated by the inclusion

in newer establishments of rooms for paying patients. Of greater importance for medical education was the establishment in the 70s of the first two hospitals that were to operate under the control of university medical schools: the University of Pennsylvania Hospital (1874) and the University of Michigan Hospital (1877). At about the same time, Johns Hopkins provided in his will funds to found a hospital and a medical school and directed (1873) that these institutions work together for the advancement of medical education.

(5) Laboratory methods had begun to play a part in clinical diagnosis.

(6) The principles and practices introduced by Lister would provide the basis for a great forward surge in operative surgery.

(7) Professional nurses with special education and training had begun to replace the uneducated, underpaid women who had previously cared for the sick.

(8) The concept of the relationship between micro-organisms and human disease was gaining credence. In 1876 Robert Koch was performing his classic experiments on the anthrax bacillus. Bancroft in Australia was demonstrating that filariae were the cause of elephantiasis; and Manson, in China, was conducting experiments that would provide the first scientific indication that a mosquito may serve as an intermediate host in the transmission of disease. However, Manson at first thought that the mosquito discharged the microfilariae of elephantiasis into water and that people acquired the disease by drinking the water.

(9) What would become the science of genetics had its experimental origin in the 1860s in the work of an Austrian monk, Gregor Johann Mendel, who demonstrated how certain characteristics were inherited by peas planted in the monastery garden. In a related field, the basic details of the manner in which cells divide so as to reproduce themselves were first worked out by Walter Flemming in Germany in 1876.

(10) In Washington, D.C., John Shaw Billings was organizing medical literature in a systematic fashion that would make it more accessible to research workers and clinicians.

(11) State governments were beginning to show serious interest in medical licensure.

The practice of medicine during the nation's second century would be profoundly influenced not only by the advances in medical science and other intramedical developments but also by a number of nonmedical discoveries and inventions of the latter part of the first century: the telephone, electric lighting, petroleum products, the internal combustion engine, the typewriter, and photography. Medical practice would also be affected by the various procedures which had been introduced to protect or enhance the health of the individual: better water supply; better disposal of waste; refrigeration in the home and in the transportation of food; more abundant and better quality milk in the cities; more abundant protein foods, derived chiefly from western cattle; and year-round availability of seasonal foods made possible by the canning industry. The health of future generations would also be influenced by a new type of law, which was first adopted by Massachusetts in 1874. This law limited the hours of work of women and children employed in factories to 10 hours per day! In 1876 there was still some uncertainty as to whether such a law should or could be enforced.

99

THE FIRST CENTURY ENDS Viewed from one aspect, the decade of the 70s was a period of unusual richness in scientific discovery and technical invention. Fortunately these were the factors which would have a cumulative and enduring influence upon the future of the nation. However, the American breathing the air of 1876 was more affected by the national turmoil which seemed almost to deprive him of the advantages of citizenship: political corruption and graft, economic depression, greedy industrialists, unemployment and underpaid workers, impoverished farmers, and devalued currency. These were the aspects of the national scene which the voter had in mind when he went to the polls for the presidential election of that year.

The election of 1876 was bitterly contested. The pressures for political reform were mounting. Samuel J. Tilden, the Democratic candidate, had won his reputation as a reformer by leading a successful fight against the corrupt Tweed Ring in New York. Rutherford B. Hayes, the Republican candidate, had been a general in the Union Army, and it was suspected that he might perpetuate the practices of his predecessor in office. President Grant, in a patently partisan move, sent federal troops to South Carolina, Florida, and Louisiana to "protect the Negro voters from the Ku Klux Klan." It was believed that if the Negroes were permitted to get to the polls they would almost certainly vote the Republican ticket. In spite of such measures to defeat him, Tilden won the majority of the popular votes. However, the electoral votes of the three "protected" states were challenged. The matter was settled by a special Electoral Commission of fifteen members, eight of whom were Republicans and seven Democrats. By voting along strictly party lines the Commission decided that each of the contested electoral votes should be cast for Hayes. These political shenanigans did little to restore confidence and to quell the turmoil in which the nation entered its second century.

PART TWO

Period of
Scientific
Advance–1876-1946

IO

The National Scene

The thoughts of men are comparable to the leaves, flowers, and fruit upon the innumerable branches of a few great stems, fed by commingled and hidden roots. These stems bear the names of the half-dozen men, endowed with intellects of heroic force and clearness.

(T. H. Huxley)

As the nation entered its second century, the wounds inflicted by the Civil War were beginning to heal. In the first year of his administration President Hayes withdrew federal troops from the only three Southern states in which they were still stationed, and he appointed a Southerner, a former Confederate officer, to his cabinet. For their part, the states of the South, welcoming the end of Reconstruction, were striving to develop new industries to strengthen their old cotton-tobacco economy.

In the years 1876 to 1912 the number of states in the Union increased from 38 to 48, and there was an increase of about 50 million in the population. About 10 million of the people were blacks born in America, of whom 90 per cent lived in the South. During these years some 20 million immigrants entered the country. In the decade 1900 to 1909, immigration averaged over 800,000 per year, reaching a maximum of just under 1.3 million in 1906.

With the growth in population there was a gradual shift from agrarian to industrial dominance. In 1870 only 25 per cent of the people lived in the cities, but by 1900 the city dwellers had increased to 40 per cent and by 1946 to 60 per cent of the population. Between the end of the Civil War and 1900, while the value of farm products had increased threefold, the value of manufactured goods had increased fourfold.

The trend of industrial growth, for the most part steadily upward until World War I, was temporarily retarded by two economic depressions, the first trailing away from the panic of 1873 and the second ushered in by the panic of 1893. The entire period between these major episodes was one of low wages and low prices for both farm produce and manufactured goods.

103

From 1897 to World War I there was almost continuous prosperity, punctuated in 1898 by the short-lived Spanish-American War and in 1907 by a brief recession. The frenzied prosperity of the 1920s was followed by the Great Depression of the 1930s.

THE EARLY YEARS OF THE SECOND CENTURY

The typical social unit of the early years of the second century has been described concisely by E. T. Neumann (Knowles, 1965):

The American family at the turn of the [nineteenth to the twentieth] century had a structure easily understood by all. There was no question that the father was the head of the family. In subsidiary position was his wife who had promised in their marriage ceremony to love, honor, and obey him—and in that era very likely meant every word of it. In the most subsidiary position came the children. The aphorism of that day, "Children are better seen than heard," provides the best clue to assessing their situation. Orders went down this structure to the children. Any discussion of these orders by the children was apt to be considered "backtalk" requiring a "summary court martial" on the spot. Articulate, imaginative children in those days were considered undisciplined and probably brought more shame than praise to their parents. And, furthermore, the children of the average American family completed their schooling in the fourth grade. From that point on, whether in the city or rural area, the children worked in some way and contributed to the welfare of the family. How this contribution was to be utilized by the family was largely determined by the father.

It might be added that the father was the only member of the social unit who had a vote in electing presidents, members of Congress, and other political figures. Since most fathers of that period were in favor of maintaining the status quo, their votes usually were cast for conservative members of one or the other political party.

The presidents from Hayes to McKinley were for the most part unimaginative and unprogressive men who exercised little initiative or power. Even as leaders of their respective political parties the presidents were relatively ineffective. When they tried to succeed themselves in office they invariably failed. Grover Cleveland served two (nonconsecutive) terms, but when he ran for office at the end of his first term (1888) he was defeated by Benjamin Harrison, and at the end of his second term (1893–1897) his bid for renomination was rejected by his own Democratic party in favor of William Jennings Bryan. McKinley, who defeated Bryan in 1896, was re-elected by a large majority in 1900, but his success was in a sense paradoxical, since his popularity resulted from the victorious Spanish-American War and the nation's territorial expansion overseas, both of which he had originally opposed.

During most of the first quarter of the second century, the Congress was more strongly conservative than the presidents. However, it did succeed in adopting three important acts of reform legislation: the Pendleton Act (1883), which placed certain civil service appointments on a merit basis; the Interstate Commerce Act (1887) for the purpose of effecting reasonable and equitable railway rates; and the Sherman Antitrust Act (1890) prohibiting combinations "in restraint of trade."

Many developments in the early part of the second century had a significant though sometimes indirect effect upon medicine. The expansion of railroads, the improvement of highways, and the increased speed and volume of waterborne travel, by river, canal, and ocean, served to break down the relative isolation of many communities and thus to aggravate problems in the control of communicable diseases. Problems that once had been local or confined to two or three states became national or even international in scope. The United States had to keep a sharp eye on diseases in foreign lands because of the unremitting flood of immigrants. An additional but in this case beneficial effect of improved transportation was the widening of the service area of rural physicians.

The organization of labor also had an effect upon health. During the first century, labor had been poorly organized, and its efforts to obtain higher wages and better working conditions were defeated almost regularly. The first labor organization to have a national impact was *The Noble Order of the Knights of Labor*. This organization was founded in 1869 as a secret society, its principal objective being "to secure to the toilers a proper share of the wealth which they create." The membership of the Noble Order, open to unskilled as well as to skilled workers, was too small to have any significant influence prior to 1876. In the 1880s, the Knights shed their secrecy and campaigned openly for new members, and in 1885 they conducted a successful strike against the Gould railroad lines. In 1886, the Knights joined several other labor organizations in initiating a strike in Chicago for an eight-hour work day. Several days after the strike began, while police were trying to disperse a mass meeting held in Haymarket Square, a bomb exploded, killing 7 policemen and wounding 60 other persons. The adverse public reaction was so violent that before a year had passed the Knights had disintegrated, and for many years thereafter it was difficult to arouse public sympathy for striking workers.

The *American Federation of Labor,* though founded in 1881, remained rather obscure until after the Haymarket incident. In 1886 it was reorganized under the leadership of Samuel Gompers, who was to be its President until his death in 1924. The membership of the Federation was limited to skilled craftsmen. This gave the newer organization an advantage: threat of a strike by the Federation had to be taken more seriously, because the skilled workers could not be replaced easily.

Under the far-sighted leadership of Gompers, the American Federation of Labor won a greater degree of public respect by announcing that it favored the capitalistic system. It fought for the principle of collective bargaining and for higher wages, shorter working hours, and better working conditions. Initially the Federation refused to take part in any except strictly local political activities. In 1908, it changed its policy and made an effort to influence the platforms adopted by the major political parties. Since it received more favorable treatment from the Democrats than from the Republicans, the Federation urged its members to vote the Democratic ticket. When the Republicans won the election, the Federation's backing of the "wrong party" served temporarily to weaken its political impact.

The progress of organized labor was to have a considerable influence in

105

the health field. Its successful efforts to eliminate children from the labor force, to shorten the hours of work for both men and women, and to eliminate hazards and improve conditions in factories, mines, and other working areas certainly had a beneficial effect upon the nation's health. Moreover, looking ahead, as organized labor gained in political power and social influence, it acquired a decisive voice in such matters as social security legislation, health insurance, and other programs that were to have an impact upon medicine.

The growth of the cities with their congested slums presented problems in housing, sanitation, nutrition, water supply, and the disposal of sewage and other wastes. Some of these problems, with which physicians, health officers, and city officials had to deal, were recognized in the first century, and means were developed for dealing with a few of them. The technical advances that had been so numerous in the 1870s began to bring practical results to the cities in the 1880s, while new and useful inventions continued to multiply. As the cities expanded, the introduction of steel-frame construction, electrically powered elevators, and central heating, all of which became available in the 1880s and 1890s, permitted the erection of buildings of increasing height. The first of the super-skyscrapers, the 60-story Woolworth Building, was completed in New York in 1913. A bare 25 years had been required for the development of the structural methods, the materials, the machinery, and the technical devices that made this fantastic building possible.

Progress was made in the early years of the second century in improvement of water supply and sewage disposal, in provision of better housing and more nutritious foods, and in partial or even total elimination of the more devastating of the epidemic diseases; but many of these improvements took place in the better sections of the city while the slums remained relatively unaffected. Moreover, the changes came about slowly. In the early years of the twentieth century even the more affluent portions of some of the larger cities, including New Orleans and Baltimore, still had to depend upon the gutters in their streets for disposal of household sewage.

In the last years of the nineteenth century the Spanish-American War and the acquisition of territories overseas, particularly in tropical regions, presented numerous new medical problems. These problems were for the most part tackled by the Army Medical Corps. Some of the outstanding results include the discovery of the manner in which yellow fever is transmitted, the identification of the bacteria that cause dysentery, and a brilliant demonstration in Panama of how the spread of certain communicable diseases may be prevented.

Changes in public education, which began to take place in the 1870s, were to have both a direct and an indirect effect upon medical education. In a landmark decision in 1874 the Supreme Court of the state of Michigan affirmed the right of the city of Kalamazoo to tax its citizens for the support of the high school. At about the same time, the University of Michigan announced that it would accept for admission, without examination, any graduate of the high schools of the state. The Kalamazoo decision, which was quickly accepted by other states, made possible a rapid increase in tax-supported high schools. Between 1870 and 1915 the number of high school students in the United States increased from 80,000 to 1.3 million. The decision of the University of Michigan to admit high school graduates without examination led other universities to follow suit and thus gave greater prestige to the high school diploma.

The number of students attending colleges and universities increased from about 50,000 in 1870 to 400,000 in 1915. Part of this increase was due to the Morrill Act, which Congress adopted in 1862. Under this act large tracts of the public domain were ceded to various states, with the proviso that the funds derived from the land grants should be used to establish and operate colleges that would offer courses "related to agriculture and the mechanic arts." Morrill's purpose in sponsoring this act was to replace the traditional classical education offered by the colleges with a type of education which he considered to be of greater practical use.

The land-grant colleges became popular particularly in the Middle West and other rapidly growing areas. Although the curriculum at these institutions was directed toward a career in agriculture or engineering, the students also were given courses in some of the arts and sciences that contribute to a modern liberal education. The combination of land grants with increasingly liberal appropriations by the states made higher education, including medical education, available to many young people at relatively little expense.

PERIOD OF REFORM During the period from 1895 to World War I the atmosphere of the United States seemed to vibrate with reform. The spirit of *laissez-faire* that had characterized the nineteenth century was being replaced by a spirit of responsible concern. Reformers were demanding new standards of honesty in politics and business and firmer governmental control of industry and finance. They were demanding also that government exercise closer surveillance of the way people lived, including the conditions under which they worked, the privies that they used, the water and milk that they drank, and the food that they ate. Organized labor, encouraged by favorable decisions in the courts and by an improving public image, was moving steadily toward what were considered to be its more radical objectives. Many of the social and political reforms had a strong moral tone—concern for the poor and underprivileged and outrage at the "dishonesty and self-interest" of politicians and business executives.

In addition to the social and political reforms, there were profound changes in the whole manner of American life. The farmer driving his Model-T Ford was no longer so isolated, and his seclusion was further reduced by the rapidly spreading web of telephone and electrical lines. More and more people were moving from the country to the cities and were becoming dependent upon industry for their livelihood. The wheels of industry and commerce were turning more rapidly, as gasoline, steam, and electrical power replaced hay, oats, and water power.

Significant reform movements got under way in the late years of the nineteenth century, when civic groups in many cities began to agitate for more responsible government. Magazines and newspapers, taking up the cause, gave publicity to specific examples of dishonesty and inefficiency in

107

government and to the baneful influence upon local politics of ethnic conflicts and the power of corporations. In 1902 and 1903, Lincoln Steffens published a series of articles (later gathered together in the classic *Shame of the Cities*) exposing dishonesty and corrupt practices in many cities. Groups advocating responsible government succeeded in electing reform mayors in Detroit, San Francisco, and Toledo in 1897, and in New York and Cleveland in 1901. Other cities soon took similar action, freeing their city halls from the control of entrenched and unscrupulous political machines. Unfortunately the reform administrations rarely remained in office for more than one or two terms, but their accomplishments had a longer and more lasting effect, leaving the cities with publicly owned utilities, cleaner public markets, better hospitals, improved public health, and other important advances.

Steffens and the other authors engaged in exposing corruption became known as the *Muckrakers*. Their accounts, sometimes more lurid than the facts warranted, were not restricted to the cities. State and national governments also came under fire. The reforms at state level were aimed not only at the elimination of corruption but also at the development of a more efficient governmental machinery and a political process more responsive to the needs and wishes of the electorate. The term "progressive" was applied to these reforms.

Wisconsin was the state in which the Progressive movement had its greatest influence. There the leader of the movement was Robert M. LaFollette, who was elected governor in 1900. By the time LaFollette resigned the governorship in 1906 to become a United States Senator, the Wisconsin legislature had enacted sweeping reforms under his leadership. These included the following: the direct primary; a corrupt practices act; an anti-lobbying bill; an industrial safety act; workmen's compensation; acts to regulate the labor of women and children, income and inheritance taxes, and railroad and utility commissions; increased support for public schools; the establishment of extension services by the state university; and a pure-food law.

By 1910 at least eight states of the Middle West and five states of the Far West had elected Progressive governors. In the East the Progressive fervor was more subdued, but its effect was appreciable in a few states. In 1906, Charles Evans Hughes, who had exposed irregularities in the management of life insurance companies, was elected governor of New York. Woodrow Wilson, elected governor of New Jersey in 1910, provided a Progressive administration that won him the support of the liberal members of his party.

President McKinley's re-election in 1900 came about because of the unplanned but "happy" events of his first administration: the winning of a popular war, the acquisition of an overseas empire, the arrival of an era of unprecedented prosperity, and a reduction in taxes. When the conservative McKinley was assassinated in September, 1901, he was succeeded in office by a man whom many considered to be a radical.

Theodore Roosevelt was young (42 years of age), energetic, aggressive, outspoken, and a student of history. Soon after his graduation from Harvard College (1880), Roosevelt entered politics and served for a time in the New York state legislature. In 1884, he opposed the nomination of James G. Blaine for the presidency, and when Blaine won the nomination, Roosevelt withdrew from politics and bought a ranch in North Dakota. In 1888 he returned to politics and served on the United States Civil Service Commission. In 1895 he was appointed Police Commissioner of New York City. In the latter office he tried strenuously to stamp out dishonesty and corruption, thus establishing his reputation as a reformer.

During McKinley's first term, Roosevelt was Assistant Secretary of the Navy. When the trouble with Spain began, the President prayed for peace while the Assistant Secretary prayed for war. Roosevelt had long favored the expansion of the United States into the Pacific area, and he had a rather boyish attitude about the glamor of armed conflict. In May, 1898, soon after war was declared, he resigned as Assistant Secretary and recruited a cavalry regiment which became known as the Rough Riders. When the exaggerated and sentimentalized news dispatches from Cuba seemed to indicate that the Rough Riders had won the war, their leader, Colonel Roosevelt, became a national hero. On the strength of his war record Roosevelt was elected governor of New York in 1898 and was nominated for the vice-presidency in 1900.

When Roosevelt succeeded McKinley, he gave the country a type of strong leadership that it had not experienced since the death of Abraham Lincoln. He immediately took steps to overcome what he considered to be the evil influence of large corporations. In 1902 the administration, acting under the Antitrust Act, succeeded in dissolving a powerful trust headed by J. P. Morgan. Roosevelt also used his influence to break a coal strike. When he threatened to have the United States Army seize and operate the mines, the mine owners agreed to have the strike arbitrated. This was the first time that a president had publicly supported organized labor.

After his election to a second term by a substantial majority, Roosevelt was in a stronger position to carry out his program. He took steps to enforce stricter regulation of corporations, including the railroads and insurance companies. Working closely with Gifford Pinchot, head of the Bureau of Forestry, he added more than 150 million acres to the National Forest Reserves, and he arranged for the conservation and better development of water resources, power sites, and mineral lands. Roosevelt's influence was weakened in 1907, when the long period of prosperity gave way to a depression. The conservative elements in the Congress were quick to attribute the depression to the President's policies.

Though Roosevelt's many staunch supporters urged him to run for a third term in 1908 he declined to do so, but he used his power and influence to persuade the Republican party to nominate William Howard Taft as its candidate.

Taft had resigned a federal judgeship in 1901 to accept appointment as the first United States Governor-General of the Philippine Islands. He was Secretary of War during Roosevelt's second term. As President he was more conservative than Roosevelt, but he supported many of the reforms initiated by his predecessor.

In 1910, when Roosevelt returned from an extended hunting trip in Africa, it became apparent that he still had the strong support of the Progressives. At the party convention for nomination of presidential candidates in 1912 the Republican party nominated Taft over the strong opposition of the Progressives. The Democratic convention nominated Governor Woodrow Wilson of New Jersey. About two months before the election a group made up largely of dissatisfied Republicans met in Chicago, founded the Progressive party, and nominated Roosevelt for the presidency. Owing to the split in the Republican ranks Wilson won the election with only 41 per cent of the popular vote.

It will be seen in subsequent chapters that great reforms in medicine coincided with the great sociopolitical reforms of the early twentieth century. The connection between the two movements is not easy to discern; either might have occurred without the other. Nevertheless, both were impelled by similar forces: (1) a more broadly educated citizenry; (2) extraordinary advances in science and technology; (3) a pent-up need to break away from entrenched and long outmoded traditions; and (4) enlightened, bold leadership.

WORLD WAR I   Though basically an austere intellectual, Wilson became a popular leader. He was an eloquent and persuasive public speaker, able to arouse enthusiastic support for the causes he espoused. In the early years of his presidency, concentrating on domestic problems, he persuaded Congress to reduce tariffs and to adopt the Federal Reserve Act, the Clayton Antitrust Act (which Gompers hailed as "labor's charter of freedom"), and a new pure-food law. In an attempt to protect American interests in Mexico he ordered General John J. Pershing to lead what proved to be a fruitless military expedition into that country.

During Wilson's second year in office, World War I erupted in Europe. For the first two years of the war the President strove to keep the United States from becoming involved. When he ran for re-election in 1916 his party's slogan was "He kept us out of war." In this election many of the Progressives voted the Democratic ticket, and owing to their support Wilson defeated his Republican opponent, Charles Evans Hughes, by a narrow margin.

Though American sentiment during the first two years of the war had favored neutrality, this posture was gradually undermined by the activities of the German U-boats. In January, 1917, the German government announced that the U-boats would sink at sight any American or other neutral vessel, armed or unarmed, that entered the war zone. Wilson responded by breaking diplomatic relations with Germany, hoping that this might induce the German government to reconsider its decision. There was no retraction on the part of the Germans, and on March 18 three unarmed American merchantmen were sunk without warning and with heavy loss of life. On April 2, 1917, Wilson, asserting that "the world must be made safe for democracy," asked Congress to declare war on Germany. Within the next four days both houses of Congress, by overwhelming majorities, joined in such a declaration.

The short-range advantage to the Allies of the American entry into the war was more than offset by the almost simultaneous collapse of the Russian imperial government. This allowed the Germans to shift large forces from the eastern to the western front in a desperate effort to achieve victory before significant American forces arrived in Europe. By July, 1918, the German offensive had spent itself, and American units were streaming across the Atlantic in greatly increased numbers. An Allied offensive during August, September, and October, in which large American forces participated for the first time, convinced the German leaders that a military victory was no longer possible. On November 9, Kaiser Wilhelm II abdicated, and two days later the war was brought to an end by the signing of an armistice.

Wilson approached the peace negotiations in a spirit of idealism and conciliation that was not shared by the leaders of Britain, France, and Italy. In the early stages of the negotiations Wilson enjoyed an immense popularity in virtually all of the belligerent nations. However, at the peace table he was forced to settle for less than he had promised, and as a result his popularity faded. Nevertheless, Wilson succeeded in achieving his most cherished objective, the adoption of a Covenant for a League of Nations. On Wilson's insistence the League Covenant became an integral part of the Treaty of Versailles.

When Wilson returned to the United States, he found it incomprehensible that certain senators failed to exhibit enthusiasm for the League. When changes in the Covenant were suggested, Wilson obstinately refused to accept any modifications. During a speaking tour in September, 1919, Wilson strove eloquently to arouse popular support for the League, but he suffered an apoplectic stroke and was unable to exert effective leadership from then until the end of his term as President. In this interval the Senate cast its vote regarding the Treaty of Versailles and was unable to muster the two-thirds majority required for ratification.

MEDICINE AND SURGERY DURING THE WAR

In the fields of medicine and surgery the United States was far better prepared for World War I than it had been for the Spanish-American conflict. In a small measure this was due to better organization; in a larger measure to better anticipation of the problems that would arise; and in the largest measure to the vast improvement in medical education, medical skills, and medical resources.

In 1916, foreseeing the probability of United States involvement in the war, President Wilson appointed a Council of National Defense. Dr. Franklin Martin of Chicago was the medical member of the Council, and he headed its medical division. Dr. Martin did a very effective job in organizing the medical profession of the country, with the full cooperation of the American Medical Association and the American College of Surgeons. After war had been declared, much of the work of the Medical Division was planned and controlled by its Executive Committee, which consisted of the three Surgeons-General, Gorgas of the Army (chairman), Braisted of the Navy, and Blue of the U.S. Public Health Service; together with Dr. Martin, Dr. W. H. Welch of Baltimore, Dr. Frank Simpson of Pittsburgh, Dr. William Mayo of Rochester, Minnesota, and Dr. Victor C. Vaughan of Ann Arbor, Michigan.

Dr. Vaughan was in charge of problems relating to communicable diseases, one of the most important medical assignments during the war. The greatest challenges in this field were presented by the 32 training

111

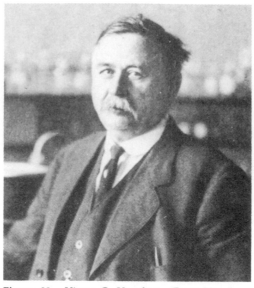

Figure 23. Victor C. Vaughan. (From Vaughan, Victor C.: A Doctor's Memories. Indianapolis, The Bobbs-Merrill Co., 1926.)

camps, each accommodating some 30,000 to 40,000 soldiers, including many raw country-boys previously unexposed to the common contagious diseases and therefore lacking immunity. It was inevitable that the city-boys would bring into every camp every disease then prevalent in the areas from which they came.

Measles and its complications presented one of the major problems of the camps; there were thousands of cases, in some camps 100 to 500 cases per day; and of every 1000 men with measles, 44 developed pneumonia and 14 died. There were also large outbreaks of mumps and of cerebrospinal (meningococcal) meningitis with distressingly high mortality. Pneumonia, occurring either as a primary disease or as a complication of other diseases, was the main cause of death: in the calendar year 1917 there were 8479 cases with 952 deaths. In the winter months of 1917–18, there were 13,393 cases of pneumonia with 3110 deaths. During the autumn months of 1918, when influenza entered the picture, the cases of pneumonia jumped to 61,199, with 21,053 deaths.

The control of venereal diseases in the camps and among the troops in Europe presented serious problems. The availability of arsphenamine for the treatment of syphilis made the long-term effects of this disease less devastating than they might otherwise have been. It is of interest that the wartime experience with venereal disease problems served as the stimulus for the first substantial federal appropriation for medical research: the Congress adopted the Chamberlain-Kahn Act of 1918 for the study and control of venereal disease.

Better sanitation in the camps and better control of water supplies, together with the routine use of typhoid vaccine, virtually eliminated typhoid fever as a serious wartime problem. The treatment of combat wounds was vastly improved as a result of more sophisticated surgical methods, better antisepsis, the use of x-rays, tetanus antitoxin and blood transfusions, and more rapid evacuation of the wounded by motorized ambulances to hospitals where they could receive definitive surgery.

Of approximately 1.4 million United States soldiers and sailors who saw active combat service, 53,400 either were killed in action or died as a result of wounds and another 204,000 were wounded in action. Yet, as in previous wars the deaths from disease, of which there were 63,000, exceeded those from wounds. The high mortality from disease occurred chiefly in the camps in the United States and was attributable, in large part, to the influenza epidemic of 1918. Had it not been for the influenza, the death rate from disease in the military forces would have been unusually low. When the mortality from influenza is included, 54 per cent of the total deaths were due to disease; this compared with 61 per cent in the Union forces in the Civil War and 84 per cent in the Spanish-American War. Among the troops of the American expeditionary force in Europe, where influenza was as serious a problem as in the United States, the number of deaths from disease was actually only about half that of the deaths from wounds.

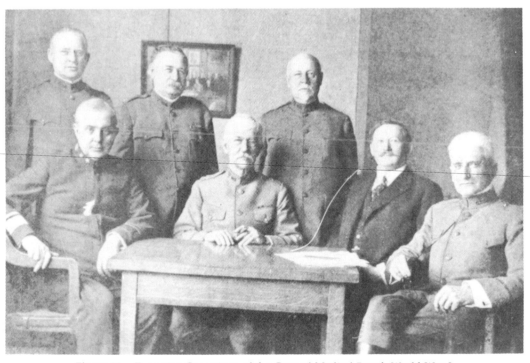

Figure 24. Executive Committee of the General Medical Board, World War I. Standing, left to right: Dr. Frank Simpson, Professor Vaughan, Professor Welch. Seated, left to right: Surgeon-General Braisted, Surgeon-General Gorgas, Surgeon-General Blue, Dr. Franklin Martin. (From Vaughan, Victor C.: A Doctor's Memories. Indianapolis, The Bobbs-Merrill Co., 1926.)

Base hospitals organized and staffed by medical schools and civilian hospitals in the United States were a new feature of the Army's medical services for troops in the field. A number of these units were organized (on paper only) at the request of Surgeon-General Gorgas before the United States entered the war. Initially they were considered to be Red Cross hospitals, but when they were called to duty after war had been declared they became components of the Army. The communities in which the parent institutions of the base hospital units were located took great pride in them and collected relatively large funds to equip them.

The organizations sponsoring base hospitals included Presbyterian Hospital (New York), Lakeside Hospital (Cleveland), Washington University (St. Louis), Harvard, Northwestern University (Chicago), and Pennsylvania Hospital (Philadelphia). Base Hospital #18, which was organized by the Johns Hopkins Hospital and Medical School, will serve as an example of how these units were put together and utilized. Like the others, this hospital was organized, on paper, as a 500-bed unit. In early April, 1917, at about the time that the United States entered the war, a group of Baltimore businessmen raised $30,000 to equip the unit. The purchase of beds and other equipment was supervised by the administrative office of the Hopkins Hospital. All surgical dressings, operating gowns, sheets, pillowcases, and towels were made by Baltimore women volunteers. A little more than a month after the declaration of war, having had no training and almost no warning, the unit was called to duty, and after hastily pulling itself together, it boarded a troop ship on June 9 and set sail for France. The medical officers, of whom there were 24, were led by Dr. John M. T. Finney. The nurses were all Hopkins-trained, and the 148 enlisted men included 32 medical students from the third-year class.

Early in July, Base Hospital #18 took over from the French a 1000-bed hospital in the Vosges. The unit had nothing important to do until mid-1918, during the latter phases of the great German offensive and the Allied advance which followed. A period of intense day-and-night activity occurred in September and October, when American troops vere heavily engaged and the unit was close enough to the front to provide primary surgical care to the wounded, who arrived at the hospital by ambulance after having had no more than first-aid treatment. While the unit was still in France, the medical students, who had volunteered as enlisted men toward the end of their third year and who had received a unique type of clinical instruction and experience at the base hospital, were awarded their M.D. degrees. Two of these degrees had to be awarded posthumously: one student died of scarlet fever, and another, oddly enough, died of typhoid fever (Turner, 1974).

**BETWEEN
TWO WARS**

During the first two years after the war the leaderless nation went through an ugly period of hate and restlessness. Discharged soldiers and those who had worked in the munitions factories and shipyards drifted aimlessly, trying to find work and to adjust to a peacetime existence. The unemployed and the unhappy sought to find a scapegoat for their predicament. There were waves of anticommunism, anti-Semitism and anti-Catholicism. The Ku Klux Klan was revived, and with all its bigotry and hate it became a political force. Many Southern blacks who had moved north to work in the war industries had to compete for peacetime jobs with returned soldiers and other white workers. As a result there were racial disorders, including a particularly bloody race riot in Chicago.

With the hate and restlessness there was also a return of a strong spirit of isolationism. Many people felt that the great sacrifices of the war had accomplished nothing; that the European nations on both sides of the conflict had returned to their old selfish ways. Americans of German, Irish, and Italian background believed that the countries of their origin had been betrayed in the peace negotiations. On the other hand, there were some who believed that the Treaty of Versailles was a step toward international peace, and they lamented the fact that the United States had not become a member of the League of Nations.

In the presidential election of 1920 the Democratic party was overwhelmingly defeated, and the Republican candidate, Warren G. Harding, moved into the White House. The Harding cabinet contained three strong and able men: Charles Evans Hughes, Andrew W. Mellon, and Herbert C. Hoover. The rest of the cabinet was made up largely of a group, who together with their cronies in lesser government posts, became known as the "Ohio gang." Harding died in August, 1923, of complications following food poisoning. Shortly thereafter, it became known that the Secretary of the Interior and the Secretary of the Navy had been involved in a corrupt agreement to turn over to private interests valuable oil deposits that were being held in reserve for the Navy. These unsavory transactions, known as the Teapot Dome scandal, led to the resignation of the two Secretaries and a jail sentence for one of them.

Calvin Coolidge finished out Harding's uncompleted term and was then elected in 1924 for another term. When he announced that he did "not choose to run" again in 1928, Herbert C. Hoover was nominated by the Republicans and won the election by a large margin over the Democratic candidate, Alfred E. Smith. During the 12 years (1921--1933) of successive Republican administrations there was a crescendo of prosperity, which came to a crashing end with the economic collapse of 1929 and the long depression that followed.

During the period of prosperity in the 20s there was some superficial improvement in international relations, but beneath the surface Hitler was fanning the embers of another world conflagration. While Hitler was thus engaged, on the other side of the world, the Japanese moved an army into Manchuria in 1931 and initiated the chain of events that would lead them to Pearl Harbor.

In the United States during the 20s almost every industry prospered; the automobile industry moved toward a top position in the economy, and in its wake the oil companies flourished, and a web of macadamized highways spread across the nation. While automobiles and trucks were stealing business from the railroads, a new form of transportation was dramatized by Charles A. Lindbergh's thrilling flight across the Atlantic from New York to Paris in 1927.

Though *Prohibition* was instituted by the adoption of the Eighteenth

115

Amendment during the second Wilson administration, its evil effects reached their height during the three Republican administrations that followed. Prohibition gave birth to a host of illegal activities: illicit stills for the manufacture of whiskey, rum-running into the harbors and beaches along the coast, speakeasies which took the place of the old saloons and hotel bars, and many other devices to make alcoholic drinks readily available. The law was so unpopular, and so many people took delight in breaking it, that enforcement was virtually impossible.

Those who gained the most from the Eighteenth Amendment were the members of the underworld. The sale of "bootleg" liquor in most of the large cities was controlled by gangs such as the Al Capone gang of Chicago. In spite of the lawlessness that it engendered, most politicians believed that Prohibition was favored by the majority of Americans, and they were afraid to take a stand against it. The first politician of national stature to voice opposition was Alfred E. Smith, and he was defeated for the presidency by Hoover.

The prosperity of the 1920s had a solid foundation in industrial growth, but on top of this foundation there had arisen a superstructure of false values created by speculation in stocks. Worthless stocks acquired fictitious value and honest stocks were forced to prices far above their worth. As the speculative structure grew taller it grew more fragile, and in October, 1929, when there was a drop in stock prices, the structure teetered and then collapsed. After the crash, stock prices continued to slide downward until 1932. The Dow-Jones average, which had reached a high of 381 in 1929, reached a low of 41 in 1932. The stock market crash ushered in a long period of depression which affected all nations and from which only a slow recovery was in progress when World War II began.

The presidential election of 1932 was held in the depths of the depression. Franklin Delano Roosevelt, the Democratic candidate, had served as Assistant Secretary of the Navy under Wilson and had been the Democratic vice-presidential candidate in 1920. In 1921 he suffered a crippling attack of poliomyelitis, but he had recovered sufficiently by 1928 to be elected governor of New York.

Roosevelt's opponent in the national election, Herbert Hoover, had been renominated by the Republicans on a platform which seemed to add up to little more than *business as usual* and a continuation of Prohibition. Roosevelt called for a "New Deal" in government, bold and aggressive leadership, repeal of Prohibition, new measures to stimulate employment and to help the farmer, and a reduction in governmental expenses. The voters gave Roosevelt more than 85 per cent of the electoral vote, making it obvious that they favored a *New Deal*, wherever that might lead.

In his stirring inaugural address the new President voiced a cautious optimism—"the only thing we have to fear is fear itself," but "only a foolish optimist can deny the dark realities of the moment." The day after his inauguration Roosevelt called Congress into special session, and in order to give himself time to deal with the financial situation he proclaimed a national bank holiday. During the next 100 days, he pushed through more than a dozen legislative acts and adopted innumerable administrative measures to combat the depression. Perhaps the most revolutionary step taken during this period was the abandonment of the gold standard.

116

The repeal of Prohibition came earlier than expected. It was made easier by the need to create new industry and new jobs and to give the farmer additional markets for his grain. In February, 1933, before Roosevelt took office, Congress approved the Twenty-first Amendment, repealing the Eighteenth Amendment.

During his first term, most of Roosevelt's energies were directed toward coping with the depression. In this he relied to a considerable extent upon the advice of a group of bright young liberals who became known as the *Brain Trust*. This group was responsible for the act creating the Securities and Exchange Commission (June, 1934); it was also involved in framing the Social Security Act of 1935, which was to have far-reaching effects during the years ahead.

In foreign affairs the Roosevelt administration recognized the communist government of Russia. Foreign trade was increased considerably as a result of reciprocal trade agreements negotiated by the Secretary of State, Cordell Hull.

During the second Roosevelt administration, labor made great strides forward. A new labor group, the Congress of Industrial Organizations, under the leadership of John L. Lewis, acquired a membership of some 4 million. In 1938 Congress passed the Fair Labor Standards Act, which prescribed a maximum work week of 40 hours and a minimum wage of $.40 an hour. A drastic reduction in the rate of immigration removed from the labor force an element which had served to keep wages down.

Though Roosevelt had failed even to mention foreign relations in his inaugural address in 1937, this issue had become his primary concern before the second term ended. When the Japanese sank a United States naval gunboat in the Yangtze River in December, 1937, it became clear that they intended to resist any American effort to thwart their conquest of China. Any lingering doubt as to the design of the Japanese was dispelled in 1939, when they captured Shanghai and proceeded to disrupt the international settlement in that city. In response to this aggression, Roosevelt decided to apply economic pressure by terminating the existing treaty of commerce with Japan. While Japan was making things difficult in Asia, Hitler and Mussolini were strutting about Europe and North Africa, making things even more difficult there.

MEDICAL ADVANCES   Prior to World War I the chief advances in medicine had been in the basic medical sciences, in surgery, and in preventive medicine. In the period between the wars, new methods of therapy began to blossom. Vitamins were discovered that could prevent or cure diseases that were particularly prevalent among the poor: vitamin D for rickets and nicotinic acid (one of the B vitamins) for pellagra. Also discovered were vitamin K, which controls bleeding in certain hemorrhagic disorders, and a substance contained in liver (eventually known as vitamin B_{12}) that could cure pernicious anemia. Insulin, first extracted from the pancreas in 1922, brought relief to thousands of individuals suffering from diabetes. The "sulfa" drugs (sulfonamides) were found to have powerful antibacterial properties and were

117

employed with great effectiveness in the treatment of many bacterial diseases, including streptococcal infections, lobar pneumonia, cerebrospinal meningitis, and gonorrhea.

An important occurrence in the interwar period was the decline of German medicine. World War I had left the German universities and research institutes with greatly reduced staffs and outdated equipment. These effects were compounded by the postwar inflation, which caused a drastic reduction in the funds available for education and research. Recovery was just getting under way when Hitler came to power and dealt the universities another serious blow with his anti-Jewish, anti-intellectual policies. As a result, many of Germany's best scientists fled to other countries including the United States. At about the same time the international tide of medical students and physicians-in-search-of-training, which formerly had been directed toward Germany, now began to move toward the United States, where funds were more plentiful and where there was a more favorable climate for educational and research activities.

In the early 1930s two important studies of American medicine were published: The *Report of the Commission on Medical Education* (1932) and the *Report of the Committee on the Costs of Medical Care* (1932). Both reports directed attention to certain inadequacies in the provision of medical care. The Committee on Costs made specific recommendations for overcoming these deficiencies: (1) that there be greater development of group practice centered around hospitals; (2) that the cost of medical care be covered by insurance and/or taxation; (3) that each state and community form a specific organization to study, evaluate, and coordinate its health services; and (4) that three new types of medical workers be trained: nursing attendants, nurse-midwives, and hospital and clinical administrators.

In the eyes of organized medicine these recommendations were wildly radical and wholly unnecessary. The editor of the Journal of the AMA, bristling in defense of the status quo, called the recommendations steps toward communism and "incitement to revolution." On the other hand, President Roosevelt and some of the members of Congress harkened to the implications of the reports; the United States Public Health Service was directed to make a National Health Survey, in the course of which a house-to-house canvas of 800,000 families was made during 1935 and 1936. The survey confirmed the results of the previous studies and emphasized that the amount of medical care received by a family was usually directly related to family income. Those who received the most inadequate care lived either in the poor sections of a city or in rural areas.

Shortly after this, in 1937, there appeared a two-volume report of the American Foundation Studies in Government, entitled *American Medicine; Expert Testimony out of Court*. The evidence brought together in this study indicated that many people lacked the medical care they needed; that there should be better integration of the services of general practitioners and specialists; and that group practice seemed to offer enough advantages to patients to warrant a more extensive trial. Evidence was also presented concerning the relative merits of state medicine and voluntary health insurance as means of assuring comprehensive medical care for all levels of the population.

Within a few months of the publication of *Expert Testimony*, a self-ap-

118

pointed group of medical men headed by a prominent New York physician, Russell L. Cecil, formulated and made public a set of *Principles and Proposals* designed to improve medical education, medical research, and medical care. This document, which was signed by about 700 doctors, stated the following (Means, 1953):

Principles

1. *That the health of the people is a direct concern of the government.*
2. *That a national public health policy directed toward all groups of the population should be formulated.*
3. *That the problem of economic need and the problem of providing adequate medical care are not identical and may require different approaches for their solution.*
4. *That in the provision of adequate medical care for the population four agencies are concerned: voluntary agencies, local, state, and Federal governments.*

Proposals

1. *That the first necessary step toward the realization of the above principles is to minimize the risk of illness by prevention.*
2. *That an immediate problem is provision of adequate medical care for the medically indigent, the cost to be met from public funds (local and/or state and/or Federal).*
3. *That public funds should be made available for the support of medical education and for studies, investigations, and procedures for raising the standards of medical practice. If this is not provided for, the provision of adequate medical care may prove impossible.*
4. *That public funds should be available for medical research as essential for high standards of practice in both preventive and curative medicine.*
5. *That public funds should be made available to hospitals that render service to the medically indigent and for laboratory and diagnostic and consultative services.*
6. *That in allocation of public funds, existing private institutions should be utilized to the largest possible extent, and that they may receive support so long as their service is in consonance with the above principles.*
7. *That public health services, Federal, state, and local, should be extended by evolutionary process.*
8. *That the investigation and planning of the measures proposed and their ultimate direction should be assigned to experts.*
9. *That the adequate administration and supervision of the health functions of the government, as implied in the above proposals, necessitates in our opinion a functional consolidation of all federal health and medical activities, preferably under a separate department.*

The publication of the *Principles and Proposals*, which today seem logical and certainly less extreme than some current proposals, gave rise to a bitter controversy within the medical profession. An editorial in the Journal of the AMA accused the signers of being virtual traitors to their fellow physicians. The controversy and the reports which preceded it served to direct public attention to some of the deficiencies in medical care. They also made the public aware of the fact that the AMA did not speak for all physicians and that there was a large group of distinguished medical educators, researchers, and practitioners who believed that American medicine was in need of improvement.

In 1938, while the controversy was at its height, President Roosevelt

119

convened a *National Health Conference* in Washington at which there was broad representation of both providers and consumers of health services. The conference confirmed the existence of serious inadequacies in medical care, but there were sharp differences between the representatives of organized medicine and the consumer representatives as to how the deficiencies could be overcome.

Though the delegates reached no consensus, President Roosevelt concluded that there was a need for a "National Health Program" to achieve more equitable distribution of high quality medical care. He suggested, among other things, that the program should include some form of social insurance to reimburse workers for the loss of earnings during an illness. This was not a new idea — between 1911 and 1935 all except four states had adopted workmen's compensation laws — but the suggestion that a redistribution of medical services be combined with a national social insurance scheme led organized medicine to mobilize all its artillery to shoot down what it stigmatized as a plan to introduce "socialized medicine" on a national scale. The battle to prevent the "socialization" of medicine was joined in earnest when, in 1939, Senator Robert Wagner introduced a bill to provide a National Health Program through grants-in-aid to states that agreed to meet standards prescribed by the federal government. The Wagner bill was defeated, but this was only one of the early skirmishes in a long and bitterly fought war which continued for the remainder of the second century.

One of the effects of the depression was to heighten the interest in prepayment for medical care. For many years certain commercial insurance companies had offered policies that provided part-payment for medical expenses, chiefly those incurred in a hospital. Similar prepayment schemes were provided by a variety of lodges, fraternal orders, labor unions, and industries. The number of persons covered by such programs was relatively small even in the prosperous 20s, and it declined during the depression years. In the 1930s the hospitals were particularly hard hit by a reduction in endowment income and charitable gifts and by the high rate of unemployment which made it necessary to provide free hospital care for a larger proportion of patients.

The plight of the hospitals led to the organization of the Blue Cross plans. Subscribers to these plans, the first of which was organized in 1933, paid a relatively small monthly fee, and the hospitals agreed to provide for the subscribers full care in semiprivate accommodations for three weeks at a prearranged daily rate to be paid by Blue Cross. The Blue Cross plans differed from the prevailing type of hospital insurance in that initially they covered the entire hospital bill for a specified period. Physician's and surgeon's fees were not covered. Blue Shield plans were organized somewhat later to take care of the doctor's bills, but unlike the Blue Cross plans, Blue Shield did not undertake to cover the entire bill.

A few prepayment plans providing more comprehensive coverage of doctor's bills, hospital charges, and other medical expenses were organized during the inter-war period. These included the plans offered by (1) the Ross-Loos Clinic in Los Angeles, in 1929; (2) the Mary Imogene Bassett Hospital, in a rural area of upstate New York (Cooperstown), in 1930; (3) the Permanente Health Plan, which was organized shortly before World

120

War II to provide comprehensive care for the workers at the Grand Coulee Dam.

WORLD WAR II   After the Italians had extended their North African possessions by occupying Ethiopia, and the Germans had bullied Austria and Czechoslovakia into submission, the world was startled by the announcement that Stalin had signed a nonaggression pact with Hitler. This announcement was made on August 24, 1939, and exactly one week later, using new blitzkrieg tactics, the Germans overwhelmed Poland from the south and west. After the lapse of another two weeks the Russians, in less spectacular fashion, marched in to take possession of eastern Poland. By the end of September, Warsaw was in ruins and Poland no longer existed as a nation.

Two days after the invasion of Poland began, Great Britain and France, honoring their treaties with Poland, declared war on Germany. They were not in a position to give direct aid to Poland; and it was soon evident that their ground and air forces had neither the training nor the equipment to withstand the new German tactics. As they had done in World War I, the British sent a large army to France, but throughout the winter of 1939–40 there was no fighting along the French-German border. New German activity began in April with the invasion of Norway and Denmark. Then in May, Hitler turned his blitzkrieg machine toward the west and quickly overwhelmed Holland and Belgium and invaded northern France. The British Army was cut off and surrounded along the Belgian and French coasts, but 300,000 of the troops miraculously escaped to England. On June 14, the German Army entered Paris, and on June 22, France surrendered. The Italians joined the German side in June, shortly before the surrender of France.

Fortunately for the British their Navy still held control of the North Sea and the English Channel, and Hitler decided to try to beat the British to their knees by bombing London and other British cities. This campaign reached its height of fury in the autumn of 1940, and it was defeated principally by the gallantry and skill of the British fighter pilots and by a new invention of British scientists, *radar*, which provided advance warning of the flight of the German bomber squadrons. By the late spring of 1941, the Germans had turned their attention to trying to shut off British supplies by stepping up the activities of the U-boats. Then in June, 1941, Hitler made his most serious miscalculation by turning against his reluctant ally, Stalin, and invading the Soviet Union.

In the early phases of the war in Europe, public sentiment in the United States seemed to be strongly in favor of maintaining neutrality. With the passage of time, however, there were increasing fears about what might happen in the Western Hemisphere if Hitler and Mussolini won the war. In September, 1940, the United States turned over to the British 50 American destroyers to assist them in their fight against the German blockade.

Prior to the presidential election of November, 1940, it had become abundantly clear that Roosevelt, who was running for a third term, was determined to give all-out support to the British "short of war." Wendell Willkie, Roosevelt's Republican opponent, was a colorful individual. He conducted a lively campaign, but he was at a decided disadvantage, since he strongly favored Roosevelt's foreign policy and much of the New Deal domestic policy. In the election Roosevelt's victory was impressive, and he concluded that the public favored his foreign policy.

During the period of the election campaign, tension had been mounting in the Far East. After the French had surrendered to Hitler, the Japanese had moved south from China into French Indochina and were building airfields there. They were talking more and more truculently about Japan's "Greater East Asia Co-prosperity Sphere," and it was feared that the next Japanese target might be the Philippines or Singapore. In July, 1941, President Roosevelt appointed General Douglas MacArthur commander of all United States Army forces in the Far East. In October, the Japanese demanded that the United States stop reinforcing the Philippines and terminate its aid to President Chiang Kai-shek of China. When it became apparent that the United States had no intention of meeting these demands, the Japanese Navy carried out its highly successful sneak raid on Pearl Harbor on December 7.

The dazzling early successes of the Japanese armed forces continued for only about six months. Their Navy was soundly defeated in the Battle of Midway Island in June, 1942, and before the end of the year the southward advance of the Japanese Army had been blocked at Guadalcanal and in New Guinea.

In the Atlantic, the British and American navies had their hands full in trying to deal with the stepped-up campaign of the German U-boats. Between January and April, 1942, almost 200 ships were sunk along the Atlantic and Gulf coasts of the United States and in the Caribbean, many of them tankers carrying much-needed fuel. By the autumn of 1942, new ships were being constructed at a rate exceeding that of the sinkings.

In the winter and spring of 1942–43, British and American forces waged a successful campaign against German and Italian forces in North Africa, and in August, 1943, the Allies occupied Sicily. These military reverses forced Mussolini to resign, and the Italians made it known that they were ready to get out of the war. To prevent such a move the Germans sent large reinforcements into Italy, and it was only after eight months of savage fighting and thousands of casualties that the Allies finally occupied Rome on June 4, 1944.

Hitler's invasion of Russia got off to a good start in the summer of 1941, but it was unable to reach its major objective, Moscow, before it became immobilized by the Russian winter. During the winter, the Russians reoccupied large areas west of Moscow. In the summer of 1942 the Germans resumed the offensive with the hope of seizing the oil fields of the Caucasus. They almost succeeded in this endeavor, but in November the Russians mounted a major counteroffensive which trapped the German Sixth Army in front of Stalingrad and forced the Germans to withdraw from the Caucasus.

In the Pacific the extraordinary capacity of the United States to produce ships and planes finally gave the Americans the upper hand on the sea and in the air. In mid-1943 General MacArthur began to move northward and westward along the New Guinea coast, employing his famous leapfrog strategy. At the same time Admiral Halsey's forces were moving up through the Solomons, while combined naval, air, and ground forces were capturing bases in the Gilbert, Marshall, Caroline, and Mariana islands.

Germany's fate was sealed when the Allies crossed the English Channel and landed in force in Normandy. While the Allies were moving ahead in France, the Russians were sweeping across the Ukraine and Poland, and by occupying Romania deprived the Germans of their one remaining source of crude oil. By April, 1945, the Russians were approaching Berlin from the east while Allied forces were marching through Germany from the south and west. On the last day of April, Hitler committed suicide, and a week later the war in Europe came to an end when the commander of the German forces signed an unconditional surrender.

In 1944 and early 1945 things were also going badly for the Japanese. General MacArthur's forces landed in the Philippines in October, 1944, and the American troops in the central Pacific occupied Iwo Jima in February and Okinawa in April. In the meantime the Japanese Navy had been rendered ineffective by heavy losses in the Battle of Leyte Gulf, and the Japanese Air Force had lost so many planes and personnel that they were reduced to the suicidal tactics of kamikaze pilots. Plans were being made for the invasion of Japan when on August 6 the first atomic bomb was dropped on Hiroshima, and three days later a second bomb was dropped on Nagasaki. On August 14, the Japanese emperor announced his nation's surrender.

President Roosevelt did not live to celebrate the victory. He died suddenly of a cerebral hemorrhage on April 12, 1945, and was succeeded by Harry S. Truman.

MEDICINE AND SURGERY DURING THE WAR

From a medical viewpoint World War II was the most successful war in which American military forces had ever been engaged. Soldiers and sailors who took part in that conflict will never forget the number of times their skin was either scratched or punctured to protect them from some kind of disease: smallpox, tetanus, typhoid fever, yellow fever, cholera, and typhus fever. If they were in a malarious area, every day they had to swallow a little yellow pill containing atabrine (quinacrine). The Japanese, by their conquests in the southwest Pacific area, had shut off the supply of quinine, which until then had been the standard drug for the prevention and treatment of malaria. The troops also had to carry gas masks to protect them from noxious fumes, and in the tropics they had to wear uncomfortably hot coveralls impregnated with a chemical to protect them from ticks, mites, and other insects that might be carriers of disease. There were also strictly enforced sanitary measures for disposal of feces and other wastes and for protection of food from flies. Oil sprays were used to prevent the breeding of mosquitoes, and in the latter part of the war DDT was used extensively to kill flies and mosquitoes and the lice which are responsible for the transmission of typhus fever.

The preventive vaccines used during World War II produced many sore

123

arms and occasional fever, usually mild. The one serious consequence was the occurrence of hepatitis following yellow fever vaccination. This was due to the presence of the hepatitis virus in some of the lots of vaccine which were used early in the war. Fortunately the hepatitis attributable to the vaccine usually was not severe, but there were more than 50,000 cases with attendant loss of time from active duty.

One of the effects of World War II was to give impetus to coordinated undertakings in medical research and development by many different agencies working together to reach a common objective. In the summer of 1941, looking forward to the day when the United States might become a belligerent, President Roosevelt decided that an organization should be created which would bring the best scientific minds together to consider how to deal with the problems of war and national defense. By executive order, the Office of Scientific Research and Development (OSRD) was created with Vannevar Bush, an electrical engineer with broad academic and administrative experience, as its director.

The Committee on Medical Research (CMR) was established as one of the component units of the OSRD, and Alfred Newton Richards was appointed its chairman. Richards was at that time Professor of Pharmacology at the University of Pennsylvania and Vice-President for Medical Affairs of the university. He and the other four civilian members of the Committee on Medical Research were experienced, imaginative, and highly respected medical scientists: Alphonse R. Dochez, Professor of Medical and Surgical Research at The College of Physicians and Surgeons, New York; A. Baird Hastings, Professor of Biochemistry at Harvard; Chester S. Keefer, Professor of Medicine at Boston University; and Lewis H. Weed, Professor of Anatomy at Johns Hopkins. In addition to the civilian members, the government

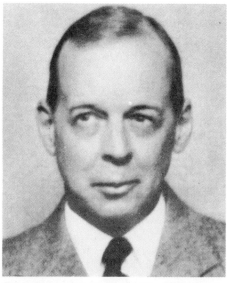

Figure 25. A. N. Richards. (From Riesman, David (ed.): History of the Interurban Clinical Club, 1905–1937. Philadelphia, The John C. Winston Company, 1937.)

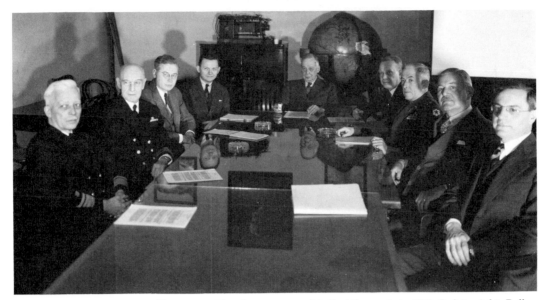

Figure 26. The Committee on Medical Research in 1945. Left to right: Rolla E. Dyer, Asst. Surg.-Gen., U.S. Public Health Service, and Director, National Institute of Health; Rear Adm. Harold W. Smith; A. B. Hastings; C. S. Keefer; A. N. Richards, Chairman; L. H. Weed, Vice-Chairman; Brig.-Gen. J. S. Simmons; A. R. Dochez; Irvin Stewart, Secretary. (Reproduced from photograph 94277 of the Army Medical Museum. National Library of Medicine, Bethesda, Maryland.)

services were represented on the committee by medical officers who had had research experience: Rolla E. Dyer of the U.S. Public Health Service, Director of the National Institutes of Health; James Stevens Simmons, Chief of the Preventive Medicine Service of the U.S. Army; and Harold W. Smith of the U.S. Navy.

This committee made many important contributions to the war effort; and they initiated, coordinated, and funded several large research and development projects that resulted in the production of therapeutic agents which not only were valuable to the military forces but which also have saved, and will continue to save, thousands of civilian lives. Two of the most successful projects were (1) the large-scale production of penicillin and (2) the development of new drugs for the prevention and cure of malaria. The chairman of the committee, Dr. Richards, is given credit for having guided these undertakings to a successful conclusion and for the skill and tact with which he induced government agencies, pharmaceutical companies, universities, and hospitals all over the country to work together in harmony to attain a common goal (Keefer, 1969).

The massive effort to achieve large-scale production of penicillin is described in Chapter 23. The second large undertaking of the Committee on Medical Research was directed toward the discovery of more effective antimalarial drugs. Large numbers of American troops were exposed to malaria in several combat areas. The only antimalarial drug which was available in adequate amounts for use in these areas was atabrine (quina-

125

crine). Atabrine was quite effective in suppressing malaria, but it did not cure the disease, and it could not be depended upon to prevent it. Military personnel who had acquired a malarial infection had no symptoms of the disease as long as they were taking their regular dose of atabrine, but when they stopped taking the drug the symptoms might appear, sometimes after an interval of several weeks or months. If atabrine were given at this time it might again suppress the malaria but only as long as the drug was being taken. Obviously it was desirable to find a drug which would be more effective in preventing and curing the disease. This was such an important matter that a special board within the framework of the CMR was appointed to deal with the problem. The program carried out under the direction of this board was by far the largest, the most expensive, and at the same time one of the most successful undertakings of the CMR.

In the course of the antimalarial research, more than 14,000 chemical compounds were prepared or synthesized, and most of them were tested for their ability to prevent, suppress, or cure malaria. It would have been impossible to test all of these compounds on troops in the field. Fortunately, birds are subject to malaria, and it was possible to utilize birds in the laboratory to carry out preliminary screening tests on almost all of the compounds that had been prepared. Only those compounds which were found to be effective against bird malaria and which did not produce toxic symptoms in other experimental animals were finally tested on soldiers in this country and in the malarious theaters.

The results of this huge program, which involved many research workers, many laboratories, and many hospitals, in this country and in England, were highly successful. New compounds were developed which not only would suppress malaria but also which would prevent or cure it. After the war these compounds were available for the prevention and treatment of malaria throughout the world.

Not only was the death rate from disease greatly reduced during World War II but also the death rate from wounds was only about half what it had been in World War I. This was due to a number of factors, including better organization, better-trained personnel, the availability of blood and plasma for the treatment of hemorrhage and shock, the use of sulfa drugs and penicillin for the treatment and prevention of wound infections, more rapid transportation of the wounded by motor ambulance and airplane to hospitals where they could receive the most expert surgical care, and the use of mobile surgical teams and well-staffed hospital ships in the island-hopping operations.

As in the case of World War I, various civilian hospitals and medical schools had organized and staffed general hospitals which were called into service soon after the United States entered the war. These hospitals were sent to every battle front, sometimes close to the action, sometimes farther back in the chain of evacuation, and they performed invaluable functions until the war came to an end.

The disease problems varied with the location of the troops. In the camps in the United States there were the usual outbreaks of the common contagious diseases, but the more serious complications of these diseases, such as pneumonia and streptococcal infections, usually could be treated successfully with the sulfa drugs and, later on, with penicillin. Hepatitis was a problem in all areas, and it produced the most prolonged disability and the greatest threat to life. Subacute gastroenteritis (Delhi belly) was a common cause of disability in the India-Burma theater. Amebic dysentery was encountered in several areas; at one time many of the hospital beds on the Island of Leyte were occupied by patients with amebic infections. Skin diseases were relatively common in the tropics, where soldiers were exposed for long periods to mud and wet clothing, and they sometimes led to prolonged disability. Malaria also created problems, not among troops who were taking atabrine but among those who had contrived not to take the drug or who had stopped taking it after leaving a malarious area. This happened among men returning to the United States, and among the Marines and other troops who were sent to Australia for rest and relaxation after fighting on Guadalcanal or in New Guinea. The United States military forces also encountered diseases with which they had not previously been familiar. For example, scrub typhus (tsutsugamushi fever) presented a problem in the islands north of New Guinea, and *schistosomiasis japonica* was met in its rarely observed acute form among troops on the Island of Leyte.

II

Medical Education

We cannot contemplate with any great satisfaction the early history of medical education in America. Probably medical education had nowhere, at any time, fallen to such a lowly state as it did during a large part of the last century in our country.

(William Henry Welch, 1915)

THE UNIVERSITIES BEGIN TO TAKE HOLD Lack of funds made it virtually impossible for American medical schools to follow the example set by the state-supported schools of Europe. Under the proprietary system, with the bulk of the student fees going directly to the professors, there was little left to meet other expenses. Endowments, even small ones, were rare. Funds simply were not available to build, equip, and operate modern laboratories and teaching hospitals or to pay even part-time salaries to qualified teachers of the basic medical sciences.

When Charles W. Eliot became President of Harvard University in 1869, the medical school had only a small endowment and its financial support was derived almost wholly from student fees. The old two-year medical course was replaced by the new three-year curriculum in 1871. It was expected that this would result in at least a temporary decline in enrollment and a consequent reduction in the income from student fees. Under the new arrangement, the medical school had become a genuine department of the university, and thus the student fees were paid directly to the university rather than to individual professors. The university, in turn, undertook to pay part-time salaries to the faculty, the amount to be more or less commensurate with the amount of time that each faculty member devoted to his work at the school. Since it was apparent that the student fees alone would not be adequate to meet the faculty payroll, in 1870 Eliot began in his annual reports and in various speeches to call for donations to build up the endowment of the medical school. He knew that this would require time, for as he repeatedly stated, "The first step toward obtaining an endowment is to deserve one."

The expected decline in the medical school enrollment *did* occur, but it

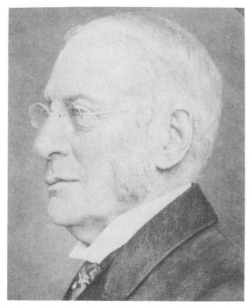

Figure 27. Charles W. Eliot. (New York Academy of Medicine.)

was less than the pessimists on the faculty had predicted, and it lasted for only a few years. In 1877, Eliot reported that not only was the student enrollment at a satisfactory level but also that there had been a significant improvement in the quality of the student body: in the year 1876–77, 44 per cent of the students had entered the school with bachelor's degrees in either the arts or sciences. This proportion of college graduates was almost twice what it had been in 1869–70. In 1881, Eliot was able to point with pride to the fact that "since 1871, when the Harvard Medical School ceased to be a private venture and became a constituent department of the University, it has received by gift and bequests $270,000." This was about five times the amount that the medical school had received for endowment in the entire century prior to 1871.

It is of interest that in his effort to raise the funds which would make it possible for the medical faculty to devote a greater proportion of their time and effort to their teaching duties, President Eliot placed no emphasis on time for research. Unlike President Gilman, who was soon to select the Johns Hopkins faculty with his eye always focused on scholarly achievement and research ability, Eliot was interested primarily in devotion to pedagogy. The following anecdote related by his biographer, Henry James, clearly reveals the order of priorities in Eliot's mind (James, 1930):

> *Professor C. L. Jackson relates that when he was a young teacher of chemistry in the seventies he asked Eliot if he might be relieved of the duty of teaching one class in order to prosecute certain investigations. The President, in his stately manner, propounded a question to which an answer can seldom be given—"What will be the result of these investigations?" They would be published, was the reply. The President wanted to know where. Mr. Jackson named a German chemical journal. "I can't see that that will serve any useful purpose here," said Eliot, and therewith dismissed the matter.*

The experience of the Harvard Medical School had shown within a decade that the preliminary educational requirements for medical students could be raised and the medical course could be lengthened from 8 months to 27 months, without significant loss of students and with improvement in the quality of the student body. Furthermore, the conversion of the school from a private venture to a true university department had removed objectionable commercial attributes which apparently had stood in the way of gifts to endowment; at any rate, the gifts began to flow in as soon as the change in status occurred, and the flow was to continue.

The size of the Harvard Medical School endowment was exceptional. In 1892 the United States Bureau of Education reported that the "productive funds" in the hands of *all* medical schools amounted to only $611,214. This contrasted with endowments of $17,599,979 for schools of theology; and whereas there were 171 endowed chairs of theology, there were only five endowed chairs of medicine (Welch, 1894).

The developments at Harvard encouraged emulation. Two other established university medical schools, those of the University of Pensylvania and the University of Michigan, which had stood hesitatingly upon the threshold of change for several years, could now stride more confidently into a three-year graduated curriculum. In addition to the change in curriculum that took place at Pennsylvania in 1877 and at Michigan in 1880, each of these schools had succeeded in establishing a new hospital under university control. This accomplishment surely must have aroused the envy of President Eliot, who had repeatedly expressed concern about the fact that the Harvard Medical School had no hospital of its own. This deficiency had made it necessary for the university to select for appointment to its clinical faculty men already holding staff positions at Boston hospitals. As President Eliot put it, "More than once this limitation of choice has proved unfortunate. More than once the school and the community have lost an important medical reinforcement because the school was not in a position to offer to the desired person an adequate hospital appointment as well as a professorship."

In addition to the efforts of the individual medical schools such as Harvard, Northwestern, and the universities of Pennsylvania and Michigan to raise the standards of medical education, other agencies began to exert a favorable influence in the early part of the second century. The American Medical Association, which had worked cautiously and certainly ineffectually toward this end for 36 years, finally found its voice in 1883, when it began the publication of its *Journal*. In 1894 the *Journal* began a series of articles exposing fraudulent medical institutions. These articles attracted national attention to the degraded state of medical education.

The Association of American Medical Colleges, which had been founded in 1876, with 22 medical schools as members, was also trying to promote better educational standards. However, it had no success in achieving a consensus among its member colleges, most of which were of the old proprietary type. After six years of fruitless debate, the Association decided to suspend its activities, and no meetings were held in the years 1882 to 1889. The Association might have remained dormant for a longer period had it not been for a *Circular* issued by five medical schools of the city of Baltimore and "the staff of the Johns Hopkins" (presumably the staff of the Johns Hopkins Hospital, since the Johns Hopkins Medical School had not yet been opened). The *Circular,* dated March 20, 1890, was addressed "to the medical colleges of the United States" and it appealed to them to send representatives to a conference to consider "medical education in this country and measures for its improvement." The circular suggested as subjects "most likely to come up for discussion: (1) A three year course of six-months sessions. (2) A graded curriculum. (3) Written and oral examinations. (4) A preliminary examination in English. (5) Laboratory instruction in chemistry, histology and pathology."

The influences responsible for the issuance of this *Circular* were not made public, but it is probable that the *Circular* was prompted, at least in part, by an address delivered in 1889 at a meeting of the *Medical and Chirurgical Faculty of the State of Maryland* by William Osler. Osler was then Professor of Clinical Medicine at the University of Pennsylvania. The subject of this address was *The License to Practice,* and in it he spoke fearlessly about the disgraceful state of the American *system* of medical education (Osler, 1889):

> *It makes one's blood boil to think that there are sent out year by year scores of men, called doctors, who have never attended a case of labor, and who are utterly igno-rant of the ordinary everyday diseases which they may be called upon to treat; men who may never have seen the inside of a hospital ward and who would not know Scarpa's space from the sole of the foot. Yet, gentlemen, this is the disgraceful con-dition which some school-men have the audacity to ask you to perpetuate; to con-tinue to entrust interests so sacred to hands so unworthy. Is it to be wondered, con-sidering this shocking laxity, that there is a widespread distrust in the public of professional education, and that quacks, charlatans and imposters possess the land?*

The meeting called for by the *Circular* was held on May 21, 1890; the subjects enumerated above were discussed, and the Association of American Medical Colleges was reactivated for the purpose of bringing together the medical colleges for consideration of, and joint action on, educational matters. Prior to 1900, some 50 to 70 medical colleges—less than half the number then in existence—were represented in the Association. The Association moved slowly and cautiously, but by 1900 it had gained enough self-confidence to require of its member colleges that they have a graded curriculum at least three years in length and that they matriculate only students who possessed a high school diploma or who had "passed a thor-ough examination in all branches usually taught" in high schools. Though these requirements seem modest enough, they represented a major advance in the collective thinking of those who ran the medical colleges.

REVOLUTION IN MEDICAL EDUCATION—THE JOHNS HOPKINS MEDICAL SCHOOL

In the whole history of education it is hardly possible to find another Institution whose influence was so far reaching as Gilman's Johns Hopkins University and Medical School.

(Abraham Flexner, 1946)

In commenting on the development of medical education in the United States, Shryock wrote in 1967 that "Mr. Johns Hopkins founded in Baltimore the first real university in the United States in 1876, and his bequest endowed a modern hospital there in 1889. In 1893 this hospital was coordinated with a new medical school patterned after its German prototype. For several decades thereafter 'The Hopkins'—more than any other single institution—became the model for medical reform."

Before describing the development of this institution, it might be well to enumerate its contributions to the advancement of medical education:

(1) A baccalaureate degree, or its equivalent, with emphasis on preliminary education in the sciences and modern languages, was required for admission to the medical school.

(2) Both men and women students were accepted.

(3) A four-year graded curriculum was provided.

(4) The faculty in the basic medical sciences (anatomy, physiology, physiological chemistry, pharmacology, and pathology) were placed on a full-time salaried basis. These positions were filled after a search for the best men available in the United States or elsewhere. This was a departure from the tradition of employing local practitioners, on a part-time basis, to fill the preclinical chairs. (This tradition was firmly fixed in all but a few schools, among them Harvard, Yale, and the University of Michigan.)

(5) Medical research by both faculty and students was fostered as part of the educational process.

(6) After completing two years of education in the basic medical sciences, students were instructed in the art of medicine and were given close contact with sick individuals. In their senior year they spent most of their time, day and night, working in the wards of the hospital, taking an active part in the care of patients.

(7) At the opening of the hospital, Osler introduced a graded system of postgraduate education for interns and residents which became a model for the postgraduate clinical education of the twentieth century.

No one knows just how Johns Hopkins acquired the knowledge that enabled him to plan so wisely for the role which his university and hospital were to play in reforming medical education in the United States. He was a man of limited education, none of it professional, and he had devoted his life to the world of business. Nevertheless, when he devised his bequest in 1867 for a university medical school and a hospital with interlocking boards of Trustees, he recognized the importance, which was then only dimly perceived by many medical educators, of having a medical school organized as an integral department of a university and of having the clinical education of medical students carried out in a hospital closely connected with the medical school. It is believed, on the basis of circumstantial evidence, that Patrick Macauley, a physician who lived near Mr. Hopkins in Baltimore, may have influenced the latter's views. In 1823, Macauley addressed the Medical and Chirurgical Faculty of Maryland on the subject of *Medical Improvement*. In this address he dwelt upon the use of hospitals for clinical instruction. Macauley died in 1849. From 1847 to 1849 he and Hopkins served together on the Board of Directors of the Baltimore and Ohio Railroad. Whether Macauley ever discussed medical education with Hopkins is not known; but it is of interest that Mr. Hopkins's library was found, after his death, to contain books on medical subjects which had belonged to Dr. Macauley (French, 1953).

133

In his will, written in 1867, Hopkins provided for two boards of Trustees, one to preside over the university, the other over the hospital. In 1873, several months before his death, he sent to the Trustees of the hospital, for which as yet no plans had been prepared, a letter of instruction (Chesney, 1943) in which he noted that he had provided 13 acres of land on which the hospital was to be built, and directing, among other things, that

It will be your special duty to secure for the service of the hospital surgeons and physicians of the highest character and of the greatest skill. I desire you to establish in connection with the hospital a training school for female nurses.

In all your arrangements in relation to this hospital you will bear constantly in mind that it is my wish and purpose that the institution should ultimately form a part of the medical school of that university for which I have made ample provision in my will.

The estate which Hopkins bequeathed to the university and hospital was valued at approximately $7 million, a huge sum for those days, to be divided equally between the two institutions.

THE JOHNS HOPKINS UNIVERSITY

In 1875 the Trustees selected Daniel C. Gilman as President of the University. In his inaugural address at the opening of the university in 1876, Gilman, after sharply criticizing the educational standards of existing medical schools, went on to say prophetically, "We may rejoice that the morning has dawned which will see endowments for medical science as munificent as those now provided for any branch of learning, and schools as good as those now provided in any other land." Gilman observed that a period of years would elapse before the opening of the hospital, and that in the intervening time it was his intention to offer a course of undergraduate study which "shall train the eye, the hand, and the brain for later study of medicine." In 1878 he announced that the premedical course would include the study of chemistry, biology, physics, modern and ancient languages, and other subjects leading to a bachelor of arts degree. This was far in advance of the admission requirements of existing medical schools, and it is significant that the course outlined by Gilman a century ago would meet the current admission requirements of all medical schools of first rank in this country.

Gilman was extraordinarily successful in his choice of professors to head the science departments of the new university. Ira Remsen in Chemistry, Henry A. Rowland in Physics, and H. Newell Martin in Biology all had received excellent training, all were first-rate teachers, all were under the age of 30 at the time of their appointment, and all were to achieve the highest distinction in their respective fields. These men played a role in formulating the plans for the medical school, and in addition to them, from 1876 onward President Gilman had the advice and assistance, in medical matters, of John Shaw Billings. Billings unquestionably had a better grasp of the deficiencies and potentialities of American medical education than almost any man of that period, and Gilman rarely made a move in laying the groundwork for the medical school without first consulting him.

134

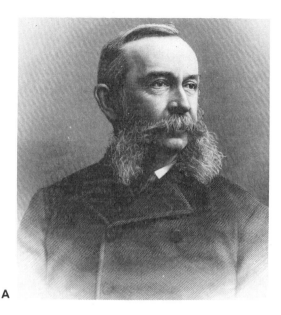

A

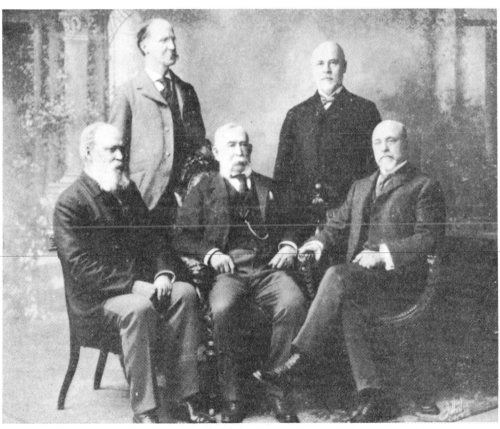

B

Figure 28. *A*, Daniel C. Gilman. *B*, President Gilman in 1901 surrounded by his chief advisers in the early faculty. Seated, left to right: Gildersleeve, Gilman, and Remsen; standing, Rowland and Welch. (*A*, From Archives of the Johns Hopkins University. *B*, From French, John C.: A History of the University Founded by Johns Hopkins. Baltimore, Johns Hopkins University Press, 1946. Reproduced with permission.)

135

An interesting description of the interim period between the opening of the Johns Hopkins University in 1876 and the opening of the medical school in 1893 was given by Henry M. Thomas, who later became Professor of Neurology at the medical school. In the early 1880s, Thomas took the premedical course announced by President Gilman, and in 1886, having received his M.D. degree from the University of Maryland, he took a course in pathology under Welch. He writes that the Hopkins University in those days was "a small compact body, made up for the most part of young, active faculty, surrounded by a group of advanced workers called fellows, other post graduate students, and a few rather over-powered undergraduates" (Thomas, 1919). It was Professor Martin, the biologist, who provided the greatest stimulation and inspiration for those who were interested in a medical career. In addition to his regular biological courses, Martin gave lectures to medical students and to practitioners of the city; and graduates of medicine entered his laboratory for special work.

Though the university could function with a reasonable degree of efficiency in temporary quarters, this was not so in the case of the hospital. Here new buildings were absolutely essential. In March, 1875, the Trustees sent a letter to five experts in hospital construction, specifying the size and type of hospital which they wished to have built and asking each expert to submit plans for construction, heating, ventilation, and administration. The plans submitted by John Shaw Billings, who was then a Lieutenant Colonel in the United States Army, were considered to be the best and were accepted by the Trustees. Billings's plans were accompanied by an essay which set forth his views on the ideal relationship between a hospital and a university medical school.

Billings's knowledge of hospital construction was derived largely from

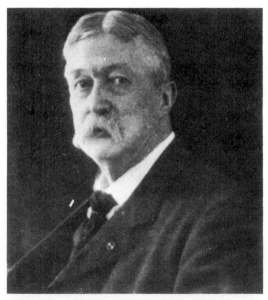

Figure 29. John Shaw Billings. (From Garrison, F. H.: John Shaw Billings, A Memoir. New York and London, G. P. Putnam's Sons, 1915. Reproduced with permission.)

his experience as an Army officer during and following the Civil War. He received his M.D. degree from the Medical College of Ohio in 1860 and then had taught anatomy at his *alma mater* while starting the practice of medicine in Cincinnati. He entered the Medical Corps of the Union Army in 1862 at the age of 24. During the war he won a reputation as a fine organizer and administrator as well as a skillful surgeon. After the war, while serving on the staff of the Surgeon General, he was delegated to make a survey of the Marine Hospital Service, and the report of this survey, together with a report on *Army Barracks and Hospitals,* which appeared in 1870, won for Billings a reputation as an authority on hospitals. The experience gained during and subsequent to the war had taught him that hospitals of the pavilion type, composed of multiple, well-ventilated, single-story buildings connected only by open-air corridors, served to minimize the spread of wound infections among the patients and provided a more healthful environment for convalescents. The hospital that Billings designed for the Hopkins embodied an extension and elaboration of the principles derived from this experience.

Billings's thoughts on medical education, which had been expressed in the essay appended to his architectural plans, went back to the days when he was successively student and teacher at the Medical College of Ohio. Daniel Drake was the founder of that college, and Billings had read with admiration the essays on medical education which Drake had written in the 1830s. In the 1860s the college no longer adhered to Drake's precepts, and Billings looked upon his own education as having been very deficient. After the war Billings made a study of the medical education systems of the European countries, giving thought to ways in which the standards in the United States might be raised. The ideas that he expressed in his essay of 1875 were further elaborated in his paper entitled *A Review on Higher Medical Education,* which was published in 1878 (Billings, 1878).

From 1876 to 1889 Billings supervised the construction of the Johns Hopkins Hospital, a prolonged and tedious process. The job was expected to cost $1.2 million, and construction was not permitted to proceed more rapidly than the income from the endowment would allow. During this period Billings remained in the Army as the officer in charge of the Surgeon-General's Library, and he continued his work on the Index Catalogue of that library. During part of this period he also served on the faculty of The Johns Hopkins University, giving lectures on hygiene, medical education, the history of medicine, and medical jurisprudence, and he continued to be President Gilman's principal advisor on medical matters. As the hospital construction was nearing its termination the Trustees offered Billings the position of Director of the hospital. He refused this offer but remained on for a time with the title of "Consulting Director."

Throughout his association with the Johns Hopkins institutions Billings had constantly in mind the creation of a new type of medical school dedicated primarily to developing practitioners of medicine "better trained and more skillful than those of other schools, but still practitioners." He considered the study of disease in the living human subject to be the essential ingredient of medical education. He presented telling arguments in favor of the conduct of research in a medical school: "What is desired is that the medical faculty shall increase knowledge and should fit its students to

137

increase knowledge, and that its attempt to do this shall not be restricted or limited by the fact that a part of its work is to teach the practical applications of this knowledge....We shall have the means to do work which is not only desirable, but which cannot be done elsewhere."

Billings advocated a four-year course of medical study: the first two years were to be devoted to study of the basic medical sciences and the last two years to study of disease in living patients in the wards and outpatient department of the hospital. He considered a baccalaureate degree to be an indispensable prerequisite for the study of medicine, and he envisioned the student body as being made up of a small group of carefully selected scholars.

In order to bring the students more closely in touch with the day-to-day problems of sick individuals, Billings incorporated, in his plan of the hospital, living quarters to accommodate the members of the senior medical class. He believed that they should live at the hospital and should share the responsibilities for the care and study of the patients. The integrated collaboration of university and hospital in the educational program proposed by Billings existed nowhere else in this country at that time; and his plan of a four-year medical course to be entered only by students who had previously acquired a bachelor's degree was to set the pattern of American medical education for the future.

THE HOPKINS MEDICAL FACULTY BEGINS TO ASSEMBLE

At the time of *William H. Welch's* appointment in 1884 as Professor of Pathology, the construction of the hospital had not been completed, but it was expected that the opening of the medical school would be made to coincide with that of the hospital. With this in view, a temporary medical faculty had been appointed, consisting of Gilman, Welch, Billings, Remsen, and Martin. In 1887, when the Baltimore and Ohio Railroad got into financial difficulties and ceased paying dividends on its common stock (of which the Johns Hopkins University held almost 15,000 shares), the plans for opening the medical school had to be suspended indefinitely. Nevertheless, provision had to be made for the supervision of the clinical services in the hospital that was soon to open.

Welch had been on the job in Baltimore since 1885. He had graduated from The College of Physicians and Surgeons, New York, in 1875. He was a scholarly young man, far more interested in laboratory work than in the practice of medicine. He hoped to pursue an academic career, but the prospects did not seem bright, for in those days in order to become a professor at a medical school one first had to become a successful practitioner.

While in medical school Welch had heard about the plans for the Johns Hopkins University and Hospital, and in 1875 he called on President Gilman to inquire about possible openings there. He was unable to see Gilman, but he did learn that the new university was not to be primarily an educational center for undergraduates but rather a true center of learning and that its faculty would be made up of scholars capable of performing original research and of guiding graduate students along the path of cre-

138

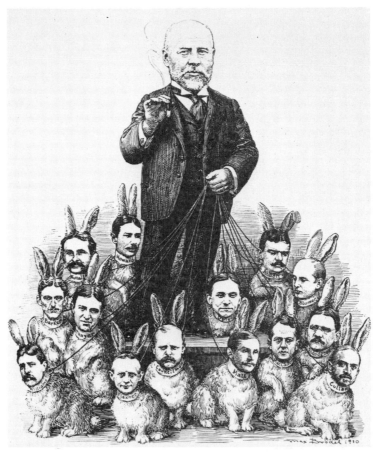

Figure 30.   William H. Welch: Some Welch Rabbits. (By Max Broedel.)

ative scholarship. From this time on Welch was hopeful of having an opportunity to join the Hopkins faculty.

In view of his lack of interest in medical practice, Welch was advised by his professors in New York to spend a year of study in Germany; he might thus prepare himself to become a teacher of histology (microscopical anatomy), a subject of growing importance which at that time was not taught in American medical schools. This advice Welch accepted with alacrity. He sailed for Germany in April, 1876, on what has been characterized as a "voyage of exploration of medicine in Europe that was in its results perhaps the most important ever taken by an American doctor" (Flexner and Flexner, 1941). He did not return to the United States until February, 1878.

While abroad Welch concentrated on the study of microscopical anatomy and pathology under some of the masters in these fields. At the same time he learned a great deal about German laboratory methods and the organization of the schools for instruction in medical science. While he was at work in Leipzig, Welch met Billings, who was then traveling in Germany in connection with his plans for the Johns Hopkins Hospital and Medical School. Welch accompanied Billings on a tour of the Leipzig medical build-

139

ings, and in the evening the two men met for a long conversation over beer at Auerbach's Keller. Billings was so profoundly impressed by young Welch that he resolved to keep him in mind as a potential candidate for the faculty of the new school.

It was while Welch was in Germany that Robert Koch announced the isolation and identification of the bacterium causing the disease *anthrax*. Though he realized that bacteriology held promise for the future, Welch was so involved in his other studies that he had little time to devote to this new subject before returning home.

Welch had been back in New York for only a short time when he established at the Bellevue Hospital Medical College the first laboratory course in pathology ever given in an American medical school. His course was popular, and when the first class ended he was induced by eager applicants from the three principal medical schools in New York City to start another course. In 1879 Welch's course was so sought after that he found it necessary to teach two sections. Three years later the Bellevue Hospital Medical College provided funds to enlarge his laboratory.

One day early in 1884, Billings appeared at the door of Welch's workroom and asked whether Welch would mind if he watched him conducting his class. The next day Billings appeared in the amphitheatre while Welch was demonstrating an autopsy. Following the demonstration Billings asked Welch what he would like most to do if adequate facilities were placed at his disposal. Welch replied that he would like to carry on original research with his own hands in a laboratory similar to those in which he had worked in Germany. After this meeting Billings wrote to President Gilman, saying that he considered Welch to be the best man in the United States for appointment as Professor of Pathology at Johns Hopkins. He believed that Welch probably had greater potential for development than the two or three German professors who were being considered for the position. President Gilman also had received letters of recommendation from some of the scientists with whom Welch had worked in Germany. In March, 1884, Gilman offered Welch the professorship. Chesney (1943) says, "That appointment unquestionably constituted one of the most important single events in the history of both the school and the hospital."

Prior to assuming his responsibilities in Baltimore, Welch spent an additional year in Germany in order to bring himself abreast of the most recent developments in pathology and bacteriology. During most of the year he worked under leading bacteriologists, including Koch, trying to master the technical procedures employed in this specialized field. After his year in Germany he returned to Baltimore well prepared to initiate work in both pathology and bacteriology. He was then 35 years old.

When Welch arrived in Baltimore, the Pathology Building, the first of the buildings which were to constitute the hospital, was being constructed. He and his assistants moved into the new building in November, 1885, before it had been completed.

Early in 1886 Welch gave a series of public lectures on bacteriology, which were well attended by the physicians of Baltimore. The following autumn Welch and his senior associate, William T. Councilman, offered laboratory courses in pathology and bacteriology for the students of the university. At the same time it was made known that the laboratory was ready to receive those who wished to undertake special research in pathology or bacteriology. Welch also offered fellowships to carefully selected, properly qualified individuals.

From the very outset an extraordinary amount of research of high quality was carried on in Welch's laboratory. There were problems: the cultures of bacteria used for study and instruction had a way of dying out, and on one occasion, in 1886, Welch had to make a hurried trip to Koch's laboratory to obtain new cultures. Since the pathology laboratory was functioning without a hospital, there were also problems in obtaining the autopsy material needed for the course in pathology. Fortunately, Councilman, Welch's associate, was Pathologist to Bay View Hospital, a relatively large public hospital on the outskirts of Baltimore, and he transported the much-needed pathological specimens in pails suspended from the handlebars of his tricycle, which he pedaled from Bay View to the laboratory, a distance of several miles. In spite of some shortcomings, Welch's pathology laboratory had far more to offer to those interested in medical science than did any other institution in the United States, and a flood of eager young doctors came there to receive a baptism in medical laboratory research. Those who worked in the laboratory under Welch prior to the opening of the medical school included many who subsequently distinguished themselves in some field of medicine. Among them were Simon Flexner, George M. Sternberg, Walter Reed, James Carroll, Alexander C. Abbott, William S. Halsted, Christian A. Herter, Franklin P. Mall, Henry M. Thomas, and Lewellys F. Barker. Of the original work which Welch himself carried on in the laboratory, that which attracted the greatest attention was his discovery of the bacillus that causes gas gangrene and which became known as the *Bacillus welchii*. Unlike the great German professors, who directed the research of their students and staff along lines which they thought would be most productive, Welch never set a student to work on a specific problem, seeming rather to avoid any such commitment. It was his belief that men did not work well on assigned tasks. In this same spirit he once stated "that students in our American medical schools suffer from over-teaching." Welch had the broad knowledge and the laboratory experience needed to guide his associates. In addition, he provided the environment and the enthusiasm which struck fire in young people.

William Osler, the first clinician to be appointed to the staff of the hospital, was a Canadian. He began his higher education at Trinity College, Ontario, where he developed an interest in biology and became proficient in the use of the microscope. In 1868 and 1869 he attended the Toronto Medical School and then transferred to the McGill Medical School, from which he received his M.D. degree in 1872. McGill had the advantage of being closely associated with the Montreal General Hospital, and the clinical experience which the students were afforded was better than that available at the schools in the United States. Osler gives the following account of his early clinical education (Cushing, 1926):

> When I began clinical work in 1870, the Montreal General Hospital was an old coccus-and-rat-ridden building, but with two valuable assets for the students — much acute disease and a group of keen teachers. Pneumonia, phthisis, sepsis, and dysentery were rife. The services were not separated, and a man for

141

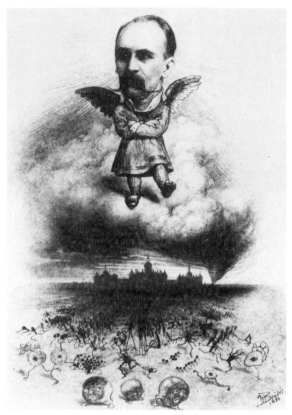

Figure 31. William Osler—The Saint—Johns Hopkins Hospital. (By Max Broedel.) (Reproduced with permission of Mrs. Charles Austrian.)

three months looked after medical and surgical patients, jumbled together in the same wards. The physic of the men who were really surgeons was better than the surgery of the men who were really physicians, which is the best that can be said of a very bad arrangement....Scottish and English methods prevailed, and we had to serve our time as dressers and clerks, and, indeed, in serious cases we very often at night took our share in the nursing.... The bedside instruction was excellent, and the clerking a serious business. I spent the greater part of the summer of 1871 at the hospital, and we had admirable outpatient clinics from Dr. Howard, and a small group worked in the wards under Dr. MacCallum.... I left the old general hospital with a good deal of practical experience to my credit.

Until 1870 the McGill Medical School had been run on a proprietary basis, and the teaching was almost entirely in lecture form and given by general practitioners.

The member of the faculty to whom Osler was chiefly indebted was R. Palmer Howard. Like his colleagues, he was a practitioner of surgery as well as medicine, but he differed from the others in having an intense interest in morbid anatomy. It was Howard who succeeded in arousing in Osler an interest in this subject.

Following his graduation from McGill Osler spent two years studying in Europe. In 1875, shortly after returning to Montreal he was appointed Professor of the Institutes of Medicine (largely physiology and pathology).

Though Osler had no official appointment at the Montreal General Hospital, he volunteered for work in the autopsy room and gradually took over most of the post-mortem examinations. He bought and personally paid for 12 microscopes for his students to use. He also took over the supervision of a smallpox ward, a very busy place at that time. In an 18-month period, 260 cases of smallpox were admitted to this ward, and of these, 24 patients died. Osler's work on the smallpox ward came to an end in December, 1875, when he himself came down with the disease. The $600 which he received for this work was used largely to clear up his debt for the microscopes he had purchased. In 1879 he was appointed Physician to the Montreal General Hospital. He devoted almost all of his time to work on the wards and in the autopsy room, and in both of these places he attracted a following of students.

Osler remained in Montreal until 1884. While there he exhibited habits of work and of mind which, years later (1925), were so beautifully summed up by Welch:

Osler's type of mind, early made manifest on the scientific side, was distinctively that of the descriptive naturalist, and so it remained to the end, even in his study of disease — interrogating nature by keen, accurate observation rather than by experiment, asking 'what' rather than 'why' or 'how,' delighted with the study of form and obvious function without concern for explanations, theories and speculations, addicted to the collection of specimens.

While in Montreal, Osler did, indeed, collect specimens — rare botanical and zoological specimens; rare books for his library; but most of all he collected specimens from the autopsy room, which when correlated with observations made at the bedside, gave new insights into the manifestations and natural history of a variety of diseases. His papers on clinical and pathological subjects attracted more and more attention. Though he taught physiology at McGill he had neither taste nor aptitude for experimental investigations. "I never could," he said, "get my drums and needles and tambours to work in harmony." In 1881 Osler attended the International Medical Congress in London at which Pasteur, Koch, and others presented papers describing their exciting bacteriological discoveries, but Osler did not appear at this time fully to grasp what he heard. In writing to his colleagues at home, he merely stated that "there was an abundant discussion about germs."

In May, 1884, William Pepper gave up his position as Professor of Clinical Medicine at the University of Pennsylvania in order to accept the senior chair as Professor of Medicine. Osler was chosen to succeed him in the clinical professorship. He was then 35 years old and was considered young for such an important position in America's oldest and most prestigious medical school. An unusual feature of Osler's appointment was that he was given a salary which made it possible for him to devote his time to teaching and research without having to practice medicine.

In speaking of Osler's early days at the University of Pennsylvania, Cushing writes (1926):

So far as the students were concerned, there can be no doubt that their first impression was one of disappointment. No polished declamations with glowing word

143

pictures of disease, such as they had listened to from Stillé and Pepper, came from this swarthy person with drooping mustache and informal ways, who, instead of arriving in his carriage, jumped off from a streetcar, carrying a small black satchel containing his lunch, and with a bundle of books and papers under his arm; who was apt to pop in by the back door instead of by the main entrance; who wore, it is recalled, a frock coat, top hat, a flowing red necktie, low shoes, and heavy worsted socks which gave him a foreign look; who, far from having the eloquence of his predecessor, was distinctly halting in speech; who also insisted on having actual examples of the disease to illustrate his weekly discourse on Fridays at eleven, and, as likely as not, sat on the edge of the table swinging his feet and twisting his ear instead of behaving like an orator—this at least was not the professor they had expected.

[However,] it was a horse of a different color when the students came in contact with Osler in the wards, for the bedside instruction such as he was accustomed to, was an undeveloped feature in the Philadelphia school....[Pepper, though the head of the medical department, was engaged in a large private practice, and he was also the Provost of the University], rarely appeared except to give his accustomed lectures, so that Osler had three wards almost to himself; and in them, with an increasingly enthusiastic group of students about him, he was to be found the larger part of each morning. [These wards were in the new University Hospital.]

The University of Pennsylvania had only recently introduced its three-year course of medical study, and the senior students of 1884 had been the first of whom an entrance examination had been required. All of the professors with the exception of Osler and Joseph Leidy, the Professor of Anatomy, were actively engaged in the practice of medicine. Osler's disinclination to engage in general practice was mystifying to his medical colleagues, who were accustomed to hold afternoon office hours and to engage in house-to-house practice. Instead Osler's afternoons usually found him at Blockley (the municipal hospital), making post-mortem examinations.

While at the University of Pennsylvania, Osler's stature in the medical world rose steadily, and in 1885 he was invited to give the Goulstonian Lectures in London. In spite of his success as a teacher Osler was not altogether satisfied with his experience at the University of Pennsylvania. In 1915, looking back on his life there, he said: "Twenty-five years ago there was not a single medical center worth the name in the United States. A most pernicious system prevailed—bad for the teacher, worse for the pupil. At the University of Pennsylvania, Pepper held a Saturday clinic and gave two didatic lectures weekly. I gave one clinic, and...held classes in physical diagosis, which were good enough in their way, but the student had no daily personal contact with patients. There was abundant material, and ... I was for five years very nearly a full-time man. There was no clinical laboratory, only an improvised room under the amphitheater." When Osler was offered the position as Physician-in-Chief of the Johns Hopkins Hospital he foresaw that this would make it possible for him to develop his own ideas about medical education, unfettered by the traditions of an established institution, and he jumped at the opportunity.

Some years later Osler recalled the manner in which the position at the Hopkins was offered to him by Billings, who had been sent to Philadelphia for this purpose by President Gilman: "Without sitting down he asked me abruptly: 'Will you take charge of the medical department of the Johns Hopkins Hospital?' Without a moment's hesitation, I answered 'Yes.' Billings then said, 'See Welch about the details. We are to open very soon. I'm very busy today. Good morning.' And he was off, having been in my room not more than a couple of minutes."

Shortly after Osler's appointment *William S. Halsted,* one of the group of brilliant young postgraduate students who had been working in Welch's laboratory, was asked to take charge of the Surgical Service of the Hospital and to organize the Dispensary. However, the term of Halsted's appointment, unlike that of Osler's, was for one year only, and his titles were to be Surgeon-in-Chief to the Dispensary and Acting Surgeon to the Hospital. Whereas Osler's salary was to be $5000, Halsted's was set at $1000 per annum. There were probably several reasons for the temporary nature of this appointment. Halsted was young and relatively inexperienced, and a search was still in progress for a more senior surgeon. In fact the position had already been offered to, but had been declined by, William Macewen, Professor of Surgery at Glasgow, Scotland. There also may have been some question about Halsted's addiction to cocaine.

After graduation from Yale College in 1874, Halsted entered The College of Physicians and Surgeons in New York City. He had a brilliant record there, leading his class and winning the competitive examination for the appointment to Bellevue Hospital as Surgical Intern. During his medical school period, two of his professors, Sands and Sabine, aroused in him an interest in surgery. After a year as House Physician at New York Hospital, in 1878, Halsted went to Europe for two years of graduate study. There he visited all of the prominent surgical clinics and was particularly impressed by the experimental work then being carried on by the German surgeons.

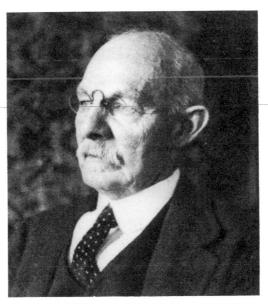

Figure 32. William S. Halsted. (From MacCallum, W. G.: William Stewart Halsted, Surgeon. Baltimore, The Johns Hopkins University Press, 1930. Reproduced with permission.)

145

According to Osler, Halsted came back home "very much *verdeutsched* and held that there were only three or four good surgeons in the world and all of them were German."

Back in New York, Halsted became a member of the staff of Roosevelt Hospital. There he organized a highly successful outpatient department and at the same time carried on a quiz course for medical students in both anatomy and surgery. He had staff appointments at The College of Physicians and Surgeons and at a number of hospitals including the Presbyterian Hospital and Bellevue Hospital as well as the Roosevelt Hospital. He reorganized the operating rooms in which he worked to meet the needs of the new antiseptic technique and gave early evidence of his devotion to clinical and laboratory experimentation. In 1881, he performed an indirect blood transfusion, possibly the first in America to be succesfully carried out. Since nothing was then known about blood groups, success in this venture required luck as well as boldness. The patient was Halsted's sister, who was in a state of collapse from postpartum hemorrhage. "I transfused my sister with blood drawn into a syringe from one of my veins and injected immediately into hers. This was taking a great risk, but she was so nearly moribund that I ventured it and with prompt results."

Halsted read in the *Medical Record* of October 11, 1884, that Dr. Koller of Vienna, had been experimenting with a new drug, cocaine, and that he had demonstrated the extraordinary anesthetic effect that a few drops of a solution of cocaine had on the tissues of the eye (cornea and conjunctiva). Realizing that Koller's observations might have other applications, Halsted immediately sent for a supply of cocaine and began a series of experiments on himself and some of his young associates. It was soon found that cocaine injected into the trunk of a sensory nerve anesthetized the area supplied by that nerve. Injections of the inferior dental nerve were made for the first time in late November, 1884, in order to extract a sensitive tooth painlessly.

Halsted's development of neuroregional anesthesia was one of his most brilliant performances. He was also the first to inject an anesthetic drug (cocaine) into the meninges and was therefore the originator of spinal anesthesia. His pioneer work on nerve-block anesthesia had been forgotten by most physicians when, in 1922, he was honored by the American Dental Association for his development of an anesthetizing procedure which had been such a boon to dentists and their patients.

Halsted and his associates who injected their own nerves in the experiments with cocaine unfortunately fell victims to the drug, the habit-forming properties of which were not known at that time. Several of them became hopeless addicts and after leading miserable lives succumbed to their addiction. For a year Halsted gave up his practice, his teaching, and his experimental work and struggled to overcome his problem. He was having little success when Welch, who had become his friend when they were both on the staff of Bellevue Hospital, sensed the drift of the situation and invited Halsted to come to Baltimore to live with him and to work in his laboratory. The invitation was accepted, and for the next three years Halsted immersed himself in experimental work.

From 1886 to 1889 Halsted enjoyed a peaceful interlude in Welch's laboratory. His only patients were laboratory animals, but in carefully planned experiments on them he worked out some of the principles and methods which form the foundation of modern surgery. In speaking of these early studies in the laboratory, Councilman, who was Welch's assistant at the time and frequently watched Halsted at work, said, "It is difficult to think of surgery more carefully conducted than was this experimental surgery by Halsted. The dog was treated as a human patient, there was the same care in anesthesia, the same technique in operation and in the closure of wounds." When the hospital opened, Halsted was ready to apply the principles and methods that had been developed in the laboratory.

At the time of Halsted's limited appointment to the staff of the hospital, Osler (1969) recalled, "He had been living in Baltimore for two years working with Dr. Welch and struggling to recover from the cocaine and morphia habit that he had acquired in New York. . . . With a morphia record and an uncertainty as to the cure, the trustees could not do more than put him on trial."

There is an intimation in these comments that the Trustees were aware of Halsted's addiction, though other evidence indicates that only Welch and Osler knew about it. Osler's statement (1969) also reveals that Halsted had become addicted to morphine as well as cocaine before coming to Baltimore. Just when or how morphine entered the picture is a mystery, but from 1890 onward it had replaced cocaine in all references to Halsted's addiction.

After a year in tentative status, Halsted was given the permanent appointment as Surgeon-in-Chief. Osler states (Holman, 1971):

> *When we recommended him as full surgeon [Surgeon-in-Chief] to the hospital in 1890 I believed, and Welch did too, that he was no longer addicted to morphia. He had worked so well and so energetically that it did not seem possible that he could take the drug and do so much. About six months after the full position had been given I saw him in a severe chill, and this was the first intimation I had that he was still taking morphia. Subsequently I had many talks about it and gained his full confidence. He had never been able [up to Osler's departure from Baltimore in 1905] to reduce the amount to less than 3 grains daily. On this he could do his work comfortably and maintain his excellent physical vigor. . . . I do not think that anyone suspected — not even Welch.*

Actually Welch was better acquainted with what was going on than Osler realized. Many years after Halsted's death in 1922, Welch revealed that

> *Although it has been reported that Halsted conquered his addiction this is not entirely true. As long as he lived he would occasionally have a relapse and go back on the drug. He would always go out of town for this and when he returned he would come to me, very contrite and apologetic, to confess. He had an idea that I could tell what he had done. I couldn't, but I let him go on thinking so because I felt it was good for him to have someone to talk it over with.*

The story of Halsted's long and semi-controlled addiction is a remarkable one. "Miraculously," as Holman (1974) has said, "despite the long addiction, there was no deterioration of self, of health, or of mentality." Even his closest friends, if they were aware of the problem — and many were totally unaware that it had ever existed — believed that he had overcome it. MacCallum, whose biography of Halsted appeared (1930) before publication of the statements by Osler and Welch cited above, believed that Halsted

147

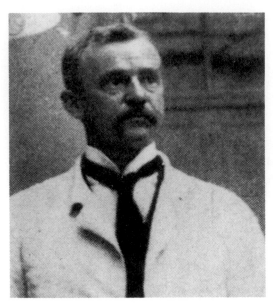

Figure 33. Howard A. Kelly. (From the Archives Office, The Johns Hopkins Medical Institutions.)

had *conquered* his addiction through "superhuman strength and determination and came back to a splendid life of achievement."

The third person to be appointed to the clinical staff of the Hopkins was *Howard A. Kelly,* who arrived in June, 1889, to take over the work in obstetrics and gynecology. Kelly was a native of Philadelphia, and while he was still a child he had developed a keen interest in natural history. He entered the University of Pennsylvania in 1873 when he was only 15 years old. In 1877, the year of his graduation from college, he was a speaker at the commencement exercises, his subject being "The Modern Drift of Natural Sciences." During this same year, Kelly matriculated at the Medical School of the University of Pennsylvania. He was a member of the first class to enter the school after the course had been extended from two sessions to three sessions of five months each. Kelly's class consisted of 136 students, of whom only 19 possessed college degrees. While in medical school, Kelly kept up his interest in natural history. He spent much of his spare time in collecting specimens of flora and fauna, his chief interest being the Reptilia.

After receiving his medical degree, Kelly began a 16-month rotating residency at the Episcopal Hospital in Kensington, near Philadelphia. During this period, he became interested in gynecology and actually started a small clinic for the treatment of gynecological cases. Kensington was an industrial community, the population of which was made up mostly of poor people, and Kelly considered that it offered unusual opportunities for a young surgeon; so he decided to remain in Kensington and open an office there. After a year's time his practice had become so large that he opened a small private hospital, chiefly for the treatment of gynecological problems. Kelly said that his work in Kensington "was the final touch necessary to convert all of my interests to my profession." His skill and ingenuity as a surgeon attracted not only patients but also medical practitioners who wanted to observe his methods. Osler, who was then in Philadelphia, made several visits to Kensington to watch Kelly operate. He said, "I had never seen anybody do abdominal work with the same skill."

In his early years in Kensington, Kelly employed Lister's antiseptic technique based on the use of carbolic acid dressings and sprays. However, he was disturbed by the irritation of wounds sometimes caused by the carbolic acid, and when several deaths from carbolic acid poisoning had been reported, he decided to give up this method. In 1886 he wrote an article, *Asepsis not Antisepsis; a Plea for Principles, not Paraphernalia,* which appeared in the *Maryland Medical Journal.* This article, one of the earliest to favor *asepsis* as opposed to *antisepsis,* attracted attention not only in the United States but in foreign countries as well.

In 1886 Kelly made his first brief trip to Europe to observe the surgeons there at work. He made a second brief trip for the same purpose in 1888. In the latter year when the chair of Obstetrics fell vacant at the University of Pennsylvania, Osler initiated a campaign to have Kelly appointed to fill the vacancy. Osler stated that he was "backing a dark horse—a Kensington colt." The campaign was successful, and Kelly was appointed to the chair. A year later, again owing to the initiative of Osler, Kelly was appointed to the position at the Johns Hopkins Hospital. Osler said later, "His success was immediate and marked. He organized his department with great ability, and very soon his clinic was frequented by surgeons from all parts of the country. He was a bold, rapid and exceptionally ingenious surgeon. Nothing contributed more to the reputation of his department than the full encouragement given to young men, and the freedom with which he spent money to facilitate work." Kelly did not confine his work to the Johns Hopkins Hospital. A few years after he arrived in Baltimore (1892) he opened a private hospital, which according to Osler, "he kept full with patients from all parts of the country."

THE JOHNS HOPKINS HOSPITAL OPENS

When the Johns Hopkins Hospital was formally opened, on May 7, 1889, President Gilman was its Director. This position had been offered to Billings in 1888, and when the offer was refused, Gilman, at the request of the hospital Trustees, added to his duties as university president those of hospital director. He was not relieved of the many organizational and administrative responsibilities of this post until Henry M. Hurd, who had been appointed Superintendent of the hospital in June, arrived in August, 1889, to assume his position.

Hurd, then 50 years of age, was the oldest member of the original professional staff of the hospital. He had received his B.A. and M.D. (1866) degrees from the University of Michigan. After working for four years as a general practitioner, he joined the staff of the Michigan Asylum at Kalamazoo, and thereafter his chief medical interest was psychiatry. When the new Eastern Michigan Asylum was opened at Pontiac in 1878 he became its first Superintendent. In this position Hurd proved himself to be an outstanding organizer and administrator. When he was recommended for the position at Hopkins, Gilman wrote to President Angell of the University of Michigan to

149

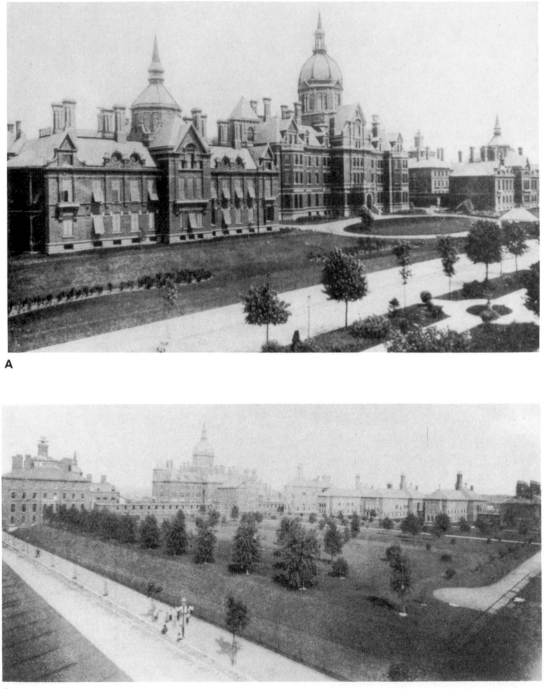

A

B

Figure 34.   *A*, The Johns Hopkins Hospital in 1889. Front view. *B*, View of the hospital buildings from the southeast, 1889.

Illustration continued on opposite page

150

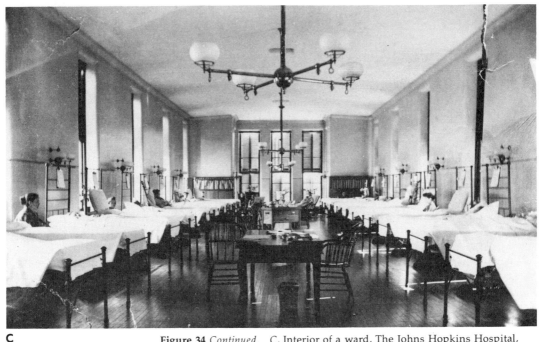

C

Figure 34 *Continued.* *C*, Interior of a ward, The Johns Hopkins Hospital, 1889. (*A* and *B*, from Chesney, A. M.: The Johns Hopkins Hospital and The Johns Hopkins University School of Medicine, a Chronicle. Vol. 1, 1867–1893. Baltimore, The Johns Hopkins University Press, 1943. *C*, From the Archives Office, The Johns Hopkins Medical Institutions.)

ask his opinion of Hurd. Angell replied: "I think it would be no mistake . . . if you should appoint him. . . . We have tried more than once to persuade him to take a medical chair here. He is refined, scholarly, gentlemanly, conciliatory in manner, capable of managing men pleasantly. He is a man of noble and elevated character." This evaluation was certainly borne out in Hurd's long career at Hopkins. An additional characteristic, not mentioned by Angell, was Hurd's intense interest in medical education and his understanding of how the hospital could contribute to the educational process. When the medical school opened he became Professor of Psychiatry, but he continued to be Superintendent of the hospital, and it was in the latter capacity that he made his greatest contribution to medical education.

The training school for female nurses, called for in Mr. Hopkins's letter to the Trustees, opened in October, 1889. Osler (1969) gives an amusing account of how the choice was made of a person to head both the Training School and the Nursing Service of the hospital:

From among the scores of applicants for the position of head of the Training School, Mr. King [Francis T. King, President of the Board of Trustees] and Dr. Billings had selected the four most promising to come to Mr. Gilman's office at different hours for inspection: Miss Parsons, an English nurse, Miss McDowell, an Irish nurse, Miss Caroline Hampton (the future Mrs. Halsted), from the New York Hospital, and Miss Isabel Hampton, a Canadian, superintendent at the Cook County Hospital, Chicago. As Miss Isabel Hampton left the room Mr. King looked approvingly at Mr. Gilman, who smiled (and posterity should know that the first President of the University had a series of most expressive smiles) assent at Dr. Billings. I whistled gently the first two bars of the tune of "Conquering Kings their titles take—from the foes they captive make," as it was quite plain that a commanding figure, a sweet face, and a sweeter voice had in the short space of fifteen minutes settled the election of the head of the Training School.

151

Osler, Halsted, and Kelly appointed to their respective staffs young men in training who lived in the hospital and who were known as Resident or Assistant Resident Physicians or Surgeons. These men not only supervised the care of patients under the direction of their chiefs but also they undertook original research and assisted with the instruction of the few postgraduate students who worked in the hospital prior to the opening of the medical school. Osler, for one, became very restive during this interval. He disliked what he called "the dry bones of postgraduate teaching," and he intimated that unless something were done to expedite the opening of

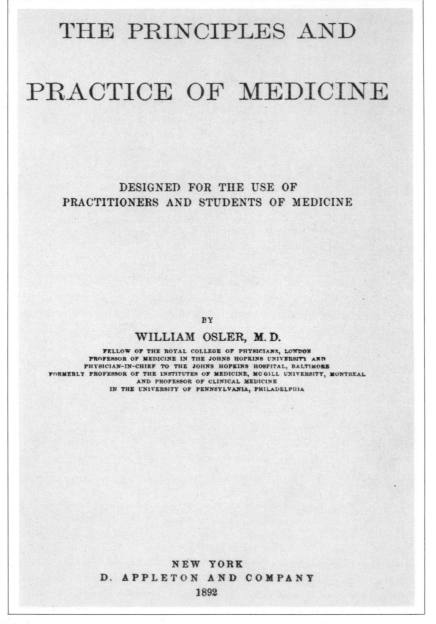

THE PRINCIPLES AND

PRACTICE OF MEDICINE

DESIGNED FOR THE USE OF
PRACTITIONERS AND STUDENTS OF MEDICINE

BY

WILLIAM OSLER, M.D.

FELLOW OF THE ROYAL COLLEGE OF PHYSICIANS, LONDON
PROFESSOR OF MEDICINE IN THE JOHNS HOPKINS UNIVERSITY AND
PHYSICIAN-IN-CHIEF TO THE JOHNS HOPKINS HOSPITAL, BALTIMORE
FORMERLY PROFESSOR OF THE INSTITUTES OF MEDICINE, MCGILL UNIVERSITY, MONTREAL
AND PROFESSOR OF CLINICAL MEDICINE
IN THE UNIVERSITY OF PENNSYLVANIA, PHILADELPHIA

NEW YORK
D. APPLETON AND COMPANY
1892

Figure 35. Title page of the first edition of *The Principles and Practice of Medicine*, by William Osler.

the school, he might be forced to go elsewhere in order to have some "real medical students" to teach.

During the year 1890, after Osler had the medical service well organized and could entrust its routine operation to his assistants, and while he was fretting about the lack of real medical students, he began writing his textbook, *The Principles and Practice of Medicine*. He had thought of writing such a book when he was in Philadelphia and in fact had written several unsatisfying chapters. He wrote that he "continually procrastinated on the plea that up to the fortieth year a man was fit for better things than textbooks." Osler crossed that dateline in 1889, and when he returned in September, 1890, from a refreshing four-month trip to Europe he decided to address himself to the textbook. He was writing the first chapter in leisurely fashion when an agent of *Appleton,* the publisher, paid him a visit and offered him a contract for the book. "We haggled for a few weeks about terms and finally, selling my brains to the devil, I signed the contract." Though he did not neglect his private patients, his consultations, and his attendance at medical meetings, Osler allowed his assistants, Lafleur and Thayer, to take the ward work off his hands so that he could devote as much time as possible to writing the book which he liked to call his *Practice.* He gave up his house and moved into the Residents' Quarters at the hospital, where throughout the year 1891, he labored in a shambles of papers and reference books. By January, 1892, the job was finished.

The *Practice* was an immediate success. It was written in a simple, clear style, easy to read and easy to understand. It was based largely on Osler's personal experience at the bedside and in the autopsy room. As each disease was taken up, consideration was given to its cause, natural history, clinical manifestations, diagnosis (with the aid of the newest laboratory methods), underlying pathology, and treatment. Some of Osler's older contemporaries criticized the *Practice* because its sections on treatment did not contain the list of elaborate prescriptions which one then expected to find in a textbook. The omission was deliberate, for Osler had decided not to clutter his work with traditional but worthless remedies. He made no effort to disguise the facts when either the cause or the cure of a disease was unknown.

Osler's *Practice* soon came into worldwide use. Rarely has the popularity of a textbook been so long sustained. The seventh edition, which appeared in 1909, was the last to be written by Osler without the assistance of a co-author. Before Osler's death in 1919 three more editions had been written with Dr. Thomas McCrae as co-author. The sixteenth and last edition was revised and brought up to date by Dr. Henry A. Christian in 1947.

THE MEDICAL
SCHOOL OPENS

The opening of the medical school, which finally took place in 1893, might have been delayed for a longer period had it not been for the activities of a group of women who were interested in promoting higher education for the members of their sex. These women offered $100,000 to the Trustees of the university for the establishment of the medical school with the proviso that women would be admitted to the school on the same terms as men.

153

The Trustees accepted this offer but stated that the medical school would not be opened until an endowment of $500,000 (including the $100,000 offered) had been secured. In 1892, Miss Mary E. Garrett, who had been the principal contributor to the original women's fund, added $306,977 to her gift to complete the endowment which the Trustees considered necessary.

Once the endowment had been provided and a tentative date had been set for the opening of the medical school, the university was faced with the problem of securing professors to head the departments in the basic medical sciences. Welch, who was serving as Dean of the Medical Faculty as well as Professor of Pathology, was the only head of a preclinical department already on the job. A search had to be conducted for the Professors of Anatomy, Physiology, Pharmacology, and Physiological Chemistry. It was not easy to find in the United States scientists in these fields who qualified, both as teachers and as original investigators, for the faculty sought by Gilman, Billings, and Welch. Nevertheless, the result of the search was to bring to Johns Hopkins three young, well-trained men who were to add renown to the school and were to achieve preeminence in their fields.

Franklin P. Mall, who was appointed Professor of Anatomy, graduated from the University of Michigan Medical School in 1883. After graduation he went to Germany, where he remained for three years, carrying on research in embryology under Wilhelm His and in physiology under Karl Ludwig. He returned to the United States in 1886 and worked in Welch's laboratory as the first Johns Hopkins Fellow in Pathology. Following this, for a short period, he was on the faculty of Clark University and then went to the University of Chicago as Professor of Anatomy. When he took his position on the Hopkins faculty he was just 31 years old.

John Jacob Abel, who was appointed Professor of Pharmacology and Physiological Chemistry, had been both an undergraduate and graduate student at the University of Michigan, from which he received his Ph.D. degree in 1883. Then for a year he had been a graduate student in biology and physiology at Johns Hopkins under Professor H. N. Martin. Following this, he spent seven years in Europe, where he studied under many of the foremost scientists in Germany and Austria. He received his M.D. degree from the University of Strasbourg in 1888. In 1891 he returned to the University of Michigan to become Professor of Materia Medica and Therapeutics. When he was called to Hopkins two years later, he was 36 years old.

William H. Howell, who was appointed Professor of Physiology, had received both his bachelor's degree and his Ph.D. in biology from Johns Hopkins, the latter in 1884. He then joined Professor Martin's staff in the Department of Biology, progressing there to the rank of Associate Professor. In 1889 he was called to the University of Michigan, where he remained until his appointment as Associate Professor of Physiology at Harvard in 1892. During his stay at Michigan he was awarded the M.D. degree. When he joined the Hopkins faculty in 1893, he was 33 years old.

It is of interest that the three newly appointed professors had all either received their medical degree from, or had served on the faculty of, the University of Michigan. In addition to these three, Dr. Hurd, the first Superintendent of the hospital, received both his arts and his medical degree from the University of Michigan.

The class that entered the medical school in the autumn of 1893 con-

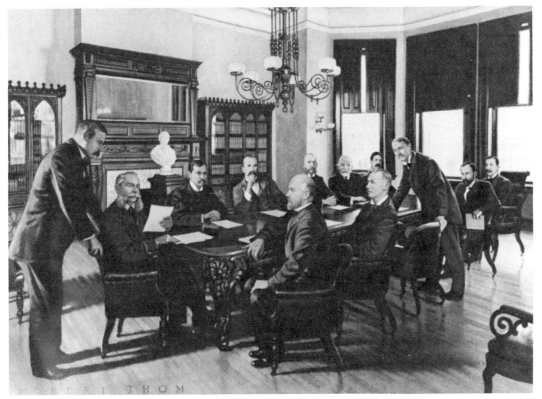

Figure 36. The Advisory Board of the Johns Hopkins School of Medicine in 1893. Standing left, Billings. In the foreground, Gilman, Kelly, Osler, Welch, Halsted, and Mall (standing). In the background (left to right), Hurd, Remsen, Williams, Abel, and Howell. (Thom portrait.) (From Great Moments in Medicine, Parke, Davis and Company. Detroit, Northwood Institute Press, 1966. Stories by George A. Bender. Courtesy of Parke, Davis and Company © 1962.)

sisted of 17 students, including 3 women, all of them college graduates. After two years of stimulating experience under the young and enthusiastic teachers of the preclinical faculty, the students entered the hospital in their third year to work first in the dispensary and then on the wards. At this stage they received additional stimulation from Osler, whose genius as a teacher of medicine was reaching new heights. He saw to it that the students came into close contact with the patients both in the dispensary and on the wards; and he organized the wards in a manner which enabled the senior students to play an essential role in the management of the patients assigned to them. In looking back at this period some years later, Osler remarked: "I hope my gravestone will bear only the statement: 'He brought medical students into the wards for bedside teaching.' "

Osler's organization of the medical clinic of the Johns Hopkins Hospital was one of the classic contributions to medical education. Here, for the first time in the United States, was a well-endowed hospital designed to serve as an essential educational component of a well-endowed university. Funds were provided for salaries for the medical faculty just as they were for the faculty of other university departments. The senior members of the clinical staff were allowed to devote part-time to a consulting practice, but the preclinical faculty and the younger members of the clinical faculty were ex-

155

pected to devote their entire time to teaching and research and (in the case of the clinicians) to work in the dispensary and on the wards.

Henry M. Thomas, whose description of the early days of the Johns Hopkins University has been mentioned previously, also discussed the methods of teaching introduced by Osler and his colleagues at the new hospital. He contrasted the experience of the Hopkins students with his own experience as a student at the University of Maryland, from which he received his M.D. degree in 1885. The Maryland school had a long and honorable history and was looked upon as one of the better medical schools of the 1880s. Thomas stated that he had had good professors at Maryland but that the instruction was based on the old two-year course of lectures. His only laboratory experience had been in the dissecting room and in a new chemical laboratory. The students had almost no opportunity for close observation at the bedside of sick individuals. Thomas was graduated without ever having been instructed in the physical examination of patients, and he received the prize in obstetrics without ever having seen a woman in labor (Thomas, 1919).

SENIOR STAFF AND
HOUSE STAFF

Osler and his senior associates lived outside the hospital. They carried on a limited counsulting practice and cared for a few patients in the private ward of the hospital. However, most of their time was devoted to work in the dispensary and on the public wards, supervising the care of patients, teaching students and house staff, and carrying on research in their fields of special interest. The Resident Physicians, the Assistant Resident Physicians, and the medical interns lived in the hospital and were in close contact with their patients, always during the day and, to the extent necessary, at night. The interns were appointed for only a single year, and they usually began their period of service soon after graduation from medical school. The Resident and Assistant Residents were appointed for an indefinite period, and they were chosen by Osler from among those whom he considered to be men of great promise. They had usually completed an internship and had signified their desires to enter upon a more or less prolonged period of additional training. This upper echelon of the house staff was made up partly from Hopkins interns who had done outstanding work and partly, to prevent inbreeding, from promising young men who had begun their clinical training at other hospitals. The position of Resident Physician (he would now be called Chief Resident) carried with it large responsibilities and opportunities, and it was a prize to be won only by men of exceptional promise. The early Resident Physicians held their positions for a period of years, and the subsequent careers of these men illustrate, on the one hand, the wisdom of Osler in selecting them, and on the other, the growth-promoting influence of the duties and authority attached to the office. The resident staff, supported by interns and senior medical students, not only formed a full-time group of enthusiastic young internists for development under ideal conditions but also afforded an excellent working force for carrying on the routine of the wards, the laboratories, and the outpatient department. This left the Physician-in-Chief and his associates on the senior staff free to devote time not only to supervising and controlling the

156

practice in the clinic but also to carrying on the teaching and research activities in which they were engaged.

In appraising Osler's contributions to medical education, one must place high on the list his graded system of residency training. A number of hospitals had interns, and a few offered house staff positions for training at a somewhat higher level; but none had provided a graded system that afforded appropriate education and training at all levels, from the senior medical students serving as clinical clerks, to the Chief Resident, a man of four or five years' postgraduate training and of mature judgment. A vital aspect of this system was the fact that it was under the control of a single individual who served as both Physician-in-Chief of the hospital and Professor of Medicine at the medical school. A similar residency system was also instituted in the Department of Surgery and the Department of Obstetrics and Gynecology. This system eventually was adopted in other institutions and has become the standard method of training in all of the special fields of medicine and surgery.

In his organization of the medical clinic and in his teaching Osler stressed the value of careful history-taking and meticulous physical examination. He also introduced a systematic course in the application of the laboratory methods of chemistry, physics, and biology to the study of patients. Students in the third year were taught the principles of these methods, and for two or three afternoons each week were drilled in putting them to practical use. Before their senior year, the students had become proficient in the laboratory examinations of blood, urine, feces, stomach juice, and cerebrospinal fluid. Osler's emphasis upon the part played by the laboratory in the complete study of the patient led some of the medical students to search for previously unrecognized manifestations of disease. As a result, a number of excellent papers based on clinical investigations came out of the medical clinic in the early days. For example, a medical student, Thomas R. Brown, was the first (1897) to discover that in patients suffering from trichinosis, a disease acquired by eating inadequately cooked pork, there was an increased number of eosinophil cells in the blood, a discovery which became useful for the diagnosis of this condition.

Another feature of Osler's teaching was the close contact that he insisted that every student should have with the progress of disease in patients. In the fourth year each student spent three months as a clinical clerk, giving all of his time to work on the medical wards. There, under the direction of the resident staff, he took the histories of new patients, assisted the interns in making the initial physical examination, performed all the clinical laboratory tests on his patients, and accompanied the Chief on morning ward rounds. During these rounds the clinical clerk gave orally an epitome of the findings of the case, watched the professor in his examination of the patient, and participated at the bedside in discussions of the anatomical, physiological, pathological, and etiological factors involved.

A brief glimpse of Osler in action is provided in Alice Hamilton's autobiography (1943). In 1896, Dr. Hamilton (later to become an authority on Industrial Medicine and Professor at the Harvard School of Public Health) was a graduate student in Welch's laboratory:

> *...sometimes I would drop work for an afternoon and attend Dr. Osler's clinic, just for the pleasure of seeing how admirably he conducted it. He was freer from what*

157

the English call swank than almost any other great man I have known. His manner with the students was that of an equal, and he always fretted against the hospital etiquette which required a nurse to stand in the presence of a doctor. That was, of course, the absolute rule in Johns Hopkins Hospital, and it was with real trepidation that the clinic nurse would sit down when he bade her. He told me with much irritation that he had once had to pass repeatedly by a nurse who was rolling bandages, and each time he did so she rose to her feet. "Such a silly waste of time and strength." He used to bring in out-of-the-way references in his talks with the students which would lead them far afield from their narrow medical path. Once it was "What is the best way to stop a hiccough?" And after an array of approved, scientific methods had been offered him, "Well, how about making the victim sneeze? Don't you remember—the physician in Plato's Symposium *cures Aristophanes that way?" Another time it was "Why do we call lead poisoning 'saturnism'? That goes back to the days when the ancients knew only eight elements, and they believed that the eight great heavenly bodies were each composed of one of these—the sun of gold, the moon of silver, Jupiter of copper, Mars of iron, Venus of tin, Mercury of quicksilver, Saturn of lead, Vulcan of sulphur. That is why we call quicksilver mercury and silver nitratre lunar caustic. And when we treat rubber with sulphur we call it vulcanizing."*

Dr. Osler was adored by his assistants and all his students, so that many of them could not help trying to imitate him, his walk, his gestures, his accent, his expression. Often I would find myself watching a little crowd of semi- and semi-demi Oslers. I liked it; I knew that the copying was not merely superficial, but that the young men had taken as their ideal a great leader.

While Osler was developing his unique medical clinic, his surgical colleague was originating what soon became known as the Halsted School of Surgery. Halsted was no less careful than Osler in the selection of his interns and residents, and following Osler's lead he instituted a similar type of gradual promotion from intern to Resident Surgeon. In the selection of house staff he usually gave preference to men who had a taste for research. According to Crowe, "The questions which Dr. Halsted put to the students were not intended to test their recollection of what they had read. On the contrary, he was trying to evaluate the young man's ability to observe, to reason, and to formulate a supportable conclusion from the known facts. The exceptional man was thus brought to Dr. Halsted's attention." In evaluating the members of the house staff for advancement up the residency ladder, Halsted had an opportunity to observe them in action over a period of many months: their management of patients, and the care, skill, and orginality that they exhibited in the operating room and in the experimental laboratory.

Halsted initiated a surgical technique at Hopkins which was far ahead of that of other large hospitals, and he made many other major contributions to surgery; but in the opinion of Crowe (1957),

The most important contribution of the Halsted School to American surgery was the Residency Training System. The house officers selected by Halsted were men of the highest type. He gave them every opportunity to become good surgeons and distinguished teachers, and a surprisingly large number went into academic medicine as soon as they had completed their hospital training. . . . In university medical schools throughout the country these men transmitted to their students and assistants not only the Halsted technique, but also the desire to raise the standards of surgical science through carefully and thoughtfully conducted research.

That men trained in the Halsted school displayed a predilection for the academic life is shown by the following figures: Of the 17 Resident Surgeons trained by Halsted, 7 became professors of surgery at leading university medical schools; 6 went to other medical schools, 4 of them at professorial levels; 1 became Surgeon-in-Chief of the Henry Ford Hospital; and only 4 went into private practice. Of 55 Assistant Resident Surgeons who had been on Halsted's house staff for one to three years, 4 remained at Hopkins to take charge of newly established subdepartments of surgery under Halsted; 41 turned to teaching—15 professors, 5 clinical professors, 5 associate professors, 3 assistant professors, 5 assistant clinical professors, and 8 instructors in surgery. Only 14 of the 55 entered private practice (Carter, 1952).

MEDICAL ART A notable feature of many of the papers, monographs, and textbooks written by the surgeons and other members of the Hopkins faculty was the excellence of their illustrations. Howard A. Kelly is often given credit for having brought the first medical artist to Baltimore. Actually, it was F. P. Mall who was responsible

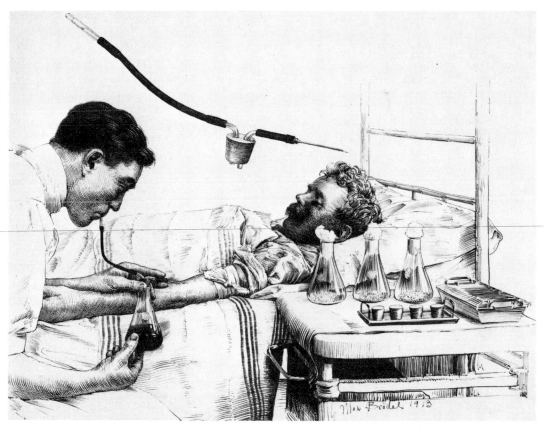

Figure 37. Early drawing of a blood transfusion in which the artist, Max Broedel, has depicted himself as the patient. (From The Broedel Collection, Department of Art as Applied to Medicine, The Johns Hopkins School of Medicine.)

for this important event. While in Leipzig in 1891, Mall was attracted by the work of a young artist, Max Broedel, then only 21 years old. Mall, who was about to move from Clark University to the University of Chicago, offered Broedel a job as artist in the Department of Anatomy at Chicago. After a delay of two years, Broedel decided to accept the offer, but by that time Mall had moved to Baltimore and was too busy with other matters to provide work for an artist. However, he knew that Kelly was seeking an artist to prepare the illustrations for the two-volume work on *Operative Gynecology* which he was then writing. Mall therefore suggested to Kelly that he employ the young German as his illustrator. Broedel arrived in Baltimore in 1894 and soon won the admiration and affection of his Hopkins colleagues. At first he worked exclusively for Kelly, but he was soon performing, with great ingenuity and success, a wide variety of illustrative tasks. In 1905 he was given academic rank as Instructor in *Art as Applied to Medicine,* and he began the instruction of a succession of young artists who were on their way to becoming medical illustrators. Broedel's Department of Art as Applied to Medicine was the first university department of medical art to be established in the United States. The work of the artists in this department did much to enhance the value of many contributions to the medical literature.

EDUCATIONAL REFORM

In the early years of the twentieth century the *Journal of the American Medical Association* in several editorials directed attention to the inferior state of medical education in the United States as compared to that in Europe. Emphasis was placed particularly on the poor quality of clinical training not only for medical students but also for those who were serving internships. During its annual convention in 1904 the Association created a Council on Medical Education which supplanted its old Committee on Medical Education. The Council was directed to take stock each year of American medical education and to submit annual reports to the House of Delegates of the Association, summarizing their findings and offering suggestions for improving the standards. A few months later the Journal of the AMA suggested that the Council on Medical Education should pay particular attention to (1) the educational requirements for admission to medical schools; (2) the relation between the actual performance of medical schools and the claims announced in their catalogues, and (3) the access of medical schools to clinical material which could be used for teaching. The Journal also called for more adequate state requirements for medical licensure. In 1905 the Council on Medical Education held a conference in Chicago, which was attended by delegates from most state and territorial licensing bodies and by committees from the Association of American Medical Colleges and the Southern Medical College Association. Following this meeting the Council presented to the House of Delegates an "Ideal Standard" for medical education. A high school education, including a year's training in several basic science courses, was recommended as a prerequisite for admission to medical school, and this was to be followed by a four-year medical school curriculum and a year's internship. Over a period of several years the

Council made tours of inspection of medical institutions and gathered a substantial amount of material concerning each medical school. The schools were grouped in four classes, "A" to "D," and efforts were made to persuade the states not to license graduates of the "D" schools. *Essentials of an Acceptable Medical College,* which was to serve as a guide for those medical schools which were attempting to raise their standards, was published and distributed to all medical schools. At the same time the Council also made available the draft of a model bill which states could adopt to license medical practitioners.

Perhaps even more important than the American Medical Association's own contributions to the betterment of medical education was the assistance that its Council on Medical Education gave to Abraham Flexner in the investigation of American medical schools which he carried out for the Carnegie Foundation for the Advancement of Teaching. The secretary of the Council, N. P. Colwell, gave Flexner access to the material that had been gathered by the Council and accompanied him during his visits to some of the medical schools (Burrow, 1963).

BLUNT DOCUMENTATION BY ABRAHAM FLEXNER   The Flexner report, entitled *Medical Education in the United States and Canada,* appeared in 1910 and has been looked upon for many years as the document that changed the course of American medical education. This report did indeed play a decisive role. However, the American Medical Association deserves a fair share of the credit. The Journal of the AMA and the Council on Medical Education had done much to prepare the medical profession to accept the recommendations made in the Flexner report; and

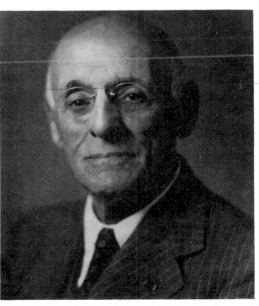

Figure 38.   Abraham Flexner. (National Library of Medicine, Bethesda, Maryland.)

161

after the report appeared, the Council on Medical Education, with the backing of the AMA and the collaboration of the Association of American Medical Colleges, saw to it that the recommendations were carried out.

The Flexner report is divided into two parts. The first part recounts the history of medical education in the United States, describes its existing status, and suggests how it can be improved. The presentation of the various topics is clear, even eloquent. The second part presents, state by state, a description of each medical school—its founding, its entrance requirements, its enrollment, its teaching staff, its general resources, its source of funds, its laboratory facilities, its clinical facilities, and the date on which the school was visted by Flexner. At the end of the section for each state and for Canada there is a presentation of general considerations and recommendations. It is important to note that the data gathered by Flexner were based not on hearsay but on a personal visit to each institution.

Flexner's report presents data regarding 155 medical schools, 7 of which were in Canada. Of the 148 in the United States, 116 were of the regular type (including 7 schools that accepted only black students and one school that accepted only women), and 32 were sectarian schools. The sectarian schools included 15 homeopathic, 8 osteopathic, 8 eclectic, and 1 physiomedical. All of the sectarian schools with the exception of two homeopathic schools (those at the University of Iowa and the University of Michigan) had no income except from student fees. The average student fee for the 1341 osteopathic students was $151, whereas the average fee for the 391 eclectic students was $91 and for the 973 homeopathic students, $103. In only 21 of the regular medical schools did the income from other sources exceed the income from student fees: 15 of these were the schools of state universities, and most of their support came from governmental funds; only 6 of the many private schools had an income from endowment sufficient to place them in this favored category (Harvard, Yale, Washington University in St. Louis, Cornell, Western Reserve, and The College of Physicians and Surgeons in New York).

Among the regular medical schools, those with the largest enrollment were the University of Louisville, Kentucky, with 600; Jefferson Medical College, Philadelphia, 591; and University of Pennsylvania, 546. The sectarian school with the largest enrollment was the American School of Osteopathy in Kirksville, Missouri, 560. The three regular medical schools with the largest enrollment were wholly dependent upon student fees with the exception of the University of Pennsylvania, which had a small additional income from the general funds of the university. The schools with the largest endowment were as follows: Harvard, $3,327,000; Washington University, St. Louis, $1,500,000; The College of Physicians and Surgeons, New York, $832,000; Western Reserve, $785,000. In the year of the survey the endowment income of the Johns Hopkins Medical School was $19,687, but part of the expense of this school was carried by the income from the large endowment of the Hopkins Hospital. At some medical schools, for example Yale and Cornell, which had very modest endowments, the university made a substantial contribution toward operating expenses from the university's general funds.

In the introduction to the Flexner report, acknowledgment is made of the "constant and generous assistance from Dr. William H. Welch of Johns

Hopkins University and Dr. Simon Flexner of the Rockefeller Institute" as well as the chairman and secretary of the Council on Education of the AMA and the secretary of the Association of American Medical Colleges. It seems probable that Abraham Flexner, who was not himself a physician, received valuable assistance from his brother Simon. Simon Flexner had seen medical education at both ends of the spectrum. He had seen it at close to its worst when he was a student at the University of Louisville, the largest of the American schools, which turned out physicians with little regard for their competence. He had also seen it at its best when he was at Johns Hopkins and while visiting the schools of Europe. Of his education in Louisville he said (Flexner, 1937):

It was a school in which the lecture was everything. Within the brief compass of four winter months the whole medical lore was unfolded in discourses following one another in bewildering sequence through a succession of long days; and lest the wisdom imparted should exceed the student's power of retention, the lectures were repeated precisely during a second year, at the end of which graduation with the degree of Doctor of Medicine was all but automatic.

The impact of the Flexner report was due not only to its revelation of the shameless incompetence of the great majority of medical schools but also to the vivid and uncompromising language which was employed to describe the deficiencies in the medical curriculum, the facilities, the equipment, the faculties, and the financial resources of the schools; and the weakness and inconsistencies of the system of state board examinations.

Flexner was also keen enough to perceive that the once formidable medical sects (homeopathy, osteopathy, and eclecticism) were losing ground and were inevitably moving toward absorption by the regular profession:

In the year 1900 there were 22 homeopathic colleges in the United States; today there are 15; the total student enrollment has within the same period been cut almost in half, decreasing from 1909 to 1009; the graduating classes have fallen from 413 to 246. As the country is still poorly supplied with homeopathic physicians, these figures are ominous; for the rise of legal standards must inevitably affect homeopathic practitioners. In the financial weakness of their schools, the further shrinkage of the student body will inhibit first the expansion, then the keeping up, of the sect.

Logically, no other outcome is possible. The ebbing vitality of homeopathic schools is a striking demonstration of the incompatibility of science and dogma. One may begin with science and work through the entire medical curriculum consistently, exposing everything to the same sort of test; or one may begin with a dogmatic assertion and resolutely refuse to entertain anything at variance with it. But one cannot do both. One cannot simultaneously assert science and dogma; one cannot travel half the road under the same banner, in the hope of taking up the latter, too, at the middle of the march. Science, once embraced, will conquer the whole. Homeopathy has two options: one to withdraw into the isolation in which alone any peculiar tenet can maintain itself; the other to put that tenet into the melting-pot. Historically it undoubtedly played an important part in discrediting empirical allopathy. But laboratories of physiology and pharmacology are now doing that work far more effectively than homeopathy; and they are at the same time performing a constructive task for which homeopathy, as such, is unfitted. It will be clear, then, why,

163

when outlining a system of schools for the training of physicians on scientific lines, no specific provision is made for homeopathy. For everything of proved value in homeopathy belongs of right to scientific medicine and is at this moment incorporate in it; nothing else has any footing at all, whether it be of allopathic or homeopathic lineage.

Flexner predicted quite correctly that all four sects which then had their own schools would be forced by the advances in medical science to join forces with the regular profession. He said that none of the eight eclectic schools had decent clinical facilities and that most of them were "without exception filthy and bare." Of the eight osteopathic schools he said that they "fairly reek with commercialism. Their catalogues are a mass of hysterical exaggerations, alike of the earning and of the curative power of osteopathy." The osteopathic schools "now enroll over 1300 students, who pay some $200,000 annually in fees. The instruction furnished for this sum is inexpensive and worthless." Of the physiomedical sect, he said it "can be dismissed in a note. It had three schools in 1907,... only one today."

Flexner was no less harsh in his criticisms of the majority of the regular schools. He recommended that many of them be abandoned and that others be merged into stronger institutions. He believed that far too many doctors were being produced and that the public would be better served by fewer and better educated medical graduates.

In an *Introduction* to the Flexner report, Henry S. Pritchett, President of the Carnegie Foundation for the Advancement of Teaching, summed up the principal findings as follows:

(1) For 25 years past there has been an enormous over-production of uneducated and ill trained medical practitioners. This has been in absolute disregard of the public welfare and without any serious thought of the interests of the public. Taking the United States as a whole, physicians are four or five times as numerous in proportion to population as in older countries like Germany.

(2) Over-production of ill trained men is due in the main to the existence of a very large number of commercial schools, sustained in many cases by advertising methods through which a mass of unprepared youth is brought out of industrial occupations into the study of medicine.

(3) Until recently the conduct of a medical school was a profitable business, for the methods of instruction were mainly didactic. As the need for laboratories has become more keenly felt, the expenses of an efficient medical school have been greatly increased. The inadequacy of many of these schools may be judged from the fact that nearly half of all our medical schools have incomes below $10,000, and these incomes determine the quality of instruction that they can and do offer. Colleges and universities have in large measure failed in the past twenty-five years to appreciate the great advance in medical education and the increased cost of teaching it along modern lines. Many universities desirous of apparent educational completeness have annexed medical schools without making themselves responsible either for the standards of the professional schools or for their support.

(4) The existence of many of these unnecessary and inadequate medical schools has been defended by the argument that a poor school is justified in the interest of the poor boy. It is clear that the poor boy has no right to go into any profession for which he is not willing to obtain adequate preparation; but the facts set forth in this report make it evident that this argument is insincere, and that the excuse which has

hitherto been put foward in the name of the poor boy is in reality an argument in behalf of the poor medical school.

(5) A hospital under complete educational control is as necessary to a medical school as is a laboratory of chemistry or pathology. High grade teaching within a hospital introduces a most wholesome and beneficial influence into its routine. Trustees of hospitals, public and private, should therefore go to the limit of their authority in opening hospital wards to teaching, provided only that the universities secure sufficient funds on their side to employ as teachers men who are devoted to clinical science.

As a result of the agitation for reform that was set in motion by the AMA and the Flexner report, 76 medical schools went out of existence between 1906 and 1920 either by ceasing to function or by merging with stronger institutions. In 1918 the Council on Medical Education raised its requirements for admission to medical school to two years of college work, and by 1920, 78 of the 86 medical schools then in existence had accepted this requirement. An increasing number of schools were by that time requiring a bachelor's degree for admission.

NEW FINANCIAL SUPPORT FOR MEDICAL EDUCATION

The best philanthropy involves a search for cause, an attempt to cure evils at their source.

(John D. Rockefeller, Sr.: Random Reminiscences)

By 1890 John D. Rockefeller had accumulated an unwieldy store of wealth, and the money was still coming in at a bewildering pace. Prior to that year Rockefeller's benefactions had been small in scale and widely scattered. He was a devout member of the Baptist Church and had made many small gifts to Baptist institutions and missions all over the world. In 1890 he became interested in a Baptist college which had been established in Chicago prior to the Civil War. This institution had just obtained a new charter to operate as a university. The Reverend Frederick T. Gates, a Baptist minister, was then the administrative head of the American Baptist Education Society, and Mr. Rockefeller first met him during negotiations leading up to the founding of the new University of Chicago. This school was the first major beneficiary of the Rockefeller fortune. Mr. Rockefeller financed it fully, and by 1910 he had given to this one institution a total of $35 million.

In 1892, while he was still undecided about how much to contribute to the University of Chicago, Rockefeller wrote a letter to Gates saying, "I am in trouble, Mr. Gates. The pressure of these appeals for gifts has become too great for endurance.... I am so constituted as to be unable to give away money with any satisfaction until I have made the most careful enquiry as to the worthiness of the cause. These investigations are now taking more of my time and energy than Standard Oil itself." Gates agreed to help. He moved into an office in the Standard Oil building in New York City, and from that time on he was Rockefeller's "Minister of Philanthropy."

165

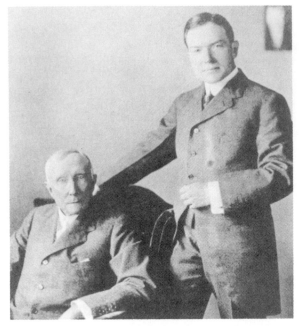

Figure 39. John D. Rockefeller and John D. Rockefeller, Jr. (From Corner, George W.: A History of the Rockefeller Institute. New York, Rockefeller University Press, 1964.)

Gates was opposed to small gifts, widely scattered. He had a "passion to accomplish some great and far-reaching benefit to mankind," and was constantly on the alert for a large undertaking which would be worthy of Mr. Rockefeller's wholehearted backing. In 1897 when he went on his summer vacation he took with him Osler's *Principles and Practice of Medicine*. In spite of the great size and technical nature of this medical textbook Gates said: "I read the whole book without skipping any of it. I speak of this not to commemorate my industry, but to celebrate Osler's charm. . . . There was a fascination about the style itself that led me on, and having once started, I found a hook in my nose that pulled me from page to page." He was particularly impressed by Osler's emphasis on the gaps in medical knowledge and on the lack of effective therapy for many diseases. Gates concluded that the best physician could offer a specific cure "for about as many diseases as there are fingers on one hand." He learned that in most instances nature performs the cures. "When I laid down this book," said Gates, "I had begun to realize how woefully neglected in all civilized countries, and perhaps most of all in this country, had been the scientific study of medicine....Moreover, while other departments of science...had been endowed very generously ... medicine, owing to the peculiar commercial organization of medical colleges, had rarely, if ever, been anywhere endowed, and research and instruction alike had been left to shift for themselves." When he returned from his vacation, Gates was convinced that the financial support of medical education and research offered the great opportunity that he had been seeking. He wrote a memorandum for Mr. Rockefeller, calling attention to the many deficiencies in medical knowledge and recommending that Mr. Rockefeller give consideration to establishing in the United States a medical research institute similar to the Koch Institute in Berlin and the Pasteur Institute in Paris. (The founding and early years of the Rockefeller Institute will be described in a subsequent chapter.)

A Rockefeller philanthropy that was to have a profound effect upon medical education was the General Education Board, which was created with an initial endowment of $1 million. The impetus for the creation of this Board was the Rockefeller family's long-time interest in the education of black people; but when the Board was incorporated in 1903 its stated purpose was improvement of education in the United States and its territories, "without distinction of sex, race or creed." Gates was appointed Chairman of the Board, but Wallace Buttrick, another Baptist clergyman, who was its first secretary, soon took over as President. In 1907 Mr. Rockefeller added to his initial gift a sum totaling $20 million. In the course of the Board's educational work in the Southern states, Buttrick learned about the prevalence of hookworm disease and the debilitating effect of this disease upon the people of many areas in the South. To deal with this problem, the Rockefeller Sanitary Commision was created in 1909 with a pledge from Mr. Rockefeller of $1 million.

The greatest of Mr. Rockefeller's benefactions occurred in 1909 when he turned over to three Trustees—his son, John D. Rockefeller, Jr., his son-in-law, Harold McCormick, and Gates—72,569 shares of the Standard Oil Company of New Jersey, valued at $50 million, to create the Rockefeller Foundation. The purposes of this huge trust were declared to be: "To promote the well being and to advance the civilization of the peoples of the United States and its territories and possessions and of the foreign lands in the

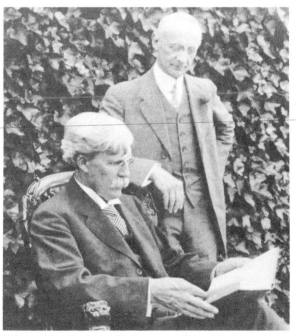

Figure 40. Frederick T. Gates and Simon Flexner. (From Corner, George W.: A History of the Rockefeller Institute. New York, Rockefeller University Press, 1964.)

acquisition and dissemination of knowledge, in the prevention and relief of suffering, and in the promotion of any and all of the elements of human progress." In the years ahead the Rockefeller Foundation would allocate large sums for the advancement of medical education and medical science throughout the world.

One of the first decisions of the Trustees of the Foundation was to make a study of the medical needs of China. As a result of this study the Trustees established the China Medical Board to oversee the work in that nation. In time the Foundation allocated large sums for the construction, equipment, and staffing of the Peking Union Medical College, which from the time of its establishment until World War II was the leading medical school of China.

The scale of the Rockefeller contributions to medical education and medical science dwarfed the gifts of all other benefactors. Nevertheless, many others—far too many to name here—gave munificent sums. A unique gift which was long in maturing was that made by Peter Bent Brigham of Boston. Brigham died in 1877 and left a fortune of $1.3 million, which under the terms of his will, was allowed to accumulate over a period of 25 years following his death. At the end of this time, the will provided, the money was to be used to found "a hospital for the care of sick persons in indigent circumstances." During the 25-year period, the bequest, by efficient management, had grown to several times the original amount. The Peter Bent Brigham Hospital was incorporated in 1902 and was built a decade later on property adjoining the handsome new Harvard Medical School buildings which had been dedicated by President Eliot in 1906. The Brigham bequest provided $1.2 million for the construction of the hospital buildings, and $5 million remained in the fund to serve as endowment. This was the first of the hospitals used for teaching Harvard medical students in which the university had a decisive voice in the selection of the medical staff.

THE MOVEMENT TOWARD FULL-TIME PROFESSORSHIPS In the first quarter of the second century the preclinical professorships in some of the better university medical schools began to be assigned, here and there, to individuals who had had special training in anatomy, physiology, chemistry, or pathology, and these professors were paid either a part-time or a full-time salary. When the Johns Hopkins Medical School opened, all of its preclinical professors were placed on a full-time university salary basis. However, even at Johns Hopkins, the clinical professorships in surgery, medicine, pediatrics, obstetrics, etc., were held by practicing physicians who were paid part-time salaries. In almost all medical schools the clinical teachers were expected to get most of their livelihood from private practice.

Agitation for full-time clinical professorships began in the 1890s, but it was 1913 before the first full-time clinical professors were appointed. In the intervening years the movement was pushed forward chiefly by four individuals: Franklin P. Mall, William H. Welch, Lewellys Barker, and Abraham Flexner.

168 When Mall was working in Leipzig, Germany, in the mid-1880s he

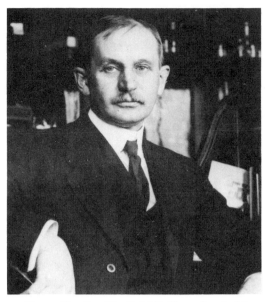

Figure 41. Franklin P. Mall. (From the Archives Office, The Johns Hopkins Medical Institutions.)

learned about a new development in clinical medicine. In 1873 Hugo von Ziemssen had organized at Erlangen a small laboratory of half a dozen rooms where the clinicians in the Department of Medicine could carry out their own resarch work. When, in the following year, von Ziemssen was called to Munich, a new hospital was built in which he created an *Institute for Clinical Research,* an innovation in that it included the first hospital laboratory to be controlled by the clinical faculty and utilized for the investigation of clinical problems. Professor Karl Ludwig, the physiologist under whom Mall was working, watched the development in Munich with great interest and applauded the fact that the clinical professors working there were able to pursue the development of new knowledge without the encroachment of private practice on their time. Ludwig often discussed his enthusiasm for this type of clinical reform with Mall. When Mall joined the Johns Hopkins faculty as Professor of Anatomy in 1893 he began quietly to talk about the advantages that might result from the creation of clinical full-time posts. Among those who frequently listened to Mall's persuasive arguments was Barker, who gave the course in neuroanatomy in Mall's department during the mid-1890s. When Barker went to the University of Chicago as Professor of Anatomy he, in turn, discussed with his colleagues the advantages of full-time clinical professorships. In an address given in 1902 which attracted wide public attention, Barker emphasized that the university-hospital clinic should be staffed by men possessed of the same talents, attainments, and personality as other professors in the university, men who had already made important contributions to knowledge; who should, like other university professors, give their full time and energy to the work of the university, to teaching, and to investigation; and who

169

should be well paid by the university so that they would not have to engage in private practice. At about this same time, Welch, who had also listened frequently to Mall's persuasive arguments, gave his presidential address to the Association of American Physicians. He pointed out that in the laboratory sciences the quality of the teaching in American schools had advanced from being one of the weakest to the strongest feature of the medical curriculum and that there were now an adequate number of anatomical, physiological, and pathological laboratories which offered students excellent training with the reasonable assurance that they could look forward to obtaining a position as teacher and director of a laboratory in one of these special fields of science. In contrast, he pointed out, young physicians wishing to fit themselves for similar careers in clinical medicine and surgery found that there were, with one or two exceptions, no comparable opportunities for training and that even if they were trained they had little chance of obtaining positions with any security for the future. In almost all medical schools clinical teachers were still being selected from among the local practitioners.

In 1904 Mall, who usually worked behind the scenes, wrote an article for *The Michgan Alumnus* in which he said (Sabin, 1934):

> There has always been a great deal of discussion of the question whether a physician's training should be scientific or practical. It appears to me that it should be both; for if he is educated only in the sciences underlying medicine, he is not a physician, while if he is educated in the practical branches only, he is likely to become a shoemaker-physician who will drift into ruts and never get out of them.

> The effort in medical education during the past 25 years has been against the production of shoemaker-physicians, by gradually introducing changes into the medical course which favor the student who is inclined to become a scientific physician. It is now clear that three steps have been taken in the reform of medical education. First, there are educational requirements which precede the study of medicine; secondly, within the medical course the sciences which underlie the more practical branches must be studied first; and thirdly, there is an ever-increasing tendency, more so in the first years of the course, in favor of teachers who are investigators.

> ...In each science there are things fundamental, and it is toward them that we should carry the student, rather than toward memorizing the endless details, even if they may be of some value to the future study of medicine and surgery. When a student has grasped some of the fundamental principles of anatomy and has acquired good habits in working, observing, and thinking, he then has a foundation of value, whether his future career is in medicine, in laryngology or in embryology. The aim should be to put him in a position in which he can find the facts as he needs them, either from specimens or books. To establish the habit of observing and reflecting, while at work with the scalpel and the microscope, is of far greater importance to the student than memorizing the subject matter for the sake of a quiz, an examination, or some subsequent clinical study. This attitude of mind is acquired only when the work has in it the spirit of research; and this kind of work is stimulated to the greatest extent when the teachers are investigators, i.e., when they are students also. Students who are thus trained are prepared to study — and in all probability will study — the cases brought before them with care and intelligence. A few of them who possess the necessary ability, zeal, and endurance, will contribute to medical knowledge. On the other hand, if the student attempts only to learn and to do the useful, he is very likely to become an empiric and get into ruts. The dif-

ference between him and a scientific physician is that the theories of the former rest upon a small collection of individual observations and a chaotic mass of reminiscences, while those of the latter rest upon the scientific investigation and experience of many minds during many centuries.

It was this type of argument—that the teacher should be an investigator and should have his full attention directed toward his students and his research without the distractions of private practice—which Mall presented in his advocacy of full-time clinical professorships.

In 1910, Mr. Rockefeller's advisor, F. T. Gates, invited Abraham Flexner to lunch. Flexner had just completed his Report on Medical Education, in which he had indicated that the Johns Hopkins Medical School was a model institution and that other schools would do well to emulate it. In the course of the conversation over the lunch table, Gates asked Flexner what he would do if he had a million dollars with which to make a start in reorganizing medical education in the United States. Flexner replied without hesitation that he would give the money to Dr. Welch to spend. Gates then asked Flexner whether he would be able to devote a few weeks to making a survey of the present medical situation at Johns Hopkins. Flexner agreed to do this, and during the academic year 1910–1911 he went to Baltimore. One day during the course of his survey Welch invited him to dinner. The other guests were Mall and Halsted. During the meal Flexner told about his conversation with Gates and asked what the Hopkins would do with this large sum of money. Mall replied: "If the school could get the sum of approximately $1 million, in my judgment there is only one thing that we ought to do with it—use every penny of its income for the purpose of placing upon a salary basis the heads and assistants in the leading clinical departments. That is the great reform which needs now to be carried through." Though Welch appeared to be noncommittal on this subject, Flexner was deeply impressed by Mall's statement (Penfield, 1967).

By this time Flexner had left the Carnegie Foundation and had become a member of the staff of the General Education Board, where he was virtually in charge of all medical affairs. A short time after his return to New York from Baltimore, the General Education Board offered Johns Hopkins a million dollars for the purpose Mall had described. For two years Welch deliberated over whether to accept the money; he did not like to have the General Education Board dictate how the money was to be used. Furthermore, he had discussed the establishment of full-time clinical professorships with his colleagues at Hopkins and had found that although the preclinical professors were in favor of such a move, the clinical faculty was divided in its attitude. After two years of cogitation Welch proposed that the full-time scheme be tried on an experimental basis in a single clinical department. He therefore asked the General Education Board, in 1919, for an endowment to provide an annual income of $15,000 for a new Pediatrics Department, including a full-time salary for the Professor of Pediatrics. Flexner, who believed that the principle should be more broadly applied, opposed Welch's request, and it was rejected by the General Education Board.

Mall continued to be active behind the scenes. In a letter written to his

171

friend Charles Minot (1911), who had just retired as Professor of Anatomy at Harvard, he said in part (Sabin, 1934):

> *We are also thinking of reform in medical education, but of the hospital side. The problem would be easy if the pork barrel were removed. Its removal would no doubt remove the exploiting medical professor and open the way for the real university professor of medicine. . . . It falls to us to demand of the last two years of medicine what they demanded of the first two and I think that the day of reckoning is at hand.*

Welch's request for an endowment for the establishment of a new full-time Department of Pediatrics (cited above) is of particular interest. Prior to 1905 the Hopkins Hospital had had a small Children's Ward and a Dispensary for Children, both of which were operated as part of the Department of Medicine under Osler's supervision. In the summer of 1905, when the hospital was having financial dificulties, the Children's Ward was closed, and it was not reopened because the hospital Trustees were then entering into an agreement to have the *Harriet Lane Home for Invalid Children,* a recently created institution, constructed on the grounds of the hospital. With the new children's hospital in the offing, the university decided, in 1906, to establish a separate Department of Pediatrics and to appoint a Professor of Pediatrics who would also serve as Physician-in-Chief of the Harriet Lane Home. In 1908, Clemens von Pirquet was appointed to this professorship. Von Pirquet was then on the pediatrics staff of the University of Vienna and was internationally recognized as an authority on acquired hypersensitivity, to which he had given the name "allergy." In February, 1909, von Pirquet and his family moved to Baltimore, where he remained for over a year, planning his new department and helping to design the layout of the Harriet Lane Home. In 1910 he was granted leave-of-absence to return to Germany to serve (temporarily?) as Professor of Pediatrics at the University of Breslau.

After several months it became apparent that von Pirquet had developed misgivings about returning to Baltimore, his objection being that the professorship was not "on a university basis." In order to remove this objection, Ira Remsen (then President of the University), in January, 1911, wrote von Pirquet a letter which set forth the first offer of a full-time clinical professorship at Hopkins. Since the terms of the offer are of considerable interest in the light of what was to follow, they are worthy of quotation (Chesney, 1963):

> *A yearly salary of $7,500 on condition that you devote yourself entirely to the care of hospital patients (both free and pay), teaching and investigation, and do not engage in private practice. . . . You will have absolute control over the admission of a specified number of free patients, the power of veto in the choice of head nurses, a specified budget for laboratory and teaching purposes, a small petty cash account, and . . . practically free choice of all your upper assistants.*
>
> *Such a position would make you eligible for a Carnegie pension, which would provide for you and your wife after retirement.*
>
> *In order to make possible for the payment of so large a salary, which will be the largest thus far paid to any professor in the University, you and your assistants will be expected to supervise the treatment of all private patients admitted to the*

172

Children's Hospital with the understanding that whatever fees are paid for such services will go into the Treasury of the Hospital and not to you.

Naturally, the pecuniary returns from such an arrangement may be much less than if you engaged in private or consulting practice; but, on the other hand, there will be certain compensations, such as uninterrupted time for work, greater facility for investigation, a regular income and finally a retiring pension.

We hope that arrangements may ultimately be made which will enable us to put the heads of the other main departments of the Hospital upon a similar basis. If this is done, the maximum salary will probably be $10,000 a year, in which you would naturally share. Even if such an arrangement does not prove feasible, we should look forward to advancing your salary to that figure, whenever the fees from pay patients in your department become sufficiently large to justify such an expenditure.

In further negotiations von Pirquet made it known that he would accept the terms of the offer provided the salary were raised to $10,000 per year. In the meantime he had been offered the highly desirable professorship of pediatrics at the Imperial University of Vienna. It was at this stage, in hopes of being able to meet von Pirquet's salary requirement, that Welch applied to the General Education Board for an endowment sufficient to produce an annual income of $15,000. In his application Welch said, "It is something of a surprise that he [von Pirquet] is willing to relinquish the leading chair of pediatrics in the world to come to Hopkins, but he was most favorably impressed with the general spirit and environment here and especially with the high class of our students." Welch's application was refused, and since the university was unable to meet von Pirquet's demands it was decided in July, 1912, to look elsewhere for a Professor of Pediatrics.

JOHNS
HOPKINS
LEADS THE WAY

There continued to be objections to the full-time scheme on the part of some of the members of the Hopkins clinical faculty, but in October, 1913, with the approval of the Advisory Board of the medical faculty and with the approval of the boards of Trustees of the university and hospital, Welch wrote to the General Education Board, requesting an endowment of sufficient size to support three full-time clinical professorships, in medicine, surgery, and pediatrics. He provided estimates of the funds needed to bring about this program. The General Education Board promptly approved a grant of $1.5 million, which was the sum needed to provide the income requested by Welch.

The reaction of the medical press to this event was mixed. Some thought it was a tremendous move forward, while others regarded it as a doubtful experiment. The powerful Journal of the AMA started out by declaring that full-time appointments "will not only elevate the standards of clinical instruction but also develop a more extensive research along the line of clinical medicine leading to a wider application of new discoveries in the treatment of disease." However, within a year the editors of the Journal had changed their minds and began to publish a series of attacks on what they termed "the Hopkins plan," contending that first-class clinicians could not

173

be expected to make the financial sacrifice of accepting university salaries. The Council on Medical Education of the AMA took a hostile attitude toward this new departure. Adverse criticism also came from distinguished members of the medical profession and from leaders in general education such as President Eliot of Harvard. Though Harvard refused to accept the scheme, two of its teaching hospitals, the Massachusetts General and the Peter Bent Brigham, adopted a less costly plan which became known as "geographic full-time." Under the latter arrangement the clinical professor derived part of his income from a salary that depended upon the amount of time he was able to devote to his teaching activities and part from patients' fees, on which a ceiling was set.

Welch felt that the best way to confound his critics was to make a success of the full-time scheme. Two of the professors in the departments to which the Rockefeller endowment was to apply, Halsted in Surgery and Howland in Pediatrics, readily accepted full-time status. However, Barker in Medicine, who had done so much to bring about this change, found that by the time the event actually occurred he was too heavily involved in practice to accept a full-time position. After Barker declined the full-time professorship it was offered to William S. Thayer, who also declined it. Finally the position was offered to Theodore C. Janeway, who was then Professor of Medicine at The College of Physicians and Surgeons in New York. Janeway accepted the offer and took up his new duties in Baltimore in July, 1914. The fact that so distinguished a physician would accept the professorship at Hopkins served to refute one of the main arguments of the critics of the full-time system: that the best qualified physicians would not be willing to work on a full-time basis.

Janeway's acceptance enhanced the prestige of the full-time movement,

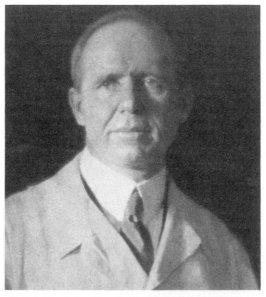

Figure 42. John Howland. (From Riesman, David (ed.): History of the Interurban Clinical Club. Philadelphia, The John C. Winston Company, 1937.)

but it remained for *John Howland,* the new Professor of Pediatrics, to prove what could be accomplished by a full-time clinical department. Howland was appointed to the professorship in July, 1912, after it had been decided that it would be impossible to meet von Pirquet's demands. Howland accepted the position at a salary of $4000 per year without any restrictions on private practice. However, from the very first Howland made it known that he favored a full-time arrangement, and he was, therefore, delighted when it was announced that the grant from the General Education Board would make this possible.

John Howland was 39 years old at the time of his appointment. A graduate of Yale, he received an M.D. degree from the New York University Medical College in 1897; but not being satisfied with his education there, he matriculated at the Cornell Medical College while working as an intern at the Presbyterian Hospital, and he received a second M.D. degree from Cornell in 1899. After serving as a resident at the Foundling Hospital (New York), he spent two years abroad, chiefly in Berlin and Vienna, studying pediatrics and pathology. He returned to New York in 1902 and became associated in practice with the nation's most prominent pediatrician, L. Emmett Holt. He also held several hospital appointments, taught at The College of Physicians and Surgeons, and finally became Chief of the Pediatrics Clinic at Bellevue Hospital. In 1910 he was called to the chair of Pediatrics at Washington University, St. Louis, the position he held at the time of his appointment at Hopkins.

Howland was enthusiastic about the opportunity afforded in Baltimore. During his first year at his new post he summed up the uniqueness of the situation (Chesney, 1963):

> *The affiliation of the Harriet Lane Home with the University marks a distinct advance in pediatrics in America. There has been up to the present time, hardly any satisfactory arrangement between universities or medical schools and children's hospitals. The condition of affairs is in marked contrast to that obtaining on the continent of Europe, especially in Germany . . . [where] the children's hospitals have not been isolated institutions but have been part of the large [university] hospital systems. . . .*
>
> *This favorable system is the one which has been adopted here. The staff of instruction of the University is the medical staff of the [Harriet Lane] Home and the Home itself is part of the Hopkins Hospital. The establishment of this system can only work for good, and must serve as an example for other institutions to follow.*

After 1913 Howland and his principal assistants all worked on a full-time basis, and the amount of first-rate research that they carried out, both in patients and in experimental animals, was prodigious. They concentrated particularly on the chemical manifestations of disease such as the acidosis associated with intestinal disturbances in children; the calcium and phosphorus metabolism in relation to tetany and rickets and to the normal growth of bone; and water and electrolyte metabolism in a variety of conditions. In order to keep his staff constantly aware of the practical problems arising in the care of sick infants and children, Howland insisted that all of his assistants devote at least half of their time to work on the wards and in the outpatient department. Perhaps it was this awareness of the practical that made so much of the work of the Pediatrics Department therapeutically productive.

175

Howland remained as head of the department from 1912 until his sudden and unexpected death from an intestinal hemorrhage while he was traveling in Europe in 1926. During those years he trained many residents and assistants who became leaders in the field of pediatrics: W. McKim Marriot, Professor of Pediatrics at Washington University; Edwards A. Park, who moved to the chair of pediatrics at Yale and then back to Hopkins as Howland's successor; Wilburt C. Davison, Professor of Pediatrics, Dean and organizer of the Duke University Medical School; Kenneth D. Blackfan, who occupied successively the chairs of pediatrics at the University of Cincinnati and at Harvard; James L. Gamble, the only member of Howland's staff finally to be given permission to devote his full time to work in the chemical laboratory and who became Professor of Pediatrics at Harvard; Grover F. Powers, Professor of Pediatrics at Yale; L. Emmett Holt, Jr., Professor of Pediatrics at New York University; A. Ashley Weech, Professor of Pediatrics at the University of Cincinnati; and others.

Turner (1974) says that "in his appeal to students, Howland seems to have filled the gap left by Osler. According to Davison, 'He was generally regarded by students as the best teacher at Hopkins.'" Further, according to Davison (Turner, 1974):

It was the reputation of Howland's department which made many educators realize that the full-time idea was sound. He was eminently qualified for the task; an able administrator, clinician, teacher, investigator, as well as a leader. He modernized pediatrics, and established a clinic, the Harriet Lane Home, which was a model from the points of view of administration, medical care, teaching and research, and spirit for those that sprang up in other medical schools. It was known all over the world, and in this country and abroad was extensively copied.

Within a few months of the apparent success of the Hopkins venture, other medical schools began to apply to the General Education Board for money to establish full-time clinical departments. Funds for this purpose were granted to Yale University and the University of Chicago; but of particular importance was the allocation of funds to Washington University in St. Louis, the University of Rochester, New York, Vanderbilt University in Nashville, and the University of Iowa. The grants to the medical schools of these institutions enabled them to attain superior status.

WASHINGTON UNIVERSITY

Robert S. Brookings, who became President of Washington University in 1905, had succeeded, in 1906, in making the University assume control and financial responsibility for the medical school, which prior to that time had operated on a proprietary basis. Following this, improvements were effected in faculty and facilities. In spite of these improvements, when Abraham Flexner visited Washington University in 1909 during the course of his survey, he "found the school a little better than the worst I had seen elsewhere, but absolutely inadequate in every essential respect" (Flexner, 1910). At about this time Brookings was negotiating with the Barnes Hospital and the St. Louis Children's Hospital with the view to establishing better facilities for clinical instruction. When Flexner wrote his report in

176

1910 he stated, "There is abundant evidence to indicate that those interested in Washington University appreciate its 'manifest destiny'; it bids fair shortly to possess faculty, laboratories, and hospitals conforming in every respect to ideal standards." He noted that "the close affiliation which has been made with the trustees of the Barnes and the Children's Hospitals revolutionizes the clinical situation of the school." In January, 1914, Brookings applied to the General Education Board for a grant to establish full-time clinical departments. In that year the Board made a grant of $750,000 (increased to $1 million in 1916), to which $500,000 was added by local donors to create an endowment of $1.5 million for full-time clinical departments in medicine, surgery, and pediatrics. The full-time departments did not actually get under way until after World War I (Robinson, 1957). It is significant that the three full-time professorships were accepted by able and distinguished men: George Dock in Medicine, Evarts Graham in Surgery, and William McK. Marriot in Pediatrics. The high tradition established by these men has continued throughout subsequent years.

VANDERBILT
UNIVERSITY

Vanderbilit University started its career under the auspices of the Southern Methodist Church, but it acquired a new govering body and a new name in the 1870s when Cornelius Vanderbilt, one of the "robber barons" who came into prominence after the Civil War, gave it $1 million to erect new buildings and to improve its faculty. In the course of the next decade Vanderbilt became recognized as the leading university of the South. Its medical school, however, continued to function as an old-fashioned lecture-course school under the proprietorship of its faculty. When young James H. Kirkland, who had received his higher education in Germany, became Chancellor of the University in 1893, he took steps almost immediately to bring the medical school under the control of the university. The course of study was lengthened to three years; the curriculum was graded; laboratory work in chemistry and bacteriology was required; and a dispensary was opened for clinical teaching. In 1899 the medical course was lengthened to four years with terms of seven months each, and students' fees were increased to provide additional funds. Since there was no endowment income, the faculty was dependent for its remuneration on student fees, and these had to be shared with the university to defray the cost of operation. In his 1910 report Flexner stated that he considered the Vanderbilt school, which then had an enrollment of 200 students, to have good prospects but that it still was not a good school. "No instructor," he said, "devotes entire time to the medical department." He noted that the income from fees amounted to $26,250 but that "this sum, adequate to provide fair laboratory instruction, is not devoted to education alone. The medical department, although organically part of the university, is under contract to wipe out with its fees the cost of the building it occupies, and meanwhile it pays the university interest at 6 per cent on the unpaid balance. . . . The school has converted the basement of its own building into a ward of 35 beds."

Flexner stated that Tennessee, with nine medical colleges, had "more low-grade medical schools than any other Southern state." Of the nine schools, six were for white students and three for black. Flexner recom-

177

mended that all of the schools be closed except Vanderbilt for white students and Meharry for black. (Of the seven medical schools for black students then operating in the United States, Flexner believed that only Howard in Washington, D.C., and Meharry in Nashville were worthy of being retained.)

Kirkland started immediately to try to overcome some of the shortcomings pointed out by Flexner. A contribution from William K. Vanderbilt enabled him to acquire new grounds for the medical school, and in 1913 the Carnegie Foundation contributed $1 million of which $200,000 was for a new laboratory building and $800,000 for endowment. Even with the improvements made possible by these gifts the school still fell short of Chancellor Kirkland's ideal. He wanted to have a school of the very highest standards. He aroused the interest of Dr. Buttrick, who was then President of the General Education Board, and of Abraham Flexner, who was then its Secretary, in developing a model medical school for the South. In 1919 the General Education Board granted the Vanderbilt Medical School $4 million, giving the following as its reasons for doing so (Robinson, 1957):

1. Not a single medical school in the entire South possesses the facilities or the personnel needed to train men to meet existing conditions or to carry on the research by means of which unsolved health problems may be ultimately mastered.

2. The strategic point for the development of such a school is Nashville, because it is situated well in the heart of the South.

3. Vanderbilt University has played a leading part in creating and maintaining scholarly standards in the South; and, finally, and perhaps most important of all, the Chancellor of Vanderbilt University, Dr. Kirkland, has the vision, energy and leadership which are required in the launching and development of an enterprise involving the establishment of a modern school of medicine.

Kirkland chose *G. Canby Robinson* to reorganize the school and to serve as its first Dean. Robinson had graduated from the Johns Hopkins Medical School in 1903; had served at the Pennsylvania Hospital from 1903 to 1908, successively as intern, laboratory worker, and Resident Physician; had spent one year in Germany working under Professor Friedrich Müller in Munich; and then had practiced medicine in Philadelphia for a year. In 1910 he went to New York to become the first Senior Resident Physician at the Rockefeller Hospital under Rufus Cole. While there, he carried out some of the earliest work in electrocardiography in this country. From 1913 to 1920 he was on the medical faculty of Washington University, St. Louis, and he was Dean of that faculty during the period when the full-time clinical departments were being organized. Though Robinson received his appointment at Vanderbilt in 1920 and immediately became involved in planning a new medical school there, he did not actually assume his position as Dean until 1925. In the interval he traveled extensively in the United States and Europe, visiting medical schools and hospitals. For part of this time he also served as Acting Physician-in-Chief of the Johns Hopkins Hospital during the period immediately following Theodore Janeway's untimely death (Robinson, 1957).

Soon after Robinson's appointment he and Kirkland decided that the existing medical school buildings, which were located two miles from the

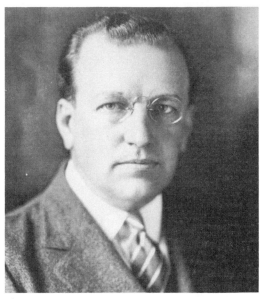

Figure 43.   G. Canby Robinson. (From the Archives Office, The Johns Hopkins Medical Institutions.)

university campus, should be abandoned and that a new building complex for the school should be constructed on the main campus. In his planning, Robinson was aiming high, and he soon came to the conclusion that the money available in the grants from the Carnegie Foundation and the General Education Board was not adequate to build and support the type of medical school that he had in mind. Therefore an appeal was made for more funds in 1921, in response to which the Carnegie Foundation and the General Education Board each contributed an additional $1.5 million. These grants were to be used to build the medical school buildings, the laboratories, and a 208-bed teaching hospital, all on the main university campus. All other funds, amounting to about $5 million, were reserved as a medical school endowment.

After a long delay, the hospital was opened in 1925, and the medical school moved to its new site on the university campus. As planned, the school began to operate with the faculty of its major clinical departments as well as all of its preclinical departments on a full-time basis. As at Hopkins and at Washington University, it was possible to fill these positions with highly qualified persons. Within a few years this school became recognized as one of the outstanding medical schools of the nation.

UNIVERSITY OF ROCHESTER   The University of Rochester, like Washington and Vanderbilt universities, has a history that goes back to the mid-nineteenth century, but it had no medical school prior to the 1920s. The university was founded as a Baptist college in 1850, but by the end of the century it was no longer under denominational control. Rush Rhees, who became President of the college in

1900, was determined to raise it to the level of a true university. At the same time, George Eastman, whose Kodak Company was the leading industry of Rochester, was determined to "make Rochester the best place in the country to live in," and with some urging from President Rhees he gave the university a large sum of money to establish a university School of Music. A few years later, the ubiquitous Abraham Flexner was responsible for suggesting that the university should also have a School of Medicine.

When Flexner became Secretary of the General Education Board in 1917, he decided that a first-rate university medical school ought to be established in upstate New York. He chose the University of Rochester as a suitable place for such an institution because he believed that President Rhees possessed the leadership to do the job. Rhees, he said, belonged "to the small group of eminent administrators who have carefully defined their objectives and who have by substantial educational success won the confidence and esteem of all critical students of higher education in America." In Flexner's opinion Rochester presented "an opening for the foundation of a medical school of the highest character." He was aware of the fact that President Rhees had won the confidence of George Eastman and other prominent citizens of Rochester and that it might be possible to raise funds locally to match a substantial grant from the General Education Board.

Flexner had several meetings with Rhees and Eastman, as a result of which Eastman agreed to contribute $5 million and the General Education Board agreed to provide a like sum for the establishment of a School of Medicine and Dentistry. (The "Dentistry" was added at the suggestion of Eastman). The announcement of the two gifts was made in June, 1920.

On the recommendation of Welch and Simon Flexner it was decided to invite the pathologist George H. Whipple to become the Dean and organizer of the new Rochester school. Whipple was then Director of the Hooper Foundation and Dean of the University of California Medical School at Berkeley, and he declined the offer to move to Rochester. President Rhees, who was determined to get his man, boarded a train for San Francisco, saying, "I don't know when I shall get back. I am not returning until George Whipple says 'yes.' " The mission was successful in making Whipple reconsider his decision, and in July, 1921, he finally agreed to accept the appointment. From then on, Whipple, with the ready support of President Rhees and the Trustees of the university, was responsible for selecting the site for the medical school, approving the plans for the buildings, and choosing the faculty for the school (Corner, 1963).

An unusual feature of the arrangements at Rochester came about because the city was preparing to build a municipal hospital at the same time that the university was planning to build the Strong Memorial Hospital as an integral part of the medical school. Owing to the combined efforts of Rhees, Whipple, Eastman, and Dr. George Goler, head of the Rochester Health Department, the city agreed to construct the new Municipal Hospital alongside the Strong Memorial Hospital and to put its medical services in complete charge of the university. According to the agreement, the Strong Memorial would provide operating rooms, diagnostic laboratories, X-ray service, pharmacy, and other special services for the patients at the Municipal Hospital. Both hospitals would be available for the clinical instruction of the students. Plans were also made to move the city Public Health Laboratory into the medical school, to be operated under the supervision of the Professor of Bacteriology. Abraham Flexner considered these cooperative arrangements between the city of Rochester and the university to be "one of the most helpful steps ever taken in this country in the direction of financing medical education on a high basis and with adequate facilities. If the other municipalities of the United States will imitate the City of Rochester we can hope to build up clinics equal to those of the great European cities."

Flexner also must have been pleased with the decision of Rhees and Whipple to place the faculty of the medical school, both preclinical and clinical, on a full-time university salary basis. As in the two schools previously mentioned, Whipple succeeded in recruiting a fine young faculty. The original heads of the departments were as follows: George W. Corner, Anatomy; Walter R. Bloor, Biochemistry; Stanhope Bayne-Jones, Bacteriology; Wallace O. Fenn, Physiology; George H. Whipple, Pathology; William S. McCann, Medicine; John J. Morton, Surgery; Karl M. Wilson, Obstetrics and Gynecology; Samuel W. Clausen, Pediatrics; and Nathaniel W. Faxon, Director of the Strong Memorial Hospital. Rhees and Whipple were criticized for having assembled what appeared to some to be a "junior Johns Hopkins faculty." It is true that five of the department heads were Johns Hopkins graduates (Whipple, Corner, Bayne-Jones, Morton, and Clausen), but only Bayne-Jones had spent his entire professional career at Hopkins. Two others, McCann and Wilson, had received part of their training at Hopkins and had served on the Hopkins faculty. In commenting on this matter, Corner said: "It would have been difficult to find in the medical world ten young men equipped, as a group, with so broad an acquaintance with the best of American and British medicine and biology."

UNIVERSITY
OF IOWA

The first large grant of Rockefeller funds to a state university occurred when the General Education Board and the Rockefeller Foundation jointly contributed $2,250,000 to the medical school of the University of Iowa. This school had been established in 1869, and in 1910 Flexner considered it to be above average in that it had full-time teachers of the basic medical sciences and that it was given relatively generous financial support by the state. At the same time, its clinical faculty and hospital facilities were considered to be very inadequate. In 1923 the university applied for a Rockefeller grant to enable the medical school to move to a new location where a teaching hospital and other facilities could be built. The state legislature had been unwilling to appropriate the large sum that was needed to make this move. Mr. Gates strongly opposed giving any Rockefeller support to state universities. He considered them to be "creatures of politics" and apparently was unaware of the liberal influences that were elevating some of the state universities to new heights of excellence. Abraham Flexner, on the other hand, was more in touch with educational developments. He took the point of view that the United States was fortunate in having two types of university—one supported by private funds, the other by state funds—which encouraged competition and made it possible to escape bureaucratic uniformity. "We are trying," he said, "to aid in the development of a country-wide, high-grade system of [medical] education in the United States. If we confine our cooperation to endowed institutions, we can practically cooperate only in the East" (Fosdick, 1952). Flexner's argument was the more persuasive, and the large grant was made to the University of Iowa Medical School, thus enabling it to change its location, build new buildings, pay full-time salaries to some of its clinical professors, and become one of the leading medical schools of the Middle West.

During the years 1913 to 1929 the General Education Board made substantial grants to the medical schools of many different universities, including Harvard, Columbia, Cornell, Tulane, Western Reserve, Rochester, Emory, University of Colorado, University of Oregon, University of Virginia, University of Georgia, and University of Cincinnati. Some of these grants were for special purposes, but most of them were to enable the institution to establish full-time clinical departments in one or more disciplines. Some of the grants were given under the condition that the institutions concerned would raise locally an equal amount of money for the same purpose.

With respect to these grants, the following is quoted from Raymond B. Fosdick's *The Story of the Rockefeller Foundation* (1952):

Surveying the General Education Board's experience in medical education over the decade and a half (1913–1929) in which the program was in active operation, it is evident that "full-time" was the point upon which opinion continued to be sharply divided. Undoubtedly, insistence on university standards for clinical departments served to swing the pendulum away from low and timid educational practices. It did more. It helped swing the whole movement for improved medical training into top-flight effort. At the same time there were those who felt that insistence on strict full-time was an unjustified intrusion on university policy.

In reviewing the efforts of the General Education Board to establish full-time departments, Alan Gregg (Director of Medical Sciences of the Rockefeller Foundation) made the following three points in 1950 (Fosdick, 1952):

(1) By its emphasis on planned professional teamwork, full-time clinical teaching has paved the way for an important form of practice today, group practice, with its economical use of costly diagnostic and therapeutic machines and instruments. (2) By diminishing the obligation of young professors, while teaching, to build up an extensive local private practice, the full-time system has opened to them a much larger choice of posts over the country, and has thus favored the growth, advancement and dissemination of able young men. Entire regions of the country can benefit from talent that otherwise would have stayed in Eastern Metropolitan Centers. (3) Few, if any, young men trained in full-time departments would now vote for the part-time teaching system, and what young men prefer has vitality for the future.

Since its early days the full-time system has spread and has become a standard feature of many of the leading medical schools. There is no longer any doubt that a full-time faculty is an absolute necessity for the basic medical science departments; moreover, it is difficult to see how the clinical

182

departments, which have everywhere grown in size and complexity, can be administered successfully by a professor who devotes anything less than full time to his job. Nevertheless, it can be argued that clinical instruction has suffered under the full-time system. According to Kubie (1971), Alan Gregg, who was one of its strongest advocates in the 1930s and 1940s, "came to dread many of the consequences . . . because he foresaw clearly how the tendency to appoint non-clinical scientists or immature clinicians to lead clinical departments would make unattainable the great goals which the full-time system had envisaged." And he deplored "the fact that older, part-time clinicians were being squeezed out of our medical faculties." Although the heads of clinical departments may have been relieved of the need to earn a living by caring for private patients, much of their time, which might otherwise be devoted to teaching, is now devoted instead to administrative duties, to supervising research activities in their departments, to attending committee meetings, to acting as advisors and panelists for the National Institutes of Health and other agencies, and to traveling to other cities and other medical centers to give lectures and attend meetings. These are important duties, and some senior person must attend to them, but at the same time there must be provision for the instruction of students and for someone to emphasize, by mature personal example, the need for continuous, sympathetic care of patients. This can probably best be provided by the part-time staff whose experience in, and enthusiasm for, the care of the patient can be an inspiration to the student.

OTHER MEDICAL SCHOOLS WITH GENEROUS BENEFACTORS

In addition to the medical schools that enjoyed the benefactions of the Rockefellers, there were several top-flight schools—including those of Stanford University and Duke University—which came into being as a result of the generosity of private benefactors. In the states of the Pacific Coast at the time of Flexner's report there were 11 medical schools—9 in California and 2 in Oregon. Of the schools in Oregon, Flexner said, "Neither of these schools has either resources or ideals; there is no justification for their existence." Of the nine schools in California, two were osteopathic, one was homeopathic, and one was eclectic. Flexner considered all of these schools and three of the five regular medical schools to be very inadequate, and one of them he characterized as "a disgrace to the state whose laws permit its existence." For the medical school of the University of California Flexner had some rare words of praise. Its entrance requirement of two years' college work was "strictly enforced." The school had a four-year medical curriculum, the first two years being conducted at Berkeley by full-time teachers and, said Flexner, "The equipment and instruction are of the highest quality." The students could elect to take their two clinical years in either San Francisco or Los Angeles; at both of these locations there were hospitals under university control. Flexner thought that the clinical facilities were inadequate and that the instruction, provided by local practitioners, was no better than average.

STANFORD
UNIVERSITY
The second California medical school in which Flexner saw some merit was that of Stanford University. This school was then in the process of moving up to a university level. Here an advance in medical education had been made possible by the philanthropy of a man of great wealth. Leland Stanford, the founder of the university, had acquired his fortune as a promoter of transcontinental railroads. The history of the institution that became the medical school of Stanford University extended back more than half a century. It had its start in 1858 as the Medical Department of the University of the Pacific and was first housed in the top floor of Dr. Elias Samuel Cooper's office in San Francisco. In 1882 this school was replaced by the Cooper Medical College under the guidance of Dr. Levi Cooper Lane, who personally provided the funds for the construction of a new school building. In 1894 the Lane Hospital, adjoining the medical school, was built with funds again provided by Dr. Lane. In 1908 David Starr Jordan, the President of Stanford University, who was himself a physician, persuaded the Board of Trustees to add a medical school to the university. A preclinical faculty of full-time professors was established at the university campus in Palo Alto, and the Cooper School and Lane Hospital in San Francisco were acquired to provide a center for the clinical instruction of students in their third and fourth years. With one exception the original clinical faculty were all part-time local practitioners who had served on the faculty of the Cooper School. The one exception was the Professor of Clinical Medicine, Ray Lyman Wilbur, who was destined to become a national leader of the medical profession, President of the American Medical Association, President of Stanford University, and Secretary of the Interior in President Herbert Hoover's cabinet.

An early addition to the preclinical faculty at Palo Alto was Hans Zinsser, Stanford's first professor of Bacteriology, who served in this capacity from 1910 to 1913. Zinsser, a brilliant teacher and investigator, subsequently moved on to head the departments of Bacteriology, successively, at Columbia and Harvard universities. Years later, he recalled joyfully his three years in Palo Alto (Zinsser, 1940):

> Golden days at Stanford! Adequate equipment, small classes composed largely of men who had worked their own ways to an educcaxion, complete independence of teaching and research. Most of the faculty, indeed, a little stodgy as usual, but among them a few brilliant spirits like Stewart Young, the physical chemist; the truly great organic chemist, Ned Franklin; Angell; Branner; Stillman; Marx; and Wilbur. . . .

> We left Stanford for Columbia with regret. Happy Stanford! The lovely Santa Clara Valley, indescribably peaceful in its golden sunshine; the fragrance of blossoms from orchards; and the evening fog streaming from the big redwoods silhouetted on the crest of the coast range. Freedom for work, freedom from urban interruptions, few— but good—students, and cheap horses.

In the period between the two world wars, Stanford added many able men to its medical faculty, and its medical school became recognized as one of the best in the country. It accepted only a limited number of students, the classes being held to 60 or less. Both the preclinical and the clinical branches became involved in an increasing amount of medical research. A serious problem, which had been foreseen by Flexner in 1910, arose from the distance that separated the clinical from the preclinical departments. As the clinicians became more deeply involved in research in which they had to use complicated scientific equipment, they felt the handicap of being 30 miles away from the scientists and the fine scientific library at Palo Alto. This problem was not solved until after World War II, when the clinical departments moved from San Francisco to Palo Alto, where a new hospital, new laboratories, and other facilities had been constructed for their use.

Duke University
In 1892 Trinity College, a small Methodist institution, moved from another location to Durham, North Carolina. In 1910 William P. Few became its President, and one of his earliest objectives was to establish a medical school as part of the college. Between 1920 and 1923 he persuaded the University of North Carolina and a local hospital (Watts Hospital) to join Trinity College in organizing a new medical school. The plans for this project were discussed with Abraham Flexner, and through him President Few obtained assurances that the General Education Board would provide $3 million for construction and endowment of the proposed school. The plan failed because President Few was unable to obtain the necessary local backing. North Carolinians could not agree as to where a new medical school should be located. Some thought that Durham (population, about 40,000) was too small to support a medical institution; some thought the funds should be used to expand the existing two-year school at Chapel Hill to a four-year school; some feared that if the school were made part of Trinity College it would be brought under sectarian control. As a result of these disagreements, the General Education Board withdrew from participation in the project. Perhaps in the end this was fortunate, for President Few, who had tried unsuccessfully for several years to arouse the interest of James B. Duke in his plan, renewed his effort in 1924, this time with success beyond his fondest hopes.

Shortly after the Civil War, Duke, who was then in his teens, had joined his father and brother in the manufacture and distribution of *Duke's Mixture,* a blend of the tobaccos grown in the vicinity of Durham. The Duke organization grew rapidly in size and wealth, and in 1890 it was incorporated as the American Tobacco Company. By 1920 Duke had accumulated a huge fortune and was beginning to consider ways of employing his wealth for the benefit of the people of North Carolina. In December, 1924, after discussions with President Few, the *Duke Endowment* was created, and Duke turned over to the Trustees of the *Endowment* a large part of his fortune, directing that some of the fund be used to establish a university and some to provide "adequate and convenient hospitals" to serve the people of rural districts. It was stipulated that $10 million was to be devoted to the university, and that of this sum $4 million was to be expended for a medical school, hospital, and nurses' home at the university. During the month in which the *Endowment* was established the name of Trinity College was changed to Duke University and the Trustees set about making plans for

185

what Duke had hopefully predicted would be "the best medical center between Baltimore and New Orleans" (Davison, 1966).

In 1927 President Few chose as Dean of the medical school Wilburt C.
Davison, a pediatrician who was then Assistant Dean of the Johns Hopkins
Medical School. Davison was responsible for overseeing the construction of
the medical school and hospital and for selecting the medical faculty. The
hospital opened in July, 1930, and the medical school three months later.
Within a few years the Duke Medical Center had gained recognition as one
of the country's outstanding institutions. In some activities it was a pioneer: (1) It developed working relations with the small hospitals and medical
practitioners in the surrounding rural communites, and it concentrated on
training physicians to work in such communities. Prior to World War II, 40
per cent of the Duke medical graduates became family doctors. (2) It was the
first medical school to offer a course in hospital administration. (3) It established the first hospital blood bank. (4) It was involved in the development of the first surviving statewide Blue Cross plan (Davison, 1966).

CONCLUSION   The admission requirements and the curriculum
in most medical schools had settled on the Hop-
kins model by 1925. There was relatively little change in this pattern until
after World War II except for internal revisions in courses to keep abreast of
developments. The vast increase in information made it necessary in most
schools to devote more curricular hours to required work and less to electives.

12

Medical Research

I have been asked on more than one occasion what have been the really great contributions of this country to medical knowledge. I have given this matter some thought and think that four should be named: 1) The discovery of anesthesia. 2) The discovery of insect transmission of disease. 3) The development of the modern public health laboratory, in all that the term implies. 4) The Army Medical Library and its Index Catalogue, and this library and its catalogue are the most important of the four.

(William H. Welch)

In the last quarter of the nineteenth century, medical science in the United States lagged far behind that in Europe. The great surge forward in bacteriology that had been led by Pasteur and Koch was involving more and more European laboratory workers, whereas almost no one in the United States had participated in the advance. The scientific education of most American physicians was so deficient and their knowledge of microscopy and other laboratory methods so limited that they could not evaluate or even understand the discoveries that were being reported from France and Germany. It was only as the system of education underwent change and the faculties of the medical schools started to focus their attention upon the basic scientific structure of medicine that Americans began to contribute to the building of the structure.

As the second century opened, some of the university medical schools permitted a few faculty members to engage in research on a small scale without actually giving them much financial support. Harvard and Yale established new laboratories and encouraged special studies in physiology and physiological chemistry. The University of Michigan had a free-standing chemistry laboratory where a limited amount of research was carried on, but for the most part it was used for a rather superior type of education in chemistry. And at the University of Pennsylvania, William Pepper made use of his popularity as a physician to secure from his admirers a few small gifts to support research. With the opening of Johns Hopkins University,

187

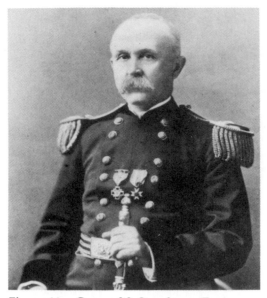

Figure 44. George M. Sternberg. (From
Sternberg, Martha L.: George M. Sternberg,
A Biography. Chicago, American Medical
Association, 1920. Copyright © 1920
American Medical Association.)

Clark University, and the University of Chicago, an orientation toward
research began to play a larger role in the selection of faculty members.
However, before the universities entered the field to any significant degree,
the groundwork for organized medical research in the United States had
been laid during and shortly after the Civil War by the United States Army
and the Department of Agriculture.

The persons principally involved in the Army's entry into medical
research were as follows: William A. Hammond, who became Surgeon-
General during the Civil War and who saw the need to promote research;
Joseph J. Woodward, whose pioneering work at the Army Medical Museum was mentioned in an earlier chapter; John Shaw Billings, who
organized the Surgeon-General's Library as a scientific resource and whose
persistent advocacy of research was largely responsible for making it an essential feature of the educational program at the Johns Hopkins Medical
School; and George Miller Sternberg, the "father of American bacteriology,"
whose systematic studies of infectious diseases attracted international attention, and who eventually, as Surgeon-General of the Army, was the
organizer of highly successful research projects including Walter Reed's
study of the transmission of yellow fever.

In 1869 the U.S. Department of Agriculture, pressed to do something to
prevent the losses caused by diseases of farm animals, invited John Gangee,
a British veterinarian, to come to Washington to study certain diseases of
cattle. The primitive state of research in this country at that time is shown
by the fact that when Gangee said that he needed a microscope, the only
one that could be found was in the Army Medical Museum. Continuing its
interest in animal diseases, the Department of Agriculture, in 1884, provided funds to create a *Bureau of Animal Industry*. It was under the auspices

of this Bureau that Theobald Smith and Daniel E. Salmon carried out their brilliant researches, which in terms of orginality and practical utility constitute America's greatest contribution of the nineteenth century to microbiology and the prevention of disease.

Basic medical research did not attract the support of wealthy philanthropists until it became apparent that it might have useful applications. This stage was reached when bacteriological research in Europe began to discover ways to prevent or cure disease. Prospective donors could then see that it might be rewarding and even exciting to fund this type of research.

During the 70s, 80s, and 90s young Americans trained in modern methods of medical research were returning home from Europe; and during this same period men of wealth were learning that medical research offered a rare opportunity for philanthropy. "This was a period when medicine, offering new hope, captivated the imagination of wealthy benefactors somewhat as religion had once done in a less secular age. Instead of building churches and monasteries, philanthropists now endowed hospitals and laboratories or set up foundations to do this for them" (Shryock, 1947b).

The conjunction of newly trained and enthusiastic investigators with newly enlightened benefactors provided the ingredients for a great leap forward in American medical research. As Henry Sigerist, the medical historian, viewed it, American medicine "rushed in a short time through all the successive stages of European development."

Nothing better exemplifies the conjunction of the scientific and fiscal forces than the founding and endowment of the *Rockefeller Institute for Medical Research.*

THE ROCKEFELLER INSTITUTE FOR MEDICAL RESEARCH

Here is an institution whose value touches the life of every man that lives.... Who has not felt the throbbing desire to be useful to the whole wide world? Here at least is a work for all humanity, which fully satisfies and fills that glorious aspiration.... Your vocation goes to the foundations of life itself.... Whatever you learn about nature and her forces and prove and incorporate into your science will be carried forward though all else be forgotten.

(Frederick T. Gates to the staff
of the Rockefeller Institute on the
tenth anniversary of the opening of the laboratories, 1914)

It may be recalled that when F. T. Gates returned to New York in 1897 after reading Osler's *Principles and Practice of Medicine,* he wrote a memorandum to Mr. Rockefeller recommending that consideration be given to establishing a medical research institute in the United States. During the next several months Gates discussed these matters at greater length with Mr. Rockefeller, Sr., and with John D. Rockefeller, Jr., who just that year had graduated from Brown University. Gates's recommendation appealed to Mr. Rockefeller, but with his usual caution in such matters he took no definite action until 1901. In the meantime, studies were made of various medical institutions in this country and abroad, and conferences were held with medical educators and researchers.

189

By 1901 Mr. Rockefeller, Sr., had decided to adopt Gates's suggestion, but he was still not convinced that the United States was ready for an institute devoted wholly to medical research. He therefore decided to proceed slowly by first offering to give $20,000 annually for at least 10 years for medical research projects and by placing in the hands of a committee of experts the arrangements for the expenditure of this money. Mr. Rockefeller asked his family physician, the distinguished pediatrician L. Emmett Holt, and another physician, Christian A. Herter, who had carried on medical research under Welch in Baltimore and who was then on the faculty of the Bellevue Medical College, to propose the names of doctors to make up the board of experts. In a letter written to Welch at about this time Herter said, "Mr. Rockefeller has expressed a strong wish that you serve on the advisory board and would be much gratified if you could see your way clear to acting as its Chairman. . . . While Mr. Rockefeller's interest in the establishment of a research laboratory is primarily humanitarian rather than scientific, I am confident that he would never allow his desire for practical results to hamper the laboratory in its direct or indirect efforts to obtain such results" (Flexner and Flexner, 1941). Welch complied with Mr. Rockefeller's request and became the first President of the Board of Directors of the Rockefeller Institute.

It was decided to postpone the establishment of a laboratory, since it was felt that for the time being, better results would be achieved by granting money for research to already existing laboratories. Grants ranging in amount from $300 to $1200 were made to individuals who became known as either research students, research scholars, or fellows of the Institute. The grants were made to Americans only, but the recipients were allowed to work in Europe as well as at home. A popular place for those who went abroad at that time was Ehrlich's laboratory in Frankfurt, Germany, which was the European center for the study of immunology and chemotherapy. The total amount of money expended for these individual grants was approximately $12,000 in 1901 and $14,450 in 1902. That these expenditures were less than the $20,000 per year which Mr. Rockefeller had offered is an indication of the lack of orientation toward research at that time.

Welch assumed almost all of the duties in getting the Rockefeller Institute started (Flexner and Flexner, 1941). He accepted no assistance, not even clerical help; every detail was attended to with his own hand, every letter handwritten. The Rockefellers were pleased by the careful, cautious manner in which Welch proceeded toward the establishment of a new laboratory. In January, 1902, he wrote to the younger Rockefeller, "I do not think the time has come to start out with a large plant with the permanent location and connections fixed, or to abandon our present plan of aiding investigations elsewhere, provided these are important, in the right field, and really need our help." He believed that before considering the establishment of a new laboratory it was necessary to have assurance that a good working staff could be secured. Most important of all was to have a topnotch scientist as Director. This position was first offered Theobald Smith, who declined because he had worked exclusively in animal pathology, and he felt that the appointment of an animal pathologist to head the Institute "might eventually arouse adverse criticism." In March, 1902, the directorship was offered to Simon Flexner, who had begun his career in medical research under

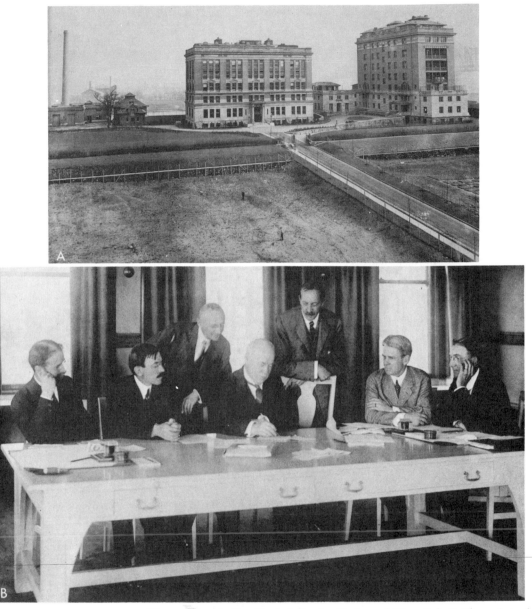

Figure 45. *A*, The Rockefeller Institute and Hospital. *B*, The original Board of Scientific Directors of the Rockefeller Institute. Left to right: Theobald Smith, Hermann M. Biggs, Simon Flexner, William H. Welch, T. Mitchell Prudden, L. Emmett Holt, Christian A. Herter. (*A*, From New York Academy of Medicine. *B*, From Corner, George W.: A History of the Rockefeller Institute. New York, Rockefeller University Press, 1964.)

Welch in Baltimore and was then Professor of Pathology at the Medical School of the University of Pennsylvania. After some delay Flexner accepted the position.

In June, 1902, Mr. Rockefeller, Sr., pledged $1 million to the Institute, to be paid out as needed over a 10-year period. In February, 1903, land was

191

purchased on the East River for a laboratory, and construction was started soon thereafter. In the fall of 1904 Flexner, who had spent a year studying biochemistry in Germany, returned to New York. The buildings on the East River still were not ready for occupancy, so a temporary laboratory was established in a converted residence. In May, 1906, the new laboratory building with its adjoining animal house and powerhouse was formally opened, and in November of the following year Mr. Rockefeller expressed his satisfaction and confidence in the new Institute by giving it $2,620,000 for a permanent endowment.

The small staff that Flexner had brought together in the original temporary laboratory consisted mostly of his friends, men whose dedication to research was known to him personally. Among them were Eugene L. Opie, a member of the first class to graduate from the Johns Hopkins Medical School, who had carried out original work on the reproduction of the malarial parasite and had written a treatise on the diseases of the pancreas; Hideyo Noguchi, who had received his medical education in Japan, had worked with Flexner at the University of Pennsylvania in pathology, and had made special studies of snake venoms; Samuel J. Meltzer, who had received his medical education and early training in physiology in Germany before coming to the United States in 1883; John Auer, who had graduated from the Johns Hopkins Medical School in 1902 and had served on the resident staff of the Johns Hopkins Hospital; and P.A. Levene, a chemist who had had excellent training in Germany before coming to the United States in 1892 and who had worked as a chemist, successively in the New York State Pathological Institute and the Saranac Tuberculosis Laboratory.

After the move into the new laboratory building, Flexner gradually began to add carefully selected individuals to the staff of the Institute. Alphonse R. Dochez, who had graduated from the Johns Hopkins Medical School in 1903 and had done some research work on the relation of iodine to the thyroid gland, joined the staff in 1906. In the same year Alexis Carrel became a member of the staff. Carrel had received his medical education in France and had come to the United States in 1905. He worked at the University of Chicago for a year before coming to New York. Peyton Rous, who joined the staff in 1909, had graduated from the Johns Hopkins Medical School in 1900 and had worked on the resident staff of the Johns Hopkins Hospital until 1906, when he became an Instructor of Pathology at the University of Michigan. Jacques Loeb, a German biologist, who had come to the United States in 1891 and had served successively on the faculties of Bryn Mawr College, the University of Chicago, and the University of California, joined the staff of the Institute in 1910.

As one looks over the background of these early members of the staff, one is struck by the fact that all of them had received their education and early training either in a foreign country or at Johns Hopkins. There is a twofold explanation for this phenomenon: (1) Flexner and his chief advisor, Welch, were familiar with the superior scientific training that was given in some of the foreign schools. (2) Medical education in the United States had been oriented toward medical practice except at the Johns Hopkins Medical School, where there had been a strong and enthusiastic emphasis on research, some of it in the basic sciences. However, the situation was

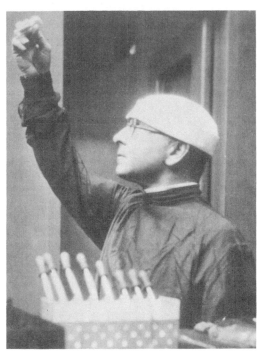

Figure 46. Alexis Carrel. (New York Academy of Medicine.)

changing rapidly as more and more schools revised their orientation. As a result, in 1910–11, when Rufus Cole was seeking out young men to carry on the research in the hospital of the Rockefeller Institute, he selected a number who had been trained at other American medical schools.

INFECTIOUS DISEASES Many diseases of man are caused by living parasites. Some of the parasites, such as the worm that produces hookworm disease and the mite that causes scabies, are visible to the unaided eye; but the parasites that are responsible for the diseases commonly classified as infectious diseases can be seen only with the aid of a microscope. These organisms are of three classes: (1) protozoa, such as the plasmodia that cause malaria and the amoebae that cause dysentery; (2) bacteria, which come in assorted sizes and shapes, including rod-shaped bacilli, spherical coccci, and spiral treponema; and (3) viruses, very minute organisms that can pass through a fine earthenware filter which holds back bacteria. Although a few of these viruses can be seen with a very high-powered light microscope, many can be seen only with an electron microscope, and some have not yet been visualized.

About 50 years ago the word *virus* acquired a new and more restricted meaning. It is an ancient Latin word which to Caesar and Cicero meant a slimy liquid or poison. According to the Oxford Dictionary, Englishmen of the eighteenth century were still using the word in this original sense: "pouring the Virus of the Asp into a wound (1702)." In 1800, it still con-

193

noted a poison but might be used to refer vaguely to the causative agent of a disease: "the pustules contain a perfect small-pox virus (1800)." In 1871 Edwin Klebs, in Germany, demonstrated that the "virus" of the disease *anthrax* (actually a bacillus) would not pass through a filter and that while the material held back by the filter would cause the disease, that which had passed through would not.

In 1892, the Russian scientist D.A. Ivanovski in the course of his studies of a disease of tobacco plants, *tobacco mosaic,* was the first to discover that a disease-producing virus could be passed through a fine filter. Six years later two German scientists, Loeffler and Frosch, demonstrated that the virus of foot-and-mouth disease of cattle could pass through the finest filter available. Walter Reed and his associates were the first to demonstrate (1901) that a major disease of man, yellow fever, is caused by a filterable virus. Subsequently, more and more diseases were found to be caused by filterable agents, but for a long time it was not known whether these were living, replicating agents or lifeless chemical substances. Gradually it was realized that filterable viruses could survive and multiply only in living cells. At first, survival of a virus could be assured only by transmitting it from one living animal to another. However, when the technique of growing cells in tissue culture (described later) had been established as a laboratory procedure, it was found that a virus would grow and multiply in the living cells of a tissue culture. This simplified the handling of viruses and was responsible for a great advance in virus research.

MICRO-ORGANISMS
AS THE CAUSE
OF DISEASE

For many decades microscopists had been observing bacteria, fungi, and other micro-organisms obtained from a variety of sources, and from time to time there had been speculation that certain diseases were caused by invisible *animalicula.* However, it was not until the 1830s that the micro-organisms and the speculation began to be brought into a meaningful association. In 1837 a Frenchman, Alexandre Donne, reported that he had seen microscopic, corkscrew-like organisms in matter taken from syphilitic chancres, and he advanced the hypothesis that the chancre was caused by the organisms. No one seemed to take his observations very seriously, and they were forgotten for three quarters of a century.

It was shortly after this (about 1844) that *Louis Pasteur* entered the field of science as a chemist. His first brilliant discovery was that tartaric acid occurs in two forms, which can be distinguished by the manner in which they rotate light. In the course of these experiments Pasteur became interested in the problem of fermentation, and he soon learned something that for a time almost no one would believe: fermentation is caused by living micro-organisms. Further, he found that different organisms (i.e., different species of yeast) produce different types of fermentation leading to the formation of different products, such as alcohol and various organic acids.

In 1863 Pasteur made a study of the spoilage of wine during storage. He found that it could be prevented or at least retarded by heating the wine to 50° C to 60° C for a few minutes and then placing it in tightly corked bottles. This procedure (which came to be known as pasteurization) prevented spoilage without affecting flavor.

Pasteur's first experience with micro-organisms as the cause of disease occurred in 1865 when he was investigating a disease of silkworms which had virtually ruined the lucrative French silk industry. He was able to demonstrate that the disease was caused by a micro-organism which infects the moth that produces the eggs from which the silkworms hatch. As a result of these studies, he was able to recommend a method by which the disease of silkworms could be prevented. But of even greater importance was the implication that this type of research, relating micro-organisms to specific diseases, might have relevance to the causes of human illness.

Pasteur suffered a stroke in 1868, which temporarily interrupted the progress of his research. During this relatively quiet period for Pasteur, Joseph Lister was investigating the hypothesis that infections of wounds are caused by micro-organisms similar to those that produce fermentation, and Robert Koch had begun his study of bacteria.

In 1876 Koch reported his epochal work on the anthrax bacillus, giving the details of how it could be grown and isolated, and how after living for several generations in a laboratory, it could still produce the disease in animals. This work aroused again Pasteur's interest in the relation of micro-organisms to disease, and within a remarkably short time he had developed a method to protect animals against anthrax. He found that this could be accomplished by injecting the animals with anthrax bacilli which had been so weakened by special treatment that they could not produce the disease, yet they could produce a state of immunity to subsequent injections with virulent anthrax bacilli. This work, which was reported in 1881, established the principle that the disease-producing properties of a micro-organism can be so attenuated that it will produce immunity without producing disease. This was, as Garrison has said, "one of the most luminous thoughts in the history of science" (Garrison, 1929). Before many years Pasteur had applied this newly discovered principle to develop a method for preventing rabies (hydrophobia) in persons bitten by rabid animals.

In the remaining years of the nineteenth century the bacteria responsible for many important diseases were discovered, including those which cause tuberculosis, cholera, typhoid fever, diphtheria, bubonic plague, cerebrospinal meningitis, lobar pneumonia, erysipelas, and gonorrhea. Americans played little part in the early discoveries in this field. However, William H. Welch, who in 1885 was largely responsible for bringing bacteriology to the United States, discovered an important bacterium, the causative agent of gas gangrene.

Though Welch was the first to offer formal instruction in bacteriology, a remarkable U.S. Army surgeon, *George M. Sternberg*, was several years ahead of him as a research bacteriologist. After the Civil War, in spite of almost constant involvement in the frontier battles with the Indians, Sternberg found time to become an expert microscopist. In 1879 he wrote a monograph on photomicrography, contributing new and ingenious methods for taking microscopic photographs. He became interested in bacteriology at an early stage in its development, and since he did not go abroad for study and had no teacher in the United States, he was in truth a self-taught bacteriologist and grew up with the new science. In 1881 he "discovered" the pneumococcus, the causative agent of lobar pneumonia, only to learn that it had been described several months earlier by Pasteur. Sternberg originally

195

found this organism in his own sputum, and he was unaware of its pathogenicity until 1885, when he "discovered" it again in the rusty sputum of a pneumonia patient. In 1881, soon after Koch described the tubercle bacillus, Sternberg was the first in America to stain and photograph it. When he learned that Welch had returned from Europe full of information about new developments in the German bacteriology laboratories, Sternberg enrolled in the first bacteriology course given in Welch's laboratory (1886). In the years that followed, Sternberg made many important contributions to the field of microbiology and was advanced to the office of Surgeon-General of the Army.

HOG CHOLERA AND TEXAS FEVER   Another major American contributor to our understanding of infectious diseases was *Theobald Smith,* who was the first to prove that a disease could be transmitted by an insect. Smith was a graduate of Cornell University (1881) and the Albany Medical College (1883). He returned to Cornell for graduate work in the Department of Physiology under Simon Henry Gage. He had been there for only a short time when Daniel E. Salmon solicited Gage's help in finding someone to assist him in a new line of research. Salmon had been chosen to organize a *Bureau of Animal Industry* within the Department of Agriculture. He expected to carry out research on some economically important diseases of cattle and hogs. Since he had to operate the Bureau on a $10,000 budget, he could not afford a salary for a well-trained, mature assistant, but he needed someone who knew

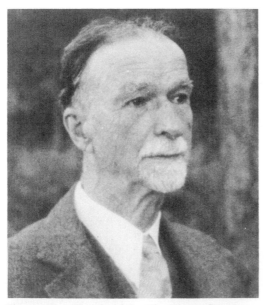

Figure 47. Theobald Smith. (From Corner, George W.: A History of the Rockefeller Institute. New York, Rockefeller University Press, 1964.)

how to use a microscope and who understood at least the rudiments of bacteriology, a science in which Salmon himself had had no training. Since his student days at Cornell, Smith had been enthusiastic about microscopes and had become proficient in using them. He had also studied German, and while at medical school he had read the reports of the bacteriological discoveries of Robert Koch and others and thus had gained some secondhand knowledge of this new science. Gage was confident that Smith had the makings of a scientific investigator; he also knew that Smith was more interested in opportunity than in salary, and he therefore recommended him to Salmon.

Smith arrived in Washington in 1884 to find that the Bureau of Animal Industry was housed in a dingy attic and that it had almost no equipment. Salmon set Smith to work on hog cholera, and in 1886 the two men together were able to report the identification of the micro-organism that causes this disease. Even more important, they were the first to discover that immunity can be conveyed by dead bacteria. Pasteur had demonstrated that immunity could be induced by attenuated but living organisms. Salmon and Smith found that pigeons, which ordinarily develop a fatal illness when injected with living cholera bacilli, could be protected from illness by being given a prior injection of killed bacilli. Utilizing this discovery, they proceeded to protect hogs against cholera by injecting them with dead cholera bacilli. For the farmer this was a highly important discovery; and 30 years later the same principle was applied on a vast scale to immunize soldiers and civilians against typhoid fever. As a result of the work on hog cholera, Salmon's name became affixed to the large and important "Salmonella" family of bacteria, which includes both the bacillus of hog cholera (*Salmonella choleraesuis*) and that of human typhoid fever (*Salmonella typhosa*).

After his very productive research on hog cholera, Smith turned his attention to a serious and widespread disease of cattle known as "Texas fever." This disease was a puzzle to cattlemen, for under some circumstances sick cattle appeared to transmit the infection to healthy cattle whereas under other circumstances sick and healthy cattle could be mixed together without evidence of transmission of the disease from one to the other. In a number of ingenious but simple experiments Smith proved that the key to the puzzle was a tick which acts as an intermediary in passing the infecting agent from sick to healthy cattle. He found that the blood that ticks sucked from the sick cattle contained the micro-organism (a protozoan) which caused the disease and that these organisms were transmitted to the next generation of ticks, which in turn carried the infection to well cattle. If ticks were not present, sick and healthy cattle could mingle with impunity. But if ticks were prevalent in the field where the cattle were mixed, the disease was transmitted from the sick to the well animals.

Smith's report of these experiments, published in 1893, is a classic. From the point of view of cattlemen, the important and practical result was that Texas fever could be eliminated by dipping cattle in a solution that would kill ticks. However, from the point of view of medical science, Smith had proved for the first time that disease could be transmitted by an insect, a principle which in time would have practical applications in the control of human disease.

197

YELLOW FEVER   In 1900 Surgeon-General Sternberg decided to set
the Army to work on some unfinished medical
business of the nineteenth century. The last of the great epidemics of yellow
fever in the United States had occurred in 1878, but in 1900 this disease still
posed a threat. It was endemic, and sporadically epidemic, in the islands of
the West Indies and in Central and South America. Concern about yellow
fever was heightened when as a result of the Spanish-American War the
United States acquired territory in the West Indies and other tropical areas.
For three years after the war, the United States kept an army of occupation
in Cuba, where yellow fever was endemic and where there was a constant
threat of an outbreak of the disease among the trooops. Since the cause of
yellow fever and the manner in which it spreads in a community were still
unanswered questions, Surgeon-General Sternberg decided to appoint a
special commission to make a study of this disease.

Before becoming Surgeon-General of the Army, Sternberg himself had
worked for some years on the yellow fever problem. As a bacteriologist he
had made extensive studies of a bacillus which was alleged to be the cause
of the disease, but he had proved that this was not the case. His own efforts
to find a causative bacterium were unsuccessful. However, the possibility of a bacterial cause was revived in 1897 when Giuseppi Sanarelli, an
Italian bacteriologist working in South America, claimed to have found the
bacillus responsible for the disease. For this "discovery" Sanarelli received
many prizes and awards.

As far back as 1881 Carlos Finley, a Cuban physician, had advanced the
theory that yellow fever is transmitted from one individual to another by
the bite of a mosquito. He had carried out some experiments on volunteers,
which he thought proved his theory. However, his experiments were not
well controlled, and they failed to convince other scientists, including Sternberg, who while working in Cuba some years earlier, had come to admire
Finley's serious purpose and integrity. Since then a British physician,
Ronald Ross, working in India in 1897–98, had proved beyond question
that malaria is transmitted by the anopheles mosquito. It seemed, therefore,
that a promising lead for the Yellow Fever Commission to follow was the one
suggested by Finley.

The members of the Commission were Major Walter Reed, Chairman,
who had already distinguished himself by his work on typhoid fever (Bean,
1974); James Carroll, a Regular Army medical officer, who, like Reed, had
studied pathology and bacteriology under Welch; Jesse W. Lazear, who
had worked on malaria and the *Anopheles* mosquito under Thayer at Johns
Hopkins; and Aristide Agramonte, a Cuban physician who had had his
medical training in the United States and was knowledgeable about the pathology of yellow fever. Agramonte had an additional invaluable qualification: he had had yellow fever and was therefore immune to the disease. The
commissioners set sail for Cuba in 1900.

The Commission first demonstrated that Sanarelli's bacillus is not the
cause of yellow fever. They proved in a thoroughly convincing manner that
the disease is transmitted by the female *Aedes aegypti* mosquito but only if
the insect has sucked the blood of a yellow fever victim during the first two
or three days of the disease. They found that the patient's blood had to
remain in the mosquito for about two weeks before the bite of the mosquito

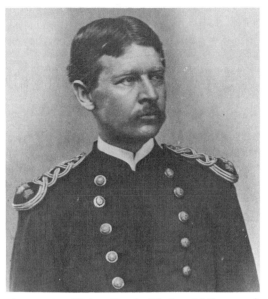

Figure 48. Walter Reed. (National Library of Medicine, Bethesda, Maryland.)

could infect a second victim. It took another three to five days after the bite before the new victim fell sick. Once a patient had recovered from the disease he could not be reinfected. If blood was withdrawn from a patient during the first three days of the disease and then injected into a nonimmune individual, it produced the disease. The same result was produced even when the blood had been filtered through an earthenware filter that held back ordinary bacteria. In brief, the Commission proved that yellow fever is caused by a filterable virus, not a bacterium, and that it is transmitted from one individual to another by a particular species of mosquito.

The work of the Yellow Fever Commission was one of the great achievements of medicine. Not only did it demonstrate how yellow fever is spread in a community but also it showed that an infectious disease could be caused by an agent that is invisible under the ordinary microscope and small enough to pass through a very fine filter. Furthermore, since a mosquito is the key to transmission, it became possible to take measures to prevent the spread of the disease. When he was informed of the Commission's findings, General Leonard Wood, who was then in command of the American troops in Cuba, ordered a vigorous campaign to eradicate mosquitoes in the region of Havana. This campaign, which was led by Major William C. Gorgas, was highly successful, and in 1902, for the first time in more than a century, there was not a single case of yellow fever in Havana. The Commission's triumph was mixed with tragedy: a member of the Commission, Jesse Lazear, died of yellow fever resulting from an accidental mosquito bite.

The studies in Cuba showed not only how yellow fever is transmitted but also how it is not transmitted. The factors such as personal contact, hygiene, sanitation, water supply, and disposal of excreta, which had been

199

found to be so important in the control of typhoid fever in Army camps, were not involved in the case of yellow fever. To prove this point the Commission selected volunteers to live in the same quarters with patients who had yellow fever. They drank the same water, ate the same food, handled the same articles, and used the same bedsheets that had been used by the patients; as long as mosquitoes were excluded from the environment, yellow fever was not transmitted to these volunteers.

RICKETTSIAS — A third major American contribution involving insects was made by *Howard Taylor Ricketts.* Ricketts graduated from Northwestern University Medical School in 1897, and after serving an internship at the Cook County Hospital in Chicago he went to Europe for further study. He returned home in 1902 to become an instructor in the Department of Pathology and Bacteriology at the new University of Chicago, where he devoted all his time to teaching and research. His early researches on blastomycosis and immunological problems were important, but it was the brilliance of his studies of Rocky Mountain spotted fever that marked him as an investigator of the first rank.

Ricketts began his studies of Rocky Mountain spotted fever in the spring of 1906 as a sort of pastime during a holiday. He promptly found that the disease could be transmitted to lower animals. He also found that a certain tick, which occurs naturally on a large number of animals in the area where Rocky Mountain spotted fever occurs, could transmit by its bite the disease from a sick to a healthy animal. He came to the conclusion that in man the disease results from the accidental bite of an adult tick carrying the infectious agent. Since only adult ticks find their way to man and since they occur only in the spring, the peculiar seasonal incidence of the disease was

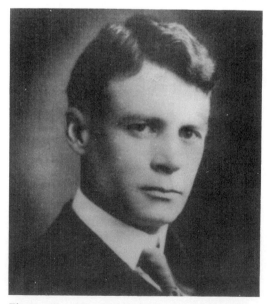

Figure 49. Howard T. Ricketts. (National Library of Medicine, Bethesda, Maryland.)

neatly explained. Finally, Ricketts discovered the micro-organism causing the disease in the blood of patients and in ticks and their eggs. (This organism is one of a family now known as *Rickettsia,* in honor of Ricketts.)

Ricketts came to realize that Rocky Mountain spotted fever resembles typhus fever, a disease that had plagued the cities of Europe for many centuries. Typhus is a highly contagious disease with a high mortality, and though it had become less prevalent in areas of improved sanitation, it still presented formidable problems. In the mid-nineteenth century, in a period of 25 years, 550 of 1230 physicians attached to institutions in Ireland died of typhus. Mexico City in the early twentieth century was still one of the important foci of the disease. In July, 1909, Ricketts decided to go to Mexico City to study typhus. He found that the disease, though similar in many respects to Rocky Mountain spotted fever, is transmitted not by a tick but by the body louse *(Pediculus vestimenti),* and he succeeded in isolating the causative organism (a rickettsia similar in appearance to that causing Rocky Mountain spotted fever) both in patients suffering from typhus and in the louse.

While he was conducting his typhus research Ricketts accepted the Professorship of Pathology at the University of Pennsylvania, but he never occupied the chair; he died of typhus fever in Mexico City on May 3, 1910, another martyr to science.

Rickettsias have now been identified as the cause of about a dozen diseases. Within a few months of Ricketts's death, Dr. Nathan Brill of New York City reported 255 cases of a typhus-like illness that he had encountered during a period of about 10 years. This disease had many of the clinical characteristics of classic typhus, but it was a much milder illness, and there was nothing to suggest that it was contagious or transmitted by insects. In only one household did more than a single case occur. It was soon demonstrated that this disease is due to a rickettsia, but the manner of its spread remained a puzzle. For a time it was known as sporadic typhus, or Brill's disease. In 1934 Hans Zinsser, Professor of Bacteriology at Harvard, reported an extensive epidemiological study of cases of sporadic typhus in New York and Boston. He was able to collect detailed records of 538 cases that had occurred between 1910 and 1933. Of these, approximately 95 per cent occurred in foreign-born individuals who had emigrated from Russia. He concluded that Brill's disease represents a recrudescence of an infection acquired abroad. He predicted that this disease probably could be transmitted by lice, and this prediction was subsequently verified. The simple explanation for the lack of transmission of the disease in the New York and Boston environments was the absence of body lice. The mildness of the disease was explained by the fact that it was a recrudescence of a prior illness rather than a new infection.

A third form of typhus, which was prevalent in the southern part of the United States, was studied extensively between 1925 and 1935 by Kenneth F. Maxcy. Maxcy was a graduate of the Johns Hopkins Medical School, and in 1921 he received the Ph.D. degree as a member of the first class to graduate from the Johns Hopkins School of Hygiene and Public Health. (He subsequently became Professor of Epidemiology in the latter school.) The disease studied by Maxcy is now known as *endemic* or *murine typhus.* In addition to carrying out extensive studies on the symptomatology and epidemiology of this disease, Maxcy in association with R. E. Dyer proved that

201

the disease is spread from rats and mice to man by a flea whose normal host is the rat.

TUBERCULOSIS
Pulmonary tuberculosis—also known as *consumption,* or *phthisis*—though less alarming than the diseases that came in spectacular epidemics, was unquestionably "the captain of the men of death" in the nineteenth century. During the first half of the century, in the cities of the United States that kept mortality records, the annual death rate from consumption was about 400 per 100,000 population; in New York City in 1812 it reached 700 per 100,000. Though the incidence of consumption was high among all classes of people, it was highest in the urban slums, where poorly nourished people were crowded together under abominable hygienic conditions.

In 1830, in the *Report of the Sanitary Commission of Massachusetts,* Lemuel Shattuck wrote: "The dreadful disease [tuberculosis] is a constant visitor to all parts of our Commonwealth, but creates little alarm because it is so constantly present, whereas the occasional visit of cholera or other epidemic disease creates alarm and, therefore, precautionary measures are taken."

This apparent blindness to the major health problem of the period was almost universal. Shryock, who examined the correspondence of a prominent and public-spirited physician over a 40-year period from 1835 to 1875, found that "he was much concerned with cholera and yellow fever as public dangers, but never referred to 'consumption' as such in all that period" (Shryock, 1966).

In addition to its constant presence there were other factors that tended to make tuberculosis less alarming: it was, for the most part, an insidious, chronic disease; its victims usually lived for months or years after contracting the disease, and while their physical condition was almost imperceptibly declining they were able to lead relatively productive lives until near the end. Occasionally the disease reached truly epidemic proportions. This was the case when it was introduced into a previously unexposed population. When the white man carried tuberculosis into the American Indian settlements, the disease spread rapidly, virtually wiping out whole tribes. In the 1890s the annual death rate from tuberculosis among the Indians on the Qu-Appelle reservation in western Canada reached the fantastic figure of 9000 per 100,000 population. In the life span of three generations, more than half the families of the tribe were eliminated. The high incidence of fatal tuberculosis among the black population of the United States has been attributed to the fact that the African Negro did not encounter tuberculosis until he left his homeland; he therefore had less racial resistance to the disease than did the white people among whom he had to live.

One of the characteristic features of tuberculosis, which has made it difficult to evaluate the effect of treatment, is its tendency to subside spontaneously or to fluctuate in intensity so that both patient and physician are misled into attributing spontaneous healing or temporary subsidence to the effect of some new form of therapy. Benjamin Rush, in about 1800, believed that phthisis could be cured by opium and an animal diet; added, of course, to his usual heroic measures. This was only one of many forms of treatment to be discarded during the first half of the twentieth century. By 1850, says Shryock, consumption "belonged to that appalling legal category known as 'an act of God.'".

For reasons which are still not fully understood, the death rate from tuberculosis gradually began to fall after 1850. This has been attributed to improvements in housing, hygiene, and nutrition that started to affect city dwellers at about that time, but the change seemed, mysteriously, to occur in all cities, good and bad, and in European countries as well as in the United States. Austin Flint, Sr., who was America's leading authority on pulmonary tuberculosis in the middle of the century, was inclined to attribute the change to more conservative methods of treatment. In 1862 Flint wrote:

> *The management of this disease twenty-five years ago was certainly not in accordance with the principle of conservatism. The measures employed, medicinal and hygienic were, indeed, directly opposed to this principle.... Blood-letting, cathartics, mercurialization, severe counterirritation were considered to be remedial, and to these were conjoined low diet and confinement within doors. Now pulmonary tuberculosis is not cured in the majority of cases, although ... there is reason to believe that the proportion of cures is considerably larger than under the treatment just referred to.... Formerly, the instances of rapid progress of the disease were more numerous, and it almost invariably advanced with a steady march, rarely occupying many months in completing its fatal career. Patients were usually confined to bed for weeks before death, lingering on the borders of the grave, suffering from extreme debility.... It was difficult to conceive of a picture more distressing and repulsive than that of a being in the last stage of consumption. Conservatism has done much towards ameliorating the condition of consumptives, even when it is hopeless as regards recovery.... Life is not infrequently prolonged and made comparatively comfortable for years.... Even when the disease is progressing to a fatal termination, the strength is usually so far preserved that a bedridden consumptive is now rarely seen, and it is not uncommon for patients to be out of doors almost up to the hour of death. I appeal to those whose medical experience has extended over a quarter of a century for the truthfulness of this comparison.*

Flint was correct: the death rate from tuberculosis had declined during that 25-year period, but the decline was not wholly attributable to the conservative type of treatment that he favored. As mentioned above, other factors, some apparent, others obscure, contributed to the more favorable outcome.

The attitude toward tuberculosis underwent a radical change when Robert Koch discovered the tubercle bacillus. William H. Welch, who was then Pathologist at the Bellevue Hospital Medical College, learned about the discovery from Dr. Flint, who, though 70 years old, relished with boyish enthusiasm every new development in medical science. Flint had shown more interest than most of his American colleagues in the *germ theory* of disease. On the morning of April 3, 1882, while Welch "lay in bed after a late evening in the dead house, the door of his room burst open and in came the old gentleman [Flint] at a run, waving a newspaper in the air. 'Welch,' he cried, 'I knew it, I knew it!' The young man must have blinked in sleepy surprise, but when Flint explained that a dispatch in the paper told of Koch's great triumph, he jumped out of bed as excited as his master" (Flexner and Flexner, 1941).

203

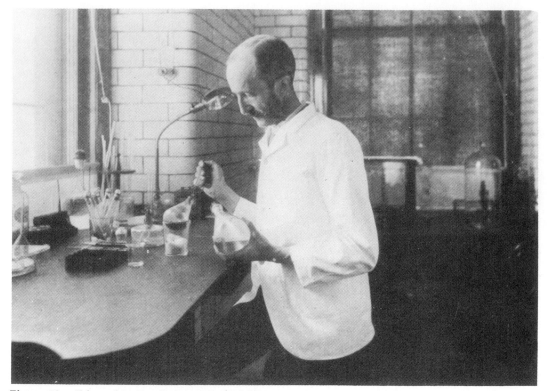

Figure 50. Edward L. Trudeau. (From Trudeau, E. L.: An Autobiography, Edward Livingston Trudeau, M. D. Garden City, N.Y., Doubleday, Page and Company, 1916. Reproduced with permission.)

The understanding of how tuberculosis spreads in a community now took a long stride foward. Studies of the sputum coughed up by patients with pulmonary tuberculosis revealed that it contained tubercle bacilli, and experiments proved that the sputum would transmit the disease to animals. It gradually became apparent that the tubercle bacillus is passed from sick to well individuals by close personal contact, particularly when the well person is exposed to the cough of the sick person. Beginning in the 1880s, patients with pulmonary tuberculosis were encouraged to wear masks when they were associating with other people and to expectorate into cups that contained a disinfectant capable of killing tubercle bacilli.

Edward L. Trudeau was one of the American physicians who appreciated the implications of Koch's discovery (Harrod, 1959). Trudeau had graduated from The College of Physicians and Surgeons, New York, in 1871, and he began the practice of medicine in New York City the following year. Soon thereafter he developed consumption, and because of this he decided to leave the city to seek a more healthful climate. He selected as a suitable place the sparsely settled Adirondack Mountain area of New York state. There he practiced medicine, studied the medical literature, and gradually regained his health. In 1884, two years after Koch's discovery, Trudeau founded the Adirondack Cottage Sanatorium at Saranac Lake, New York, for the treatment of incipient tuberculosis. This was the first tuberculosis sanatorium worthy of the name to be established in the United States.

Trudeau seems to have kept closely in touch with all developments in the field of medicine that had a bearing on the diagnosis, prevention, or treatment of tuberculosis. He followed Koch's work with intense interest and was one of the first to appreciate the value of Francis H. Williams's studies on the X-ray diagnosis of pulmonary disease. From early in its history the sanatorium had a small laboratory for diagnostic studies, in which an increasing amount of research took place. Convinced of the need for more research in this field, in 1894, Trudeau founded the Saranac Laboratory for the study of tuberculosis, the first research laboratory created for this purpose in the United States. For the next several decades, Trudeau and a succession of able young assistants (most, if not all, of whom had first come to the sanatorium to be treated for tuberculosis) carried on much important research on the tubercle bacillus, the tuberculin test, tuberculosis in experimental animals, and the use of new diagnostic methods and various medicines, diets, and other therapeutic measures in patients. Many of the leaders in the field of tuberculosis during the first half of the twentieth century got their start in the cottages and laboratory at Saranac.

Among other Americans who made important early contributions to the study of tuberculosis was Theobald Smith. In 1898 Smith demonstrated by experiments on laboratory animals that there were two quite distinct strains of tubercle bacilli: one, the bovine strain, came originally from cattle; the other, the human strain, came from patients with tuberculosis. Smith described the methods by which the two types of tubercle bacilli could be identified. Koch confirmed and praised Smith's work and claimed that there was little danger of transmission of the bovine type to man. This prediction proved to be incorrect, for in 1902, M. P. Ravenel, Bacteriologist for the State Livestock Sanitary Board of Pennsylvania, obtained an organism from a tuberculous child which he identified as the bovine type of tubercle bacillus. With this as a lead it was soon discovered that raw milk from cows infected with the bovine bacillus was a common source of tuberculous infection in children.

After the discovery of the tubercle bacillus it was hoped that means would be found to kill the bacillus within the human body or at least to make the body more resistant to its effects. In 1890 Koch thought that he had discovered a cure for tuberculosis. In that year he reported at the International Medical Congress in Berlin that he had made a substance, which when injected into normal guinea pigs, rendered them resistant to tuberculosis, and when injected into guinea pigs with advanced tuberculosis, it arrested the disease. Three months later he reported that this work had been extended to human patients with very encouraging results. Though Koch was guarded in his claims, he stated that "the experience, up to the present, indicates that in phthisis the treatment cures early cases with certainty, and that moderately advanced cases may also be cured." In neither of his first two reports on this subject did Koch describe the origin or preparation of the substance that he had used to treat the animals and the patients. It was known at first as "Koch's lymph." Subsequently it turned out to be tuberculin which had been prepared by boiling, filtering, and concentrating a broth culture of tubercle bacilli. In spite of the cautious and preliminary nature of Koch's reports, tuberculous patients from all countries flocked to Berlin for treatment. Before many months had passed, it became apparent

205

that the tuberculin treatment not only was ineffective but also was dangerous; there were severe and sometimes fatal reactions to the tuberculin.

In his second report in 1890 Koch had stated that "the generalized reaction to injection of 0.01 cc is uniformly elicited if any tuberculous process is present. Thus, it is not too presumptuous to assume that in the future this agent will become an indispensable diagnostic aid. Questionable early cases will be detectable where sputum examination and physical examination may still be negative" (Lechevalier and Solotorovsky, 1974). Although tuberculin proved to be worthless as a therapeutic agent, it came into wide use as a diagnostic agent. A minute amount of tuberculin injected into the skin will cause no reaction in individuals who have never acquired a tuberculous infection; but in patients who have had such an infection, whether it be quiescent or active, redness and swelling will develop at the site of the injection. The true nature of the tuberculin reaction was not understood until the first decade of the twentieth century, when von Pirquet and Schick reported their work on hypersensitivity and allergy. In the second decade of the century, the whole subject of tuberculin sensitivity came under intensive investigation at Trudeau's Saranac Laboratory, particularly by Allen K. Krause and Edward R. Baldwin.

Specific and effective treatment for tuberculosis did not become available until after world War II, but even before this there had been a dramatic decline in the death rate from tuberculosis. In considering mortality statistics it must be remembered that there were no national statistics during the first century. The only statistics were local, and they involved principally the larger urban centers. Statewide registration of deaths began in the latter part of the nineteenth century. By 1900, 26 per cent of the national population was included in the states in which deaths were registered. The percentage of the population in the registration area had increased to 81 per cent in 1920, and 100 per cent in 1940.

The mortality figures quoted earlier in this chapter are those of a few cities in which the tuberculosis death rate during the first half of the nineteenth century was about 400 per 100,000 population per year. The comparable tuberculosis mortality rate in the registration states was, in round figures, 200 in 1900, 150 in 1910, 120 in 1920, 70 in 1930, and 50 in 1940. This steady decline is attributable to a variety of factors, including public concern aroused by a number of individuals and organizations, of which the most important was the National Tuberculosis Association. More specifically, some of the major contributing factors were as follows: better understanding of how the disease is spread; earlier diagnosis by means of X-ray surveys and tuberculin tests; the virtual elimination of the bovine type of infection by the pasteurization of milk and the elimination of tuberculous cows from the dairy herds; and more widespread institutional care in private sanatoria and state and municipal tuberculosis hospitals, thus providing better medical supervision and at the same time removing the patient from contact with other individuals to whom he might transmit the disease.

The number of tuberculosis sanatoria and hospitals had increased to about 400 by 1910, and in the middle of the present century there were more than 100,000 beds devoted specifically to the care of tuberculous patients. Institutionalized patients received not only better medical care but also specialized forms of treatment as needed. One such form of treatment was pneumothorax, the introduction of air into one side of the chest to collapse the diseased lung on that side. This procedure, first strongly advocated in the United States by John B. Murphy, Professor of Surgery at Northwestern University, puts the diseased lung at rest, reduces the cough and gives the tissues a better opportunity to overcome the infection. A surgical procedure known as thoracoplasty also was used in selected cases to collapse a diseased lung.

With the fall in mortality there was also a fall in the prevalence of tuberculosis in the United States as indicated by tuberculin tests, autopsies, and X-ray surveys. In the early years of the twentieth century, surveys using the tuberculin skin test indicated that virtually 100 per cent of the population had acquired a tuberculous infection prior to the age of 20. By 1940 this figure had been reduced to about 50 per cent, and by 1965, after the introduction of specific antituberculosis therapy, only 5 to 10 per cent of young adults reacted to tuberculin (except in some urban areas), whereas 50 to 80 per cent of persons over the age of 50 gave positive reactions (a reminder that the disease had been more prevalent when they were growing up).

In the early work with the tubercle bacillus, researchers hoped that it might be possible to do with it what Pasteur had done with the anthrax bacillus; namely, to develop an attenuated strain that could be used to immunize individuals against tuberculosis. Trudeau was among the first to develop, quite accidentally, a partially attenuated strain of tubercle bacilli. His experience demonstrates how, in biological research, a flight of human hope can be dashed by the caprice of a lowly bacterium. This story was told by Krause in 1919:

> In 1891 Dr. Trudeau isolated a culture of human tubercle bacilli by passing through a rabbit material that had been obtained from the cadaver of a man who had died of miliary tuberculosis. At the time of isolation and for a short time afterwards it exhibited what might be called standard virulence for guinea pigs; but after about two or three years of incubator existence it underwent a very noticeable diminution in its capacity to infect these animals. This lessened invasiveness was as difficult of explanation as are other similar instances that are not infrequently noted by all experimental workers with tubercle bacilli, namely, that after a certain period of vegetative life away from the animal body, cultures not uncommonly lose something of their original infectivity. Having lost much of its former virulence this culture of Dr. Trudeau's in the years that followed showed another peculiarity that is common to tubercle bacilli. This was that its diminution of virulence was not progressive to the vanishing point. It retained a certain degree of infecting power for guinea pigs that during the last 20 years has not changed one way or the other. From time to time numerous attempts were made to enhance its virulence by means of successive animal passage . . . by Dr. Trudeau, by Dr. Baldwin and by the author, . . . but these efforts always were unsuccessful. It appeared that its newly acquired inherent infectiousness was a fixed and static matter resisting all ordinary methods that aimed to change it.

While the work at the Trudeau Laboratory was in progress, two French bacteriologists, Albert Calmette and Camille Guerin, were having greater success in work of the same type at the Pasteur Institute in Lille, France. In 1908 these scientists began to grow a strain of bovine tubercle bacilli on po-

207

tato cooked in bovine bile, with the hope of obtaining an attenuated strain for vaccinating cattle against tuberculosis. After 13 years, during which the bacillus was transferred every two weeks to a new batch of the potato and bile medium, the organism was completely nonvirulent, even at high doses, for all animal species. When calves two weeks old were injected subcutaneously with this attenuated bacillus they became immune to subsequent injections with virulent bovine tubercle bacilli. Fifteen months after vaccination, the animals were still resistant to a virulent strain capable of killing all the controls of the same age in less than two months. The authors designated their modified bacillus with the initials BCG. Between 1921 and the publication of their report in 1924, 217 infants in families where there was heavy exposure to tuberculosis had been vaccinated with BCG. Follow-up information indicated that these children were healthy and that they showed no evidence of tuberculosis in spite of their heavy exposure. These experiments seemed to indicate that BCG was safe to administer to infants and was effective in preventing tuberculosis.

Over the next few years BCG was used on an increasingly extensive scale with what appeared to be a high degree of success. However, BCG immunization received a serious setback in 1929 as the result of a dreadful experience in Lubeck, Germany. There 252 children were vaccinated with BCG, and a few weeks later 71 of the children were dead from a serious tuberculous infection. At first it was thought that this catastrophe was due to a sudden increase in virulence of the BCG strain. However, this proved not to be the case. It was found that the BCG vaccine had been contaminated with a virulent strain of tubercle bacilli in the Public Health Laboratories of Lubeck prior to injection into the children (Lechevalier and Solotorovsky, 1974). After this temporary setback, BCG came into wide use in many countries to protect children from tuberculosis, but its use in the United States has been rather limited.

The first antituberculosis program was proposed in 1889 by Hermann M. Biggs. He submitted to the Health Department of New York City a report in which it was recommended that the authorities require inspection of cattle in order to eliminate infection from bovine sources. The report also recommended disinfection of rooms or hospital wards occupied by tuberculous patients and that the public be educated about the need for precautions against the spread of infection. No action was taken on the first two of these recommendations, but the Health Department did issue an educational journal, the circulation of which opened a campaign which was soon to become widespread. In 1892 Biggs succeeded in establishing the first Health Department Diagnostic Laboratory, and the following year he urged that all hospitals and physicians be required to report cases of tuberculosis and that special hospitals be established for the segregation of tuberculous patients. These proposals were opposed by physicians who held that registration would violate the privacy of doctor-patient relationships. Nevertheless, the public antituberculosis campaign that had been set in motion soon gathered momentum. This was the period in which political reform was beginning to gain public support, and between 1890 and 1897 other cities and states began to follow the lead of New York City. In Massachusetts in 1890, Vincent Y. Bowditch established the Sharon Sanatorium, which five years later became the first state tuberculosis hospital in the country. The first municipal tuberculosis hospital was established by the city of Cincinnati in 1897.

An important individual in the early years of the antituberculosis movement was *Lawrence F. Flick* of Philadelphia. He was discouraged by the apathy of the medical profession toward the establishment of facilities for the care of patients with consumption, and he therefore turned to the public for support. In 1892 he arranged with a group of friends, mostly laymen but including several physicians, the founding of the Pennsylvania Society for the Prevention of Tuberculosis. For the next 15 years this society issued, and its members distributed personally, a series of pamphlets designed to educate the public. In 1893 the society urged the Philadelphia Board of Health to require registration of tuberculous patients, but this move was strongly opposed by the medical profession. The matter came to a head in a famous debate at the College of Physicians, Philadelphia, during which many of the city's most prominent physicians and surgeons rejected and ridiculed the idea. Flick read a letter of support from John Shaw Billings. William Osler, who participated in the debate, backed Flick but qualified his position by holding to the old view that the disease is inherited. The meeting made it apparent that registration was overwhelmingly disapproved by the profession, and the Board of Health decided to postpone action. In spite of this rebuff, Flick continued his antituberculosis campaign, and finally in 1901 the Pennsylvania legislature provided funds for establishment of a free hospital for poor consumptives at Whitehaven, under the direction of Flick.

A wealthy citizen of Pittsburgh, Henry Phipps, was attracted by the work at the Whitehaven Hospital and became interested in the antituberculosis movement. Flick met Phipps in 1902, and the two men toured Europe together, visiting hospitals, sanatoria, and research institutes. They were impressed by the need for further scientific research on tuberculosis, and when they returned to the United States Phipps provided an endowment for a research institute in Philadelphia, which opened in 1903. The institute had small wards for the care of inpatients, a dispensary, and a pharmacy, all of which were to be oriented toward scientific investigation. Unlike the Rockefeller Institute, the Phipps Institute was devoted to the study of a single disease, and its staff not only conducted scientific investigations but also participated in a program of public education. Furthermore, they played a role in founding additional tuberculosis hospitals and in obtaining legislation for the control of tuberculosis and the care of tuberculous patients.

In most European countries, health and welfare programs were funded by the government, but in the United States both the federal and the state governments were slow to become involved. Because of this reluctance on the part of government and because of the lack of support from the medical profession, the antituberculosis movement was conducted largely by laymen. Societies such as the one that Flick had established in Pennsylvania were formed in a number of other states. The fervor displayed by these societies was sometimes intense, but they did not proceed blindly; there were always enough medical practitioners and scientists who favored their cause to provide scientific guidance.

In 1903 the Committee on the Prevention of Tuberculosis of the Charity

209

Organization Society of the City of New York undertook a study to obtain more accurate information concerning the extent of the tuberculosis problem and of the institutions available for the care of tuberculous patients. It was shown that the problem was indeed a serious and extensive one; that it involved particularly people in poverty areas; that the annual cost of tuberculosis to the nation, direct and indirect, totaled as much as $330 million; and that at a time when there were 40,000 deaths from tuberculosis each year, there were only 8000 beds available in tuberculosis institutions. The great need, of course, was for free beds, and although 5000 of the 8000 available beds were for nonpaying patients, most of these were concentrated in five states. The study also brought out the fact that although tuberculosis presented a health problem of the first magnitude, the national attitude toward it was one of inertia and indifference.

In 1902 a Commission on Tuberculosis was established in Maryland at the instigation of Drs. Welch and Osler and Dr. John F. Fulton of the State Board of Health. This Commission held a major meeting and exhibit in Baltimore in 1904. The meeting was well planned and brought together for the first time the really effective leaders in the tuberculosis movement from all parts of the country. The participants included Osler, E. C. Janeway, Theobald Smith, the statistician Frederick Hoffman, Flick, Ravenel, Trudeau, and V. Y. Bowditch, among many others. A committee of 15, with Osler as Chairman, was given power to act in the matter of forming a National Antituberculosis Association. The committee held two meetings, one in New York City and the other at the Phipps Institute in Philadelphia. At a meeting held in March, 1904, the committee adopted a motion proposed by Flick that "we here assembled do now organize ourselves into a United States Society for the Study of Tuberculosis." With the adoption of this resolution the National Tuberculosis Association came into being. At the first general meeting of the new Association, Trudeau was elected President, Osler and Biggs, vice-presidents, H. B. Jacobs, Secretary, and George M. Sternberg, Treasurer. A headquarters office was rented in New York City for $10 a month, and Dr. Livingston Farrand became the Association's first Executive Secretary.

At the first annual meeting of the National Tuberculosis Association in 1905, it was agreed that the only way to deal with a disease such as tuberculosis was to attack it simultaneously with both scientific and social weapons. The dedication and enthusiasm of the members made it clear that the organization had a serious purpose, and after the meeting the press applauded the objectives of the new Association and signified its willingness to give publicity to its campaign.

As time passed it became clear that the Association considered its role to be chiefly promotional and advisory rather than directive. It would not locate cases, provide relief, or found hospitals; but it would encourage other bodies to do all these things. The ultimate goal was a public health program; but in order to accomplish this end, the public first had to be aroused. With this in view, efforts were made to form local voluntary societies, which would then campaign for the necessary laws and institutions. A way had to be found to defray the expenses of a long-term illness, which the consumptives themselves were unable to meet. If this were not done, families of even moderate means would be forced into indigency, or, alternatively, they would refuse to cooperate in the important matter of case-finding and hospitalization. An active campaign to find cases early in the course of the disease was necessary because many of the poor did not see doctors until advanced illness forced them to do so.

At about the time of the organization of the National Tuberculosis Association, methods of case-finding were improving rapidly. The tuberculin skin test, the examination of sputum for tubercle bacilli, and X-ray pictures of the chest all were available, but they involved expense greater than many individuals could bear. The Association hoped that state and local governments, through their public health services, might be persuaded to take over at least part of this expense. In relation to its efforts to influence government, the Association acquired a powerful political ally when President Theodore Roosevelt became its honorary vice-president, a position he held for 15 years.

By 1917, every state and territory had its own tuberculosis society. As a result of the activities of the state societies, the traveling exhibits, newspaper publicity, and political pressure, the proportion of public funds expended for tuberculosis rose steadily, reaching 50 per cent by 1909 and going rapidly higher thereafter.

Until about 1910 the National Association had very little money. In 1903 a Danish postmaster conceived the idea of selling Christmas stamps as a means of raising funds to care for Danish children ill with tuberculosis. Jacob A. Riis, a Danish-American leader who had lost six brothers as a result of tuberculosis, began to publicize the Christmas stamp idea in the United States. In 1907 he wrote a glowing account of the program in the magazine *Outlook*. This article was read by Miss Emily T. Bissell, who was seeking funds to maintain an open-air "shack" for consumptives near Wilmington, Delaware. Miss Bissell designed a Christmas seal and borrowed $40 to have the seal printed on 50,000 stamps. With the cooperation of the local post office these stamps were put on sale at a penny apiece two weeks before Christmas, 1907. The stamps were sold in envelopes each containing 25 stamps. The message printed on the envelope was, "These stamps do not carry any kind of mail, but any kind of mail will carry them." The sale brought in $3000 and aroused so much enthusiasm that Miss Bissell urged the American Red Cross to undertake a nationwide sale the following year. This suggestion was adopted, and the sale of Christmas seals brought in $135,000 in 1908 and $250,000 in 1909. The National Tuberculosis Association became a joint partner in this venture; the Red Cross preparing the stamps and the National Association providing publicity and arranging the sale. Ultimately the National Tuberculosis Association took over the entire program which provided its first reliable and sizable income.

Questions were raised as to whether the work of the Association was playing any part in the decline in the death rate from tuberculosis. To answer such questions it was decided to adopt a proposal made by Lee K. Frankel of the Metropolitan Life Insurance Company, who wanted a demonstration of what could be accomplished in a community by utilizing the most advanced techniques for finding and controlling cases of tuberculosis. The town chosen for this demonstration was Framingham, Massachusetts. The demonstration began with an extensive survey of the incidence of disease, followed by a program directed toward improving the general

211

(Rates per 100,000 population)

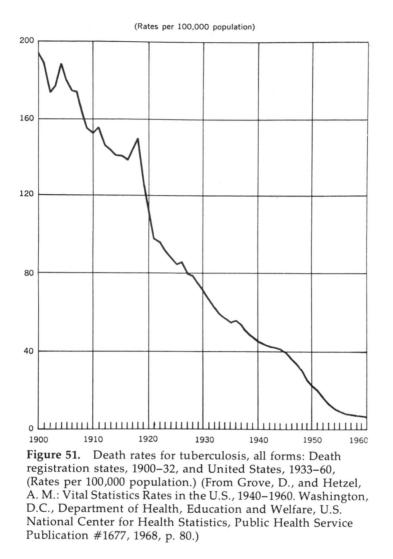

Figure 51. Death rates for tuberculosis, all forms: Death registration states, 1900–32, and United States, 1933–60, (Rates per 100,000 population.) (From Grove, D., and Hetzel, A. M.: Vital Statistics Rates in the U.S., 1940–1960. Washington, D.C., Department of Health, Education and Welfare, U.S. National Center for Health Statistics, Public Health Service Publication #1677, 1968, p. 80.)

health of the community. The immediate benefits of the demonstration were apparent in comparative death rates. Infant mortality dropped from an average of 76 per 1000 live births in 1916–17 to 49 in 1922–23. But even more striking than this effect was the drop in the tuberculosis death rate: it fell from an average of 121 per 100,000 population for the decade 1907–1916 to only 38 in 1922–23. When compared to similar communities in which no health campaign had been undertaken, the death rate in Framingham declined more than twice as rapidly.

The National Association devoted very little money to research prior to 1920, though it did provide part of the support for the excellent basic studies of the anatomy of the lungs that were carried out by William Snow Miller at the University of Wisconsin. After 1920, support was given to a variety of research activities including studies of the growth, metabolism, and chemical composition of the tubercle bacillus. Of great practical importance was the research conducted by Esmond R. Long and Florence B. Seibert on the preparation of a purified standard tuberculin, which became known as PPD. Dr. Seibert worked with two pharmaceutical concerns, Sharp and Dohme and Parke, Davis and Company, shortly before World War II, to prepare PPD for general distribution. This product has served as a stable and reliable international standard tuberculin for all comparative testing. Although the National Association contributed funds for a number of research projects, the total amount expended, in present day terms, was extraordinarily small; only $121,715 between 1926 and 1947.

One of the great problems in dealing with tuberculosis in the United States was the high susceptibility of the black population to this disease. In the northern states the mortality rate for blacks was some six to seven times that for whites living in the same areas. Tuberculosis case-finding was particularly difficult in the black population, but case-finding improved in the 1930s and 40s, when PPD became available for skin testing of school-age children. Mass screening by X-rays was also started in a number of industries and selected communities.

The standard treatment for active pulmonary tuberculosis up to the end of World War II was sanatorium care, a good diet, balanced rest and outdoor exercise, and special procedures such as pneumothorax and thoracoplasty when needed. Specific chemotherapy for tuberculosis will be discussed in a subsequent chapter.

HISTOPLASMOSIS   A wholly different kind of pathogenic microorganism, the *Histoplasma capsulatum,* was discovered by an American, Samuel Taylor Darling, on the Isthmus of Panama in 1906. Darling observed the organism in sections of tissue taken post-mortem from three cases. It was not known at the time whether the organism had caused the disease from which the patients had died. In fact, many years passed before it was realized that histoplasmosis, the disease caused by the fungus *Histoplasma capsulatum,* is a quite common infectious disease in North America. In retrospect it seems certain that Darling's patients died of histoplasmosis, but no other case of the disease was recognized until 1926, when Drs. Cecil J. Watson and W. A. Riley of the University of Minnesota reported a case originating in that state, the first case to be reported in the United States. In 1934, W. A. Demonbreum at Vanderbilt University demonstrated conclusively that the *Histoplasma capsulatum* can be grown by cultural methods in the laboratory and can be transmitted to animals. The prevalence of histoplasmosis was not recognized until after the histoplasmin skin test had been developed. This test allows one to diagnose histoplasmosis just as the tuberculin test allows one to diagnose tuberculosis (Christie, 1951).

In 1945, Amos Christie and J. C. Peterson of Vanderbilt University Medical School and Carroll E. Palmer of the U.S. Public Health Service demonstrated that in a number of patients who were believed to have pulmonary tuberculosis, the tuberculin test was negative while the histoplasmin test was positive, leading to the conclusion that the lung disease was due to histoplasmosis rather than to tuberculosis (Christie, 1951).

In many respects histoplasmosis resembles tuberculosis, and many cases of the former were unquestionably mistaken for the latter prior to the use of the differentiating skin test. It is now known that the incidence of histoplasmosis is very high in some parts of the eastern and midwestern United States. There are areas in which the histoplasmin skin test is positive in 80 to 90 per cent of the population. Fortunately, many of these individuals have never suffered any ill effects of the disease, but some show evidence of having had histoplasmosis of the lungs, and occasionally the disease manifests itself in an acute and fatal form. In most individuals histoplasmosis is a benign disease; there are virtually no symptoms and no special treatment is required. In the mid-1950s an antibiotic *amphotericin B,* was discovered which is effective against the histoplasma in the more acute forms of the disease. Interestingly, this antibiotic was derived from another fungus which was originally recovered from the soil of the Orinoco River region of Venezuela.

INFLUENZA During the four autumn months of 1918 a great pandemic of influenza caused 21 million deaths throughout the world; nearly half a million of them occurred in the United States. There are records of two other major epidemics of influenza in North America during the past two centuries. The first of these occurred in 1789, the year in which George Washington was inaugurated President. The first steamboat did not cross the Atlantic until 1819, and the first steam train did not run until 1830. Thus, this outbreak occurred when man's fastest conveyance was the galloping horse. Despite this fact, the influenza outbreak of 1789 spread with great rapidity; many times faster and many times farther than a horse could gallop. The attack rate was high, and the disease affected chiefly middle-aged persons. The mortality rate was low, and the few deaths that occurred may well have been due to the "heroic" therapeutic measures used in those days. Robert Johnson described this epidemic in his inaugural dissertation for the degree of Doctor of Medicine at the University of Pennsylvania in 1793. He attributed the spread of the disease to a "vicious quality of the air," the same factor that was held responsible at that time for the spread of malaria and yellow fever. The information regarding this epidemic is important because it demonstrates that influenza spread with unbelievable rapidity before fast modern transportation was available.

The second great epidemic of influenza in the United States occurred in 1889–90. This was a worldwide pandemic, which apparently began in Turkestan in May, 1889; by November it involved most of Europe, and in December it had become widespread in England and North America. The epidemiological and clinical characteristics of this illness were much like those of the pandemic influenza of 1918 except that the symptoms were less severe and the mortality rate was considerably lower. Since bacteriological discoveries were being made at a rapid rate at the time of this epidemic, an intensive effort was made to find a bacteriological cause for influenza. Professor Ludwig Pfeiffer in Germany believed that he had discovered the influenza bacterium *(Haemophilus influenzae),* and for the next 30 years it was generally believed that the cause of influenza had been found.

The epidemic that occurred in 1918 extended into 1919, during which time the world was deeply preoccupied by war; thus its early phases attracted little attention. In the late winter of 1917–18, ill-defined acute respiratory disorders were observed more or less simultaneously in Europe, Asia, and America. By April these disorders were spreading among troops and civilians in France. At this time the disease was recognized as influenza. During the summer, influenza was seen widely in western Europe, in India, and elsewhere. It became known as "three-day fever," a rather mild illness characterized by lassitude and generalized aching that soon gave way to an uneventful convalescence.

In August the disease began to take on a more serious character, and the death rate in France began to climb. Though the illness frequently began with the mild symptoms previously noted, an increasing number of cases developed complications, usually a severe pneumonia, and it was the latter that was responsible for the deaths. In early October the more serious form of the disease crossed the Atlantic. Boston was the first city to be seriously affected; a week later it was New York; the following week, Washington and Chicago; next, New Orleans; and then the cities of the West Coast. In the Army camps, where soldiers were crowded together in barracks, the incidence was particularly high. The death rates everywhere soared to new peaks. Emergency hospitals were created in schools, churches, town halls, and other buildings. So many people were ill that the whole economy and business of the country were thrown out of gear.

Two notable features of this epidemic were that the disease occurred more frequently among children from 5 to 14 years of age and that the greatest number of cases and nearly half the total number of deaths occurred in people less than 40 years old. The case fatality rate in the autumn months of 1918 in the cities of the United States ranged from 3.1 per cent in New London, Connecticut, to 0.8 per cent in San Antonio, Texas. Military personnel in the camps in the United States were the hardest hit; in the four autumn months about 25 per cent of the soldiers contracted influenza, and of these, approximately 6 per cent died. Stated in other words, about 1 soldier out of every 67 in the camps lost his life as a result of influenza.

In spite of intensive efforts, no bacterial cause of the epidemic could be discovered. From the information gathered it seemed clear that Pfeiffer's bacillus was not responsible. It was not until 1933 that Smith, Andrews, and Laidlaw, in England, isolated a filterable virus from the throat washings of a patient with influenza. These investigators took an important step foward when they found that the virus was capable of infecting ferrets, and this was the means by which they isolated it. Later work showed that mice and fertile chicken eggs could be infected also. The information which has been gathered since then has proved that influenza is caused by one of several closely related filterable viruses. A simple diagnostic test has now been developed for recognizing influenza and for determining which strain of virus is involved. Since the virus causing the 1918 epidemic was never isolated, it is not known just how this virus compares with the viruses that caused more recent epidemics.

At the height of the pandemic in the autumn of 1918, a new disease appeared among swine in the Middle West. Millions of swine became ill, and thousands died. J. S. Koen of the United States Bureau of Animal Industry was the first to recognize that this was a new disease. He was impressed by the fact that it had occurred simultaneously with human influenza and that

215

the symptoms in the hogs resembled those in the human patients. He believed that the hogs had contracted the disease from people. Koen's theory was not given much publicity, because it was not proved and because it was feared that the public might become alarmed and give up eating pork.

Epidemics of swine influenza continued to occur annually, and in 1928 Paul A. Lewis and Richard S. Shope of the Department of Animal Pathology (Princeton branch) of the Rockefeller Institute began a systematic search for the causative agent of this disease. They soon demonstrated that a filterable virus played a role in the causation, but it did not appear to be the sole factor, because when the virus was administered alone, it produced a disease that was clinically much milder than the true swine influenza that occurred naturally. Further study indicated that the full-blown disease occurred only when a hog was infected with two organisms: the filterable virus and a bacillus somewhat similar to Pfeiffer's bacillus. After it had been shown that human influenza is caused by a filterable virus, it was found that the virus of swine influenza is almost identical to the human virus. This gave support to the belief that swine influenza had indeed originated with the

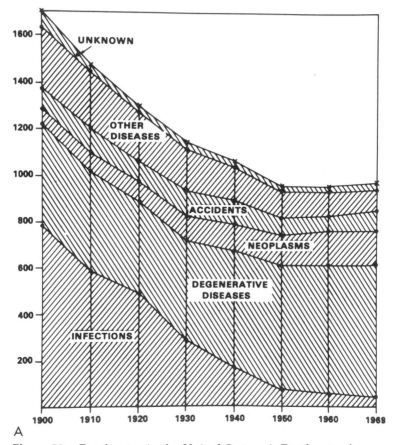

A

Figure 52. Death rates in the United States. *A*, Death rates from all causes (1900–69); *B*, Death rates from infections (1900–69). (From Peery, Thomas M.: The new and old diseases. A study of mortality trends in the United States, 1940–1960. Ward Burdick Award Address. Reproduced with permission from Am. J. Clin. Pathol. *63*:453, 1975.)

216

Illustration continued on opposite page

TABLE 1. ANNUAL U.S. DEATH RATE, 1900 AND 1950*

	1900	1950
All causes	1719.1**	963.8
All infectious diseases	785.1	82.0
Intestinal infections	194.9	7.8
Meningitis	40.6	1.8
Measles	13.3	0.3
Diphtheria and croup	40.3	0.3
Influenza, bronchitis, pneumonia	228.4	33.0
Tuberculosis	195.1	22.5
Other	72.5	16.3

*Adapted from Peery, 1975.
**Per 100,000 population.

epidemic of human disease. It also offered a plausible explanation of the mild and severe phases of the 1918 pandemic.

THE DECLINE OF INFECTIOUS DISEASES   The decline in the importance of infectious diseases as causes of death may be stated concisely in statistical terms. There were no accurate national statistics prior to 1900. Table 1 displays what happened between 1900 and 1950 in the registration states. It should be noted that the death rate had started to fall before this period.

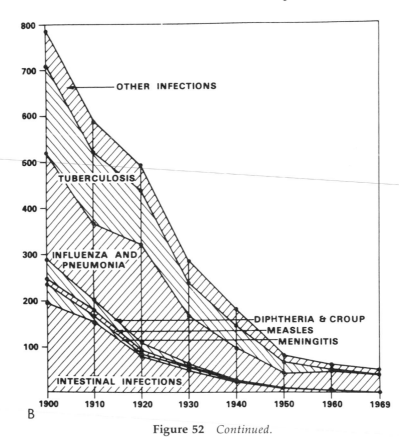

Figure 52 *Continued.*

NONINFECTIOUS DISEASES

In the 25 years leading up to 1900, so much attention had been atttracted by the triumphs of microbiological research that all other types of medical investigation were cast into the shadows. Infectious diseases had long been the major spoilers of life, but now that ways were being found to prevent or cure them, people began to hope that all diseases were caused by "germs" so that they could be controlled by one of the newfangled methods — sanitation or vaccines or antitoxins or chemicals.

These wishful individuals — and many doctors were among them — failed to see that while the microbiologists were performing their magical feats, investigators in other fields of medicine were quietly plowing virgin soil, where they were finding that many diseases had no relation to microbes. Indeed, in some of these maladies the cause was not a positive one, such as a bacterium, but a negative one, a deficiency of some substance required to maintain health. These diseases fell into two main categories: (1) those in which there were deficiencies of substances normally generated within the body (hormones); and (2) those in which there were deficiencies of substances normally entering the body through the digestive tract (nutrients, vitamins, and minerals). American research workers were among those who played leading roles in plowing this new ground.

HORMONES

Hormones are natural secretions of the endocrine glands. They are potent biological substances that serve as the chemical messengers of the body. Together they make up a large family of chemicals that activate, coordinate, and regulate the phenomena of life. (The name *hormone* was first used by two British physiologists, Bayliss and Starling, in about 1905; it is derived from a Greek word meaning "I arouse to activity" (Bayliss, 1924). The endocrine glands are composed of cells that manufacture hormones and release them into the circulation as needed to perform specific regulatory functions. A unique feature of the hormones is that their effect is not upon the tissue from which they arise but upon tissues in other parts of the body or upon general metabolic and nervous activity. Examples of endocrine glands are the *thyroid* and the *pituitary,* each of which is a single structure; the *adrenals,* of which there are two; and the *parathyroids,* of which there are four. Some endocrine glands, such as the parathyroids, produce a single hormone; others, such as the pituitary and the adrenals, produce several different hormones, each of which has its own specific function. Not all hormones are produced in discrete endocrine glands; the catecholamines, for example, including the powerfully vasoactive norepinephrine, are synthesized and stored in widely scattered nerve cells.

Diseases attributable to the endocrine glands are basically of two types: (1) diseases in which there is overproduction of a hormone, usually due to a tumor of the gland, or to an overgrowth or overactivity of a particular type of cell in the gland; (2) disorders in which there is underproduction of a hormone, usually caused by absence, atrophy, destruction, or lack of appropriate stimulation of a gland or of a particular type of cell in the gland. In some instances, deficient production of a hormone is due to a diet which lacks an ingredient essential for the synthesis of the hormone.

218

Our knowledge of hormones and of endocrine function has been acquired for the most part within the period of the second century, and American clinical and laboratory workers have made important contributions to our understanding of this complex subject.

Some of the anatomical and physiological effects of castration were well recognized in ancient times. Eunuchs, for obvious reasons, were employed as keepers of the harem. Up to the middle of the eighteenth century the most favored operatic singers were eunuchs, the so-called *castrati*. Their soprano voices possessed great power because their vocal cords, resembling those of a woman, were combined with the lungs of a man. It was not known then that the anatomical and physiological effects of castration were due to the lack of an internal secretion (hormone) normally supplied to the body by the testes. The first published experimental evidence of a physiologically active internal secretion by the testes appeared in 1849, when Arnold A. Berthold of Göttingen reported that when the testes were removed from a rooster he lost the characteristic cockscomb and feathers. If then the testes of another rooster were implanted in the castrated fowl, the original male features reappeared.

The Thyroid. Except for the testes, the only endocrine glands whose functions were at least partially recognized before 1876 were the thyroid and the adrenals. Goiter (enlargement of the thyroid gland) was described as far back as the days of the Roman Empire. In 1602, Felix Platter noted that in certain regions of Switzerland goiter was common and was associated with stunted growth and feeble-mindedness. We now know that this condition, which is called *cretinism,* is due to a lack of iodine in the food and water of the region in which the disease occurs. Iodine is an essential component of the chemical structure of the thyroid hormone. Lacking iodine, the thyroid gland grows larger, but it is unable to manufacture the thyroid hormone, without which normal bodily growth and mental development do not occur.

In 1850, a disease similar to cretinism was observed by Thomas B. Curling of London in two children in whom autopsy revealed a total absence of thyroid tissue. In these cases the disease was due not to the deficiency of an essential dietary ingredient but to the lack of the entire chemical factory (the thyroid) which normally makes the hormone. In adults when the secretion of the thyroid hormone becomes deficient a condition known as *myxedema* develops. This condition was first described by William W. Gull of London in 1873. Gull designated this state *cretinoid* because so many of the features were the same as those observed in cretins. He observed these patients only during life, and he had no opportunity to examine the thyroid glands. We know today that myxedema (sometimes called Gull's disease) is due to lack of the thyroid hormone, resulting from degeneration and atrophy of the thyroid gland during adult life. A similar condition can be produced by surgical removal of the thyroid.

Myxedema was the first endocrine-deficiency disease to be treated successfully. In 1891, an English physician, George R. Murray, prepared a glycerin extract from the thyroid gland of a freshly killed sheep and injected it subcutaneously, twice a week, into a woman with typical myxedema. The patient's appearance reverted toward normal, and her symptoms gradually subsided. This therapeutic experiment provided the first proof that a substance (it was not yet called a hormone) manufactured by an endocrine

219

gland of another animal could be substituted for the substance normally manufactured by the corresponding gland in man.

Hyperthyroidism, also known as *exophthalmic goiter, thyrotoxicosis,* or *Graves' disease,* was the first condition to be described in which the symptoms were due to overproduction of a hormone. In this disease, which is characterized by extreme nervousness, loss of weight, protruding eyes, rapid heart action, and other symptoms, the thyroid is enlarged, but it differs from the common type of goiter in that the thyroid is less prominent and softer.

The thyroid was the first endocrine gland to be removed or reduced in size by surgery because it was believed to be overactive. Prior to 1860, surgical excision of all or part of a goiter had been attempted about 100 times. The reason for operation in these cases was almost always a mechanical one; a large goiter had made breathing or swallowing so difficult that something had to be done. In more than half the cases the operation led to the death of the patient, frequently from hemorrhage or postoperative infection. In speaking of the operation for goiter, Samuel D. Gross, then one of America's leading surgeons, said in 1866, "The question arises, is such a procedure proper or justifiable? In a word, can the thyroid gland, when in a state of enlargement, be removed with a reasonable hope of saving the patient? Experience emphatically answers, no" (Halsted, 1919).

In the 1870s, though surgeons were becoming bolder, thyroidectomy was still an operation which most surgeons wished to avoid. Halsted said that during the years 1879–80 when he was working in Billroth's large surgical clinic in Vienna and attending the operations regularly, he did not see a single operation for goiter. After returning to New York, Halsted knew of only one operation on the thyroid in that city during a six-year period (1880–86), and that was a simple procedure for the removal of a small tumor.

In Europe during the 1880s, particularly in the German, Austrian, and Swiss surgical clinics, improved surgical technique and the use of antiseptic procedures made operations on the thyroid less hazardous, and they were performed with greater frequency. As a result of better surgery, more patients survived the operation. With the increased number of survivors, a new type of postoperative complication came to light. Within the first day after operation some patients developed tetany (extreme nervous irritability and muscular spasms). This in itself might lead to death wihin a few days, or it might continue for weeks, or it might gradually subside. If the patient survived for an additional period of weeks or months he often developed the characteristic features of myxedema. The Swiss surgeon Theodor Kocher recognized myxedema in one of his postoperative patients only three years after Gull had first described this disease. As more thyroidectomies were performed, more of these complications were encountered. Kocher reported that myxedema had occurred in 30 patients out of 100 on whom he had performed a thyroidectomy. Both tetany and myxedema were observed more frequently in those cases in which the most complete extirpation of the thyroid had been accomplished.

Until the 1890s it was believed that both the tetany and the myxedema that followed thyroidectomy were caused by thyroid deficiency. The phase of tetany was called *acute thyroid deficiency,* and myxedema was considered to be due to *chronic thyroid deficiency*. In 1896, two Italians, G. Vassale and F. Generali, demonstrated that the acute phase is due not to thyroid deficiency but to removal of the tiny and inconspicuous parathyroid glands. These glands were not discovered until 1855 (Remak), and their function remained obscure until 1896. Since the four parathyroid glands are attached to the posterior surface of the thyroid, one or all of them might be damaged or removed during the course of a thyroidectomy. In fact, since surgeons were unaware of the parathyroids until 1896, it was only a stroke of good fortune when enough parathyroid tissue was left behind to prevent the occurrence of tetany. Fortunately, not much parathyroid tissue is required. Halsted performed some experiments on dogs, in which the parathyroids were removed and a small portion of one of them was implanted in the animal's tissues. "We made the startling and hardly believable observation that the life of a dog may be maintained by a particle of parathyroid tissue only one-quarter of a millimeter in diameter and extinguished by tetany on its removal."

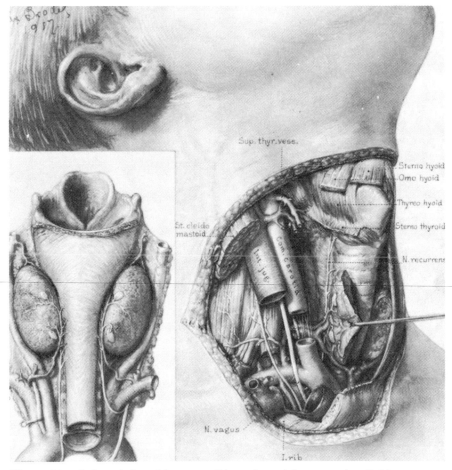

Figure 53. Subtotal thyroidectomy: Dissection of the operative field (by Max Broedel). (From the Broedel Collection, Department of Art as Applied to Medicine, The Johns Hopkins School of Medicine.)

221

It was only after surgeons had learned that they had to take care not to damage or remove the parathyroids and that at least a small amount of thyroid tussue must be left behind to prevent the development of myxedema that the surgical treatment of exophthalmic goiter (hyperthyroidism) became feasible. Since it was not known at first how much of the thyroid gland would have to be removed to correct the overproduction of the thyroid hormone, the earliest operators removed only one half (one lobe) of the gland. This proved to be inadequate in most cases, and finally, through trial and error, a standard operative procedure known as *subtotal thyroidectomy* was adopted for use in cases of hyperthyroidism. The operation most widely used was developed by Halsted between 1900 and 1910, and the background of its development is described in Halsted's monograph, *The Operative Story of Goitre* (1919), in which the instruments used and each step in the operation are beautifully portrayed by drawings executed by the incomparable Max Broedel.

It remained for an American biochemist, Edward C. Kendall, to isolate and identify chemically the thyroid hormone. Kendall received his Ph.D. in chemistry from Columbia University in 1910. He then worked for a year as a research chemist for Parke, Davis and Company in Detroit, where he was assigned the task of isolating the essential hormone of the thyroid gland. He was not happy with his experience in a commercial laboratory, because he felt that closer association with physicians and patients was desirable for

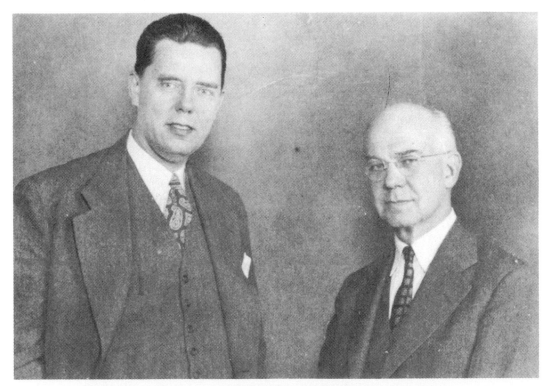

Figure 54. Edward C. Kendall (right) and Philip S. Hench. (From Samter, Max (ed.): Classics in Allergy. Columbus, Ohio, Ross Laboratories, 1969.)

research on medical problems. He therefore obtained a position as head of the new biochemical laboratory at St. Luke's Hospital, New York, where he continued his work on the thyroid.

Sixteen years before Kendall went to St. Luke's Hospital, Eugen Baumann, a German scientist, had found that a unique feature of thyroid tissue was its high content of iodine. In his search for the thyroid hormone Kendall was, therefore, looking for a substance containing iodine. He was proceeding with this work and had obtained a substance from thyroid tissue that contained 33 per cent iodine, when St. Luke's Hospital ran out of funds to support his research. In 1914, Kendall wrote to Louis B. Wilson, chief of the Laboratory Division of the Mayo Clinic, asking whether Wilson would be interested in having a chemist who wanted to study the thyroid gland. Kendall was offered a position as biochemist at the Mayo Clinic, where he found that several members of the medical staff were greatly interested in thyroid disease, including Henry S. Plummer, the chief of the Department of Medicine. In less than a year after taking up his work at the Mayo Clinic, Kendall succeeded in isolating the pure crystalline thyroid hormone containing 65 per cent iodine, to which the name *thyroxin* was given. Kendall reported his accomplishment in May, 1915, at a meeting of the Association of American Physicians, before whom so many important medical discoveries have been announced (Hench, 1952).

The Parathyroids. The physiological function of the parathyroid hormone, which had been brought to light by thyroid surgery, was clarified in 1909 when W. G. MacCallum and C. Voegtlin at Johns Hopkins found that in animals with tetany resulting from removal of the parathyroids, the calcium level in the blood was considerably below normal and that tetany could be prevented by the injection of calcium salts. In 1925 James Bertram Collip, then at the University of Alberta, Canada, isolated the parathyroid hormone to which he gave the name *parathormone*.

It is now known that the principal function of the parathyroid hormone is to regulate the calcium and phosphorus metabolism of the body. When there is a deficiency of the hormone, the calcium level in the blood falls and tetany results. On the other hand, when there is an excess production of the hormone, as occurs with tumors of the parathyroid glands, calcium rises to a level higher than normal in the blood. In the latter circumstance, calcium, the mineral which gives bone its strength, is withdrawn from the bones, and a bone disease known as *osteitis fibrosa cystica* results. At the same time, calcium is excreted in the urine in excessive amounts, and renal stones develop. Fuller Albright, Walter Bauer, and their associates at the Massachusetts General Hospital, in 1930s and 1940s, did much original and valuable work in relation to the pathogenesis, diagnosis, and treatment of both hyper- and hypo- parathyroidism and other conditions affecting the metabolism of calcium and phosphorus.

Insulin. The disease *diabetes mellitus* has been known for centuries. Originally it was diagnosed by tasting the urine and finding that it was sweet. In the latter part of the eighteenth century, crude chemical tests demonstrated that the sweet taste of the urine and blood plasma of diabetic patients was due to the presence of sugar. Prior to 1920 the only treatment for diabetes was strict control of the diet, with severe limitation of carbohydrate intake. In spite of the most rigid dietary restrictions, the disease fre-

223

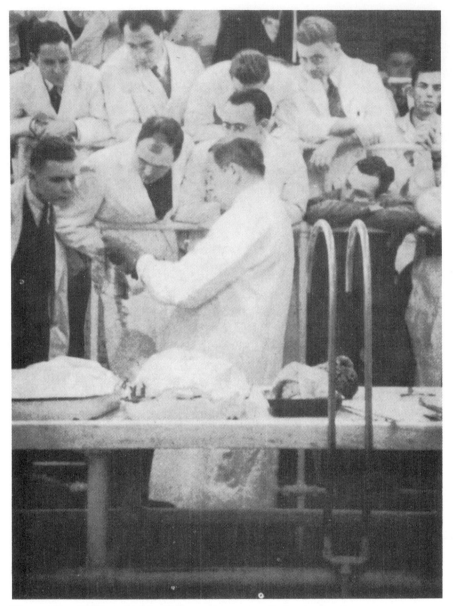

Figure 55. William G. MacCallum (foreground) demonstrating pathological specimens to students of medicine. (From the Archives Office, The Johns Hopkins Medical Institutions.)

quently was fatal. It tended to be milder in older individuals, but young diabetics rarely survived for more than a few years.

In 1889 two scientists in Germany, Joseph von Mering and Oscar Minkowski, were carrying out some investigations on the digestive function of pancreatic juice. When they removed the pancreas of a dog in order to keep the pancreatic juice from entering the intestine, they discovered much to their surprise that the animal developed diabetes. It was thus revealed that the pancreas produces not only a digestive juice (which had long been known) but also another substance which is required for normal

224

carbohydrate metabolism. In further experiments Minkowski found that if the pancreatic duct was tied off so that the digestive secretion of the pancreatic acinar cells could not reach the intestine, the animal could not digest its food. It became emaciated and eventually died, but it did not develop diabetes. Minkowski concluded that a non-acinar component of the pancreas produced an antidiabetic internal secretion.

When Eugene L. Opie was a student in the first class to graduate from the Johns Hopkins Medical School, he had the following experience: "During the laboratory course in Pathology I found in a section of the pancreas a strange body which I showed to Dr. Welch when he made his unhurried rounds of the class. He told me it was a structure described by Langerhans in 1869. 'Find out all you can about the islets of Langerhans,' Welch said to me." After graduation Opie became a member of Welch's department and concentrated his attention on diseases of the pancreas. In the course of his studies he discovered and reported that in some cases of diabetes the islet cells showed evidence of degeneration.

Several years after Opie had begun his study of the pancreas, his classmate and fellow member of the Department of Pathology, William G. Mac-Callum, performed an ingenious experiment on a dog. He separated the tail of the pancreas from the rest of the gland and tied off its secretory duct but left the pancreas in place. Seven months later it was found at operation that the separated tail portion of the pancreas had shrunk to such an extent that it was scarcely detectable as a discrete body of tissue. At this point the intact part of the pancreas, which appeared to be quite normal, was removed. The animal did not develop diabetes. Three weeks later the small remnant of the tail section was removed, and large amounts of sugar appeared in the urine. Microscopic examination of the remnant showed that it was made up largely of cells of the islets of Langerhans. MacCallum concluded that these cells produced something that prevented the occurrence of glycosuria.

MacCallum's experiment, which was reported in 1909, was carried out on only a single dog, but his results soon were confirmed by other research workers. The evidence seemed to point clearly to the islet cells as producers of an antidiabetic hormone, but all efforts to extract such a hormone from the pancreas were unsuccessful until 1920, when Frederick G. Banting, a young Canadian surgeon, provided the clue that solved the problem.

Banting was born in 1891 near Toronto. His medical education at the University of Toronto was hurried by the onset of World War I. After graduation in 1916, he joined the Canadian Army Medical Corps in France and was severely wounded six weeks before the war ended. He returned to Canada and settled in London, Ontario, opening an office for the practice of orthopedic surgery. He also held an appointment as Demonstrator in the Department of Physiology at the University of Western Ontario. While looking up material in the library for a lecture on diabetes that he was preparing, he found an article in the October, 1920, issue of the journal *Surgery, Gynecology and Obstetrics*. This article, by Moses Barron of the Department of Pathology of the University of Minnesota, reported four cases of diabetes in which microscopic examination of the pancreas disclosed varying degrees of degeneration of the islets of Langerhans. Though Barron's article contained no original observations, it gave an excellent brief

225

review of the work of von Mering and Minkowski, Opie, MacCallum, and others and stated that the "present study bears out the conclusion that the islets secrete a hormone... which has a controlling power over carbohydrate metabolism."

Barron's article gave Banting an idea that so excited him that he could not sleep that night, and at 2 A.M. he made the following entry in his notebook: "Ligate the pancreatic ducts of dogs. Wait six to eight weeks for degeneration. Remove the residue and extract." This note conveys Banting's notion that previous attempts to obtain the antidiabetic principle from the intact normal pancreas had failed because of the destruction of this principle by the digestive enzymes of the pancreas during the course of extraction. The experiments of Minkowski, MacCallum and others had suggested a way to eliminate the cells that produced the digestive enzymes.

The facilities at the University of Western Ontario were inadequate for the type of experiments that Banting had in mind, so he decided to seek the aid of Professor J. J. R. MacLeod, Director of the Department of Physiology at the University of Toronto and an authority on carbohydrate metabolism. MacLeod at first tried to discourage Banting from undertaking what he considered to be a naive and unpromising project. However, Banting was persistent, and MacLeod finally agreed to provide some experimental animals and to allow Banting to use one of the research laboratories during the summer months.

Recognizing that Banting lacked chemical training, MacLeod suggested that Charles H. Best, a medical student who was approaching graduation and who had received training in both physiology and biochemistry, join Banting to provide assistance with the chemical aspects of the project.

Banting and Best tied off the pancreatic duct of several dogs and waited patiently in the hot summer weather for the enzyme-producing tissues to atrophy. Toward the end of July they succeeded in obtaining pancreatic tissue in which only the islet cells were in healthy condition, and an extract was made of this tissue. When they injected this extract into a diabetic dog on the night of July 30, 1921, the animal's elevated blood sugar was definitely lowered. Over the next few weeks they repeated their experiment several times until they were certain that the substance they were obtaining from the pancreas could lower the blood sugar and prolong the life of their diabetic dogs. When the results were reported to Professor MacLeod he was skeptical about the claims of these inexperienced investigators, and he made them repeat the experiments over and over. By late 1921 even MacLeod was convinced that the substance extracted from the islet tissue—"insulin"—was effective against the experimental diabetes of dogs. At this juncture, MacLeod arranged for Professor J. B. Collip of the University of Alberta, who had experience with the chemistry of hormones, to join the group in order to devise a method for preparing a pure form of insulin. Before January, 1922, Collip had prepared an insulin that was considered pure enough to use on human patients.

A dramatic scene was enacted in a Toronto hospital in January, 1922. The central character was now not a dog but a 14 year old boy. He was little more than a skeleton, weighing but 65 pounds. He was a victim of diabetes, which had progressed in spite of a rigid diet, and his blood and urine were loaded with sugar. This boy, on the verge of coma, was given a hypodermic

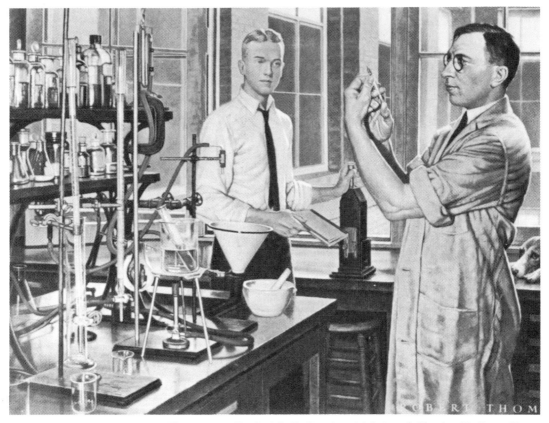

Figure 56. Frederick G. Banting (right) and Charles H. Best. (From Great Moments in Medicine, Parke, Davis and Company, Detroit, Northwood Institute Press, 1966. Stories by George A. Bender.)

injection of insulin in a very weak solution. Two or three hours later, tests of the blood and urine showed definite improvement, and more insulin was cautiously injected. Within two weeks, on daily doses of insulin, the youngster once again looked and acted like an individual in good health. The possibility existed that some unknown factor rather than the insulin was responsible for the improvement. The only way to clear up any doubt about this was to withhold the insulin for several days just as had been done in the experiment on the dogs. For 10 days, therefore, insulin was withheld. The boy's condition deteriorated rapidly, and he once again displayed all the distressing symptoms of uncontrolled diabetes. There could now be no doubt about it: insulin had done the trick. As soon as injections were resumed, the patient again regained his health.

In May, 1922, Banting and his co-workers reported the results of their experiments on dogs and on diabetic patients at a meeting of the Association of American Physicians. However, even before insulin had been tested on a single patient, the press had heard about the research, and diabetics from all parts of the world began to clamor for this new substance. It was not until several years after the discovery that the supply of insulin began to meet the demand. Banting and Best refused to profit directly from their

227

discovery. They applied for a patent on insulin but arranged to have the University of Toronto assume responsibility for administering the patent and for assuring the quality of the insulin produced. In 1922, Eli Lilly and Company entered into an agreement to undertake the commercial production of insulin.

In 1923 Banting and MacLeod were awarded the Nobel Prize in medicine for the discovery of insulin. Since they felt that their associates deserved recognition, Banting gave half of his share to Best, and MacLeod gave half of his share to Collip. At the outbreak of World War II Banting gave up everything that he cherished to devote himself wholeheartedly to the Canadian war effort. Tragically, in 1941, he lost his life in the crash of a bombing plane off the coast of Newfoundland.

Professor John J. Abel of Johns Hopkins, who had narrowly missed isolating pure epinephrine in 1899, succeeded in isolating pure crystalline insulin in 1926, and he proved that it is a protein. Abel was 69 years old at the time of this great achievement.

As in the case of other hormones, it has been found that illness may be caused by overproduction as well as by underproduction of insulin. The first case of the former type was reported in 1927 by Russell M. Wilder and co-workers of the Mayo Clinic. Their patient had a cancer of the pancreas composed of cells of the islets of Langerhans. The blood sugar was extremely low, and unless the patient was given large amounts of sugar, he was in an almost perpetual state of insulin shock. After the patient died, analysis of the tumor revealed that it contained insulin. Since then similar cases have been reported. Fortunately, not all insulin-secreting tumors are malignant. When the tumor is a benign one, a dramatic cure can be effected by surgical removal.

The Adrenals. In 1849 Thomas Addison, at Guy's Hospital, London, described the disease now known as Addison's disease. It is characterized by weakness, debility, feeble heart action, and a peculiar pigmentation of the skin. Addison attributed the disease to destruction of the adrenal glands, which he had observed in autopsies on these patients.

After Murray's success in treating thyroid deficiency with a thyroid extract, efforts were made to prepare an extract of the adrenal glands for the treatment of Addison's disease. Osler was among those who made the attempt. In 1896 he published a paper entitled "Six cases of Addison's disease with a report of a case greatly benefited by the use of suprarenal extract." His extract was made from pigs' adrenal glands, chopped up and thoroughly powdered in a mortar, to which pure glycerin was added. This material was then filtered and administered in small doses each day to a patient with classical Addison's disease.

The treatment was continued in the hospital for almost four months, during which the patient showed progressive improvement: he gained 19 pounds; the pulse strengthened and the pulse rate fell toward normal; and the patient's energy and spirits improved. He left the hospital in excellent condition. When the patient was examined four months later, he said that he was as well as he had ever been in his life, and he showed no evidence of Addison's disease except for persistent pigmentation of the skin. This was perhaps the first successful treatment of Addison's disease. Glycerin, which was used in the extraction process, is now known to be an effective solvent

228

for some of the adrenal hormones. In spite of Osler's apparent success, the results that he reported were not reproduced until almost 40 years later.

The adrenals are far more complex organs than the thyroid: they produce many different hormones, and it is not surprising that the early efforts to prepare an extract suitable for the treatment of patients were unsuccessful.

An adrenal gland is made up of a central portion, the *medulla,* and an outer portion, the *cortex.* The first hormone to be extracted from the adrenal was *epinephrine* (Adrenalin), which was given its name in 1899 by John J. Abel of Baltimore. In 1895 G. Oliver and E. A. Schafer of the University College, London, had obtained an extract from the adrenal glands of animals which had a powerful effect in raising the blood pressure. Abel set about trying to isolate this substance in pure form. He did not succeed in this attempt, but he did obtain a highly active monobenzoyl derivative of epinephrine. Jokichi Takamine, a Japanese chemist who had visited Abel's laboratory, thought he saw a way around the difficulties that Abel had encountered. By introducing some relatively simple changes in the chemical procedures, he succeeded in 1901 in isolating epinephrine in pure crystalline form. It is now known that this hormone is produced by the adrenal medulla.

After epinephrine had been isolated by Takamine, some researchers thought that it might be effective in the treatment of Addison's disease (adrenal insufficiency), but this proved not to be the case. Attention therefore turned to the adrenal cortex as the possible source of an effective substance.

Adrenal insufficiency can be produced in animals by removing the adrenal glands, and in 1927 F. A. Hartman and his associates at the Univer-

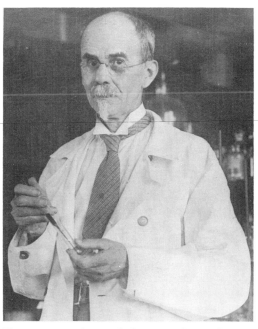

Figure 57. John J. Abel. (From the Archives Office, The Johns Hopkins Medical Institutions.)

sity of Buffalo succeeded in making an adrenal cortical extract that prolonged the lives of adrenalectomized animals. They named the unidentified active substance in this extract *cortin*. In 1930 two improved extracts were made, one by Hartman and his associates, the other by W. W. Swingle and J. J. Pfiffner of the Department of Biology at Princeton University. Not only did these discoveries make it possible to treat Addison's disease but also they initiated intensive efforts by many investigators to isolate and identify the active substance or substances in the adrenal cortex. In 1930 E. C. Kendall, who had isolated thyroxin, turned all the resources of his laboratory at the Mayo Clinic to this problem. Others had the same objective, and a dramatic scientific race began, the chief competitors being O. P. Wintersteiner and J. J. Pfiffner at the Department of Biochemistry at Columbia University and Reichstein and his associates in Switzerland.

While this race was in progress two groups of Americans, George A. Harrop and his colleagues at Johns Hopkins and Robert F. Loeb and his colleagues at The College of Physicians and Surgeons, New York, discovered almost simultaneously that in adrenal insufficiency the kidneys fail to retain sodium. As a result, sodium is lost from the body, and the level of sodium in the blood serum is reduced. This and other related disturbances in mineral metabolism account for some of the major physiological abnormalities observed in Addison's disease. It was found that both in dogs from whom the adrenal glands had been removed and in patients with Addison's disease, marked temporary improvement resulted from the administration of sodium chloride. This important discovery also made it possible to utilize measurements of mineral metabolism to determine the effectiveness of various substances obtained from cortical extract. At about this same time it became apparent that adrenal insufficiency is also accompanied by a

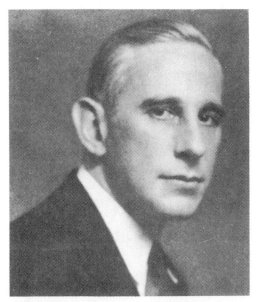

Figure 58. Robert F. Loeb. (From Riesman, David (ed.): History of the Interurban Clinical Club, 1905–1937. Philadelphia, The John C. Winston Company, 1937.)

disturbance in carbohydrate metabolism: poor glycogen storage, a tendency toward low blood sugar, and an increased sensitivity to insulin are present.

By 1934, Kendall's group at the Mayo Clinic had separated from adrenal extract a small amount of crystalline material that was soon found to be a mixture of closely related compounds of uncertain chemical composition and physiological potency. From that point on, crystals began to be precipitated out of cortical extracts almost simultaneously in New York, Minnesota, and Switzerland.

By 1942, 28 crystalline compounds had been isolated, but it was not easy to determine which of these was responsible for the cortin-like activity, because 3000 pounds of adrenal gland were needed to produce about 1 gram of the crystalline materials. In addition, after the crystals had been removed from the extract, even greater activity for maintenance of life was found in the amorphous fraction that remained. The crystalline compounds were steroids derived from cholesterol, and at least five of them were biologically active. Of these five, 11-desoxycorticosterone had the greatest effect in controlling the mineral metabolism, and *compound E* had the greatest effect on carbohydrate metabolism. Kendall was concentrating his efforts on isolation and purification of *compound E*.

In 1942, George W. Thorn reported that he and his associates at Johns Hopkins and a group of cooperating physicians had employed synthetic 11-desoxycorticosterone obtained from Reichstein for the treatment of Addison's disease in 158 patients. The treatment corrected the mineral metabolism, and most of the patients gained in strength, vigor, and weight. Many of them were able to return to work. However, the carbohydrate metabolism was not corrected, and the pigmentation of the skin was unaffected. Thorn stated that treatment with the synthetic steroid was not as effective as that with cortical extract, but it certainly prolonged life and had the advantage of being simpler, less expensive, and less disturbing to the patient (Thorn et al., 1942).

During World War II, Merck and Company devoted a great part of their research effort to the development of adrenal steroids. They found that *compound E* could be made from desoxycholic acid of bile. They developed, on a pilot scale, a method for greatly increasing the yield of this compound; however, there was very little demand for *compound E*, and while it was being made on a small scale in 1949 its price ($200 per gram) made it too expensive to be generally useful.

Meanwhile new developments were taking place at the Mayo Clinic. Philip S. Hench (see Fig. 54) of the clinic staff was making a study of rheumatoid arthritis. In most cases this disease is relentlessly progressive; but Hench had noted that if patients with rheumatoid arthritis developed jaundice or became pregnant there might be a remission in the arthritis which was sometimes quite impressive. Hench and his colleagues attempted to reproduce the effects of jaundice or pregnancy by various means. These included the transfusion of blood from jaundiced or pregnant donors to arthritic patients; the administration of female hormones and various biliary products; and the production of jaundice experimentally by the administration of several different chemical agents. None of these artificial procedures seemed to have any appreciable effect on the arthritis.

Hench also had been impressed by the fact that the weakness, fatigue,

231

and low blood pressure exhibited by many patients with rheumatoid arthritis were similar to the symptoms of Addison's disease, and he began to wonder whether the antirheumatic substance might be an adrenal hormone. As a result of conferences with Kendall in early 1941, it was decided to administer *compound E* to rheumatoid patients, but the amount of this substance which was then available was almost negligible; hence it was decided to try some of Kendall's rather crude extract, *cortin*. This had no beneficial effect. Further work along these lines was not undertaken until after World War II.

In 1948 Kendall obtained from Merck and Company a part of their small supply of *compound E,* which by that time had been renamed *cortisone.* The effect of this compound on rheumatoid arthritis was tested by administering it in a daily dose of 100 milligrams intramuscularly to a severely arthritic patient. Within three days the patient had shown dramatic improvement. This was the first evidence of the anti-inflammatory action of cortisone.

Diseases due to overproduction of adrenal hormones have undoubtedly existed for centuries, but they have been recognized only within the past 50 years. The adrenals produce a number of different hormones, each with its own physiological function, and the symptoms depend upon which particular hormone is being overproduced. Overproduction of epinephrine was the first of these conditions to be recognized. In 1922, Labbé, Tinel, and Doumer, in France, directed attention to a condition in which there were upward surges in the blood pressure (paroxysmal hypertension) such as might result from intravenous injection of epinephrine. Labbé and his associates related this disease to a tumor found during autopsy in one of the adrenal glands.

The first case in which a cure of paroxysmal hypertension was effected by surgical removal of a tumor of this type was reported in 1927 by Charles H. Mayo of the Mayo Clinic. In this case the correct diagnosis was not made before operation. The first case in which a correct preoperative diagnosis was made and the tumor removed with highly successful results was reported in 1929 by Maurice C. Pincoffs of the University of Maryland. This was also the first case in which it was definitely proved by biological tests that the tumor contained large amounts of epinephrine. It was evident that the cells of the tumor were manufacturing epinephrine and releasing it periodically into the blood. These tumors, known as pheochromocytomas, are uncommon, but it is important to diagnose them correctly, since removal of the tumor will promptly relieve a condition that otherwise would terminate fatally. A number of tests are now available to aid in making the diagnosis, and many patients suffering from the effect of pheochromocytomas have been restored to normal health.

As has already been noted, the adrenal cortex produces steroid hormones which regulate mineral and carbohydrate metabolism. It also produces another group of steroids known as androgens or male hormones, which exercise control over sexual development and function. Harvey Cushing, at the Peter Bent Brigham Hospital, was the first to recognize a disease caused by overproduction of adrenal cortical hormones. In this rare condition, described by Cushing in 1932 and now known as *Cushing's disease,* mineral and carbohydrate metabolism and sexual function are disturbed to varying degrees. The disturbance may be caused by tumors of one or both adrenals, either benign or malignant, made up of cortical cells. It also may be caused by overgrowth (hyperplasia) of the cells within intact adrenal glands or by overstimulation of the cortical cells by basophil adenomas of the pituitary, leading to the production of excessive amounts of hormones. The treatment for Cushing's disease depends upon the cause: a tumor may be removed surgically; bilateral hyperplasia of the adrenals is now treated by removing both adrenal glands and treating the patient for adrenal insufficiency (which can be treated medically with a high degree of success, although there is no satisfactory medical management for overproduction of cortical hormones). Overstimulation of the adrenal by a basophil tumor of the pituitary gland may be corrected by surgical removal or by irradiation of the pituitary. The methods for diagnosing and treating Cushing's disease have, in large measure, been perfected in the United States.

The Pituitary (Hypophysis). The pituitary gland is a small body of tissue situated at the base of the brain. Although it weighs less than a gram, it produces a host of highly active and important hormones. In the 1890s an extract of pituitary tissue was injected into animals and was found to have a powerful effect in raising the blood pressure. During the first two decades of the twentieth century it was discovered that pituitary extracts also cause strong contraction of the uterus and are capable of reducing the flow of urine in patients having *diabetes insipidus,* a malady characterized by excessive production of urine. It was gradually learned that the substance producing these effects was made by the posterior portion of the pituitary.

In an effort to isolate the active principle of the posterior pituitary, John J. Abel at Johns Hopkins succeeded in contracting the activity into an extremely small mass; the material he obtained was so powerful that it would stimulate the uterus in a dilution of 1 part in 20 thousand million. Abel mistakenly concluded that a single hormone of the posterior pituitary is reponsible for the effects on blood pressure, urine secretion, and uterine contraction. It subsequently became clear that two hormones, closely related chemically, are involved; one, *oxytocin,* being responsible for the effect on the uterus, the other, *vasopressin* — sometimes called *antidiuretic hormone (ADH)* — being responsible for the effect on blood pressure and urine production. These two hormones were fully identified chemically, and in the early 1950s Vincent duVigneaud of the Cornell University Medical College performed the remarkable feat of synthesizing them, for which he was awarded the Nobel Prize in chemistry in 1955.

The anterior lobe of the pituitary gland produces a greater variety of hormones than does the posterior portion. The first of its hormonal activities to be recognized was its effect on growth. A condition known as acromegaly, described by the French neurologist Pierre Marie in 1886, is characterized by enlargement of the hands, feet, jaw, tongue, lips, and certain internal organs. Several years after first describing this condition, Marie reported that autopsies had revealed that it is associated with enlargement of the pituitary gland. In 1901, Alfred Fröhlich in Germany reported the case of a teen-aged boy in whom an enlargement of the pituitary gland was associated with an entirely different type of abnormality. There were none of the features of acromegaly; the boy had a peculiar type of obesity, infantile testes, and lack of secondary sexual development.

233

Just how Marie's and Fröhlich's observations were to be reconciled was a puzzle. Physiologists had made repeated efforts to gain a better understanding of the function of the pituitary by removing the gland surgically in experimental animals. Surgical removal had been utilized to clarify the function of other endocrine glands, including the testes, thyroid, the adrenals, and the parathyroids; but removal of the pituitary, hidden as it is beneath the brain, was a far more difficult surgical undertaking. Very few animals survived the operation, and when they did survive it was usually found that the pituitary had not been removed completely. Some research workers had concluded that the pituitary is essential for life; others believed that it performs no important physiological function. This was the situation when Harvey Cushing entered the picture about 1905.

Cushing was a highly skilled surgeon with a special interest in surgery of the brain, and he had the advantage of a well-equipped and well-staffed experimental surgery laboratory at Johns Hopkins. By 1909, with the assistance of Samuel J. Crowe and John Homans, Cushing had carried out a remarkable series of observations on 50 dogs subjected to various degrees of extirpation of the pituitary gland (Crowe, Cushing, and Homans, 1910).

At about this same time Charles H. Mayo of the Mayo Clinic sent Cushing a patient suffering from acromegaly. Several surgeons had previously attempted to remove the pituitary in acromegalic patients, but the operation had been successful in only a single case, that reported by Hermann Schloffer of Germany in 1907. In March, 1909, Cushing operated on Mayo's patient. He found the anterior lobe of the pituitary to be considerably enlarged, and he removed about one third of it. The patient made a rapid recovery from the operation, and the evidences of acromegaly, with the exception of the enlargement of the bones, gradually subsided. The patient lived a relatively normal life for the next 21 years.

The observations on the animals from which various portions of the pituitary had been removed and on the acromegalic patient, together with a study of the reports in the literature, gave Cushing an extraordinarily clear and advanced perception not only of the role of the pituitary (hypophysis) but also of the interrelated function of the endocrine system. Cushing's observations made it easy to reconcile the disease described by Marie with that described by Fröhlich: he concluded that acromegaly is due to an overgrowth (adenoma) of the secreting cells of the pituitary and that the obesity with infantile sexual characteristics is due to overgrowth of a different type of tissue, one which compresses and destroys the secreting cells. Since Cushing's animal experiments were performed on puppies as well as adult dogs, they gave some insight into the effect of pituitary destruction at differing age levels (Cushing, 1909b, 1910):

Two conditions, one due to a pathologically increased activity of the pars anterior of the hypophysis (hyperpituitarism), the other to a diminished activity of the same epithelial structure (hypopituitarism), seem capable of clinical differentiation. The former expresses itself chiefly as a process of overgrowth — gigantism when originating in youth, acromegaly when originating in adult life. The latter expresses itself chiefly as an excessive, often a rapid, deposition of fat with persistence of infantile sexual characteristics when the process dates from youth, and a tendency towards a loss of the acquired signs of adolescence when it appears in adult life.

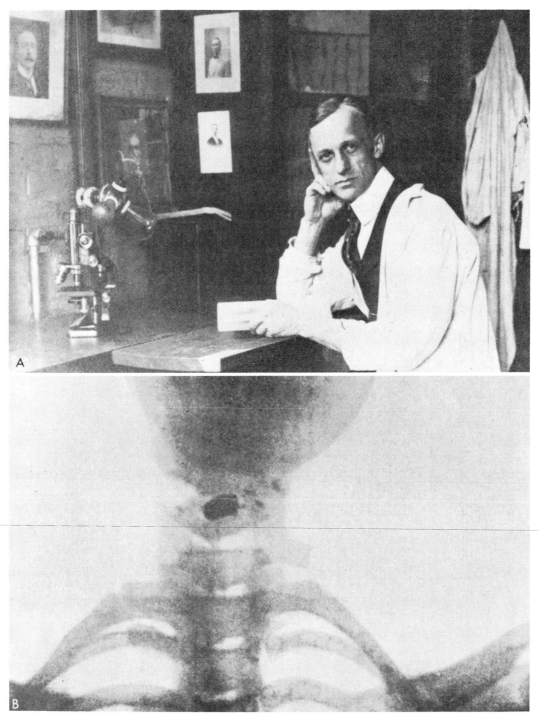

Figure 59. *A,* Harvey Cushing. *B,* First X-ray taken by Cushing at the Johns Hopkins Hospital. (From Fulton, John F.: Harvey Cushing, A Biography. Springfield, Ill., Charles C Thomas, Publishers, 1946. Reproduced with permission.)

235

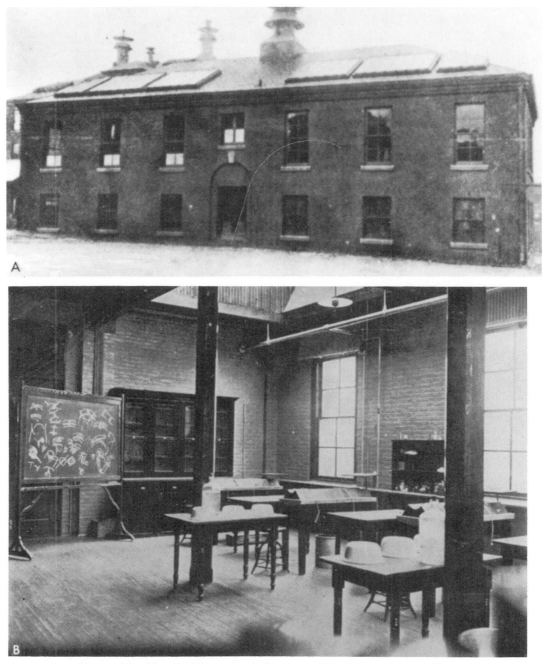

Figure 60. The old Hunterian Laboratory. The first experimental laboratory for surgical research, Johns Hopkins Medical School. *A,* The building; *B,*Corner of students' operating room. (*A,* From Chesney, A.M.: The Johns Hopkins Hospital and the Johns Hopkins University School of Medicine, A Chronicle. Vol. 3. Baltimore, The Johns Hopkins University Press, 1943. *B,* From the Archives Office, The Johns Hopkins Medical Institutions.)

Experimental observations show not only that the anterior lobe of the hypophysis is a structure of such importance that a condition of apituitarism is incompatible with the long maintenance of life, but also that its partial removal leads to symptoms comparable to those which we regard as characteristic of lessened secretion (hypopituitarism) in man. A tumor of the gland itself, or one arising in its neighborhood and implicating the gland by pressure, is naturally the lesion to which one or the other of these conditions has heretofore been attributed, though it is probable that over-secretion from simple hypertrophy or under-secretion from atrophy, will be found to occur irrespective of tumor growth when examination of the pituitary body becomes a routine measure in the postmortem examination of all cases in which the conditions suggest one or the other of the symptoms-complex described. When due to tumor, surgery is the treatment that these conditions demand, and at present there are reasonably satisfactory ways of approaching the gland.

It may be said that the pituitary body is a double organ in the sense that the secretion of its anterior and solidly epithelial portion discharges into the blood sinuses which traverse this part of the gland. . . . Though possessing a physiologically active principle, as shown by the results of injection, the secretion of the posterior lobe does not seem to be so vitally essential to physiological equilibrium as that of the anterior lobe, the total removal of which leads to death with a peculiar train of symptoms which set in at an early date in adult and after a longer interval in younger animals. . . .

In view of the apparent interrelation of many of the glands of internal secretion it is quite probable that certain of these symptoms known to accompany hypophyseal disease may be consequent upon a secondary change in other glands which follows the primary lesion of the hypophysis. These changes are seemingly more outspoken and more widespread after a lesion of the pituitary body than after a corresponding lesion of any other individual member of the group of ductless glands, and in view of its unusually well-protected position one might have conjectured that it must represent a vitally important organ.

The thought expressed in the last paragraph of the foregoing quotation — that the pituitary exerts its effect by influencing the activity of other endocrine glands — was a brilliant inference supported by only a few scattered facts, but time would prove it to be remarkably accurate. Prior to Cushing's interest in the subject there had been talk about the interrelation of the endocrine glands, but as late as 1924 the distinguished British physiologist William M. Bayliss considered such talk to be no more than "elaborate theories" based on "slender evidence." The final proof of Cushing's hypothesis had to await the identification of anterior pituitary hormones, whose effect upon other endocrine glands could be demonstrated in experimental animals and in man.

Herbert M. Evans had done special work as a student under Cushing in the experimental surgery laboratory and was a member of Mall's Department of Anatomy while the studies on the pituitary were in progress. In 1915 he went to the University of California (Berkeley) as Professor of Anatomy. In 1921 Evans and an associate, J. A. Long, were the first to identify the growth-stimulating (GH) and gonadotropic (sex-gland—stimulating) properties in an extract of the anterior lobe of the pituitary. For a time it was believed that the anterior lobe produced only these two hormones. In 1927–30, P. E. Smith (in work started at Stanford University and completed at The College of Physicians and Surgeons, New York) carried out a series of experiments on rats in whom hypophysectomy had been performed, and he demonstrated that in the absence of the pituitary gland not only do failure of growth and atrophy of the sex glands occur but also there is atrophy of the thyroid and adrenals.

Within the next five years the following anterior pituitary hormones were identified, all of them in experiments conducted by Americans: (1) thyroid stimulating hormone (TSH), by Leo Loeb and R. B. Bassett of Washington University, St. Louis; (2) adrenal stimulating hormone (ACTH), by J. B. Collip and his associates at McGill University, Montreal; (3) mammary-gland–stimulating hormone (prolactin or LTH), by Oscar Riddle and co-workers at Cold Spring Harbor, New York; (4) the follicle-stimulating (FSH) and luteinizing (LH) hormones, which have specific effects upon the ovaries and testes, by H. L. Fevold, F. L. Hisaw, and others at the University of Wisconsin. These hormonal substances were first identified in rather crude form, and the isolation of more refined products did not take place until after World War II, when new chemical methods utilizing columns of ion-exchange resins and other methods became available. ACTH was isolated in pure form in 1953 by W. F. White and W. L. Fierce of the Armour Laboratories, Chicago.

It is now possible to measure many of the hormones present in human blood and urine. This has made it possible to gain a better understanding of the interrelation of the endocrine glands and to detect underproduction or overproduction of particular hormones. Cushing's hypothesis that the anterior pituitary hormones exert their effect by influencing the secretion of other endocrine glands has been borne out, but the situation is much more complicated than he imagined. The release of the pituitary hormones is controlled by the hypothalamus (the inferior portion of the brain, to which the pituitary gland is attached), and regulation is effected by various feedback mechanisms, which serve to maintain equilibrium and to prevent hormonal excesses. The studies of the anterior pituitary hormones have brought to light new therapeutic procedures and have resulted in the production of powerful substances for the treatment of endocrine diseases and other abnormalities. For example, the administration of ACTH stimulates the adrenal cortex to secrete cortisol and corticosterone, and it is therefore a very useful anti-inflammatory agent; there is no more dramatic therapeutic effect than that of growth hormone on certain types of dwarfism; and various sexual abnormalities can be alleviated by the gonadotropic hormone.

NUTRITION
AND METABOLISM

Nutrition is the process by which any living organism, plant or animal, takes in food, absorbs it, and uses it. Plants require inorganic chemicals, air, and sunlight, whereas animals require not only inorganic materials, such as minerals, but also organic substances manufactured by plants and other animals. *Metabolism* comprises all the processes by which the body transforms food into living tissue and energy. We now know that in order to maintain human life, the environment must provide proteins, carbohydrates, fats, water, oxygen, minerals, and vitamins; but in the first quarter of the nineteenth century almost nothing was known about nutritive requirements or the chemical processes by which nutrients are metabolized.

Our present understanding of nutrition and metabolism began with research conducted in Europe, principally in Germany, in the mid-nineteenth century. Justus von Liebig (1803–1873), Professor of Chemistry at the University of Giessen, Germany, was the first to classify the organic foodstuffs and to attempt to determine in a qualitative manner the roles played by protein, carbohydrate, and fat in the body's metabolism. In addition, he was the first to recognize the importance of chemical transformations within the body; to stress that the interaction between organic matter, derived from food, and oxygen, derived from the air, leads to a series of chemical reactions that result in the production of heat and motion; and to clarify that the end products of these transformations are carbon dioxide, eliminated through the lungs, and nitrogen, excreted in the urine. In Liebig's view, if one measured continuously over a period of time the carbon dioxide in the expired air and the organic nitrogen (chiefly urea) in the urine, one could form an accurate quantitative estimate of the chemical transformations that occur in the body.

Carl Voit (1831–1909) of Munich, who had been both a student and an assistant of Liebig, undertook to gain a better understanding of the metabolic processes through the use of more precise analytic methods. He devoted many years to this endeavor. In collaboration with Max von Pettenkofer, he constructed an apparatus for measuring the gas-exchange rate in man; and a *calorimeter* to measure the number of calories of heat generated by metabolism during the period of an experiment.

Three Americans who had been students in Voit's laboratory achieved distinction in the field of metabolic research: Wilbur O. Atwater (1844–1907), Graham Lusk (1886–1932), and Francis G. Benedict (1870–1957). Atwater, the eldest of this trio, was Professor of Chemistry at Wesleyan University (Connecticut) from 1873 until his death. Benedict, after his return from Germany, was a member of Atwater's Department of Chemistry from 1896 to 1907, and from 1907 to 1937 he was Director of the Nutrition Laboratory of the Carnegie Institution of Washington. When Lusk returned from Germany in 1891 he joined the Physiology Department at Yale, where he rose to the rank of professor in 1895. He spent the major part of his scientific career as Professor of Physiology at the Cornell University Medical College in New York.

In 1892, Atwater, with financial assistance from the United States government, began the construction of a calorimeter. E. B. Rosa, a physicist, assisted with the design and was responsible for the technical perfection of the apparatus. Associated with the calorimeter was an apparatus for measuring the carbon dioxide produced by the individual whose heat production was being determined. Several years later a still better calorimeter was devised by Atwater and Benedict. With the new model (1907), it was possible to measure, along with the measurement of heat production, both oxygen consumption and carbon dioxide elimination.

Two of these calorimeters were constructed, one at the Cornell Medical College, the other at Bellevue Hospital, both in New York City. Using these instruments Benedict and Lusk, together with Eugene F. Dubois and other collaborators, were able to determine the basal metabolism of normal individuals and to measure the effect of various diseases upon the metabolic

239

rate. For example, they were able to determine precisely the increase in metabolic rate caused by various levels of fever. Dubois developed an improved formula for expressing the basal (minimal) metabolic rate in calories produced per hour per square meter of body surface. As a by-product of his calorimetric studies, Benedict devised a simple apparatus for measuring oxygen consumption in resting patients. Utilizing this apparatus and Dubois's formula, one could determine whether a patient's basal metabolism was above or below normal. For many years, this was the method used in diagnosing hyperthyroidism (in which the basal metabolism is above normal) and hypothyroidism (in which the basal metabolism is below normal). Measurement of the basal metabolism was used for determining the effectiveness of treatment as well as for diagnostic purposes.

One of the features of the calorimeter is that it allows one to determine not only the total energy expended by an individual under controlled conditions but also the amount of energy contributed by each of the energy-producing components: protein, carbohydrate, and fat. Benedict carried out studies (1907) on the effect of starvation and made the important discovery that in a starving individual, glycogen (carbohydrate) is first utilized to supply energy but that when the glycogen stores in the body run low, the body begins to derive its energy from the combustion of protein. In other words, as long as glycogen is available, protein is spared, but a point is reached during starvation at which the individual begins to destroy his own tissues (protein) to keep the metabolic fires burning. Benedict was able to calculate the amount of protein destroyed each day and the amount of glycogen and fat utilized.

In 1903, Atwater and Benedict began a series of studies to determine the metabolic effect of exericse, and they concluded that fats and carbohydrates, but not proteins, are utilized to supply the energy. In these experiments the subject performed a measured amount of work by riding a stationary bicycle set up inside the original Atwater-Rosa calorimeter. Years later, utilizing the new calorimeter, Benedict and Cathcart employed a professional cyclist to ride the bicycle until he was too exhausted to ride any longer. The energy produced by the rider was fairly constant at 600 calories per hour. This appeared to be about the limit of sustained muscular effort for a human subject. The metabolic calculation indicated that the rider had reached the point of exhaustion when he had consumed his body's supplies of glycogen.

Lusk and R. J. Anderson, in 1917, were able to show that when energy is produced in the body, it makes little difference whether it is produced by the combustion of fat or carbohydrates. The caloric content of a food is the important factor in energy production.

In addition to those who began their metabolic research under Voit, there was another group of American investigators whose tradition was established at the laboratory of Professor Willy Kühne at the University of Heidelberg. It may be recalled that at the end of the first century, a laboratory of physiological chemistry, the first to be established in this country, was founded at Yale University, with *Russell H. Chittenden* (1856–1943) as its Director. The laboratory was not opened until several years after its founding, because Chittenden, still in his early 20s, was a student at Heidelberg. At that time Kühne was engaged in a study of the chemical aspects of nutri-

240

tion. He was particularly interested in a group of chemical substances which in very minute amounts were able to expedite (catalyze) chemical reactions such as those occurring during the process of digestion. Since these substances behaved much like the material in yeast which causes fermentation, Kühne gave them the name *enzymes,* from Greek words meaning "in yeast."

In Kühne's laboratory Chittenden began a remarkable series of chemical studies of the intermediate products in the digestion of food by the enzymes in the stomach and intestinal tract. After he returned to Yale, he continued to work on problems in digestion, nutrition, and metabolism, and he and his students made a number of important contributions. Chittenden was the first to isolate glycogen, the chemical form in which carbohydrate is stored in the body. He also did extensive work to determine the minimum nutritive requirement of the body in relation to its capacity for work and nitrogenous equilibrium. Chittenden was Professor of Physiological Chemistry at Yale from 1882 to 1922. His research laboratory was not in the medical school but in the Sheffield Scientific School, and he was involved in the training of chemists rather than of physicians. In addition to his work at Yale, Chittenden reorganized and modernized the course in Medical Chemistry at The College of Physicians and Surgeons, Columbia University, in 1898 and spent one day each week in New York supervising this course.

Many of Chittenden's students, though trained primarily as chemists, carried on significant basic medical research in chemistry, physiology, and pharmacology. For example, one of his protegés, Alfred Newton Richards, while Professor of Pharmacology at the University of Pennsylvania, illuminated the whole field of renal physiology by his brilliant and ingenious studies of the manner in which urine is filtered from the blood by the glomeruli of the kidneys. However, Chittenden's students did most of their outstanding work in the field of nutrition; three of them, Mendel, Osborne, and McCollum, were involved in the discovery of *vitamin A* and helped to elucidate the biological functions of vitamins B and D.

Vitamins A and B. Since the eighteenth century it had been known that health cannot be maintained unless a small amount of a substance of unknown chemical composition is present in the diet. This was first demonstrated in the case of the disease *scurvy,* which had been the cause of illness and many deaths among sailors engaged on long sea voyages. It was found in the eighteenth century that scurvy could be prevented or cured by a small amount of the juice of a citrus fruit.

Along these same lines it was shown in the late nineteenth century that the incidence of *beriberi* in the Japanese Navy could be reduced by providing a more liberal diet for the sailors. Shortly after this, Christian Eijkman, a Dutch physician in Java, demonstrated that individuals who developed beriberi while subsisting largely on polished rice could be cured of their disease by adding to the diet the rice polishings (i.e., the material removed from the rice in the process of polishing). In 1911 Casimir Funk, a Polish biochemist working in Germany, found that a nervous disorder of pigeons that occurred when they were fed polished rice could be cured by feeding the birds the rice polishings. Funk made a concentrate of the polishings and was able to obtain a water-soluble crystalline material, which in very small amounts could cure the disease of pigeons. It was de-

241

termined that the crystalline substance contained nitrogen, and it was believed to be an amine. For this reason, Funk gave his crystals the name *vitamine*. It was soon demonstrated that *vitamine* in small amounts would cure beriberi in human patients.

While Funk was discovering *vitamine,* an Englishman, F. Gowland Hopkins, was carrying out another type of dietary experiment. He fed young rats a mixture of pure protein, fat, carbohydrate, and salts, and he found that the rats ceased to grow, although the nitrogen content and the energy value of the diet were quite sufficient for growth. When a minute quantity of fresh milk was added to the diet, growth resumed and progressed rapidly. These results were reported in 1912, and in the following year two groups of American scientists, Thomas B. Osborne (1859–1929) and Lafayette B. Mendel (1872–1935) at Yale, and Elmer V. McCollum (1879–1967) and Marguerite Davis at the University of Wisconsin obtained a fat-soluble substance from cream and butter, which in minute amounts would provide the growth-promoting material lacking in Hopkins's diet. This substance became known as *vitamin A.* In 1916 McCollum and Kennedy found that two substances actually are required for normal growth in young rats: fat-soluble vitamin A and another substance, which they designated vitamin B (Mendel et al., 1932). It is now known that vitamin B is made up of a number of water-soluble vitamins, each of which is designated by a number. For example, the anti-beriberi factor, which has been identified chemically as *thiamine,* is known as vitamin B_1; whereas the growth-promoting factor, with which McCollum was concerned, has been chemically identified as *riboflavin* and is known as vitamin B_2. Since then a number of other B vitamins have been identified, some of which will be mentioned later.

In 1919, Harry Steenbock, who was then Associate Professor of Agricultural Chemistry at the University of Michigan, made the astute observation that the vitamin A content of vegetables varies with the degree of pigmentation of the vegetable, and it was subsequently demonstrated that vitamin A is derived from the plant pigment carotene.

Vitamin D. Americans also played a vital role in the discovery of the cause of rickets and the curative effect of vitamin D. Rickets is an ancient disease; Thersites, a soldier in the Greek ranks before the walls of Troy, was bowlegged, with rounded shoulders that almost met across his chest. Several fifteenth and sixteenth century paintings show the Christ child with bow legs, square head, chest deformities, and other stigmata of infantile rickets. However, it was not until 1650 that Francis Glisson, Regius Professor of Physic at Cambridge University, wrote his famous treatise giving a full and excellent description of rickets.

Cod-liver oil first came into use as a medicine in the latter part of the eighteenth century, and rickets was soon listed among the many diseases that the oil was alleged to cure. A short treatise on cod-liver oil, written in 1855 by the Dutch physician L. J. deJongh, listed other diseases for which the oil should be prescribed: rheumatism, migraine, gout, skin diseases, and tuberculosis. Like quinine, which was used for every type of fever until its specificity for malaria was revealed, cod-liver oil was used for every type of bone and joint disease until its specificity for rickets was revealed.

In 1919 Edward Mellanby, an Englishman, proved convincingly that rickets is caused by a deficient diet, and he demonstrated that the deficiency could be overcome and the disease prevented or cured by adding to the diet certain fats, notably cod-liver oil. Mellanby drew the conclusion that the antirachitic factor was probably identical with fat-soluble vitamin A. One year later, F. G. Hopkins, at Cambridge University, found that when oxygen was passed through heated butterfat or cod-liver oil the vitamin A in both substances was destroyed but that the cod-liver oil retained its ability to protect animals against rickets. Following this lead, McCollum and his associates (1922) at Johns Hopkins passed a stream of oxygen through hot cod-liver oil and found that though the oil had lost its vitamin A effect, it retained its potency not only to prevent but also to cure rickets in experimental animals. This was clear proof that vitamin A and the antirachitic factor were not identical, and McCollum named the antirachitic factor remaining in the oxygenated oil, fat-soluble *vitamin D*. Within a few months McCollum and his associates had developed a method for the assay of vitamin D in foods (McCollum, 1957).

In 1921 Paul G. Shipley, who with Edwards A. Park of the Department of Pediatrics at Johns Hopkins had been studying the bone disease associated with rickets, observed that rats fed a diet that normally would produce rickets showed no sign of the disease if they were exposed to sunlight; whereas rats on the same diet that were kept indoors and away from the sun developed the expected changes in bone. This was not an entirely new idea. For many years rickets had been vaguely associated with unhygienic city living and lack of fresh air and sunshine. Moreover, a German physician, Kurt Huldschinsky, working in Berlin during and after World War I, had reported in 1918 that ultraviolet radiation was a specific cure for rickets.

How these observations on the effect of sunlight were to be reconciled with the experiments on vitamin D posed a problem. The puzzle began to resolve in 1924 when, almost simultaneously, Alfred F. Hess of New York and Harry Steenbock of Wisconsin reported that antirachitic potency could

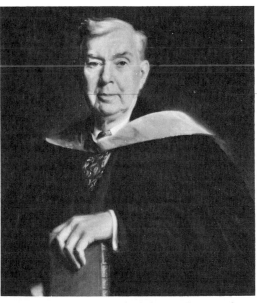

Figure 61. Elmer V. McCollum. (Portrait by Daniel MacMorris. From the Archives Office, The Johns Hopkins Medical Institutions.)

243

be conveyed to a number of different biological materials by exposing them to the rays of a mercury-vapor lamp. Further investigation disclosed that the substance in food that was activated by ultraviolet radiation was not fat, as initially believed, but a substance associated with fats, an obscure sterol called *ergosterol*. This substance occurs in the antirachitic oils and fats; and it is of particular interest that it is present in measurable amounts in human skin. The probable explanation of the antirachitic effect of sunlight is that the ultraviolet beam forms vitamin D from the ergosterol in the skin; the vitamin then passes into the blood and is carried to the bones and other tissues where it is needed. Pigmentation of the skin reduces its permeability to ultraviolet light, and this helps to solve another clinical riddle: the fact that black babies develop rickets more frequently than do white babies living under similar conditions. Black infants can be protected from rickets by ultraviolet radiation, provided it is of sufficient intensity and duration. It is now known that ergosterol is not the only sterol that can be activated by ultraviolet light, but it is still one of the most useful.

There are several forms of vitamin D. The term vitamin D_1 was applied to the first antirachitic substance to be isolated from irradiated ergosterol. A second form, also isolated from irradiated ergosterol, is *calciferol* or vitamin D_2. Vitamin D_3 is obtained by irradiating another substance, 7-dehydrocholesterol. Vitamins D_2 and D_3 are the ones commonly used, and they have approximately the same physiological effect. Vitamin D is not the only dietary factor required for normal development of bone in growing children. The principal minerals involved in building solid bones are calcium and phosphorus. These must be present in the diet in adequate amounts and proper proportions. The importance of the latter factor was established in a series of experiments carried out under the supervision of John Howland, Professor of Pediatrics at Johns Hopkins.

Amino Acids. As progress was made in the study of nutrition, interest began to focus in the 1890s on the structure of the protein molecule and its relation to metabolism. It was known that the protein molecule contains amino acids, and in 1898 Albrecht Kossel, Professor of Physiology at Marburg, Germany, predicted that eventually it would be found that proteins are composed of polypeptides, which in turn are made up of a number of amino acids joined together. A year later the brilliant German chemist Emil Fischer began to combine amino acids to form polypeptides. By 1906 he had succeeded in linking together 18 amino acids, but he got no closer than this to the formation of a protein. Up to this time, the role that the amino acids play in mammalian metabolism was unknown; they had not been demonstrated in the blood, and there was no proof that they were absorbed from the intestinal tract as a sequel to the digestion of dietary protein.

In 1906, William H. Howell, at Johns Hopkins, was the first to demonstrate, by a rather crude method, that amino acids appear in the blood. Six years later, two groups of American scientists—Otto Folin, Professor of Chemistry at Harvard, and his colleague, Willey G. Denis, biochemist at the Massachusetts General Hospital; and Donald D. Van Slyke and his colleague, Gustav M. Meyer, at the Rockefeller Institute—demonstrated that amino acids are absorbed from the intestine and that they appear in the blood and tissues. Van Slyke and Meyer found that when a fasting dog was given a protein meal there was a marked rise in the amino acid level of the blood. The microchemical methods developed by both Folin and Van Slyke in the course of these experiments subsequently became widely used in clinical work throughout the world for the determination of the chemical constituents of blood. Prior to that time, multiple chemical determinations required larger amounts of blood than could be drawn safely from any one patient. With the new micromethods it became possible to carry out multiple determinations on a single small sample.

The first actual isolation of specific amino acids from blood was carried out at Johns Hopkins by John J. Abel and his associates (1913). To accomplish this task Abel devised an ingenious method known as *vividiffusion,* which took advantage of the fact that amino acids will pass through the minute pores of a collodion membrane. Abel withdrew blood from the artery of a living animal and passed it through collodion tubes immersed in salt solution. After passing through the tubes, the blood flowed back into a vein of the animal so that it was not lost to the body, and the vividiffusion could be continued for a relatively long time. The amino acids were identified in the salt solution through which the blood in the collodion tubes had passed.

One of the results of the work on amino acids, in which Hopkins, Osborne, Mendel, McCollum, and their co-workers all participated, was to show that the body can manufacture certain of the amino acids but that it is unable to manufacture certain others (tryptophane, for example) which are required for normal protein synthesis.

During the period when the vitamin and protein studies were being carried out, there were other important American contributions to the study of metabolism. Walter R. Bloor, a biochemist who worked successively at Harvard, the University of California, and Rochester University, made significant contributions to an understanding of fat metabolism. Charles D. Woods and E. R. Mansfield, in 1904, published a study of the diet of the lumbermen of Maine, showing that the average daily diet per man contained 8083 calories, about three times the number of calories required by those engaged in sedentary occupations. This appeared to be about the maximum caloric requirement for men engaged in heavy daily work. During World War I, John R. Murlin, a colleague of Graham Lusk, made a study of the food requirements in the United States Army and found that the average Army cavalryman needed 3633 calories per day. Atwater and Lusk drew up tables showing the food requirements in terms of calories for males and females at different ages.

Vitamin K. The use of vitamin K to treat a particular type of hemorrhagic disorder in man was the result of the convergence of several lines of research. Henrik Dam, a Danish biochemist who had received part of his early training at the Rockefeller Institute, discovered in 1929, while working at the University of Copenhagen, that chicks fed on a diet containing almost no fat developed a tendency to bleed. Dam believed at first that the hemorrhagic tendency was due to a lack of vitamin C, but the addition of vitamin C and other known vitamins to the diet failed to prevent the bleeding. In 1934 it was discovered by Dam and his collaborators that if hemp seeds were included in the diet, the bleeding did not occur. It was apparent that the hemp seeds contained a substance that afforded protection against this particular type of hemorrhagic disorder. This factor, which appeared to

245

be necessary for normal blood-clotting, was named vitamin K (koagulation vitamin). H. J. Almquist, an American biochemist, and C. L. R. Stokstad, working at the University of California, Berkeley, found in 1935 that vitamin K is a fat-soluble substance and that it is present in liver fat and in alfalfa. Subsequently it was discovered by Almquist and his associates that the vitamin is present in large amounts in the feces of most animals and that it is formed in the intestinal tract by the activity of bacteria.

While Dam, Almquist, and their colleagues were working on vitamin K, William B. Hawkins and George H. Whipple at the Rochester University Medical School found in animal experiments that when the bile formed in the liver was diverted by a fistula (side-tract) so that it did not enter and pass through the intestines, the animals were likely to develop excessive bleeding. In the same year, Armand James Quick and associates at Marquette University Medical School in Wisconsin reported that the bleeding tendency of jaundiced patients, which had long been unexplained, was due to a decrease in prothrombin (a coagulation factor) in the blood. In the following year W. B. Hawkins and K. M. Brinkhous (University of Rochester) showed that the bleeding in animals whose bile had been side-tracted was likewise caused by a deficiency in prothrombin and that the bleeding could be prevented by feeding bile salts to the animals. In 1938, H. R. Butt and co-workers at the Mayo Clinic and E. D. Warner and associates at the Rochester University Medical School reported that a combination therapy consisting of bile salts and vitamin K was effective in relieving the hemorrhagic tendency in patients suffering from jaundice. It thus became apparent that vitamin K and adequate function of the liver are linked to the clotting of blood, which is necessary for the prevention of hemorrhage.

The clotting of blood is the result of a series of events: a fine mesh of fibrin is formed by the action of the enzyme thrombin upon a protein, fibrinogen, in the blood. Thrombin is derived from prothrombin, a substance formed in the liver. Dam's work demonstrated that vitamin K is essential for the formation of prothrombin. In certain liver and intestinal diseases there is an insufficient supply of vitamin K for the formation of an adequate amount of prothrombin. Hence there is poor clotting of the blood, and hemorrhage occurs. This deficiency can be remedied by the administration of vitamin K.

In 1939, Dam and Paul Kirrer, a Swiss chemist, reported that they had been able to prepare pure vitamin K from green leaves. In that same year Edward A. Doisy, Professor of Biochemistry at the St. Louis University School of Medicine, and his co-workers isolated vitamin K from alfalfa, determined its chemical composition, and succeeded in synthesizing it in the laboratory; thus making it readily available in pure form for the treatment of patients.

In the 1940s the pieces of the complicated puzzle first posed by vitamin K began to fall neatly into place. This fat-soluble vitamin is essential for normal clotting of blood. It may enter the body in the diet, or it may be formed in the intestine by bacterial activity. In either event, it cannot pass through the intestinal wall and enter the blood unless bile is also present in the intestine. When the bile ducts, which convey the bile from the liver to the intestine, are blocked by gallstones or a tumor, vitamin K, though it may be present in the intestine in large amounts, cannot gain access to the

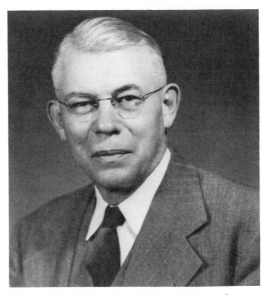

Figure 62. Edward A. Doisy. (National Library of Medicine, Bethesda, Maryland.)

blood. It is therefore not delivered to the liver, where it is essential for the formation of prothrombin. The deficiency of prothrombin results in poor blood clotting, which in turn leads to bleeding.

The medical importance of this work is that the bleeding tendency in patients with blockage of the bile ducts can be counteracted successfully by administration of vitamin K directly into the circulation. Bleeding in such patients had for years presented a serious hazard in operations for gall-stones or other types of obstruction of the bile ducts. Now surgeons, before an operation, can determine whether there is a deficiency of prothrombin and if so can administer vitamin K to correct the situation.

In 1943, Dam and Doisy were awarded the Nobel Prize in medicine for their work on vitamin K.

Pellagra. One of the great achievements in vitamin research was, at the same time, an intriguing adventure in scientific detective work. The disease pellagra, which is characterized by a peculiar form of dermatitis, digestive disorders including diarrhea, and nervous and mental abnormali-ties, had been recognized in Europe since the eighteenth century. It was first described in Spain in 1735. During the nineteenth and early twentieth centuries it was prevalent in many European countries including Italy, Spain, Portugal, Greece, Turkey, and the Balkan states. It was also encoun-tered in parts of Asia, Africa, and South America, and in the islands of the East and West Indies. Over 100,000 cases were reported from Italy in 1881 and a similar number from Romania in 1906.

In the mid-nineteenth century, it was generally believed that pellagra was somehow associated with a diet of maize ("Indian corn"). This belief probably went back to Barnino, who in the early seventeenth century described a disease that resembled pellagra and that occurred among the maize-eating tribes of American Indians. The disease seemed to affect those populations in which Indian corn was a dietary staple. For example, it was

247

widespread in southern Egypt, where maize was the common cereal but was rare in northern Egypt, where millet was eaten. In spite of its apparent relation to diet, it was generally believed that pellagra was an infectious disease.

Pellagra was first clearly described in the United States during the Civil War. It was probably one of the causes of the high death rate in the Southern prison camps, but it was not until 1907 that the work of James W. Babcock focused attention upon the prevalence of the disease among the civilian population in the southeastern states.

Between 1909 and 1913 two extensive surveys confirmed the fact that pellagra was widespread in the South and also seemed to support the view that the disease was infectious in origin. Since statistical studies indicated that the incidence of pellagra was increasing, and since it was believed to be contagious, the United States Public Health Service decided to investigate the matter. In 1914, *Joseph Goldberger* (1874–1929) was selected to take charge of the study.

Goldberger was born in Hungary, but at the age of 7 his family brought him to the United States. When he was 16 he entered the City College of New York, intending to become a civil engineer. After two years in college his interest shifted from engineering to medicine, and he entered the Bellevue Hospital Medical College, from which he graduated in 1895. After two years as Resident Physician at Bellevue he entered private practice in Wilkes-Barre, Pennsylvania. In 1899 he gave up his practice to join the United States Public Health Service. From 1900 to 1905 he was assigned to work on yellow fever in Puerto Rico, Mexico, and elsewhere. During this

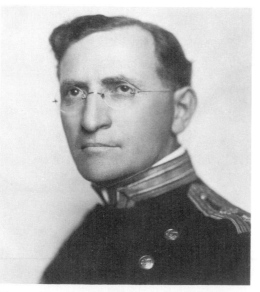

Figure 63. Joseph Goldberger. (National Library of Medicine, Bethesda, Maryland.)

period he contracted yellow fever and narrowly escaped death. Following this he devoted his attention to parasitology for several years, doing some outstanding work in that field. In 1909 he accompanied Howard Taylor Ricketts on his trip to Mexico City to study typhus fever, and Goldberger is credited with having pointed out that Mexican typhus and Rocky Mountain spotted fever are different, though closely related, diseases.

When Ricketts contracted typhus in Mexico City, Goldberger also came down with the disease, but unlike Ricketts he had the good fortune to recover. After his Mexican experience Goldberger continued to work on typhus fever and other infectious diseases. Among other things he was the first to succeed in transmitting measles to monkeys. It was because of his long record of productive research in the field of infectious diseases that Goldberger was chosen to supervise the pellagra investigation (Parsons, 1931).

Early in the course of his studies Goldberger investigated the occurrence of pellagra at two orphanages in Mississippi. In each of these institutions, in spite of good general care, reasonably good housing, and a diet that was nutritious by the standards of that day, more than half of the children had pellagra. Goldberger decided that the disease was not likely to be infectious: the adult attendants did not have pellagra; not all of the children had the disease; some had more than one attack in the course of a single year; and there was no evidence of transmission from the affected to the healthy children or adults although they lived together in close association. Goldberger noted that the disease affected principally children over three years of age and that the diet for this group, though adequate in terms of calories, was deficient in meat and other protein foods. Those under the age of three received plenty of milk, but this was not included in the diet of the older children. The adult attendants who did not have pellagra received meat as part of their diet. Goldberger obtained funds from the Public Health Service to supplement the diet of the children, and in the ensuing months pellagra disappeared.

In 1915 Goldberger turned his attention to a state sanatorium in Georgia where pellagra had been observed frequently. He selected two groups of patients for study. Both groups were kept under similar conditions except that one group continued to receive the regular institutional diet while the other group was given a diet supplemented as it had been for the orphans. During a nine-month period of observation about half of those on the regular diet developed pellagra, but the disease failed to occur in the group receiving the supplement. While this experiment was in progress, 12 volunteers among the convicts at a state prison farm in Mississippi were placed on a diet deficient in protein and similar to the institutional diet provided in the orphanage and prison. By the end of six months, five of the convicts had developed obvious signs of pellagra.

Goldberger and his associates were unable to produce pellagra by any means other than a deficient diet. They attempted to transmit it to volunteers with materials obtained from patients who had the disease in its most florid state. These materials included nasal secretions, capsules containing feces and urine, and injections of blood. It therefore seemed inescapable that the disease was dietary rather than infectious in origin. Goldberger believed at first (1922) that it is caused by the lack of certain amino acids

249

contained in protein foods; but when he found that it could not be prevented by feeding the protein *casein* but that it could be prevented quite successfully by adding dried yeast to the diet, he concluded that some factor other than amino acids is responsible. He named this factor (1926) the P-P (pellagra-preventive) factor. Further investigation revealed that the P-P factor is associated with water-soluble vitamin B; but whereas the anti-beriberi vitamin is destroyed by heat, the P-P factor was found to be heat-resistant. In 1929 the latter factor was designated vitamin G as a tribute to Goldberger, who died that year. For a time it was believed that vitamin G was closely related to vitamin B_2, but vitamin B_2 has since been chemically identified as riboflavin, and in 1937 Conrad Elvehjem of the University of Wisconsin identified the pellagra-preventive substance as nicotinamide, a separate factor of the vitamin B complex.

Thus Joseph Goldberger, who had undertaken the study of pellagra expecting to find that it is caused by a micro-organism, ended his study by proving that it is attributable to a dietary deficiency and that this disease, which had killed thousands of people in various quarters of the globe and had had disastrous consequences for millions of others, could be prevented by the simple expedient of adding dried yeast to the diet. More recent studies of the use of nicotinamide for the treatment of pellagra have indicated that the disease is due to a multiple dietary deficiency and that when it is present in full-blown form it cannot be completely cured by the use of this one chemical alone.

Pernicious Anemia. Prior to 1926, pernicious anemia, as its name suggests, was an inexorably fatal disease. Those affected rarely lived more than two or three years after the first symptoms appeared. The disease is sometimes called Addisonian anemia because it was so clearly described in 1855, long before doctors knew how to make blood counts, by Thomas Addison of Guy's Hospital, London. Addison's concise but remarkably full description of the clinical and post-mortem features of what he called "idiopathic anemia" was written "as a preface to my subject"—his subject being the classic description of the disease of the adrenal glands now called *Addison's disease.* The description of the anemia was, in a sense, a classic within a classic.

Pernicious anemia was not a very common disease, nor was it a rarity; before 1926 every large hospital was caring for several of its victims in various stages along the road to death. It was easy to recognize the typical victim: he was a man of about 45 years, with blue eyes and prematurely gray hair, appearing to be well nourished but with an unhealthy lemon-yellow pallor of the skin. The anemia was often profound, the number of red blood cells being reduced to about one third or one fifth or even one tenth of normal. In addition to the anemia, the disease usually affected the nervous system, and the stomach was invariably affected. When a tube was introduced into the stomach, either no gastric secretion could be withdrawn or there was a small amount of stomach juice which lacked the hydrochloric acid normally present.

Many theories as to the cause of pernicious anemia had been proposed, but none withstood the test of time. Likewise many forms of treatment were advocated, and some for a brief period seemed promising, only to be discarded as failures a year or two later. After World War I the popular form of therapy was blood transfusion, but transfusion had no more than a transitory effect on the anemia and no effect on the other symptoms of the disease.

This was the situation when *George Richards Minot* (1885–1950) entered the picture. He had graduated from the Harvard Medical School in 1912. In his senior year as a student he had become interested in the microscopic examination of blood, and in this he had been encouraged and given assistance by J. Homer Wright, Professor of Pathology. The following year he was a House Pupil (intern) at the Massachusetts General Hospital. This was the year in which David Linn Edsall came to Boston, the first outsider to be appointed to two top positions in the Harvard medical community: Jackson Professor of Clinical Medicine at the Medical School and Chief of the Medical Service at the Massachusetts General Hospital. This was also the first time that the occupant of these important positions was given a salary sufficient to let him devote most of his time to teaching and research. Edsall was one of the original *Young Turks* (members of the American Society for Clinical Investigation) and a keen exponent of clinical investigation. He spent much of his first year in Boston trying to find space in the hospital for research laboratories and encouraging the young members of the staff to pursue their problems from the bedside to the laboratory and back again to the bedside. Minot found this new atmosphere stimulating, and though his routine duties kept him too busy for research he continued his interest in

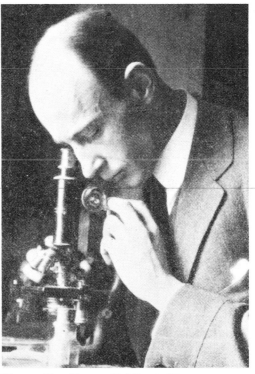

Figure 64. Geroge R. Minot. (From Rackemann, Francis M.: The Inquisitive Physician. Cambridge, Mass., Harvard University Press, 1956.)

251

diseases of the blood and seized every opportunity to examine blood specimens in the laboratory.

Toward the end of his internship Minot talked with Dr. Edsall about his future. Edsall advised him to go away from Boston and find work in a new place where he could learn different methods of medical research and could pick up some new ideas. He said that if Minot would like to go to Johns Hopkins for a year or two the time would be well spent, and he offered to write a letter of recommendation to William S. Thayer, Clinical Professor of Medicine at Hopkins. Minot discussed the matter with his friend Francis W. Peabody, who had spent a year (1908–09) in Baltimore as Assistant Resident in Medicine. It was during this time that Barker, with his new ideas about clinical science, was reorganizing the Hopkins Medical Clinic, and Peabody had found his experience there to be so exciting and instructive that he urged Minot to accept Edsall's advice. This Minot did, and he spent the year 1913–14 working as Assistant Resident in Medicine under Thayer.

Soon after arriving in Baltimore, Minot wrote to a close friend (Francis Rackemann) in Boston, comparing the situation at the Hopkins Hospital with that at the Massachusetts General Hospital. He said that he was "snowed under with work" and complained about the maid service in the residents' quarters: "When the wash comes up you have to put it away yourself!" "There is no ice or crackers in the living room, and no fireplace." He said that his clinical duties involved looking after six or seven private patients of Dr. Thayer, and "I act as a regular resident over the two house officers (interns) and the colored ward which holds about twenty-four patients" (Rackemann, 1956).

While in Baltimore, Minot kept up his interest in the blood, and because of this interest Dr. Thayer asked Dr. William H. Howell whether he could give his young assistant some working space in the physiology laboratory. Howell was then doing research on the factors responsible for the failure of blood to clot—work which several years later was to lead to the discovery of the anticoagulant *heparin*. Minot was given space in Howell's laboratory, and there he got his introduction to organized experimental research under a master. He worked in partnership with G. P. Denny, and the two of them together wrote a paper on "The origin of antithrombin." While Minot was in Baltimore he wrote his first paper on pernicious anemia. The treatment of this disease was then going through a phase in which removal of the spleen was in vogue, and Minot's paper, which appeared in the *Bulletin of the Johns Hopkins Hospital* in 1914, was entitled "Nitrogen metabolism before and after splenectomy in a case of pernicious anemia."

Particular attention has been given to these early years in Minot's medical career because they were formative years and because during this period Minot came under the influence of five of the seven men who in his Nobel Prize address, in 1934, he credited with having "taught me how science provides the means by which human suffering may be alleviated and [having] aided me to understand fundamental knowledge and clinical problems." The five men were Wright, Thayer, Peabody, Edsall, and Howell; the other two were his close associates in Boston, Drs. Roger I. Lee and Edwin A. Locke.

After his year in Baltimore, Minot returned to Boston and spent most of his time studying blood diseases at the Massachusetts General Hospital. He

252

learned about the overactive state of the bone marrow in pernicious anemia (which had first been described by William Pepper of Philadelphia in 1875), and he learned how to distinguish between old and new red blood cells in the circulation. Dr. Wright taught him how to use a new stain, which showed strands of reticulum in some of the red cells, and he identified these reticulated cells as young cells. His studies indicated that the percentage of these reticulated cells in the circulation increases when the bone marrow is actively producing new blood cells. For a time, Minot turned his attention to leukemia, a malignant disease of the white blood cells, and Francis Peabody persuaded him to continue his work in this field at the Huntington Hospital, which specialized in the study and treatment of cancer and other malignant conditions.

While he was in the midst of his research at the Huntington Hospital, in 1921, Minot developed diabetes. He was then 36 years old, and at that age, in those years, diabetes usually was fatal within a few years. Minot placed himself under the care of Dr. Elliott P. Joslin of Boston, one of the world's foremost specialists in diabetes. The treatment that Joslin advised was in effect a starvation diet. This was the best treatment that could be offered at the time, and initially Minot's condition seemed to improve. After about a year, however, his symptoms increased, and his weight fell to 120 pounds (Minot was 6'1½" tall).

It has been said that Banting, Macleod, and their associates, who were responsible for the discovery of insulin, were also responsible for the discovery of the cure for pernicious anemia. Banting made his dramatic report on the discovery of insulin at a meeting of the Association of American Physicians in May, 1922. Prior to that time a very small amount of insulin had been made in the research laboratory, no more than enough to treat a few patients. In April, 1922, the Eli Lilly Company had not yet started the large-scale production of insulin. In August, Joslin received a small amount of insulin to test on one of his patients, but it was January, 1923, before he obtained a slightly more liberal amount to begin the treatment of George Minot. On the first day of treatment Minot received a total of only six units; by April the insulin supply had increased so that the daily dose could be raised to 14 units. From this point onward the Lilly Company was producing insulin on a commercial scale, and the dosage could be adjusted to meet the patient's needs. By this time Minot had gained in weight and vigor and felt much improved.

At about the time that the diabetes was brought under control, Minot began to reconsider a thought that had first entered his mind during his intern days: that pernicious anemia is caused by a dietary deficiency. His renewed interest in this subject was aroused by the work of George H. Whipple.

Whipple graduated from the Johns Hopkins Medical School in 1901, and after graduation he remained at the school as a member of Welch's Department of Pathology. He was Associate Professor of Pathology during the time that Minot was in Baltimore. In 1914 Whipple left Baltimore to become Director of the Hooper Foundation for Medical Research in San Francisco. There he began a series of experiments on the influence of diet on hemoglobin production in dogs which had been made mildly anemic by

253

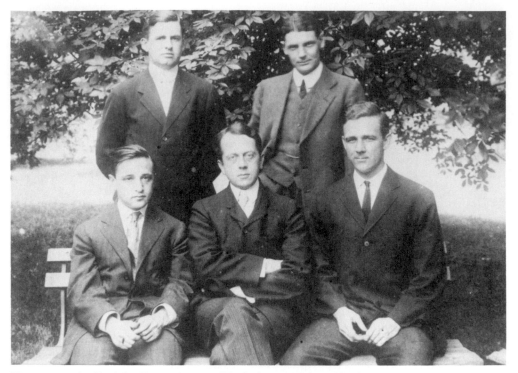

Figure 65. Staff of the Department of Pathology at Johns Hopkins, 1908–1909. Standing: Dr. J. T. King (left), Dr. Stewart; seated (left to right): Dr. M. C. Winternitz, Dr. W. G. MacCallum, Dr. George Whipple. (From the Archives Office, The Johns Hopkins Medical Institutions.)

the withdrawal of blood. He found that liver was one of the best foods for rebuilding the hemoglobin and overcoming the anemia.

In 1923 Whipple moved to Rochester, New York, to become Professor of Pathology and Dean at the new Medical School of the University of Rochester. He continued his work on the dietary treatment of anemia in dogs, using an improved technique for the measurement of hemoglobin production, and again demonstrated the superiority of liver as a dietary factor (Corner, 1963).

In 1924, with Whipple's experiments in mind and with the assistance of Dr. William P. Murphy, Minot began to feed liver to some of his patients suffering from pernicious anemia. The effect of the liver diet on the symptoms and on the condition of the blood was closely followed and recorded. The initial results were so encouraging that more patients were placed on the liver diet and the ration of liver was increased to between a half-pound and a pound a day. By early 1926, 45 patients had been treated on this special diet, and the results were uniformly good; in only one patient had the anemia relapsed and that occurred in a patient who refused to continue the diet. It was found that a rise in the reticulocyte count in the blood was a particularly sensitive and early indication of improvement. The rise occurred usually between the fifth and tenth day after the liver diet was started. Coincident with the rise in reticulocytes, a gradual and steady climb in the number of red blood cells and the hemoglobin began, and after about two months the anemia disappeared and the patient was feeling quite fit. However, it was noted that there was little or no improvement in any neurological abnormalities that existed before treatment began and that the liver diet had to be continued in order to prevent a relapse of the anemia.

In May, 1926, just four years after Banting had announced the discovery of insulin, Minot announced the successful treatment of pernicious anemia to the same audience, the Association of American Physicians.

It was realized that a diet containing such large amounts of liver was difficult for many patients to consume and was inedible for some. Minot saw that if the specific factor that counteracted the pernicious anemia could be isolated from the liver and administered to patients, this would greatly simplify the treatment. To accomplish this he sought the aid of Edwin J. Cohn, Professor of Physical Chemistry at Harvard, who had wide experience in protein chemistry. Professor Cohn found almost at once that it was possible to eliminate the large mass of liver protein and to retain the active principle in a relatively small residue, which became known as "Fraction G." This fraction was found to be highly effective when tested by Minot and his associates on patients suffering from pernicious anemia. The question soon arose as to how the liver extract was to be manufactured and made available to practicing physicians. In order to control the manufacture of Fraction G and to assure its quality, it was decided that a patent should be applied for in the name of Harvard University. The Eli Lilly Company was given exclusive rights to manufacture Fraction G. A special committee was appointed at Harvard to supervise the arrangements for quality control of each batch of extract that was put on the market. In the course of this work it was found that the extract could be given intravenously and that it produced maximal effects in small quantities.

Important new light was cast on the nature of pernicious anemia in

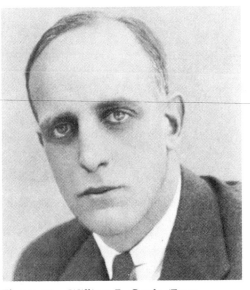

Figure 66. William B. Castle (From Riesman, David (ed.): History of the Interurban Clinical Club, 1905–1937. Philadelphia, The John C. Winston Company, 1937.)

255

1928 by the work of William B. Castle, a young associate of Minot. Castle believed that the cause of pernicious anemia was probably related to the well-known deficiency in the secretion of gastric juice. To test this theory, he ate some beef, allowed it to remain in his stomach long enough for the gastric secretion to act on it, then withdrew the digested beef from his stomach and introduced it into the stomach of a patient having pernicious anemia. He found that the beef under these circumstances had the same effect as liver. He concluded that two factors are involved in the development of the material that is effective against pernicious anemia: one is an *intrinsic factor* supplied by the normal stomach, the other, an *extrinsic factor* supplied by the diet. Subsequent work has verified Castle's hypothesis. It is now known that the intrinsic factor combines with the extrinsic factor in such a way as to promote its absorption from the intestinal tract. Once it has been absorbed, the effective factor travels in the blood to the liver and is stored there, to be used as needed to promote the maturation of the red blood cells in the bone marrow (Castle, 1961).

In 1934 George R. Minot, William P. Murphy, and George H. Whipple were awarded the Nobel Prize in medicine for the discovery of the liver treatment for anemia.

Shortly before Minot's death in 1950, a group of workers at the Merck Institute in New Jersey isolated in pure crystalline form the factor that counteracts pernicious anemia and identified it as *cyanocobalamin,* which is now generally known by its simpler name, vitamin B_{12}. This vitamin is both the extrinsic factor and the anti–pernicious-anemia principle of the liver. On a weight basis, vitamin B_{12} is the most potent of the known vitamins. It can be supplied in pure form for clinical use at relatively low cost. A patient suffering from pernicious anemia can be maintained in good health on an extraordinarily small dose of vitamin B_{12}: 30 micrograms injected intramuscularly once a month is sufficient.

TOOLS OF RESEARCH

TISSUE CULTURE

Many dramatic developments in medicine have resulted from the discovery or invention of a new tool or technique. No technical advance has been more impressively productive than the discovery of the method by which living cells removed from their parent organism can be made to grow in an artificial medium. The technique by which this is accomplished is known as *tissue culture* or *cell culture.* It has had a far-reaching effect in many fields of science, and today it is a much used and highly valued laboratory procedure.

Biologists in the mid-nineteenth century were already aware that death of the organism is not necessarily accompanied by death of its individual parts. In 1885, Wilhelm Roux, in Germany, obtained small bits of tissue from a chick embryo and succeeded in keeping them alive in an artificial medium for short periods of time. Following this, several other research workers achieved similar results, chiefly with the tissues of cold-blooded animals. In 1906 Beebe and Ewing of the Cornell Medical College succeeded in growing cells obtained from a malignant tumor of a dog. However, the first successful tissue culture in the modern sense was performed by Ross G. Harrison in 1907.

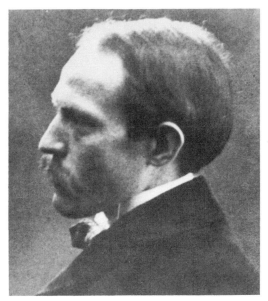

Figure 67. Ross G. Harrison. (From the Archives Office, The Johns Hopkins Medical Institutions.)

Harrison received his A.B. and Ph.D. degrees at the Johns Hopkins University, the latter in 1894. While he was working for his Ph.D. he spent a year in Bonn, Germany, under Moritz Nussbaum, and he returned to Bonn in 1899 to receive his M.D. degree. From 1896 to 1907, Harrison taught histology and embryology in Mall's department at the Johns Hopkins Medical School, where he rose to the rank of Associate Professor of Anatomy.

It was during his last year in Baltimore that Harrison developed the technique of tissue culture. He was then studying the development of the nervous system in the frog embryo, and his experiment was designed to answer a very basic question in neurology: How does an embryo construct the individual nerve fibers that connect the central nervous system with the various parts of the body? In some species these fibers are short, but in others, for example in humans, they may grow to three feet or more in length. Some embryologists believed that each fiber, short or long, grows out from a single cell; others held that the fibers are made up of a succession of short lengths, each built by local cells and somehow joined end to end. Harrison solved the problem by cutting out a bit of the spinal cord from a frog embryo and placing it in a clear drop of coagulated frog lymph, which he could observe under a microscope. In this manner he was able to watch the living nerve fibers sprout out from nerve cells and grow in length as far as the clotted medium allowed them to extend. Thus Harrison, in this simple but ingenious experiment, not only invented an important research method but also solved one of the fundamental problems of neurology. His demonstration that the entire length of the nerve fiber is produced by its parent cell changed the whole concept about the formation of the nervous system.

Soon after Harrison reported his method of growing cells in tissue culture, Alexis Carrel at the Rockefeller Institute made use of it to answer questions that had arisen in the course of his surgical research on the healing of

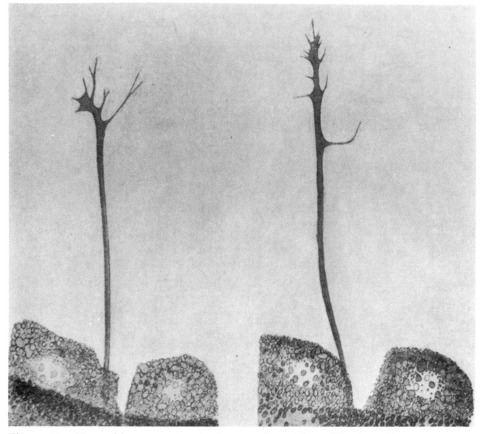

Figure 68. Nerve fibers growing in tissue culture. (From Harrison, R. G.: Embryonic transplantation and development of the nervous system. Anat. Rec 2:385, 1908.)

wounds. Carrel had been puzzled about how cells of the skin, connective tissue, blood vessels, and nerves grow out to fill the gaps and close the wounds created by disease, injury, or surgery. For years, Carrel's success in grafting tissues, in patching vital arteries with materials taken from elsewhere in the body, and in transplanting whole organs such as kidney or spleen, had given him hope that in the future surgeons might learn to keep human tissues alive in storage and possibly even to grow them as replacements for damaged elements of the body. He was, therefore, attracted by Harrison's method of cultivating cells outside the body. Without delay, he sent his assistant, Montrose T. Burrows, to New Haven to work with Harrison, who in 1907 had become Professor of Comparative Anatomy at Yale. Burrows worked in Harrison's laboratory for a number of months and not only learned his methods but also succeeded in improving the culture medium in which the tissues were grown. Using the improved medium, Burrows was able to grow cells from nerve tissue and skin and even from heart muscle. In the cultures of heart tissue he was able to answer a question about which there had been long-standing debate: Does the rhythmic beat of the heart arise within the heart muscle itself, or is it stimulated by nerve impulses? In the cultures, the heart muscle cells, free of all possible nervous connection, underwent spontaneous rhythmic contraction, thus giving visible proof that the heartbeat originates within the muscle cells. With his new technique, Burrows was also the first to observe, in cells removed from the organism, the details of mitosis (the manner in which a growing cell divides to form two new cells).

Carrel's most important contributions to tissue culture were as follows: (1) the introduction of strict surgical asepsis in the handling of tissues subjected to culture; (2) the perfection of the instrumentation for tissue culture, including his invention of a specialized flask that bears his name; and (3) the demonstration of the relative ease with which one may cultivate the tissues of warm-blooded animals. (Harrison's work had been done with frog tissue.) Carrel also was able to utilize in his experiments the great manual dexterity that won him fame as a blood-vessel surgeon and transplantor of organs (for which he subsequently won the Nobel Prize).

Carrel's rather spectacular methods and his charisma soon attracted public attention to the awesome fact that cells could be grown in "bottles" far removed from the living body and could even attain a semblance of immortality by long outliving the animal from which they originated. To convince skeptics of the potentialities of the tissue culture method, Carrel determined to keep alive cells obtained from the heart of an embryonic chick by transplanting them every two or three days to a fresh nutrient medium. He hoped to present overwhelming evidence that the cells of the culture could survive and multiply over a long period of time. Carrel's famous culture was started on January 17, 1912, and in April, when it was 85 days old, having passed through more than 30 transplantations, he reported that it was still growing vigorously. Additional reports were issued in February, 1913, and in May, 1914, after it had been transplanted 358 times. The press, for whom the "chicken heart culture" seemed to have a romantic appeal, followed Carrel's reports with rising interest. The reports were, in fact, rather misleading, for the heart muscle cells of the original tissue had died out early in the life of the transplant; the cells that were still growing in 1914 were those of the connective tissue (fibroblasts) that originally supported the muscle tissue. Nevertheless, the chicken heart culture was a great success in that it showed that connective tissue cells could be kept alive outside the body for an indefinite period of time. The cells continued to be kept alive and growing until April 26, 1946, two years after Carrel's death and 34 years after the tissue had been taken from the chick embryo.

Following the early work of Harrison and Carrel, other investigators adopted the technique, and there began a long list of experiments designed to answer a variety of basic questions in biology.

When Ross Harrison left Baltimore for New Haven in 1907, the work in tissue culture at Johns Hopkins was taken over by Warren H. Lewis. Lewis had been associated with Harrison in the Department of Anatomy since 1900, and he performed his tissue culture work in this department until 1940. From 1915 onward his studies were carried out in the new Laboratory of Embryology, which was established at Johns Hopkins by the Carnegie Institution of Washington, and in this work his wife, Margaret Reed Lewis, was his collaborator. Working together they made many improvements in the instrumentation of tissue culture and in the media in which cells are grown, and much new light was thrown on the structure and behavior of living cells.

259

They pioneered in the use of time-lapse cinephotography, which enabled them to speed up, on the screen, activities far too slow to be detected by direct observation. Their moving pictures showing how individual cells move about and ingest food and water not only were fascinating to watch but also revealed previously unobserved aspects of cellular behavior.

In 1923, the Lewises became interested in the growth and behavior of cells of malignant tumors. Working with a young colleague, George O. Gey, they demonstrated that tumor cells are permanently altered from the normal state and retain a malignant pattern of growth through many successive generations in tissue culture. Subsequently they were able to show how living malignant cells of connective-tissue origin differ from their normal counterpart, the fibroblast. Over the years, since the early work of the Lewises, the tissue culture technique has come into wide use in the field of cancer research.

Not only has the use of tissue culture contributed to our knowledge of the manner in which normal and malignant cells grow and behave but also it has provided a means for growing and identifying a number of important viruses. These viruses can be grown only in tissue culture, in the presence of living cells. Hence, this technique has become an important tool of the virologist. Two outstanding examples of the use of tissue culture for work with viruses may be cited.

(1) *Max Theiler,* a South African who had received his medical education in England, came to the United States in 1922 and for eight years worked at the Harvard School of Tropical Medicine, concentrating his attention upon the virus of yellow fever. In 1930 he moved to the Rockefeller Institute, and while working there he discovered a method to weaken the virulence of the yellow fever virus. This was accomplished by growing the virus in a chick embryo tissue culture medium and transferring it every few days to a fresh lot of the culture medium. After dozens and dozens of such transfers it was found that the virus had lost its capacity to produce yellow fever but that it still retained its ability to confer immunity. These facts were verified first in monkeys and then in human subjects. Theiler's observations led him to the development in tissue culture of a protective vaccine against yellow fever. The vaccine proved to be highly effective in field tests on large numbers of people in South America, and in the early 1940s the Rockefeller Institute began to produce the vaccine on a massive scale. It was used extensively by the United States military forces during World War II. In 1951 Theiler was awarded the Nobel Prize for his work on yellow fever.

(2) *John Franklin Enders* received his bachelor's degree at Yale and then began to work toward a Ph.D. in the Germanic and Celtic languages at Harvard. Along the way he discovered that bacteriology held a greater attraction for him than did languages. In 1929 he became an Assistant in the Department of Bacteriology and Immunology at Harvard, working under Professor Hans Zinsser. In Zinsser's laboratory during the next few years he carried out a number of important studies in the field of virology. Prior to World War II he became interested in trying to prepare a vaccine from viruses grown in tissue culture. After the war (1946) he was invited to conduct research regarding infectious diseases at the Children's Hospital in Boston. In this work he was joined by two young Fellows, Thomas H. Weller and Frederick C. Robbins, who received support from funds pro-

260

vided by the National Foundation for Infantile Paralysis. Working under Enders's supervision and utilizing tissue culture as a tool, Weller undertook some studies of the chickenpox virus while Robbins tried to track down a virus as the cause of epidemic diarrhea in infants. One morning when the three investigators were sipping coffee together and comparing notes about their work, Enders mentioned that he had some poliomyelitis virus stored in his freezer. After some further conversation it was agreed to join forces on work with this virus. Earlier attempts to grow the polio virus in various types of tissue culture had failed, though it could be kept alive in cultures containing human embryonic brain tissue. It was feared that any vaccine prepared in cultures containing brain or nervous tissue would be hazardous for human use, since it might cause a reaction damaging to the nervous system.

Employing somewhat different methods from those previously used, Enders and his associates, in 1949, reported two major advances: first, that polio virus could be grown in culture tubes containing non-nervous tissue; and secondly, that it was possible to recognize the presence of the virus by a chemical test, without injecting the virus into a test animal. For these discoveries Enders, Weller, and Robbins received the Nobel Prize in 1954. As a direct result of their work, using similar methods, Jonas E. Salk developed an anti-polio vaccine that passed its field tests in 1954 and became available for general use in 1955.

It would not be feasible to detail here all of the many ways in which tissue culture has been utilized in medical research. It has been employed to study biomedical problems in microbiology, hormone research, toxicology, embryology, pharmacology, radiobiology, the standardization of antiviral chemotherapy, the study of biochemical mechanisms in fibroblasts, the identification of the carriers of certain genetic traits, the preparation of poliomyelitis vaccine, the isolation and identification of viruses, the titration of toxins and other agents that damage tissues, titration of immune sera, and a variety of other uses. It has become such an important tool in both basic and applied research in medical science that many have felt that its impact has been as important as the introduction of the compound microscope.

The technique of tissue culture is now so simple that it can be carried out in any laboratory. In the early days when Carrel began his work, only a few highly skilled investigators were able to use it, and the necessity of doing everything under aseptic precautions made the construction and operation of laboratories for this type of work a complicated and costly procedure. All of this has changed since the advent of antibiotics such as penicillin, streptomycin, and chloramphenicol, which are added to the tissue culture medium at a concentration that eliminates bacteria but that still allows the tissue cells to grow and multiply. The end of new and fruitful uses for tissue culture is not yet in sight.

The tissue-culture story serves as an example of one of the ways in which modern medical science has advanced toward the achievement of major objectives. It was fortunate that Ross Harrison had served successively as student, instructor, and Associate Professor in Mall's Department of Anatomy. Mall's concept of anatomy was altogether different from that of his predecessors. For centuries anatomy had been taught as a frozen, immu-

261

table science. In the first century it had been looked upon largely as an introduction to surgery. *Professor of Anatomy and Surgery* was a common title in the faculties of many medical colleges. Students were drilled in anatomy by lecture, demonstration, and quiz; they learned by rote the relations of the bones, muscles, nerves, blood vessels, and other structures in the various parts of the body, chiefly to prevent them from committing some blunder in their surgical incisions and explorations. To Mall, on the other hand, anatomy was a living, pervasive science, and he taught his students and staff to view it in this light. It was not enough to say that the sciatic nerve originates in the sacral plexus of the spinal cord and supplies nerve fibers to the skin and muscles of the leg; one should inquire as to how the nerve develops in the embryo and during childhood and how it acquires its ability to conduct sensations and to make muscles contract. Mall deliberately avoided standing over the shoulders of his students, and he shunned teaching by rote; he encouraged his students to think for themselves and to seek their own explanation for problems that puzzled them. In this same spirit Mall's staff devoted more time to original investigation than to drilling anatomy into students.

It was an easy matter for critics brought up in the old school to ridicule the experiments that Harrison reported in 1907. How could a man who was being paid to teach anatomy be excused for trying to grow the nerve cells of a frog? What relevance did this have to the practice of medicine and the cure of disease? Obviously the relevance was difficult to establish; but in retrospect we see that it was there, and as the years rolled by this became more and more evident. Harrison's tissue-culture technique, which had been designed to answer a basic question in neurology, found many uses in answering other fundamental questions. In addition, it was an essential factor in the discovery of a way to prevent both yellow fever, the scourge of the first century, and infantile paralysis, a disease more feared by parents than any other childhood infection. Thus, a technique invented by a basic scientist for use in cold-blooded animals, which initially seemed to have no relevance to human disease, turned out, in the course of time, to have a profound effect upon many aspects of medical science and upon the practice of medicine.

Tissue culture, owing to its wide applicability, was certainly at the head of the list of research tools devised between 1876 and 1946. Although it will not be possible here to give attention to many other important tools, two examples will be cited; one—micropuncture and ultramicrochemical techniques— led to a major advance in physiological research; the other—the electron microscope—had far-reaching effects upon morphological studies.

MICROPUNCTURE AND ULTRAMICROCHEMICAL TECHNIQUES

In the early 1920s, Robert Chambers, Professor of Microscopic Anatomy at Cornell University Medical College, developed instruments for micromanipulation that enabled him to dissect and inject single cells under the high magnification of a compound microscope. Chambers's technique was adapted by Alfred Newton Richards and his associates at the University of Pennsylvania to the study of renal physiology. In 1921, using a micromanipulator and a micropipette, Richards and his colleague Joseph T. Wearn succeeded in collecting fluid from the glomerular capsules of frogs' kidneys. The amount of fluid that they were able to collect was minute—only about 0.0001 cubic centimeter per hour. It was believed at first that this was too small an amount to permit quantitative chemical analysis, but rather crude qualitative analyses indicated that the glomerular fluid resembled a protein-free ultrafiltrate of the frog's blood plasma. In a long series of experiments between 1921 and World War II, the group at the University of Pennsylvania extended their studies to other amphibians and reptiles and adapted and refined a number of quantitative chemical methods so that they could be employed for the analysis of infinitesimal quantities of fluid with a high degree of accuracy (Richards, 1929 and 1938).

When Otto Folin, at Harvard, in the first and second decades of the twentieth century, developed colorimetric methods that permitted accurate chemical analyses on amounts of fluid of the order of one cubic centimeter, this was considered to be a triumph of chemical methodology. However, by 1930, Richards and his associates were able to reduce Folin's procedures to fantastically small dimensions; for example, the method for analysis of uric acid was adapted to volumes of fluid ranging from 0.00003 to 0.00005 cubic centimeter containing 3 to 10 millionths of a milligram of uric acid; and the average error in these measurements was no greater than 5 per cent (Bordley and Richards, 1933).

The experiments in Richards's laboratory gave a direct and unequivocal answer to a basic question in renal physiology: they showed that the process of urine formation begins at the glomerulus, where the constituents of blood plasma, with the exception of protein, are filtered through the glomerular membrane. The experiments also indicated that as the filtered fluid passes down the tubule en route to the bladder, all of the sugar, much of the water, and some of the other chemical constituents are reabsorbed into the blood. It was believed at first that these two processes—filtration and reabsorption—were wholly responsible for urine formation. In later experiments, it became apparent that some of the substances appearing in urine actually are secreted by the cells of the tubules. This had long been suspected, and E. K. Marshall, Jr., and collaborators at Johns Hopkins had shown that in certain fish, urine formation is due entirely to tubular secretion, since the kidneys are not equipped with glomeruli. There was some question about the relevance of these findings to the formation of urine in mammals, but other experiments soon removed any doubts about the ability of the cells of the tubules to secrete substances into the urine.

In work carried on independently in 1934–35 by Richards's group and by Homer W. Smith, James A. Shannon, and their associates at the New York University College of Medicine, it was shown that *inulin,* a vegetable starch not normally present in the blood of animals, when injected into the blood, is filtered by the renal glomerulus but is not reabsorbed in its passage down the tubule. Therefore, the amount of inulin in the urine serves as a measure of glomerular filtration. If a substance, in passing from blood to urine, is concentrated to a greater degree than is inulin, its concentration must have been raised by the excretory action of the tubular cells. This was found to be true of a number of substances. For example, when either para-amino hippurate or iodopyracet (Diodrast) is injected into the circulation, its concentration by the kidney may be many times greater than that of inulin. In fact, these substances are so avidly extracted from the blood by the renal tubules that the quantity appearing in the urine in a given period of time can

263

be utilized to calculate the rate at which blood is flowing through the kidney (provided that the concentration of the substance in the blood is known and is maintained at a constant level).

While this work was in progress, Arthur M. Walker in Richards's laboratory, with the collaboration of Jean Oliver of the Long Island Medical College, an expert in the microscopic anatomy of the kidney, had advanced further with the techniques of micropuncture and microchemistry so that they could obtain and analyze fluid from various isolated segments of the tubules of mammalian kidneys and thus gain some insight into how each portion of a tubule performs its secretory or reabsorptive activities. Since that time the techniques of micropuncture and ultramicrochemical analysis have been improved and widely utilized in the investigation of normal and abnormal function of the kidney (Windhager, 1968, chapter on *Micropuncture Methodology* in Orloff and Berliner, 1973).

The extent to which the techniques and concepts that were developed in the laboratories of Richards and Smith in the 1920s, 1930s, and 1940s provided the basis for our present understanding of renal physiology may be gleaned from any comprehensive modern treatise on this subject (Orloff and Berliner, 1973). As a consequence of these fundamental studies, it is now possible to estimate with a reasonable degree of accuracy, in the living human subject, the efficiency with which the various functional components of the kidney are performing their tasks in health and in disease.

ELECTRON MICROSCOPE

The substitution of electron beams for light beams in microscopy was pioneered in Europe in the 1920s and 1930s. The resolving power of an ordinary light microscope is limited by the wavelength of light; clear resolution cannot be obtained with a magnification much greater than 2500×. Electron beams suitable for microscopy have a wavelength about 1/100,000 that of visible light, and the resolving power is therefore much greater. This principle was utilized in Germany in 1939 to visualize with a crude electron microscope the tiny discrete particles of the tobacco-mosaic virus, a filterable virus that causes a disease of tobacco plants. It was obvious that the potentiality of electron microscopy was very great, but the war was then on in Europe, and nothing further was done there to improve or exploit this new instrument. The first commercially available electron microscope was produced in the United States by the Radio Corporation of America. It was described in 1941 in the *Journal of Bacteriology* by Ladislaus L. Marton, a Hungarian physicist trained in Switzerland who settled in the United States in 1938 and became a research worker at the RCA Laboratory. Marton's article describes the optical principles, structural features, resolving power, and the utility and limitations of the RCA instrument. This was the first description of a complete, utilitarian electron microscope.

After World War II, electron microscopes were produced by several manufacturers in the United States and Europe, and they came into wide use for the study of a multitude of biological phenomena. They have added enormously to our understanding of disease-producing organisms and the tissue changes wrought by disease.

264

THE ADVENT OF CLINICAL SCIENCE IN THE UNITED STATES

. . . the disorders of the animal body, and the symptoms indicating them, are as various as the elements of which the body is composed. The combinations, too, of these symptoms are so infinitely diversified, that many associations of them appear too rarely to establish a definite disease; and to an unknown disease, there cannot be a known remedy.

(Thomas Jefferson, 1807)

In the early years of the twentieth century, medicine was moving rapidly from its old empiricism toward a new scientific base. With the greater accuracy in diagnosis made possible by the use of X-rays, chemical examinations of blood and urine, and bacteriological techniques, the practicing physician found it necessary to add to his traditional skills an understanding of how to make use of the tools of science. The changes in the preliminary requirements for medical education and in the medical curriculum were designed to equip the new generation of physicians with knowledge that would enable them to avoid the blind guesswork of older generations and to base their diagnosis and treatment upon a thorough study of their patients. The students were taught that in this study they should utilize not only time-honored methods such as history-taking and physical examination but also all appropriate scientific procedures. The more thoughtful students also learned that the science of medicine is never stationary but rather that it advances progressively as new discoveries are added to old ones; and that they might even contribute to the advance by being skeptical of old theories and taking a fresh, quizzical look at the problems presented by their patients. It was in the atmosphere of inquisitiveness created by these thoughtful students and their teachers that clinical science was established.

THE CHANGING OF THE GUARD AT HOPKINS

In his planning for the Johns Hopkins Hospital and Medical School, John Shaw Billings had a vision of the future which few others had at that time. He clearly foresaw that there was an opportunity to bring together the art and science of medicine to form a new clinical science, and it was his hope that the Hopkins institutions would lead the way toward this objective (Billings, 1889):

. . . . There is a widespread hope and expectation that these combined institutions will endeavor to produce investigators as well as practitioners, to give to the world men who can not only sail by the old charts, but who can make new and better ones for the use of others. This can only be done where the professors and teachers are themselves seeking to increase knowledge, and doing this for the sake of the knowledge itself;—and hence it is supposed that from this hospital will issue papers and reports giving accounts of advances in, and of new methods of acquiring knowledge, obtained in its wards and laboratories, and that thus .all scientific men and all physicians shall share in the benefits of the work actually done within these walls. But, however interesting and valuable this work may be in itself, it is of secondary importance to the future of science and medicine, and to the world at large, in comparison with the production of trained investigators, full of enthusiasm, and imbued with the spirit of scientific research, who will spread the influence of such training

265

far and wide. It is to young men thus fitted for the work that we look for the solution of some of the myriad problems which now confront the biologist and the physician.

Do I seem to ask too much? To be too sanguine as to what human thought, and study, and skill may accomplish? to forget that there is one event unto all; that the shadow of pain and death comes on the wise man as on the fool? I have two answers. As surely as our improved methods of prevention and treatment, based on the advances in knowledge of the last fifty years, have already extended the average duration of life in civilized countries nearly five years, have prolonged thousands of useful and productive lives, and have done away with the indescribable agonies of the pre-anaesthetic period, so surely we are on the verge of still greater advances, especially in the prevention of infectious and contagious disease, in the resources of surgery against deformities and morbid growths, and in the mitigation of suffering due to causes which cannot be wholly removed. But the second answer is more important, and it is this: It is our duty to try to increase and diffuse knowledge according to the means and opportunities which we have, and not to rest idle because we cannot certainly foresee that we shall reap where we have strewn.

Knowledge had certainly been increased and diffused during the first 12 years of the Hopkins Medical School, but by 1905 the time had come for another stride toward the blending of art and science.

In 1904 Osler accepted an appointment as Regius Professor of Medicine at Oxford University, and in 1905 he left Baltimore for England. Before his departure he stated that he had had two ambitions while at Johns Hopkins: "to make myself a good clinical physician" and "to build up a great clinic on Teutonic lines, not on those previously followed here and in England, but on lines which have placed the scientific medicine of Germany in the forefront of the world." Actually Osler's clinic in Baltimore had combined the German medicine of the 1870s and 1880s with the nineteenth century British tradition of teaching medicine to small groups of students at the patient's bedside. Osler was ahead of his American contemporaries when he insisted that laboratories be established in close proximity to the wards and that students be drilled in the use of laboratory methods. But he looked upon the clinical laboratory chiefly as an aid in the diagnosis and study of disease — the place where one could examine by microscopical, chemical, and physical means samples of blood, urine, and other substances obtained from patients. In Osler's view the clinical laboratories were for observational studies, not for experimental work. Although he encouraged original inquiries he appeared to believe that research requiring special tools and experimental methods should be carried out in the departments of physiology, pharmacology, and pathology. Those who worked in these preclinical departments were in accord with Osler's concept; they were willing to acknowledge the clinician's observational and descriptive powers and his skill in diagnosis, but they believed that he had neither the time nor the training for real laboratory research.

Lewellys F. Barker succeeded Osler as Professor of Medicine at Hopkins. He had a professional background quite different from that of Osler in that he had spent far more time in the laboratory than at the bedside. He was a medical graduate of the University of Toronto and had completed a one-year internship in Toronto before coming to Baltimore in 1891 to work in the newly opened Johns Hopkins Hospital. He spent a year working in Osler's clinic and then was appointed Fellow in Pathology under Welch.

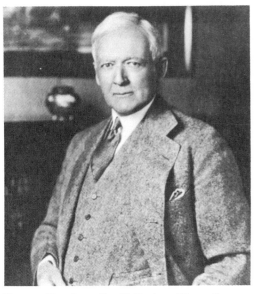

Figure 69. Lewellys F. Barker. (From the Archives Office, The Johns Hopkins Medical Institutions.)

After a year with Welch he moved to the anatomical laboratory to work with Mall, and there he enjoyed for the first time the thrill of discovery: he demonstrated the presence of iron in eosinophil cells. Except for six months spent in Leipzig in 1895, carrying out some neurological studies, Barker remained in the Department of Anatomy, rising to the rank of Associate Professor. Then, in 1899 he was appointed Resident Pathologist and Associate Professor of Pathology. In 1900 he left Baltimore to become Professor of Anatomy at the University of Chicago. This was the position he held at the time of his appointment as Osler's successor.

In 1902 Barker delivered an address entitled *Medicine and the Universities,* in which the major theme was a plea for reorganization of the clinical departments of university medical schools. It was his conviction that these departments should become centers of research as well as of teaching. He did not agree with the Oslerian view that research should be left to the preclinical departments. In addition, Barker proposed that the clinical professors be placed on a full-time salary to relieve them of the necessity to earn most of their livelihood by engaging in private practice (Barker, 1907a).

When Barker moved back to Baltimore in 1905 there were no funds to implement his plan for full-time clinical professorships. However, within a year he was able to reorganize the Department of Medicine so as to provide better opportunities for investigation of human disease problems. He created within his department three research divisions, each with its own laboratory: (1) The Biological Laboratory under Rufus Cole was to concentrate chiefly on infectious diseases. (2) The Physiological Laboratory under Arthur D. Hirschfelder was to be concerned for the most part with cardiovascular and pulmonary diseases. (3) The Chemical Laboratory under Carl Voegtlin, a native of Switzerland who had obtained his Ph.D. in

267

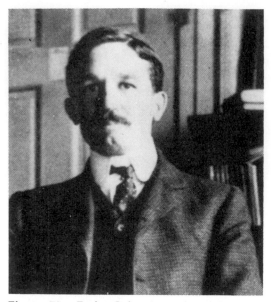

Figure 70. Rufus Cole. (From the Archives Office, The Johns Hopkins Medical Institutions.)

Chemistry from the University of Freiburg (1903), directed its efforts toward metabolic problems (Barker, 1907b).

At the time of his appointment to head the Biological Laboratory, Rufus Cole was serving as Resident Physician of the hospital. He had risen to this position under Osler, and during Osler's last year in Baltimore, Cole was his Resident Physician. He continued to hold this post under Barker until January, 1906, when he resigned in order to devote all of his time to the Biological Laboratory. Since he had served in the same capacity under both Osler and Barker, Cole had a unique opportunity to compare the style and methods of the two physicians-in-chief. He described his observations as follows (Corner, 1964; Sabin, 1934; Bondy and Brainard, 1959):

> *Under Dr. Osler the opportunities for careful observation were never better and the importance of careful study of the more superficial aspects of disease never more insisted upon. But there existed in the clinic no great incentive to learn more about the fundamental nature of disease, and facilities for making the necessary investigations were lacking. The belief was general that medicine was basically different from biology or chemistry or anatomy and could only be studied by different methods. From time to time doubts about this point of view were expressed but chiefly by workers in the underlying sciences, and they usually held the opinion that the real investigations must be carried out by workers in their laboratories, since clinicans neither had the necessary time nor did they have the adequate training for these more complicated techniques. Dr. Barker on the other hand held that a primary function of the university department of medicine should be the encouragement of research and accordingly that the professor of medicine should be freed from the burdens of a private practice and allowed to devote his time to his own investigations and those of his staff.*

Thus, Cole seems to salute the replacement of the *avant garde* of the 1880s by the *avant garde* of the new twentieth century.

Interesting and important work was done in all three of the new research laboratories of the Department of Medicine. The physical facilities of the laboratories were very primitive, and the funds available to support the work were extremely limited. Cole, Hirschfelder, and Voegtlin all were paid pitifully small salaries. Dr. Voegtlin had no secretary and no laboratory assistant. He therefore had to write everything in longhand and wash his own laboratory glassware. But the three men were all able and industrious scientists. Hirschfelder's experience in the Physiological Laboratory enabled him to write a book on *Diseases of the Heart and Aorta,* which appeared in 1910. In 1913 he left Baltimore to become Professor of Pharmacology at the University of Minnesota. Voegtlin, working with W. G. MacCallum, made the important discovery of the role which the parathyroid glands play in calcium metabolism. He eventually became the first Research Director of the National Cancer Institute.

Rufus Cole, in the Biological Laboratory, was particularly interested in developing the use of blood cultures for medical diagnosis. He had begun this work while he was still a member of the house staff. His pioneer studies of typhoid bacilli in the blood of patients sick with typhoid fever constituted the first *systematic* clinical laboratory research done at the Johns Hopkins Hospital. Cole also was interested in protective vaccines, and Frederick F. Russell, an Army medical officer who worked under Cole in the Biological Laboratory in 1906, was responsible for carrying out the first large-scale trial of antityphoid vaccination. Cole remained as head of the Biological Laboratory for less than three years. In 1908 he was placed in the enviable position of having to choose between two important jobs. He turned down an offer to become Professor of Medicine at the University of Michigan in order to accept a position as Director of the still uncompleted 50-bed research hospital of the Rockefeller Institute.

THE ROCKEFELLER
HOSPITAL

Rufus Cole saw in the Hospital of the Rockefeller Institute an opportunity to develop a program of intensive clinical investigation in an environment devoted entirely to research and free of the demands of medical practice and teaching. There would be an opportunity to train young men who would then carry the new attitudes and new scientific methods to medical schools and hospitals elsewhere.

The plan that Cole presented to the Rockefeller Board of Directors for the organization of the hospital staff was a combination of what he learned from Osler of the advantage of a full-time graded residency training program and what he had learned from Barker about the great need for full-time physicians trained for, and devoted to, clinical investigation. The plan called for a resident staff of young men of proven ability who were capable of doing independent research. Each of these men would have full control of a group of patients suffering from a disease in which he was particularly interested. Each would be provided with assistants and facilities for animal experimentation and laboratory tests. The new Hospital would be an independent department of the Rockefeller Institute and would be under the control of Cole and his staff.

Cole's plan was accepted by the Directors in January, 1909, and in the

269

general endowment Mr. Rockefeller provided funds for the employment of a salaried medical staff at the new hospital. The Hospital of the Rockefeller Institute was officially opened on October 17, 1910.

In his organization of the staff and facilities of the hospital Cole was guided by a principle which gradually has become the basic precept of academic clinical medicine throughout the United States: that the diagnosis and treatment of disease should go hand-in-hand with their study in the laboratory. In this manner the art and science of medicine would be melded; and the treatment of disease would be guided by science and knowledge rather than by ignorance and empiricism. Four senior members of the hospital staff were appointed: Alphonse Dochez to organize the pneumonia service; Homer Swift to work on rheumatic fever; Alfred Cohn in cardiology; and Donald Van Slyke in renal disease. Younger men at the resident or fellowship level who had exhibited an interest in medical research were assigned to each of the senior members to form study groups. Each group had its own beds for patients and its own laboratory facilities.

Cole himself chose to work with Dochez on acute lobar pneumonia. This disease was very common in the late nineteenth and early twentieth centuries, and it was associated with such a high mortality rate that Osler called it "the captain of the men of death," using the phrase which John Bunyan originally had applied to tuberculosis. Cole had begun his studies of pneumonia before he left Baltimore. He continued to work on this disease until his retirement in 1937; and after that the work was carried forward by his associates. The story of the pursuit of the problems presented by this one disease is a fascinating one. It is a story worth recounting briefly, for it indicates that well-directed persistence in the study of a single outstanding disease problem can bring to light a succession of unexpected discoveries, and in this case it led to the discovery of one of the most fundamental principles in biology.

Lobar pneumonia is an infection of the lungs caused by the pneumococcus that was discovered by Pasteur in 1880. Cole and Dochez began their work by trying to prepare an antiserum for the pneumococcus that could be used in the treatment of patients. They quickly discovered that there are many different types of pneumococcus and that an antiserum for one type is ineffective for other types. One of their major contributions was the development of a simple method for typing pneumococci obtained from patients. One of the types most frequently found as the cause of human pneumonia was designated *type I*. By the end of 1912, Cole and Dochez had developed in horses a serum for use against type I pneumococcus and were working toward the development of antisera for other types. In time antipneumococcal sera were being produced in quantity and were given wide distribution for the treatment of pneumonia. This form of treatment was not abandoned until the sulfonamides became available. The use of antipneumococcal serum is credited with saving thousands of lives the world over. Quite apart from these practical results, the studies of the pneumococcus opened up unforeseen areas of research in the chemistry of immunity and heredity.

Cole and his associates became interested in trying to identify the slight chemical differences that give each type of pneumococcus the ability to call forth its own particular antibody. To tackle this problem an inves-

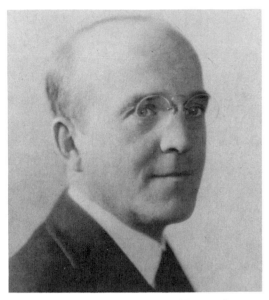

Figure 71. Oswald T. Avery. (National Library of Medicine, Bethesda, Maryland.)

tigator was needed who had a thorough knowledge of bacteriology and a background in chemistry. For this position Cole chose Oswald T. Avery, who joined the staff of the Rockefeller Hospital in 1913. Avery was a graduate of Colgate University and he had received his M.D. degree from The College of Physicians and Surgeons, New York. After working for a few years in clinical medicine, his interest shifted to bacteriology and immunology. From 1907 to 1913 he was Associate Director of the Department of Bacteriology at the Hoagland Laboratory in Brooklyn. After joining Cole's staff Avery proved to be a genius at keeping the pneumococcal research moving along productive channels. In his work he had the assistance of a series of extraordinarily able associates, including Michael Heidelberger, Walther F. Goebel, Martin H. Dawson, J. L. Alloway, René Dubos, Colin M. MacLeod, and Maclyn McCarty.

In their early work Avery and his associates found that the chemical substances responsible for the induction of specific immunity are located in the capsule that envelops each pneumococcus. This capsule is composed almost entirely of polysacccharides, sugars linked to form very complex compounds. It was found that slight differences in the polysaccharides endowed each type of pneumococcus with the specific qualities that activated specific antibodies when the pneumococci were injected into animals. In 1923 Goebel joined Avery and Heidelberger in this study, and his work established the important principle that the immunological specificity of a carbohydrate is determined by its precise molecular structure. Avery and Goebel were able to create an artificial antigen that would elicit antibodies not only against itself but also against virulent pneumococci. In 1935 Goebel was able to report that by using a derivative of a synthetic sugar he had created an artificial antigen so close to that formed by the living type III pneumococcus that when injected into rabbits, it protected them against in-

271

fection with highly virulent organisms of this type. This was the final proof of the concept that the antigenic specificity of the pneumococcus resides in the polysaccharides of the bacterial capsule. This demonstration provided one of the foundation stones of immunochemistry.

In the early 1930s Avery's interest was excited by the report of some work done by a British pathologist, Fred Griffith, in 1928. Griffith reported that when he inoculated mice with a mixture of a harmless strain of living pneumococci and the dead remains of a virulent strain, to his astonishment the mice died from infection with live pneumococci resembling in all respects the virulent strain. Since he could not believe that the killed bacteria had come to life, he had to assume that something had passed from the dead organisms to transform the living harmless strain into a virulent one. Avery asked one of his young associates, Martin Dawson, to study this phenomenon. Dawson was able to confirm Griffith's observations, but he went further and found that it was not necessary to inject the organisms into a mouse; he could obtain the same transfer of virulence by mixing the two strains of pneumococci in a test tube.

In 1932, Alloway, another of Avery's young associates, took the matter still further by demonstrating that in order to bring about a transformation of the harmless bacteria, a fluid extract made from the dead virulent bacteria served just as well as the bacteria themselves. This indicated that the transforming agent was a chemical substance. Avery himself continued this line of investigation, working first with Macleod and later with McCarty. They extracted and systematically broke apart the chemical constituents of virulent type III pneumococcus, testing the transforming power of each fraction. In 1944 they arrived at an essentially pure substance possessing the transforming power in very high concentration. This proved to be a nucleic acid of a type which Levene and Jacobs had first identified years before at the Rockefeller Institute; it was deoxyribonucleic acid—now commonly known by its initials, DNA.

Since the change in the character of the organism from harmless to virulent brought about by the DNA was inherited by subsequent generations of the transformed pneumococcus, DNA immediately aroused great interest in geneticists. The demonstration that a nucleic acid could induce a heritable change in a living organism was quite unexpected. Nucleic acids generally had been thought to be rather inert biologically. However, in the years that followed the discoveries of Avery and his group it was shown that DNA exists in chromosomes of higher animals and is a constant and characteristic ingredient of genes. Thus, the work of Avery's group on bacterial transformation brought to light a chemical mechanism of heredity that operates throughout the biological scale, from bacteria to mammals.

SOCIETY
FOR CLINICAL
INVESTIGATION
We have seen how at the Johns Hopkins Hospital and at the Hospital of the Rockefeller Institute scientific methods were applied more directly to the study of human disease. At these institutions and others that followed their example, young men were trained in clinical research, and these young men went forth to medical schools in all parts of the nation, carrying with them their enthusiasm and their methods for in-

vestigating the causes and effects of illness. As a result the medical profession began to learn that the mysteries presented by their patients should not be accepted as natural phenomena but should become the subject of active investigation.

What was needed at this time was a means of bringing together the scattered young clinical investigators so that they might present their work, obtain intelligent criticism of it, and exchange ideas. The person who recognized the need and saw how it might be met was *Samuel J. Meltzer.*

Meltzer was born in Russia in 1851, but he studied medicine in Germany and received training in physiology under Helmholz and Dubois-Reymond. From 1880 to 1883 he carried out research in Germany but was unable to obtain a suitable post there because he refused to give up his Jewish faith and submit to Christian baptism. Because of this, he decided to emigrate to the United States. His first impression of American medicine was a discouraging one. He had been trained as a research physiologist, but there were no openings for such a scientist in New York. In order to support himself he had to begin the practice of medicine, and in time he became a successful and much sought after practitioner. Nevertheless Meltzer was determined to continue his research activities. One of his earliest research projects in the United States was carried out with William H. Welch at the Bellevue Hospital in 1884. Together they showed for the first time that red blood cells can be destroyed by mechanical agitation. In spite of his growing practice Meltzer continued to spend part of each day in some sort of research activity. After seeing his patients he would perform his experiments in the physiological laboratory at The College of Physicians or in his own home, often working late into the night.

Meltzer's practical knowledge of clinical medicine and his thorough acquaintance with scientific methods and the scientific literature led him to

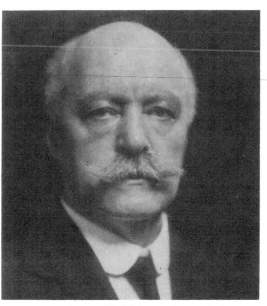

Figure 72. Samuel J. Meltzer. (New York Academy of Medicine.)

273

realize how often the results of research in a basic science can be applied to the solution of a clinical problem. His most important contributions were made in the borderland between medical science and medical practice. Though Meltzer gradually established a reputation as a first-class physiologist and investigator of clinical problems, and though he published one or more scientific papers every year, his major contributions did not come until later. When the Rockefeller Institute opened in 1903 Simon Flexner invited him to become a member of the staff. At first Meltzer agreed to do this on a half-time basis, devoting the other half of his time to his medical practice. However, in 1906 he gave up his practice and became a full-time member of the Institute.

While at the Institute Meltzer carried out many important investigations. Two may be cited to indicate how closely his research was related to practical clinical problems. Meltzer and Auer, in 1909, while studying the methods of artificial respiration that were then available, hit upon the idea of keeping the lungs inflated and aerated by a stream of air blown through a tube inserted into the windpipe by way of the mouth or nose. By this means the blood flowing through the lungs could be supplied with oxygen in the absence of the normal breathing movement of the chest. When ether vapor was added to the airstream the animal could be anesthetized for surgical procedures. This invention was quickly adopted by surgeons, for it enabled them to substitute, in operations of the face and neck, a Meltzer-Auer tube for the mask usually employed for the administration of ether. Meltzer's invention also made possible the triumphs of modern surgery of the heart and lungs. In such operations, when the chest is opened the lungs are kept inflated and aerated by a tube of the type developed by Meltzer and Auer.

Meltzer's second contribution of practical significance occurred in 1910, after Auer and Lewis, working in his laboratory, demonstrated for the first time that when anaphylactic shock is produced in guinea pigs by injecting them with a substance to which they are highly sensitive, death results from intense constriction of the bronchial tubes. Viewing this observation in the light of his clinical experience, Meltzer proposed the now universally accepted hypothesis that bronchial asthma is a phenomenon related to anaphylaxis and is caused by exposure to a substance to which the individual is sensitive.

Meltzer was a firm believer in the value of learned societies for the stimulation of creative thought and activity. In 1903 he had been the inciting force in the creation of the *Society for Experimental Biology and Medicine*, and in 1905 he strongly supported the founding of the *Harvey Society* in New York. In June, 1907, Meltzer attended a meeting of the American Medical Association in Atlantic City. While walking on the boardwalk he was engaged in conversation by some of his young admirers: David L. Edsall (a graduate of the University of Pennsylvania who later became Professor of Medicine and Dean at the Harvard Medical School), Warfield T. Longcope (a graduate of Johns Hopkins who later became Professor of Medicine successively at The College of Physicians and Surgeons, New York, and Johns Hopkins), Joseph H. Pratt (a graduate of Johns Hopkins who later became Professor of Clinical Medicine at Tufts Medical School and Physician-in-Chief of the New England Medical Center), and Wilder Tileston (a graduate of the Harvard Medical School who later became Professor of Clinical Medicine at Yale). During the course of this conversation Meltzer tossed out the idea that it would be a fine thing to have an association for those involved in clinical investigation. He suggested that such an association might be organized as a junior satellite of the distinguished Association of American Physicians, which was made up mostly of older men who were well established in university posts. The junior organization would be made up mostly of younger men who were actively engaged in clinical research. After a series of organizational meetings, the *American Society for Clinical Investigation* was formally constituted in May, 1908. The new society became informally known as the *Young Turks,* after the real Young Turks who startled the world in 1908 with a revolt against the Sultan of Turkey and instituted sweeping reforms in the decrepit Ottoman Empire. The first President of the American Society for Clinical Investigation was Samuel J. Meltzer.

The state of affairs in one of our best medical schools at the time the new society was founded has been well described by James H. Means, who was then a student at the Harvard Medical School (Bondy and Brainard, 1959):

> *The transition from the preclinical to the clinical years in medical schools involved almost as great a change in direction as that from college to professional school. The teachers of the first and second year subjects and those of the third and fourth year subjects constituted two distinct groups with quite different viewpoints, and there was limited communication between them. The clinicians brushed off the preclinical scientists as mere laboratory men who knew but little of medicine, and the scientists looked upon the practice of medicine as largely unscientific guesswork. The whole manner of life between these two groups was different. The preclinical scientists were in the mold of college teachers on the campus. They were full-time salaried people. There were no full-time clinical teachers in those days or salaries either for that matter. Small token honoraria were given by the university but nothing by the teaching hospitals. These men taught, and attended hospital patients for their livelihood in private practice. Any degree of unanimity in a faculty so constituted sure was hard to come by. This gap was later to be closed by the development of the middle estate in medicine, namely the full-time academic, salaried clinician.*

It was Meltzer's idea that the new Society for Clinical Investigation would help to close the gap mentioned by Means. It was his strong conviction that training in one of the sciences allied to medicine and extensive work in the laboratory were as essential to the development of a topnotch clinician as was his clinical training. Meltzer's ideas and the means he employed to implement them were important foundation stones in the development of the modern scientific medical practitioner.

In his presidential address at the first meeting of the Society for Clinical Investigation, Meltzer elaborated his thoughts on the relation of clinical science to preclinical science and to the practice of medicine. He believed that clinical research should be conducted in a separate department of clinical science in the medical school and "be theoretically and practically separated to a considerable degree from the mere practical interest. . . . It will be the practice not less than the science which will benefit by such a separation." He thought that efficiency in practice should be the supreme object of medicine and that the attainment of this objective was the business of the clinical scientist (Meltzer, 1909):

> *Clinical science will not thrive through chance investigations by friendly neighbors from the adjoining practical and scientific domains. For such a purpose we need a standing army of regulars. The investigator in clinical science must devote the best part of his time and intellectual energies to the cultivation and elevation of this field just as the physiologist does in his domain. . . . Without the development of such a department of clinical science, the efficiency of the practice of medicine will lag behind, no matter how progressive the allied sciences of medicine are and how great their efforts to be useful in medicine may be.*

It may be recalled that the birth of the Society for Clinical Investigation occurred almost simultaneously with the opening of the Hospital of the Rockefeller Institute. Meltzer, who was a member of the Institute, and Rufus Cole, who was the first Director of the Hospital, had almost identical concepts of the proper relation between science and medical practice. In speaking of this period Cole said (Bondy and Brainard, 1959):

> *The idea of university departments of medicine was in the air, and it was evident that this idea would soon reach concrete expression in a number of places. The [Rockefeller] hospital appeared to be the logical place in which leaders of this new movement could be trained and be given opportunities to work and be fired with the spirit of investigation which could be disseminated throughout the projected clinics. It seemed that the hospital should not adopt a policy of splendid isolation but should play its part in the reorganization of medical teaching in this country.*

As Cole had hoped, those trained at the Hospital of the Institute did indeed move on to take important positions in many different medical schools. In 1938, of the 179 people who had been on the hospital staff during the preceding 28 years, 112 occupied full-time academic positions, and many more had university affiliations of one kind or another.

13
Hospitals

The emergence of the hospital as a health center has been occasioned by the success of medical science. The doctor has seen himself change from an intuitive, independent artist far removed from the hospital as a House of Despair to a scientific social worker, heavily dependent on what is now a House of Hope with its centralization of specialists and expensive machinery.

(John H. Knowles, 1965)

It was noted in Part I that toward the end of the first century the design and purpose of hospitals were changing. Where space permitted, the newer hospitals were being built on the pavilion design developed by the Army; but in the urban centers such as New York, space was rarely available, and hospitals had to be constructed on a multistory pattern. Occasionally a ward or two of the pavilion type might be attached to the main building for handling of infected or potentially infectious cases. This was done at Roosevelt Hospital, which was one of New York's most up-to-date hospitals in the 1870s. The following is a description of that hospital and some of its functions in 1878 as seen through the eyes of a journalist, W. H. Rideing, writing for *Harper's New Monthly Magazine* (quoted from Brieger, 1972):

The Roosevelt Hospital . . . is spoken of by the eminent English surgeon Erichsen as the most complete medical charity he has ever seen. It is near the Central Park and the Hudson River, in a situation both quiet and salubrious. The material used is principally brick. It has a central administrative department with lateral pavilions, and a large detached barrack ward, which is erected in the garden and has no communication with the main structure, except by an open corridor. The administrative building contains the various offices; the apartments of the officers and their families; an apothecary's shop and a laboratory, in which all the drugs used are prepared; a very complete operating theatre; and small wards for patients requiring special accommodations. The barrack ward is devoted solely to the reception of acute surgical cases, and contains thirty-six beds, arranged two by two on each side of the in-

terspaces between the windows. . . . The garden contains, besides the barrack ward, an isolated hut for the reception of erysipelas cases, and in summer, when the flowers and shrubs are blooming, it is much frequented by convalescent patients. Sixteen hundred and seventeen cases were treated in 1876, 1,451 of which were free; 602 were Americans and 558 were Irish. The death rate of all the cases treated is 9 percent, or more than 3 percent less than that of Bellevue.

The hospital . . . was the first in this country to adopt, through the exertions of Dr. Robert F. Wier, the antiseptic method of treating wounds invented by Joseph Lister, a celebrated Scottish surgeon. The method . . . is based on the experience that the inflammation which follows a wound, such as an amputation, is due to the decomposition of the discharges that are always formed on any cut surface. . . . Lister believes he has demonstrated that the cause of the putrefaction is due to the lodgment on the wound-secretions of minute living bodies floating in the air, and he discovered, after trying many other disinfectants, that carbolic acid would kill these germs. The principle, therefore, consists in surrounding a wound from its reception to its cure with an atmosphere charged with the vapor of the acid; and to accomplish this the surgeon operates amid a thin cloud of spray made by atomizing a weak solution, in which his hands, instruments, sponges, are also immersed. The blood vessels are tied by carbolized cords, the edges of the wound closed by carbolized stitches, and, finally, layers of gauze impregnated with carbolic acid and resin are bound over the wound and a considerable part of the adjoining skin, the resin causing the carbolic acid to be evolved slowly, so that the dressing need not be changed for several days. Dr. Wier considers the success of the method proven, and states that by its use the mortality resulting from serious operations has been noticeably reduced, and that under it the closure of the most serious wounds is truly wonderful.

In the same article in which Rideing described the Roosevelt Hospital he also described, in vivid terms, New York's system for dealing with accidents and other medical emergencies. The hospitals were connected by telegraph wires to the nearest police stations. Three of the hospitals had ambulances: Bellevue Hospital, near the center of population on the East Side, had several; on the West Side the New York Hospital at Fifteenth Street had two; and the Roosevelt Hospital at Fifty-ninth Street had one. When an accident was reported to a police station, the nearest hospital was notified by a telegraphic signal, and an ambulance was sent out. The following is Rideing's firsthand account of what happened when an ambulance was summoned:

We were loitering one morning last January in the apothecary's shop of the New York Hospital, which, besides the long rows of shelves filled with glass jars and bottles, contains a dial instrument, whose imperative tinkling suddenly put an end to our conversation. "The ambulance is wanted at 18th Street," the surgeon in charge explained; and though his name was Slaughter—an obviously unfortunate one for an Esculapian—he proved himself to be one of the tenderest men that ever touched a wound. The apothecary's shop is in the basement, and from it a door opens upon a courtyard, at one side of which is a stable. A well-kept horse was quickly harnessed to the ambulance; and as the surgeon took his seat behind, having first put on a jaunty uniform cap with gold lettering, the driver sprang to the box, where we had already placed ourselves, and with a sharp crack of the whip we rolled off the smooth asphalt of the courtyard into the street. Our speed was only pardonable in view of its object. As we swept around the corners and dashed over the crossings, both doctor and driver kept up a sharp cry of warning to the pedestrians, who

278

darted out of our way with haste, or nervously retreated to the curb looking after us with faces expressive of indignant remonstrance, until they discovered by the gilt lettering on the panels what our vehicle was. The surliest cardrivers and the most aggressive of truckmen gave us the right of way and pulled up or aside to afford us passage. People in a hurry stopped to look after us and strove on tiptoe to discover whether or not we had a passenger. We rattled over the uneven cobblestones of West 18th Street, and at No. 225, where there was an iron gate before an alley-way with a small house at the end, an old man appeared and hailed us. We alighted, and followed him into the front room on the ground floor, the doctor carrying his instruments under his arm.

[The patient, an old Irishman] had slipped on entering and fractured his leg a short distance above the ankle. . . . Obtaining a candle, we found the sufferer lying on a disordered bed with all his clothes on and a pipe in his mouth, the room having neither windows nor other light or ventilation than that which struggled from the kitchen through the door. . . . The doctor energetically threw his coat and cap on the floor, regardless of the gold lettering and gold buttons, and prepared for business. Two splints were selected, and a roll of cotton bandages taken from a sachel. . . . [The doctor] raised the injured limb and applied the splints to it, packing them with oakum before binding them with the cotton ribbon. . . .

[The patient] was lifted by two burly policemen onto the stretcher, which had been brought from the ambulance into the outer room. The stretcher, like all the appliances of the ambulance, is mercifully ingenious, and devised with the object of giving the sufferer the least possible pain in transportation. It consists simply of a strip of canvas about three feet wide and seven feet long, with a tube at each side, through which the wooden poles for carrying it are slipped. . . .

The ambulance had been backed up to the curb, and the tail-board removed. We now discovered that it had two bottoms, and the upper one, which was softly padded, had been drawn off on caster wheels so that it slanted from the end of the vehicle to the sidewalk. The padding was luxuriously yielding, and when the stretcher had been placed upon it, it was pushed into the ambulance and the tailboard closed upon it. The doctor took his seat behind and we drove off. . . . We trotted under the archway of the hospital and pulled up before the door of the receiving ward, where two orderlies drew the stretcher out and deposited it on a bed . . . while Dr. Slaughter reported the case to the house surgeon, who was thence responsible for it.

During the first half of the second century the hospital gradually moved toward a central position in the care of the sick. This came about as the result of many factors, including the following: more attractive and more functional design of hospitals; better control of intramural infections by antiseptic and aseptic methods; the increase in the amount and complexity of surgery and the consequent need for well-designed, well-equipped, and competently staffed operating rooms; recognition of the importance of well-organized and skilled nursing care; the need for centralization of expensive laboratory and X-ray equipment to serve many physicians caring for many patients; the change in the hospital's image from that of a hideous death house to that of a haven where illness could be cured and lives saved; and the provision of suitable accommodations for both rich and poor.

The increase in the number of hospitals in the first two decades of the twentieth century was extraordinary. The factors just cited were not always responsible for the increase. Every community, regardless of size, seemed to believe that it must have its own hospital where its own general practitioner could perform complicated surgery (for which he was usually wholly untrained). The majority of the small village hospitals were little better than those of a century earlier, except that they avoided the crowding and the high incidence of infections, and they were designed to serve paying patients rather than the poor. The methods of diagnosis and treatment were all so new that the people and even the physicians failed to recognize the risks imposed by incompetence. The situation in the farmland of Kansas during this period was well described by Hertzler (1938):

> . . . *As to why so many hospitals sprang up through the enterprise of individual doctors, . . . I can offer no solution. . . . Likely, several factors were active with most of them. At any rate, almost simultaneously the idea of building a hospital, out where the patients originate, occurred to a number of doctors. . . . Perhaps it was because some doctor in a neighboring town had one. . . . At any rate, as the result of that something many small hospitals sprang up in small towns even when the distance from an established hospital was not great. Actual need, therefore, was not a very compelling factor. I know of one small town which had five hospitals, the number, curiously enough, being exactly equal to the number of doctors located there. . . . At one time Kansas had more "hospitals" per capita than any other state in the Union. . . .*

> *After the private hospitals became a sort of epidemic, many churches established hospitals; either by building a new one in opposition to the private hospital, or by taking over a private one and with this as a nucleus building a sizable institution. . . .*

> *Fifty years ago [this was written in 1938], only the larger cities had hospitals. Only emergency work was done by the country doctor, and at that time only the emergencies due to accident were treated by him. The conveyances in that day were such that most country patients were a long way from a hospital. For instance, this place was thirty-five miles from one, and that meant at least five hours of travel if the roads were good. If the roads were bad the distance was lengthened. By the time the family gathered and sat as a jury on the doctor's judgement that an operation was needed, many other precious hours elapsed. Because of the delay the mortality of operations, therefore, was necessarily very high. When fatalities occurred, the hospital, being the last link of the chain became, at least subconsciously, the culprit—the ultimate cause of death.*

> *As more diseases came within the range of the surgeon, the need for more convenient hospitals became emphasized. This was the more laudable excuse for the establishment of the many small hospitals. Before that excuse becomes valid, of course, a hospital needs to have a surgeon capable of doing such operations. Surgeons, I may confide, do not recognize their limitations until they outgrow those limitations, if ever they do, and look backward to their beginning. To be sure, those of us who built hospitals had no doubts on this point—at least not before the hospital was built. Afterwards, no doubt, there were moments that harassed us.*

> *Medical cases in that early day were nearly all treated at home. In fact, there was little occasion for nonsurgical patients to be taken to the hospital. The examinations known in those days could be done as well in the patient's home as in a hospital. The profusion of examinations now commonly done, notably chemical and X-ray examinations, were at that time, of course, unknown. . . .*

> *Those who started hospitals paid aplenty for the advantages they obtained, or sought to obtain, by the establishment of a hospital of their own. . . .*

> *Like most moonlight dreams it was not the first cost, but the upkeep, that became the important matter. . . .*

One of the chief services of the hospital was that it broke the patients of hospital shyness. They learned to go to the hospital for relief of minor ailments and for the beginning of the more serious ones. Patients were much more willing to go to a hospital at home near their friends, under the care of a doctor known to them, than to go long distances to a city to be placed under the charge of a strange doctor and in strange surroundings. As patients submitted to operation earlier the mortality lessened, which in turn served to decrease the fear of hospitals. This in many cases enabled the small-hospital doctor to operate with lower mortality than the city surgeon. . . .

Physically, most of these small hospitals had for the greater part a like genesis. They had their beginnings, in most instances, in a private residence. . . . Sometimes the doctor and his family lived downstairs and the wife did the cooking. The second-story rooms housed the patients. Some smart and handsome doctors married nurses, in which case the lady did the nursing and a cook was hired. I knew a number of instances in which the wife-nurse performed both functions.

Usually half a dozen or fewer hospital beds found available space in these houses. The operating room was usually the bedroom of the former cook, selected for this purpose because it was not a desirable room for a hospital bed. The kitchen stove usually supplied the heat for the sterilization of the instruments and dressings. This made it necessary for the doctor to eat an early breakfast, so that the stove could be available as a sterilizer when it came time to prepare for the operation. Operating in such hospitals was but slightly removed from the kitchen surgery of any private residence. . . .

Those of us who began in towns too small to provide a private residence of sufficient size started with specially designed buildings which, because of expense, were wooden structures of about six or a dozen rooms. Such buildings could be more nearly adapted to the need to which they were to be put than the old private residence. These small hospitals usually were fitted with a small sterilizing room and a more adequate operating room than their old residence contemporaries. Yet they were all equally primitive in every essential and all veritable firetraps.

In 1902 Hertzler built his own hospital of the type just described at a cost of $6000. He gave the following description of the staff of his hospital:

. . . The trained nurse in charge received $40 a month, the most capable nurse I ever met. . . . Two girls, each receiving $2 a week, did the cooking and the laundry. My assistant got $50 a month and boarded himself. The janitor got half this amount. . . . I got my board. This service constituted the overhead. [All] personnel at a cost of $131 a month.

. . . I resolved to charge no more than $4 a day for the patient's room and nursing, and no more than $150 for any operation. I resolved never to demand a fee in advance, never to inquire if they were or ever would be able to pay even a thin dime. . . .

[Hertzler's hospital failed partly because of his own ill health.] The struggle was long, difficult, heartbreaking. Naturally, at first only the most difficult cases, which established surgeons did not want, came to the new institution. Necessarily, the results were not always good. This, of course, works its vicious circle.

In the end Hertzler was forced by the holder of the mortgage "to sign away the very small equity I had in the hospital. It was a contemptibly cruel thing to do, because my equity was so small that it meant very little to those financially interested in the hospital." Hertzler's story does not end there;

281

in 1916 he built a new fireproof building properly designed as a hospital. This new institution with a growing staff of specialists operated successfully for many years.

Throughout the rural areas of the country, during the first half of the twentieth century, there were many small hospitals serving the patients of one or two or sometimes several general practitioners who were performing surgery that was often beyond their competence, along with their other activities. In contrast with the makeshift rural hospitals, the hospitals in the large cities, particularly those affiliated with universities, were growing in size, complexity, and scientific perfection. Two developments in New York City will serve to illustrate this trend.

In 1910 Abraham Flexner reported that there were ten medical schools in New York City. "The schools that are now called university departments grew up as proprietary institutions. They have never been adequately financed. They obtained, and still obtain, their clinical facilities at each other's expense: that is to say, what one gets, the other loses." Clinical instruction was seriously impaired by lack of cooperation on the part of the hospitals. The hospitals and the doctors on their staffs. . . .

. . . naturally refuse to yield to the universities; and until they do yield, the universities cannot freely reconstruct their clinical branches.

The major part of the clinical instruction [of the Cornell students] is given at Bellevue Hospital, directly opposite the college. [As for Columbia students], every physical and educational condition is already satisfied by Roosevelt Hospital: the scientific laboratories [of the medical school], the dispensary, the maternity hospital are on one side of the street; the general hospital [Roosevelt] on the other. Together they would form an ideally compact and complete plant. That they are not so operated cannot but be deplored as a tragic mischance. It is to the world at large no matter of consequence how they happened to drift apart. There are interests at stake that are entitled to outweigh all personal and historic considerations.

It is evident from these comments that Roosevelt Hospital and The College of Physicians and Surgeons were not comfortable allies. One reason was that the hospital Trustees appointed doctors to their medical staff without regard to the needs or wishes of the College; another source of dissension was that the hospital authorities insisted on dictating when and how the wards were to be used for the instruction of students.

Flexner (1910) believed that though the clinical facilities for Columbia and Cornell students left much to be desired, these two schools were worthy of preservation and encouragement. "Of the New York City schools, Columbia and Cornell alone have at this moment any financial strength. Neither of them, indeed, is in actual possession of sufficient endowment, but there is little reason to doubt that what is additionally requisite will be forthcoming."

Like many of Flexner's predictions this one was close to the mark. Within the next 20 years, both the Columbia and the Cornell schools had enlarged their endowments and changed their principal hospital partners. The College of Physicians and Surgeons became allied with the Presby-

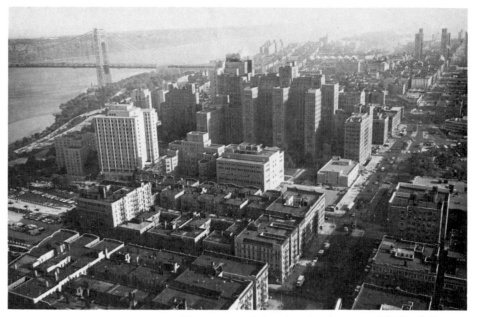

Figure 73. Columbia-Presbyterian Medical Center.

terian Hospital and the Cornell Medical College with the New York Hospital. The result of each of these alliances was the construction of a large medical center.

The first of the new establishments to come into being was the Columbia-Presbyterian Medical Center. This joint undertaking was conceived almost immediately after the appearance of the Flexner report by Edward S. Harkness, a member of the Board of Managers of the Presbyterian Hospital. With the acquiescence of his fellow Board members, Mr. Harkness made it known that the hospital would permit the nomination of its professional staff by the university and would open its wards, with almost no encumbrances, to the medical school faculty for the clinical instruction of students. This was an arrangement that the Roosevelt Hospital had refused to accept.

A formal agreement of affiliation between Columbia University and the Presbyterian Hospital was signed in 1911, and plans for a new medical center were under consideration when all planning was brought to a halt by World War I. After the war, planning was resumed, and finally, in 1922, a site for the center was selected on Washington Heights, where the colorful evangelist Billy Sunday had had his camp grounds and where many New Yorkers had "hit the sawdust trail." After a long period of construction, the Columbia-Presbyterian Medical Center opened its doors in 1928. When completed, the Center was a huge complex of buildings spread over many acres. Included in the complex were The College of Physicians and Surgeons, with its administrative, teaching, and research facilities; the Presbyterian Hospital, with its many wards and services; the Vanderbilt Clinic; the Sloane Hospital for Women; the Babies Hospital; and the Neurological Institute. In addition, the new New York State Psychiatric Institute and Hospital was built on the grounds of the Medical Center, and like all other

283

hospital units in the complex, it was to be used for the instruction of students (Rappleye, 1958).

There were many distinguished medical figures on the original staff of the Medical Center. William Darrach was Dean, and the faculty included the following professors as heads of departments: Walter W. Palmer in Medicine; Allen O. Whipple in Surgery; Herbert B. Wilcox in Pediatrics; Benjamin W. Watson in Obstetrics and Gynecology; Frederick Tilney in Neurology; Haven Emerson in Public Health; and Samuel R. Detwiler in Anatomy.

The joint undertaking of the New York Hospital and Cornell University got started somewhat later than the one just described. The early history of the New York Hospital was recounted in Part I. It will be recalled that when it was described by a visiting Frenchman in 1794, it provided accommodation for "fifty or sixty patients of both sexes," for each of whom there was a wooden bed. As the years passed the hospital grew in size, but it remained in the most congested district of the city until it moved, in 1877, into a new building on Fifteenth Street west of Fifth Avenue.

Compared with the New York Hospital, the Cornell Medical College was a "Johnny-come-lately." It was founded in 1898 when dissident members of the faculty of the New York University and Bellevue Hospital Medical College persuaded the authorities of Cornell University that a new

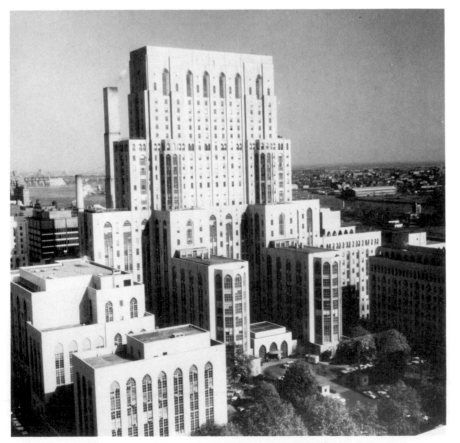

Figure 74. New York Hospital—Cornell Medical Center.

medical school was needed; and Colonel Oliver Hazard Payne, a former associate of John D. Rockefeller in the oil business, made the new venture possible by giving $1.5 million to construct and equip a medical school building. (Colonel Payne later gave the medical school $4 million for a permanent endowment.) The school opened in 1898 in a rented building on the Bellevue Hospital grounds. In its first year it had 245 students, most of whom had transferred from the New York University and Bellevue Hospital Medical College. Its new building, situated across the street from Bellevue, was designed by the distinguished architectural firm of McKim, Mead and White and was opened in 1900.

The original faculty of the Cornell Medical College included some outstanding medical personalities, among them Austin Flint, Jr., Professor of Physiology, and James Ewing, Professor of Pathology, both of whom were established investigators as well as teachers. The faculty was given a rather antique flavor by the Professor of Anatomy, who was a practicing surgeon rather than a professional anatomist. The real leaders of the school were William M. Polk, the Dean and Professor of Gynecology, and Lewis A. Stimson, Professor of Surgery.

From the first, the college endeavored to maintain the highest standards. It opened with a four-year graded curriculum, and in 1908 it made a radical change by raising its entrance requirement to three years of college work from the previous requirement of a high school diploma. The immediate effect of this change was almost disastrous: only 11 students were admitted in 1908. However, Colonel Payne, who favored the higher standards, gave assurance that he would make up the loss of revenue from reduced enrollment, and in a few years the enrollment had risen to the desired level. At about this time the college added several distinguished professors to its faculty, including Graham Lusk in Physiology and Stanley R. Benedict in Biochemistry.

In the case of the Columbia-Presbyterian affiliation it was the hospital that took the initiative, but the dominant figures in the New York Hospital–Cornell affiliation were Polk and Stimson of the Medical College. The association of the two institutions began in 1913, when the hospital agreed to make half of its public services available for teaching and to have these services placed in charge of the professors of the college. In 1927, after years of negotiation, a formal affiliation agreement was signed. The preamble of this agreement sets forth the considerations that prompted it (Robinson, 1957):

The Hospital is impressed with the importance of rendering a larger and more important service to the sick of the community and to medical science through a more intimate and organic association with the Medical College. . . . The University wishes to associate itself organically with the Hospital . . . for the purpose of developing the Medical School on advanced and steadily advancing university lines. In the teaching of students and in the development of medical research it is the common purpose of the two institutions to be in a position to offer opportunities which will attract to their staff and faculty the ablest teachers, investigators and physicians that are anywhere procurable.

Among other things the agreement stipulated that a new medical center would be built and that the associated activities would be directed by a Joint Administrative Board of seven members.

285

During the negotiations leading up to the agreement, a strong supporter of the affiliation was Payne Whitney, nephew of Colonel O. H. Payne, the original benefactor of the Medical College. Sensing that the affiliation was not far off, Mr. Whitney, in 1924, purchased land along the East River, adjoining the land of the Rockefeller Institute, and an architect was engaged to draw up preliminary plans for a medical center on this plot. The plans were all well advanced when Whitney suddenly died, just one month before the formal agreement was signed. The severe blow resulting from the loss of an active and imaginative leader was in some measure mitigated by his will: he bequeathed $12.4 million to the New York Hospital and $2.8 million to the Cornell Medical College.

The Medical Center project gained financial support not only from the Whitney bequest but also from a rapid succession of other large donations: $7.5 million from the General Education Board; $2 million from J. Pierpont Morgan; $2 million from the Laura Spelman Rockefeller Foundation; and $1 million each from George F. Baker, Sr., and George F. Baker, Jr. These large sums and others of lesser amounts were added to the endowments and other funds that the two institutions already possessed, including the $4 million endowment fund presented to the Medical College by Colonel Payne. Prior to the stock market crash of 1929, the potential resources of the hospital and Medical College were estimated to be $60.6 million; another fine example of how the generosity of the wealthy contributed to medical progress.

In 1927, G. Canby Robinson, who had been the Dean and organizer of the Vanderbilt Medical School, was persuaded to leave Nashville to become the Director of the Medical Center and Dean of the Cornell Medical College. In the meantime the plans for the Center had expanded, and more property had to be acquired along the East River. The plans were finally approved by Robinson and the Joint Administrative Board in April, 1928, and construction began in June, 1929.

When the New York Hospital opened at its new location in September, 1932, the Medical Center was one of the most imposing and beautiful structures in New York City. It was more compact and architecturally more harmonious than the Columbia-Presbyterian Center. The main tower of the hospital rose to a height of 27 stories; its "great pointed arches," as Sigerist ecstatically remarked, "reminiscent of the Palace of the Popes at Avignon." The other parts of the structure were skirts to the tower, with the offices, classrooms, and laboratories of the Medical College oriented toward the west so that the view across the East River would be reserved for the patients. The Payne Whitney Psychiatric Clinic was in a separate building, but in harmony with the rest. The bed capacity for patients was 987, and there were provisions for handling large numbers of outpatients. There were also rather elaborate quarters and recreational facilities for house staff and a residence for 500 nurses.

While the Medical Center was being constructed, Robinson was busy selecting a remarkably able group of professors to head the departments of the Medical College and the clinical services of the hospital. Appointments to these positions were made with the understanding that the heads of all major departments would give their *full time* to the hospital and Medical College without financial dependence on private practice and that the salaries would be adequate to make this possible. Some of the former members of the faculty were retained in their professorships but were placed on a full-time basis. These included Eugene Dubois, Professor of Medicine; Oscar M. Schloss, Professor of Pediatrics; Stanley R. Benedict, Professor of Biochemistry; and Charles R. Stockard, Professor of Anatomy. Both Dubois and Schloss were strongly oriented toward clinical research, and Schloss was willing to give up a large private practice to accept a full-time position that would allow him time to work in the laboratory. Other professors were brought in from more or less distant places: Eugene L. Opie in Pathology, Herbert S. Gasser in Physiology, George J. Heuer in Surgery, Henricus J. Stander in Obstetrics and Gynecology, and George S. Amsden in Psychiatry.

The New York Hospital–Cornell Medical Center had the misfortune of being conceived and built in the financially expansive days of the 20s. Construction had been started just four months before the stock market collapsed. Contracts that had been signed when stocks and bonds were selling at a premium had to be paid for when securities had shrunk to a fraction of their former value. Robinson (1929), who felt the shock of this calamity as keenly as anyone, said:

> The plans were developed without definite limitations being placed on the cost of construction and equipment. It was correctly estimated that the contemplated plant . . . would cost, including land, buildings and equipment, $30,000,000. These estimates were made in the halcyon days of finance during the boom that preceded the stock market crash of October 1929, which ushered in the dreadful depression that changed the outlook in every direction and created serious difficulties for this great medical project. . . .

> The hospital had much greater financial responsibilities than the medical college and sustained a more serious loss from the economic depression. It was obliged to liquidate a large portion of its investments to pay for the construction of the buildings, and securities had to be sold when the stock market was much depressed, incurring an estimated loss of about $15,000,000. The anticipated endowment of the hospital was thus diminished to that extent. This created a situation in which economies were imperative and operating deficits seemed inevitable, especially since the depression had decreased patients' ability to pay for their medical care.

> As a means of reducing the cost of operating the hospital, the number of beds to be put into use was cut by about 300, and the equipment of several floors was omitted. Restrictions had to be placed on departmental programs, and the financial situation created at the hospital the general feeling of insecurity which prevailed everywhere during the early days of the depression. It was an unfortunate time to launch a great medical project for which many people had high hopes and great expectations.

Robinson, who through no fault of his own had been caught in this financial squeeze, had to give up his position as Director and Dean. He retired in 1934.

Many years would elapse before the New York Hospital–Cornell Medical College Association could recover from the effects of the depression. However, its financial backers were so generous, even in periods of adversity, that it never really failed in its major missions: patients received excellent care; the instruction of students and house staff was maintained on a high level; and research went forward, though at something less than the

287

expected pace. In time both the hospital and the Medical College would be back on a firm financial base, but the flamboyant vision that was evoked in the rosy 20s will almost certainly never be brought into focus.

The large gap that separated the great urban medical centers from the makeshift hospitals of Kansas and other rural areas was filled by a variety of hospitals of assorted sizes: some, general hospitals; others, special hospitals. From the late nineteenth century onward the number of all types was increasing.

According to Corwin (1946), in the United States in 1873 there were 178 institutions providing inpatient care of the sick;* 88 of these were located in three northeastern states, New York, Pennsylvania, and Massachusetts; 17 were in Illinois, 8 in New Jersey, 7 in both California and Ohio, and the remaining 53 were scattered among 24 states and the District of Columbia. The total number of patients receiving hospital care in 1873 was 146,472. By 1943 there were 6655 hospitals with 1,649,254 beds (about one hospital bed for every 80 people in the country), and during that year 15,374,698 patients were treated in hospitals. If only registered hospitals are considered, there were in 1945 approximately 1,740,000 hospital beds. Of these, approximately 550,000 were in federal hospitals, 620,000 in state hospitals, 190,000 in other government hospitals, 330,000 in nonprofit private hospitals, and 50,000 in proprietary hospitals. In addition to the registered hospitals there were over 2000 unregistered hospitals, most of them proprietary institutions of less than 25 beds each.

The increase in the number of hospitals in the United States prior to 1946 was not governed by any systematic planning at the federal or state level. The provision of hospital facilities was regarded as a primarily local community responsibility. The federal government was concerned with special classes of individuals only, such as the military forces and veterans; whereas the states were involved principally in the care of patients with long-term illnesses such as tuberculosis and mental diseases. The increase in the number of beds for the civilian population exceeded by several-fold the increase in population. Many of the new hospitals were the result of the benefactions of those who had accumulated wealth in the period of expanding industrialization, but the principal cause of the increase was the phenomenal development of medicine and surgery and the shift from the home to the hospital for maternity care as well as for all types of serious illness, for all levels of the population. Although many kinds of hospitals were built, the general hospital remained the most important in terms of the number of patients treated. It was also the major training ground for physicians, nurses, and technical personnel, and it served as a center for the advancement of medical knowledge through research. In 1943, though general hospitals contained only about 40 per cent of the hospital beds, they admitted over 90 per cent of all hospitalized patients.

Recognition of the importance of the hospital led several private foundations to assist communities in building hospitals or improving those already in existence. In 1925, for example, the Commonwealth Fund offered to meet two thirds of the cost of building hospitals in communities that would

---

288   *Rosen (in Friedson, 1963) evidently considered only 149 of these to be hospitals (see Part I).

provide suitable sites, responsible management, necessary maintenance, and one third of the building cost. The donor required that these hospitals be community general hospitals held by local nonprofit corporations as a public trust; that patients be accepted without regard to race, creed, color, or economic status; and that all physicians in good standing in the community be allowed to admit their patients to the institution. The W. K. Kellogg Foundation, in its Michigan Community Health Program, also contributed to the extension and improvement of hospital facilities by providing X-ray and laboratory equipment. The Duke Endowment started a program of hospital assistance at about the same time as the Commonwealth Fund, which was limited to North and South Carolina, where hospital services were badly needed.

In 1931 a program was started in Maine by the Bingham Associates Fund, a cooperative organization of 26 independent hospitals within the state. This program was intended not only to upgrade the hospitals but also to provide, in increasing measure, for the self-education of physicians. The small community hospitals were to depend upon the larger regional hospitals for the services of specialists. The main center was in Boston and was associated with the Tufts Medical School and the New England Medical Center. It included a diagnostic hospital to which physicians in the affiliated hospitals could send patients who presented baffling problems.

Hospital service gradually came to be one of the major industries of the United States, with plant assets in 1943 totaling approximately $5.5 billion and with a yearly operating expenditure of about $1.5 billion. Most of the capital funds were provided on a nonprofit basis by voluntary contributions of public-spirited citizens and religious and fraternal organizations and through tax funds. By the end of World War II the principal stockholder was the American public. At that time only about 5 per cent of the total hospital investment was of a business (proprietary) character. During the economic depression of the 30s, owing to the shrinkage of private funds, government at all levels was called upon increasingly to furnish the capital needed for hospital construction. It was in this setting that Congress adopted the Hill-Burton Hospital Construction Act. This Act did not become fully effective until after World War II; one of its features was that it required each state applying for a grant under the Act to submit a plan for integrated and regionalized hospital services within the state.

To help people to meet the rising cost of hospitalization, various insurance plans became available. By 1945 approximately 30 million people were covered by insurance that paid either a part of or all hospital expenses. The Blue Cross plan has been mentioned in an earlier section; in addition, plans were offered by fraternal organizations, by commercial insurance, by medical service organizations in industry, and by individual hospitals. In 1943 there were 86 Blue Cross plans in 43 states, the District of Columbia, and Puerto Rico, with nearly 21 million subscribers. A problem that came to the fore at about this time was that Blue Cross subscribers were admitted to hospitals at a rate about 50 per cent higher than the rate for the population as a whole. It was not clear whether this was due to the fact that people who lacked hospital insurance were not getting the care they needed or because those who had insurance were demanding more care than was reasonable and necessary. Certainly physicians and hospital authorities were less hesi-

289

tant about admitting, and less anxious to discharge, patients whose bills were guaranteed by a third party. Whatever the cause, Blue Cross had to increase its rates to cover the costs of increased utilization.

The rapid increase in the number of hospitals in the early decades of the twentieth century, together with the increase in the number of laboratory tests, X-ray examinations, and surgical operations, brought about a need for better regulation of hospital practice and procedure. Richard C. Cabot and E. A. Codman, both of Boston, did a great deal to stimulate the acceptance of professional accountancy in hospital work. In 1912 Cabot wrote an article, *Diagnostic pitfalls identified during a study of three thousand autopsies,* and shortly thereafter, in 1917, Codman published *A Study in Hospital Efficiency.* Cabot put a great deal of the blame on the trustees of charitable hospitals for their exclusive preoccupation with financial matters and with an utter lack of concern for the medical results achieved in their institutions. He also admonished the medical staffs of the hospitals for their lack of interest in end results, though these were the major concerns of patients and of medical science. The criticisms of hospital practice that were so clearly and effectively stated by Cabot and Codman aroused the ire of many physicians, but they made an invaluable contribution to quality control in American hospitals.

In 1918 the *American College of Surgeons* inaugurated a very effective program of surveying hospitals to determine whether they met specified standards. This program did more than any other factor to improve the work done in hospitals. Each year the list of approved hospitals was published by the College and appeared in the newspapers of the community concerned. This enabled the people who patronized a hospital to see how it stood in the eyes of those who were competent to judge. The specific requirements were as follows: definite organization of the medical staff; accurate clinical records for each patient; the maintenance of adequate diagnostic and therapeutic facilities, including at least (1) a laboratory or laboratories for chemical, bacteriological, serological, and pathological work, and (2) an X-ray department providing both radiographic and fluoroscopic services; regular clinical staff conferences at least once a month; and a report by the pathologist on every organ removed at operation.

In 1918 a survey was made of 692 hospitals in the United States and Canada having more than 100 beds; only 12.9 per cent met all the requirements set by the American College of Surgeons. With each annual survey more hospitals were inspected, and a greater percentage met the requirements. By 1943, of 4045 hospitals surveyed, 80.4 per cent were on the approved list. However, the smaller the hospital, the more difficulty it had in meeting the requirements; whereas 93 per cent of those having more than 100 beds were approved, only 39.6 per cent of those having between 25 and 49 beds were on the approved list.

In addition to the survey made by the American College of Surgeons, a survey was made by the *Council on Medical Education of the American Medical Association* to certify hospitals for intern and residency training. The basic concept of this survey was that only hospitals under competent clinical supervision and guidance should be granted the privilege of training interns, since the internship is an invaluable part of a physician's education. In order to be accredited for intern and residency training a hospital must have a clinically competent staff organized to provide a planned educational program; a well-equipped and readily accessible medical library in the charge of a competent librarian; a system for recording and maintaining complete case histories of all patients; adequate laboratories and X-ray equipment; the services of a pathologist; and at least 15 per cent of the patients dying in the hospital must be subjected to autopsy.

In 1914 the first list of approved hospitals for intern training was published by the American Medical Association. It consisted of 508 general hospitals, with openings for 2667 interns. In addition, 60 special hospitals and 35 state institutions for the insane offered a total of 428 internships. Thus, there were in that year a total of 3095 approved internships, of which only 2527 were filled. By 1922 the number of available approved internships was about equal to the number of medical students graduating each year. However, between 1926 and World War II the number of approved internships increased at a rate greater than the number of medical graduates. This excess of available internships had at least two important effects upon postgraduate medical education: it served to attract an increasing number of foreign medical graduates; and it gave rise to competition between hospitals to make their internships more attractive. In the early years of the century interns either received no salary or a few dollars a month to use as pocket change. In 1937, 84 per cent of the interns in 534 hospitals served without salary or received $25 a month or less. By 1943 only 85 of the hospitals with approved internships paid no salary; 68 paid less than $25 a month, 158 from $25 to $49 a month, 199 from $40 to $74 a month, 89 from $75 to $99 a month, and 77 paid $100 or more. Over the years, the salaries paid to interns and residents have increased at a fantastic rate, and as the salaries have gone up the required hours of work have gone down. Before 1930 almost no interns or residents were married, but in recent years many of them not only have been married but also have one or more children to support.

As more and more physicians and surgeons confined their practice to limited specialty areas, specialty boards were created to examine and certify physicians and surgeons in various specialties and subspecialties. As the prestige of the specialty boards increased, hospitals began to require that work in special fields be done only by those possessing the appropriate certification.

The hospital can be a valuable repository of medical information, but this important source was never adequately utilized until 1913, when a monograph published by Frederick L. Hoffman demonstrated the practical value of hospital statistics, using for this purpose the experience of the Johns Hopkins Hospital for the period 1892 to 1911. In the same year Charles F. Bolduan devised a simplified method for collecting and collating hospital medical statistics. Eight years later, Raymond Pearl described in detail a procedure for assembling and presenting such statistics. With some modification, the Bolduan method was tested on a relatively large scale when in 1923, the *Hospital Information Bureau of the United Hospital Fund* of New York obtained and tabulated information on over 20,000 patients who had been discharged from six hospitals in New York City and Brooklyn. This experiment proved that much valuable information to guide medical care could be obtained by pooling the statistics from a number of hospitals.

291

A decade later, all of the hospitals in the city of New York were included in a study undertaken by the Welfare Council of New York City. In this study, approximately 575,000 discharge certificates were analyzed. Since that time (1933), the gathering and analyzing of hospital medical statistics has become a well-developed procedure and has provided much valuable information.

The *American Hospital Association*, which was founded in 1899 as the *Association of Hospital Superintendents*, adopted its present name in 1906. Originally it was a small organization that gave its members an opportunity to exchange views on administrative matters. Between 1910 and 1930 it grew rapidly, and by the end of this period its meetings were attended by over 400 delegates from more than 300 hospitals. Since then, the Association has continued to grow in size and importance, becoming an increasingly potent force in the hospital field and a representative for hospitals in national matters. Its councils and publications have done much to improve the design, administration, and services of hospitals.

14

Medical Practice

What Holmes said of law, "It is a window through which one may look out upon mankind," is certainly true for medicine.

(John Romano)

During the years 1876 to 1946 methods of diagnosis and treatment improved steadily. Some of the improvements have been discussed in other chapters, particularly in the chapter on research, in which attention was focused on diseases caused by micro-organisms, dietary deficiencies, and hormonal disturbances. The discoveries in these fields opened an entirely new world to practitioners of medicine and surgery; and laboratory methods and hospital resources became indispensable accessories to medical practice. Doctors had to learn how to cleanse and robe themselves for operations; how to use a huge new armament of instruments; how to measure blood pressure with a sphygmomanometer; how to interpret figures expressed in strange symbols such as "mg %" and "pH"; how to distinguish between an *a-wave* and a *v-wave* in a pulse tracing, and a *P wave* and an *R wave* in an electrocardiogram; how to calculate calories and electrolytes and vitamins; how to use vaccines, antitoxins, and chemotherapy; how to administer thyroxin, insulin, and other hormones when they were deficient and how to control them when they were in excess; how to tell the difference between a psychosis and a psychoneurosis; and innumerable other procedures, devices, and expressions, none of which were known in 1876. They became known gradually as the scientific base of medicine was created; and when they became known the practitioner had to master them for the good of his patients.

In this chapter we shall discuss several additional major developments that contributed to improvements in medical care: (1) a change in the manner of delivering care, pioneered by the Mayo Clinic; (2) improvements in surgery that rendered this mode of treatment safer, more effective, and far

293

more widely used; (3) the development and increasing use of blood transfusion, particularly as an adjunct to surgery; and (4) the discovery of X-rays and their use for diagnosis and treatment.

THE MAYO CLINIC

The best interest of the patient is the only interest to be considered, and in order that the sick may have the benefit of advancing knowledge, union of forces is necessary to develop medicine as a cooperative science; the clinician, the specialist, and the laboratory workers uniting for the good of the patient. . . . The people will demand, the medical profession must supply, adequate means for the proper care of patients, which means that individualism in medicine can no longer exist.

(William J. Mayo, 1910)

In 1889, the year in which the Johns Hopkins Hospital was opened, a small hospital was also opened in a sparsely populated area of the Middle West. This was St. Mary's Hospital in Rochester, Minnesota, an institution having no medical school affiliation and no expectation of engaging in medical education or research. It was established for purely practical reasons: the progress in surgery—better anesthesia, Lister's antisepsis, new instruments, new nursing techniques—had made it desirable to have a more sophisticated environment than the farmer's kitchen for the performance of surgical operations and for the postoperative care of surgical patients. In time there grew up around this small hospital one of the world's great medical centers. The Mayo Clinic, an institution with a new and unique type of organization for the delivery of medical care, was the prototype of group medical practice; in addition, it eventually became one of the great centers for medical research and medical education.

William Worrall Mayo (1819–1911) was born in Manchester, England, where he studied chemistry and physics under the eminent John Dalton and later served as a medical apprentice at the famous Manchester Infirmary. He did not remain there long enough to qualify for a medical license but sailed for America in 1845. His first job in the United States was as a chemist at Bellevue Hospital, New York, but dissatisfied there, he wandered westward through Buffalo and Lafayette, Indiana, where he became a partner in a tailor shop. By 1849 he had again started on a medical career, taking a preceptorship under a local practitioner and studying at Indiana Medical College. He eventually received a medical degree from the University of Missouri. After practicing in various places in the Midwest, he finally settled in Rochester, Minnesota, in 1863. He was soon recognized as the most competent physician and surgeon of the area, and he became actively involved in community affairs. A leader in the state medical association, he was instrumental in giving the ethical practice of medicine a legal standing in Minnesota.

Dr. Mayo had a strong influence on his two sons, imparting to them not only his love of medicine but also his sense of social responsibility. He succeeded in guiding his sons to the two medical schools in the Middle West that had pioneered in extending and modernizing their curriculum. In 1883, William J. Mayo graduated from the University of Michigan Medical

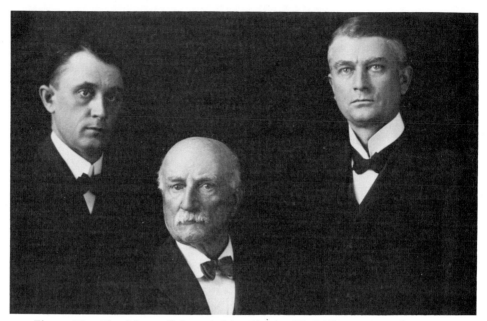

Figure 75. The Mayos (left to right)—Charles H., William W., and William J. (Courtesy of Dr. Charles Roland.)

School, and in 1888 Charles H. Mayo graduated from the Medical School of Northwestern University. Both returned to Rochester to work with and to learn from their father, who by that time had one of the largest practices in the upper Midwest.

In 1883 Rochester was hard hit by a cyclone, and Dr. Mayo was appointed by the City Council to take charge of a hospital improvised for the emergency. He recruited Mother Alfred and her teaching community of the Sisters of St. Francis to act as nurses during the disaster. This experience impressed Mother Alfred with what could be accomplished in a hospital, and she approached the elder Mayo with the idea of establishing a permanent hospital in Rochester. Dr. Mayo was not in favor of this proposal; he argued that Rochester was too small to support a hospital—the cost would bring financial disaster—and that in the eyes of the public a hospital was little more than a pest house, a place to go to die. Stunned by this emphatic veto, Mother Alfred nevertheless succeeded in extracting a promise from Dr. Mayo that should her Community raise enough money to build a hospital, he would take charge of it. The funds were raised, and in 1887 Dr. Mayo selected a site for the building. He and his son Will then toured Eastern hospitals to study architectural design. St. Mary's Hospital was built and was ready to receive patients on October 1, 1889.

When the hospital opened, the senior Mayo was 70 years of age and was ready to retire from active practice. In spite of his energy and enthusiasm, he knew that the responsibility for success of the hospital lay with his sons. He therefore appointed himself Consulting Physician and Surgeon, and his two sons, one barely out of medical school, made up the attending staff. As "Dr. Will" recalled years later, "We were a green crew in those days and we knew it." For the first two years, the entire work of the institu-

295

tion, medical and surgical, nursing, bookkeeping, and housekeeping, was carried out by the two young Mayos and the small staff of sisters. During the first year of operation, the hospital provided care for about 300 patients, and under the skillful management of William J. Mayo, the institution was self-supporting.

The growth of the Mayo's surgical practice was phenomenal. Dr. Will said later that he was convinced that "much of our success was due to opportunities existing at the time we started to practice." This was indeed a factor, for St. Mary's Hospital was opened at the beginning of the era of modern surgery. Within a few years antisepsis would be replaced by asepsis, and surgeons would learn that they could open the abdomen, the chest, or the cranial cavity with little risk of infection. Operations that previously had been performed only as sequels to accidents, or in emergencies, could now be planned ahead after careful diagnostic studies. One no longer had to wait for the appendix or the gall bladder to rupture; one could anticipate and prevent such dangerous consequences. But the Mayos did not travel in the wake of progress; they were among those who led the way. Dr. Will and his brother took advantage of what he called "the existing opportunities" and exhibited imagination and skill not only in operative surgery but also in the organization and delivery of medical care.

In 1897, eight years after St. Mary's Hospital opened, 915 surgical operations were performed; in 1900, 1823; in 1904, 3154; in 1906, more than 5000, and over one half of these were intra-abdominal. Working in their remote location without nearby competitors, the Mayos performed some operations by the hundreds, or even by the thousands of cases. Patients came to the clinic from greater and greater distances, and with the mounting volume of work the Mayos were forced to expand their facilities and obtain professional assistants. The articles that they contributed to the medical journals, describing their successes in unprecedentedly large numbers of cases, sent the Mayo Clinic soaring to worldwide prominence during the years 1895 to 1906.

When asked what contribution to surgery had made the Mayos famous, Dr. William Braasch (1969), who knew them well, stated that he had difficulty in giving a precise answer.

Their operations for umbilical hernia, varicose veins and bunions have been called "Mayo operations." Although the Mayo technique was original, these operations are of minor importance in comparison with their contributions to surgery of the gall bladder and bile ducts and surgery for pyloric obstruction, duodenal ulcer, gastric cancer and goiter. Of great importance has been their modification of techniques used by other surgeons. Most surgeons who have made notable contributions to surgery became well known because of one or two outstanding contributions, in contrast to the Mayo innovations which were made in so many surgical fields. The great number of patients coming to the Mayo Clinic meant that operations would be performed in almost every field of surgery, so that the two brothers were able to evaluate new surgical methods and then make their own modifications of them. As a result of the many improvements they made in operative techniques, the mortality as well as the morbidity rates of many operations were lowered decidedly.

In the years prior to 1900 the Mayo Clinic was essentially a well-organized private surgical practice. Two physicians had been added to the staff of the clinic, one in 1892 and the other in 1896. Neither of these men, A. W. Stinchfield and Christopher Graham, was involved in the surgery. Their function was to relieve the Mayos of the nonsurgical aspects of their practice; they served as diagnosticians, making the preoperative studies and diagnoses that would allow the Mayos to decide whether an operation should be done and, if so, what procedure should be used. It was 1905 before another surgeon was added to the staff. In that year E. Starr Judd, who had served for two years as Charles Mayo's assistant, received an operating room of his own for general surgery. Then specialists were added to the staff to perform the surgery in otolaryngology and ophthalmology. In 1905 a pathology laboratory was established under the direction of Louis B. Wilson, who had been Assistant Director of the bacteriological laboratories of the Minnesota State Board of Health. Two years later a separate laboratory was created for surgical pathology, with William C. MacCarty in charge. In 1911 a third pathologist, Arthur H. Sanford, was added to take charge of the work in bacteriology, serology, and parasitology. These various laboratories were set up for the sole purpose of aiding in the diagnosis and care of the patients.

Except for various studies in relation to operative surgery, virtually no research was carried out until Frank C. Mann, who had been Professor of Pathology at Indiana University, was appointed chief of Experimental Medicine at the Clinic and opened a research laboratory. In 1914 the chemist Edward C. Kendall was added to the research staff. (Kendall's brilliant research is noted in the section on Hormones, Chapter 12.)

Henry Plummer, who joined the staff of the clinic in 1901, proved to be an extraordinarily able and innovative physician. Dr. Will said frequently that hiring Plummer was "the best day's work I ever did for the Clinic." Plummer was a graduate of the Medical School of Northwestern University, and he early demonstrated his versatility by doing pioneer work in bronchoscopy and esophagoscopy and in the use of the electrocardiograph, but his major contribution to the advancement of medicine while he was at the Mayo Clinic was in the field of hyperthyroidism. He found that if patients with exophthalmic goiter were treated with daily doses of iodine, many of their more serious symptoms subsided temporarily, and within about two weeks they were in much better condition for surgical removal of the goiter. Plummer's preoperative treatment of patients suffering from goiter saved many lives at the Mayo Clinic, and it was soon widely adopted in other institutions.

In addition to his work in this special field, Plummer introduced X-ray and laboratory diagnosis into the clinic program, and he devised a system for keeping patients' records that ultimately served as a model for many other institutions. In 1912 he persuaded the Mayos that they needed a new clinic building. Although new wings had been added to the original building in a piecemeal fashion since 1894, Plummer argued that the clinic needed a separate structure large enough to meet the needs of the group and adapted to its peculiar purposes. He was named Chairman of the Building Committee and for some months devoted much of his time to formulating a plan of organization that would coordinate and integrate the activities of the clinic group.

Several years before Plummer began to work on his plan, William Mayo

297

in 1910 had enunciated the guiding principle quoted at the beginning of this section. With this ideal in mind Plummer devised a plan for the new building which he believed would offer the advantages of specialization in medicine while at the same time avoiding its dangers.

The new building was formally opened in May, 1914. All departments were organized into divisions and sections. Each Senior Physician became the head of a section in the Division of Medicine; each Attending Surgeon was the head of a section in the Division of Surgery. With the exception of the sections in Ophthalmology, Otolaryngology, and Orthopedic Surgery, all sections came under the heading of either General Medicine or General Surgery. Dr. Will insisted that specialization should go no further than the addition of a "major interest" to general practice in each section.

The scattered laboratories were at last brought together in the Division of Laboratories, with Wilson as its director. There were four laboratory sections: Clinical Pathology, headed by Sanford; Surgical Pathology, under MacCarty; Experimental Medicine, under Mann; and Experimental Biochemistry, under Kendall.

The library, editorial office, and art studio made up a new Division of Publications under Maude Mellish, who was responsible for editing the papers submitted for publication by members of the Clinic. The Division of Records and Statistics was headed by Mabel Route, but it was under the personal supervision of Dr. Plummer. Finally, there was the business office, which was given full responsibility for investigating the financial status of the patients, determining the charge for services rendered, and collecting the accounts.

Dr. Plummer as head of the Department of General Medicine turned his attention toward raising the quality of the medical and diagnostic services to the same high level as the surgical services. With this in view he sought out men of national standing to head the various sections of his department.

The central idea represented by the new building and the new staff arrangements was cooperative private group practice. Cooperation of a sort among clinicians, surgeons, and laboratory workers was taken for granted in certain municipal, state, and university hospitals; but it was something quite new in private practice. In commenting on the major contributions of the Mayo Clinic, Rynearson stated (1964):

> *These two men created something new in the field of medicine. Almost nowhere in our country were there any physicians who were working together in private practice for the mutual advantages to patients and themselves. In most areas of our country medicine centered about universities, largely in big cities, and the pattern often followed the Prussian system of a professional pyramid with Herr Geheimrat Professor at the top. When he spoke all others listened; he led and they followed. . . . In this country there are now hundreds of voluntary groups, and the inspiration and planning for such practice began with the Mayos in Rochester.*

Another major contribution of the Mayo Clinic was in the field of graduate medical education. In 1907, when William Mayo was elected a member of the Board of Regents of the University of Minnesota, he became familiar with, and concerned about, the problems of medical education. In 1912 he

298

visited Eastern medical centers to observe facilities for graduate training. He then appointed a committee, of which Wilson was Chairman and Plummer a member, to outline a plan for the organization of a graduate school. In February, 1915, the Mayo brothers and their partners executed articles incorporating the *Mayo Foundation for Medical Education and Research,* turning over to the foundation securities valued at $1.5 million, which were placed in the hands of the University of Minnesota to be used as an endowment for the Foundation. The program in graduate medical education supported by the Foundation was administered by a committee made up of five members from the faculty of the University of Minnesota and five from the staff of the Mayo Clinic. The first faculty was composed of 31 appointees from the University Medical School and 26 from the Mayo Clinic. Those who enrolled for the graduate course were called Fellows. They were given a three-year educational experience that included work with patients, laboratory study, research, preparation of a thesis, and written and oral examinations, culminating in a University of Minnesota M.S. or Ph.D. degree. The student could choose to concentrate in any one of nine major specialty areas. From the beginning the requirements for a fellowship were put on a high level, including a bachelor's degree plus a medical degree and one year's internship. Many students took advantage of this excellent opportunity to obtain specialty training.

In time the Mayo Foundation took over the ownership of the buildings and facilities of the Mayo Clinic, and the earnings of the clinic in excess of its operating expenses were turned over to the Foundation, to be expended for the promotion of medical education and research (Johnson, 1964).

PROGRESS IN SURGERY   America's great contribution to surgery in the first century was inhalation anesthesia. In the second century, contributions were numerous and substantial. Halsted's experimental surgery led the way in the establishment of basic surgical principles, and he also developed the standard procedure for several major operations, including intestinal resection, repair of inguinal hernia, subtotal thyroidectomy for hyperthyroidism, and the radical operation for carcinoma of the breast. In addition, Halsted encouraged his assistants to develop several fields of surgery; for example, neurosurgery by Harvey Cushing and Walter E. Dandy and urological surgery by Hugh H. Young. Appendectomy became the commonest abdominal operation after an American physician, Reginald H. Fitz, had identified appendicitis and invented its name. Howard A. Kelly made many improvements in gynecological and urological surgery and pioneered in the use of radium as a supplement to surgery in the treatment of cancer. Alexis Carrel perfected the technique for anastomosing (joining) blood vessels and discovered a way to solve some of the basic problems in the transplantation of organs. In collaboration with Charles A. Lindbergh, the famed transatlantic aviator, Carrel invented a "mechanical heart" that enabled him to keep alive whole organs such as the heart or kidney by supplying them with a circulation of artificial blood. George W. Crile, Professor of Surgery at Western Reserve University, did some highly original research on surgical

299

shock and developed improved methods for the use of blood transfusion; his monograph on *Blood Pressure in Surgery* was the first treatise on this important subject.

New and ingenious techniques for a variety of operations were devised by American surgeons, among whom the Mayo brothers and their associates were prominent. John B. Murphy, Professor of Surgery at Northwestern University, was particularly inventive and resourceful in intestinal and orthopedic surgery, and he was one of the most successful vascular surgeons prior to Carrel. Rudolph Matas, Professor of Surgery at Tulane University, was the originator of a new surgical technique for the radical cure of aneurysms and was one of the first to exploit the practical applications of nerve-block and spinal anesthesia (1899).

A comparison of the number and type of operations performed at the Presbyterian Hospital, New York, in 1939 with those performed in 1889 indicates the progress of surgery during that 50-year period. During this interval, the bed capacity of the hospital increased from 130 to 587. In the earlier year, 97 beds were allocated to surgery of all types, whereas in the later year 128 beds were allocated to general surgery, with additional beds provided for surgical specialties such as urology and gynecology. In the following tabulation, only the general surgical service is included for the year 1939.

TABLE 2. NUMBER AND TYPE OF OPERATIONS, PRESBYTERIAN HOSPITAL, NEW YORK, 1889 AND 1939*

	1889	1939
Total operations	402	3259
Selected operations		
Drainage of abscess	86	60
Amputations	20	23
Hernia operations	11	245
Operations for breast cancer	6	60
Appendectomies	1	245
Gall bladder operations (cholecystectomies)	0	249
Thyroidectomies	0	294
Operations for intestinal cancer	0	144
Deaths	60	68
Mortality rate (per cent)	16.5	2.1

*Adapted from Haagensen and Lloyd, 1943.

In 1889 the abdomen was opened only 32 times, and 13 of these operations were for removal of ovarian or uterine tumors (not included in the tabulation).

ANTISEPSIS AND ASEPSIS

Antisepsis was no more than a topic of conversation among American surgeons when Joseph Lister attended the *International Medical Congress* in Philadelphia in 1876. His antiseptic system had already been approved by an enthusiastic following in Scotland and had been applied with success by a number of prominent surgeons on the continent of Europe. American surgeons, on the other hand, had not accepted the germ theory of infection and were loath to adopt the cumbersome methods recommended by Lister.

In England, Lister's methods were no better received than they were in the United States. Indeed, it was fashionable at that time in the best surgical circles of London to view Lister's theory of infection with ridicule and amusement. "The surgeon of one of the largest teaching hospitals [in London] could always raise an appreciative laugh by telling anyone who came into the operating theater to shut the door quickly, in case one of Lister's microbes came in!"

It was in part this negative attitude of the prominent and influential English surgeons that induced Lister in 1877 to give up his position in Edinburgh to accept the chair of surgery at the much smaller King's College Hospital in London. There he hoped to give his opponents a firsthand demonstration of the value of his methods.

One of Lister's first responsibilities was to deliver the introductory address of the 1877–78 session at King's College. A student who was there wrote, many years later (Thomas, 1920):

This address was delivered from behind a table covered with pipettes, glass flasks, tubes containing milk and blood, and the other paraphernalia required to demonstrate Lister's contention that neither milk nor blood had any inherent tendency to putrefaction, and that if either of these fluids was drawn and preserved under what we should now call sterile precautions, it remained free from putrefaction indefinitely. . . . I sadly confess that we students were bored and we showed it . . . we shuffled our feet and reminded the lecturer that his hour was up and that it was time for tea.

What really troubled the London surgeons was that they should have to acknowledge the superiority of a wholly new system of surgery that had originated north of the border.

Perhaps the Americans had better reasons for their backwardness, though they too had a tendency to cling to their accustomed ways. It will be recalled that the English surgeon Erichsen, who made a tour of American hospitals in 1874, found another explanation for the American surgeons' lack of interest in antisepsis. American hospitals, he observed, were better planned, better ventilated, less crowded, and cleaner than were their British counterparts; as a result infections were less likely to occur and less likely to spread and hence there was a less urgent need for antiseptic methods.

Many American surgeons virtually bypassed the era of antisepsis but were quick to embrace the aseptic technique that began to supplant it in the 1880s. Howard A. Kelly, whose paper "Asepsis not antisepsis; a plea for principles not paraphernalia" appeared in 1886, had not bypassed Lister's methods; he had tried them but disliked the "paraphernalia" and became an early advocate of the change to asepsis (Kelly, 1886).

Antisepsis was employed by Lister to *kill* germs. To this end, wounds were bathed in carbolic acid, and surgical dressings were soaked in it, and the air surrounding the patient during an operation was sprayed with it. *Asepsis* was based on a different principle. It might be called prophylactic antisepsis, and it was designed to prevent the contamination of wounds and dressings by bacteria rather than to kill the bacteria after the contamination had taken place. Most of the basic procedures of the aseptic technique were developed during the period 1885 to 1900. When asked in 1882, "What is new in surgery?", the renowned German surgeon Ernst von Berg-

301

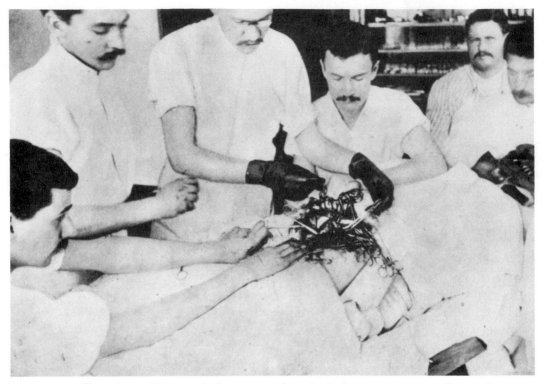

Figure 76. First surgical operation for which the operator wore gloves. Operator, William S. Halsted. (Photo by James F. Mitchell. Ann. Surg. *122*:902, 1945. Reproduced with permission.)

mann replied, "We wash our hands today *before* we operate rather than *afterwards*." It was Bergmann who took the first major step in the aseptic technique when, in 1886, he introduced steam sterilization of the surgical dressings that were to be used during and after an operation. Then came similar sterilization of the gowns which were to be worn by the surgeons and nurses at the operating table; thorough cleansing of the hands and arms by scrubbing with soap and water, followed by soaking in a solution of bichloride of mercury, for all who were to take part in the operation; cleansing and sterilization of the skin at the site of the surgical incision; sterilization of instruments in boiling water; sterilization of sutures by immersion in antiseptic solutions; and the use of sterile caps and masks by the members of the surgical team.

Along the way, as these various procedures were being incorporated into the aseptic technique, in 1889 or 1890, Halsted introduced the use of sterile rubber gloves. This was done initially not to achieve asepsis but to protect the hands of the head operating-room nurse (the future Mrs. Halsted), who was sensitive to bichloride of mercury. Hunter Robb, Associate in Gynecology under Kelly, in a treatise on *Aseptic Surgical Technique* (1894), was the first to recommend that the operating surgeon wear rubber gloves to guard against infections. The first operator to do so regularly was Joseph C. Bloodgood, then Halsted's Resident in Surgery, who invariably wore gloves from 1896 onward. Bloodgood reported that in 20 hernia operations before 1896, four wound infections occurred, but in his next 100 hernia operations, during which he wore gloves, there was only a single infection. After 1900 the wearing of rubber gloves by all members of the surgical team became an established feature of the aseptic technique.

IMPROVEMENTS
IN TECHNIQUE

Many basic improvements in surgical technique were made by Halsted during the period of his experimental work on dogs in Welch's laboratory (1886–89). He demonstrated that rough handling of tissues either by the surgeon's hands or by instruments, or crushing of tissues with clamps or forceps, led to poor healing and invited infection. He found that fine needles and fine silk thread provided more secure and less irritating sutures than did the coarse needles and catgut that were then in common use. He developed and tested new instruments to control bleeding and to minimize injury to the tissues. He learned to close surgical incisions layer by layer, without tension, for he found that tension on the skin or the underlying tissues interferes with the blood supply and retards healing.

As soon as aseptic techniques made it possible for surgeons to operate safely within the abdomen, attention was given to one of the major problems of such operations, the control of bleeding (hemostasis). Initially the artery clamps used in the United States to control hemorrhage were poorly designed, and not enough of them were available at the operating table. Halsted (1913), who early recognized the importance of hemostasis, said that on his return from Europe in 1880,

> I was impressed with the fact that our surgeons were greatly handicapped in most of their operations by lack of proper instruments, particularly of artery clamps. They were insufficient in number and design. Few hospitals, in New York at least, possessed as many as 6 artery clamps in 1880. . . . Americans, newly arrived in Austria, were greatly amused at seeing perhaps a dozen clamps left hanging in a wound of the neck while the operator proceeded with his dissection and were inclined to ridicule the method as untidy. However, it slowly dawned upon us that we in America were novices in the art as well as the science of surgery.

Halsted designed a new artery clamp to meet his own high standards of hemostasis, which has subsequently been known as the *Halsted clamp*. Sometime later Halsted wrote (1913):

> Artery clamps, adequate in number and design, undoubtedly played a very important role in the strikingly rapid progress in the art of operating made by surgeons, the world over, in the final quarter of the 19th Century. The confidence gradually acquired from masterfulness in controlling hemorrhage, gives to the surgeon the calm which is so essential for clear thinking and orderly procedure at the operating table.

Surgeons also made efforts to use blood transfusions in the treatment of shock and anemia resulting from hemorrhage. Occasionally this method was successful, as when Halsted, in 1881, gave his sister some of his own blood. It was believed and in fact had been demonstrated, as in the case of Halsted's sister, that life could be saved by transfusion of blood following severe hemorrhage. However, transfusions did not become safe and were

303

almost never employed until the discovery of the blood groups made it possible to select a donor whose blood was compatible with that of the recipient and until methods had been developed to prevent the clotting of blood as it was being transferred from donor to recipient.

Abdominal surgery made tremendous strides forward during the last quarter of the nineteenth century. In the mid-1870s surgeons in Germany, utilizing Lister's antiseptic measures, performed numerous operations within the abdomen. Vincenz Czerny, Professor of Surgery at Heidelberg, in 1879, was the first successfully to resect (remove) a cancer of the large bowel. By 1884 he had reported a total of 18 such operations with 8 fatalities.

Many of the fatalities following bowel resection were due to peritonitis: when a cancerous section of bowel was removed and continuity of the gut was restored by sewing the cut ends together, the stitches frequently pulled out, and the intestinal contents escaped into the abdominal cavity, producing peritonitis. Halsted, working with Mall in the late 1880s, discovered a way to sew up the intestine so that the stitches would not pull out. This technique, which was soon employed by surgeons everywhere, greatly decreased the hazards of intestinal surgery.

One of the most dramatic developments of this period was the clinical recognition of appendicitis and its cure by surgery. Even though our forefathers never heard of appendicitis, this condition unquestionably had caused many deaths for many centuries. In 1812 James Parkinson, the London physician whose name is best known for his description of paralysis agitans (Parkinson's disease), wrote an account of a fatal case of a ruptured appendix in a boy of five. In 1827 a young Parisian physician, François Melier, in an article on appendiceal rupture, suggested that if the diagnosis could be definitely established during life, it might be possible to treat this condition by surgery (Haagenson and Lloyd, 1943). In 1843 Willard Parker, Professor of Surgery at The College of Physicians and Surgeons, New York, successfully diagnosed, opened, and drained an abscess in the lower abdomen resulting from rupture of the appendix. He had learned to recognize this condition in its early stages, but it did not occur to him to operate earlier, because entering the abdomen in the days before antisepsis almost invariably resulted in infection and death.

The most important contribution in this field came in 1886, when Reginald H. Fitz of Boston presented at a meeting of the Association of American Physicians a report of his studies of appendicitis. Fitz was a graduate of the Harvard Medical School, and after an internship at the Boston City Hospital he went to Germany for further study. There he came under the influence of two of the world's great pathologists, Rokitansky in Vienna and Virchow in Berlin. On his return to Boston in 1870 he began teaching pathology at the Harvard Medical School, and in 1871 he was appointed "Microscopist and Curator of the Pathological Cabinet" at the Massachusetts General Hospital. In his work at the hospital he had an opportunity to observe the manifestations of appendicitis both on the wards and in the autopsy room. In 466 cases he had made the diagnosis of this disease either on clinical grounds or at autopsy. His report in 1886 clearly defined the symptoms and signs by which a diagnosis of appendicitis could be made. He recommended that treatment begin with rest, liquid diet, and sedation with

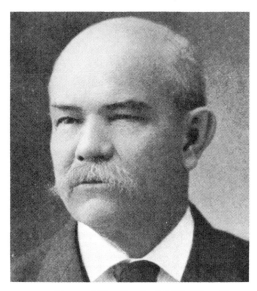

Figure 77. Reginald H. Fitz. (From Riesman, David (ed.): History of the Interurban Clinical Club, 1905–1937. Philadelphia, The John C. Winston Company, 1937.)

opium; but if general peritonitis seemed imminent at the end of 24 hours he recommended that the abdomen be opened and the appendix removed. In 1889 he reported observations on 72 additional cases and at this time was bold enough to recommend early operation, or even removal of the appendix in a quiet interval between attacks. It was Fitz himself who coined the name "appendicitis" for the disease whose clinical manifestations he had so clearly described (Fitz, 1886).

Stimulated by Fitz's studies, surgeons began to diagnose appendicitis with increasing accuracy. Drs. Thomas G. Morton and Henry B. Sands of New York were among the first (1887) to perform appendectomies. In the early reports the patients were not subjected to surgery until perforation of the appendix had occurred, but Sands became interested in the recognition of the disease at an earlier stage and in 1888 succeeded in diagnosing and removing an inflamed appendix before perforation had occurred. Sand's assistant, Charles McBurney, in 1889, first described the area of the abdomen (now known as "McBurney's point") where tenderness is most likely to be detected in cases of appendicitis. After 1890 appendectomy was a common operation, but it took several decades for medical practitioners to become alert to the possibility of appendicitis, and as a result many patients were not subjected to surgery until general peritonitis had developed. For example, as late as 1936, 16,480 deaths were ascribed to appendicitis and its complications during a single year, a mortality rate of 12.8 per 100,000 population.

Another operation that began to be performed with increasing frequency during the last quarter of the nineteenth century was that for gall bladder disease. Although the formation of stones in the gall bladder and some of the complications that result from their presence were known for many years to anatomists and pathologists, this subject attracted little atten-

305

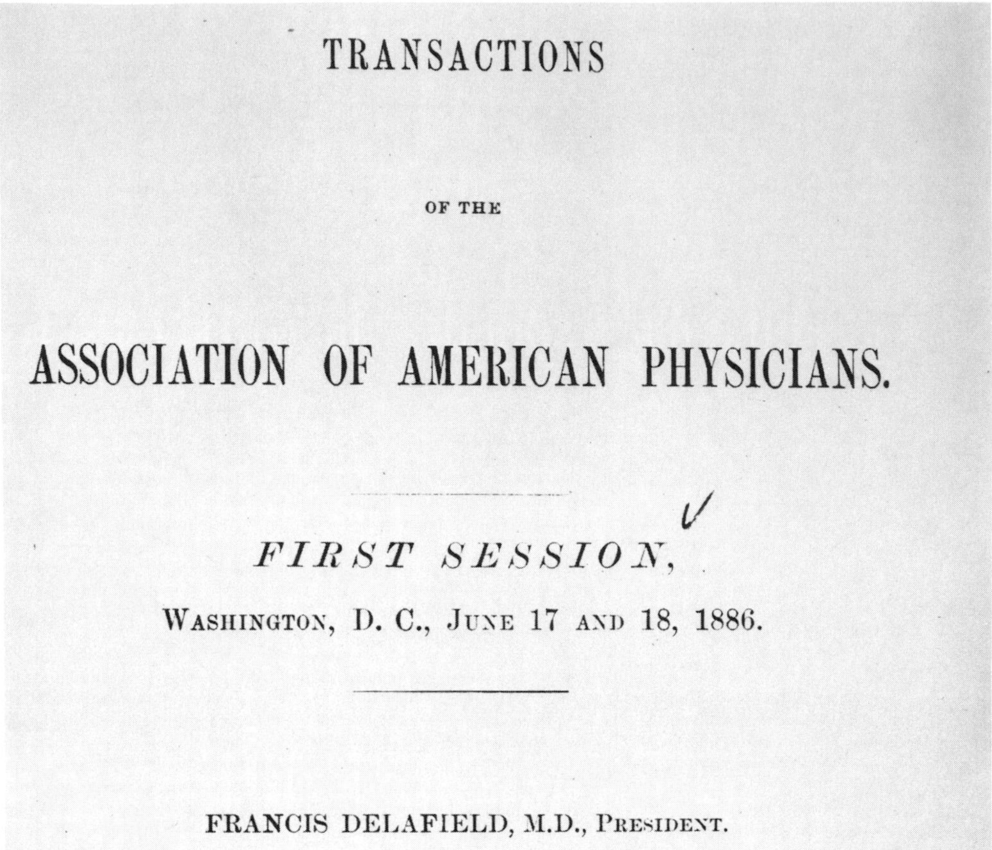

TRANSACTIONS

OF THE

ASSOCIATION OF AMERICAN PHYSICIANS.

FIRST SESSION,

WASHINGTON, D. C., JUNE 17 AND 18, 1886.

FRANCIS DELAFIELD, M.D., PRESIDENT.

JAMES TYSON, M.D., SECRETARY.

JAMES T. WHITTAKER, M.D., RECORDER.

PHILADELPHIA:

WM. J. DORNAN, PRINTER.

1886.

Figure 78. Title page of the first volume of the Transactions of the Association of American Physicians, in which Fitz's paper appeared.

tion until 1863, when a London physician, J. L. W. Thudichum, wrote a monograph describing various types of gallstones and the symptoms sometimes associated with them. He noted that in some instances the stones blocked the main or common bile duct and that fatal consequences might follow the rupture of a distended gall bladder. The first American surgeon to open and drain a distended gall bladder was John S. Bobbs of Indianapolis, in 1867. This operation was performed under the mistaken impression that a tumor that could be palpated in the right upper abdomen was an ovarian cyst. Bobbs incised the cystlike tumor and much to his surprise found that it contained bile and many gallstones. After the bile and gallstones had escaped through the surgical wound, the opening in the gall bladder was closed, and the patient recovered.

In 1878 Marion Sims, the famous American gynecologist, was the first surgeon correctly to diagnose a distended gall bladder and deliberately to drain it. Sims gave the name *cholecystotomy* to this operation. Among the earliest operations of this type was one carried out by Halsted under particularly trying circumstances. In 1881, the year after he began the practice of surgery in New York City, he was called to Albany to see his elderly mother. She was gravely ill and jaundiced and had a large mass in the region of the gall bladder. None of the distinguished consultants who saw her dared to attempt an operation. Young Halsted decided to undertake the operation himself, even though he had never performed this type of surgery. He incised the abdominal wall, found a distended gall bladder, opened it, and discovered that it contained pus and several stones. The pus and stones were evacuated from the gall bladder, and the patient recovered.

An operation devised in the 1890s for the cure of inguinal hernias is today one of the commonest surgical procedures employed. Attempts had been made sporadically during the preceding 50 years to effect a satisfactory cure for hernia, but they had usually met with failure, or at best the results were no more than partially successful. In reviewing the subject in 1890 William T. Bull, then Professor of Surgery at The College of Physicians and Surgeons in New York, concluded that the results did not justify further efforts to cure hernia by operation. He advised the use of a truss as the best treatment for this condition. Halsted had become interested in hernia before he moved to Baltimore. While in New York he made a number of careful dissections of the groin in cadavers and thus gained a thorough understanding of the anatomical structures of the area. In November, 1889, six months after the Johns Hopkins Hospital opened, Halsted presented the results of a new operation for hernia, which he had performed successfully on five patients. By a remarkable coincidence Eduardo Bassini, Professor of Surgery at Padua, had devised an almost identical operation and reported it also in 1889. Since then there have been improvements in some of the details of the operation, but the basic principles are the same today as they were in 1890.

NEUROSURGERY   The person who led the way in the development of neurosurgery in the United States was *Harvey Cushing*. Cushing was a graduate of Yale College and the Harvard Medical School. His interest in medicine was aroused during his last two years at

Yale, when he took courses in physiological chemistry under Professor Chittenden. His first exposure to neurosurgery occurred in his final year at medical school, when he had an opportunity to work with J. W. Elliot, a Boston surgeon who had been trained by Victor Horsley of London, the orginator of some of the early neurosurgical operations. After his internship at the Massachusetts General Hospital, Cushing went to Baltimore in 1896 to become a Resident Surgeon on Halsted's service. During four years on the resident staff he became an accomplished general surgeon. In 1900 he went to Europe, where he worked under Hugo Kronecker in Berne, Switzerland, Victor Horsley in London, and Charles S. Sherrington in Liverpool. All of these men were noted for their neurological research, but Cushing stated some years later that he had no expectation at that time of specializing in neurosurgery.

When he returned to Baltimore, in 1901, Cushing brought with him a Riva-Rocci sphygmomanometer, which he had obtained in Italy. This was the first practical apparatus for the clinical measurement of blood pressure. Cushing was responsible for introducing this instrument to the American medical profession and for stressing the importance of determining the blood pressure at regular intervals during a surgical operation.

Back at Hopkins, Cushing was assigned to neurological work in the Surgical Clinic, and in 1905, when the construction of the Hunterian Laboratory of Experimental Medicine had been completed, he took charge of the work there. This laboratory was devoted largely to experimental surgery and to the instruction of students in the fundamentals of operative surgery. Both of these activities were directed by Cushing. It was in the Hunterian Laboratory that Cushing and his assistants carried out the early experimental studies on the physiology and surgery of the pituitary gland. Cushing's treatise, *The Pituitary Body and its Disorders* (1912), was his first major neurosurgical publication. Not only did this monograph summarize the results of many experimental studies but also it documented 50 actual operations, which placed Cushing far ahead of the field in this type of surgery. The early operations for brain tumors were very discouraging, but as Cushing gained experience and developed better methods for localization of tumors, the results improved.

Cushing left Baltimore in 1912 to become Professor of Surgery at Harvard and the first Surgeon-in-Chief of the Peter Bent Brigham Hospital. He continued his neurosurgical investigations, and during World War I he had extensive experience in France with the surgical treatment of brain injuries. He retired from his positions in Boston in 1932 and, in that same year, published three major works: (1) his description of the disorder now known as *Cushing's disease;* (2) his review, in collaboration with Percival Bailey, of 2000 operations for *Intracranial Tumors;* (3) his monograph on the *Pituitary Body and the Hypothalamus.* After his retirement from Harvard, Cushing accepted an appointment as Sterling Professor of Neurology at Yale, a position he held until his second retirement in 1937.

Cushing's leadership in the field of neurosurgery was never seriously challenged until *Walter E. Dandy* appeared on the scene. Dandy graduated from the Johns Hopkins Medical School in 1910. During his last two years as a student he became a great admirer of Halsted and Cushing, and instead of moving on to the usual internship, he spent his first year after graduation in the Hunterian Laboratory working on the pituitary under Cushing's direction. In 1911 he was appointed Assistant Resident in Surgery and served for a year as Cushing's clinical assistant. Cushing offered to take Dandy to Boston with him, but before the year ended the two high-strung, temperamental personalities had had so many clashes that Cushing withdrew his offer, and Dandy was left behind with no job in sight. Having no hospital appointment, he decided to return to work in the Hunterian Laboratory, where he joined forces with the Pediatric Resident, Kenneth D. Blackfan, and carried out a remarkable series of studies on hydrocephalus ("water on the brain"). Dandy was the first to produce this condition in animals so that he could test various ways of treating it. Halsted, much impressed by this work, reinstated Dandy to a position on the resident staff, and after he had served for several years as Assistant Resident he was elevated to the rank of Chief Resident in 1916 and held this position for two years.

During his term as Chief Resident, Dandy originated a new method for localizing brain tumors by means of contrast radiography following injection of air into the cerebral ventricles. This procedure, which greatly facilitated the diagnosis and localization of brain tumors, has been characterized as "the greatest single contribution ever made to brain surgery" (Crowe, 1957). Dandy remained at Hopkins, extending his studies of neurosurgical problems, and in 1922 he became chief of the neurosurgical service. During 24 years in this position his ingenuity and dexterity as a surgeon became known internationally. He originated several important operations including those for (1) tumors of the acoustic nerve, (2) facial neuralgia, (3) Meniere's disease, (4) herniation of the intervertebral discs, (5) aneurysms of the arteries at the base of the brain.

Samuel J. Crowe, who had worked for long periods with both Cushing and Dandy and knew both men intimately, wrote in 1957: "In spite of the deep admiration and affection the writer felt for Harvey Cushing, he is compelled to acknowledge to himself that Walter Dandy to an even greater extent than Cushing, had the kind of creative imagination, intuition and persistence which we are accustomed to regard as the highest form of genius."

UROLOGY   Hugh H. Young graduated from the University of Virginia in 1893. During his years as an undergraduate, he also took the two-year lecture course in medicine then offered at Virginia. He is said to have been the only man ever to receive the B.A., the M.A., and the M.D. at the end of four years in college. After graduation he began the practice of medicine in his home town, San Antonio, Texas, but he quickly realized that he was ill prepared for practice, and he decided to apply to the Johns Hopkins Hospital for some sort of position that would enable him to improve his knowledge and gain experience. In 1894 he was accepted as a graduate student in the surgical dispensary. In addition to his work in the dispensary, he took advantage of the opportunity to spend his spare time in the laboratory, learning how to use a microscope and studying pathology and bacteriology. In the course of these studies he made the first diagnosis of an anthrax infection at the Johns Hopkins Hospital; he succeeded in culturing the anthrax bacillus, and he was able to trace the source of the infection to a warehouse that dealt in hides and hair.

In 1895, while Young was working as a graduate student, James Brown, a brilliant young surgeon who had headed the work in urological surgery, suddenly died. Brown had been the first person to catheterize the ureter in a male subject, and his loss was a severe blow to the surgical service. Shortly after Brown's death, Young was appointed Assistant Resident in Surgery, and his interest in, and aptitude for, urological work attracted Halsted's attention. In 1897, much to Young's surprise, Halsted asked him to take charge of the work in genito-urinary surgery. When Young protested that he knew next to nothing about this subject, Halsted replied, "Welch and I said you didn't know anything about it, but we both believe that you can learn." Young's first contribution to his new specialty was the construction, in 1898, of an improved type of cystoscope.

It was Young's perineal prostatectomy that won him international fame. He had performed his first prostatectomy in 1896, using a suprapubic approach, and all the prostatectomies that he performed during the next several years were by this route. However, the mortality associated with the suprapubic operation was disturbingly high—about 20 per cent—and this led Young to devise a different approach. He performed his first perineal prostatectomy in October, 1902, and in the next 14 months he performed 50 of these operations without a single fatality. In 1904 he performed his first radical operation for removal of a cancerous prostate. This was considered to be a daring and difficult undertaking, and Young persuaded Halsted to be his first assistant at the operation. The result was highly successful (Crowe, 1957). In 1906, Young published two monographs reporting his early experiences as a genito-urinary surgeon: *Studies in Urological Surgery* and *Hypertrophy and Cancer of the Prostate Gland*.

Young invented the "punch operation" for removal of tumors of the small median lobe of the prostate. In 1912, he performed·this operation so expeditiously and with such success on a wealthy patient, "Diamond Jim" Brady, that the grateful Mr. Brady provided the funds to construct and partially endow the James Buchanan Brady Urological Institute, a separate unit of the Johns Hopkins Hospital.

Young was the author of *Practice of Urology* (two volumes) and of numerous articles and monographs on various aspects of his specialty. In 1917 he founded the *Journal of Urology*. In his Institute he trained many of the outstanding urologists in the United States, and he remained a leader in this field until his death in 1945.

TRANSFUSION OF BLOOD

The transfusion of blood has become one of the most important and most widely used therapeutic procedures. It saves hundreds, perhaps thousands, of lives daily. With bottles of blood near at hand, it is now possible to perform surgical operations that it would have been folly to undertake two or three decades ago. Individuals involved in accidents that result in heavy loss of blood would die in many cases if they could not be transfused. There are many other conditions in which a transfusion can be a lifesaving measure, including bleeding from an ulcer of the stomach or duodenum; from a typhoid ulcer of the intestine; from a diverticulum of the

310

intestine; from the lungs in patients having tuberculosis; from the uterus as a complication of pregnancy or in association with tumors; from various parts of the body as a consequence of certain blood diseases.

Blood transfusion was seriously discussed as a possible therapeutic procedure as early as the seventeenth century. The first transfusions were attempted by injecting blood obtained from various animals; this effort was soon abandoned because violent, fatal reactions almost invariably followed. About the beginning of the nineteenth century occasional efforts were made to perform transfusions with human blood, but again the result was usually a severe and sometimes fatal reaction.

The first person to make a careful study of transfusion and to report a convincingly successful one was James Blundell (1790–1877), Professor of Obstetrics at Guy's Hospital, London. In 1818, Blundell successfully transfused a desperately ill patient with 12 to 14 ounces of blood from several donors during the course of half an hour, the blood being transferred rapidly from donor to recipient by means of syringes. Blundell's success was not altogether accidental. He had approached the subject of transfusion with the unbiased attitude of an experimental physiologist, and the conclusions that he reached were based on personally conducted experiments. His experience led him to enunciate several basic principles: (1) death from hemorrhage can be prevented by transfusion of blood, but the blood must be obtained from animals of the same species; (2) only human blood can be used for human transfusions; (3) passage of blood through a syringe does not deprive it of its life-giving properties; (4) venous blood is as satisfactory for transfusion as arterial blood. In 1829, Blundell reported in *The Lancet* another successful transfusion in a case of severe postpartum hemorrhage. He believed that he had saved this patient's life by administering eight ounces of blood taken by means of a syringe from the arm of his assistant. This patient made a complete recovery.

Others who tried to follow Blundell's lead had occasional success, but serious reactions were so frequent as to discourage the use of transfusions except in patients on the verge of death from loss of blood.

In the United States, transfusion was considered to be a treacherous undertaking, and it was rarely attempted before the twentieth century. There are only two records of transfusions of wounded soldiers during the Civil War. One of these was believed to have saved the soldier's life. However, since only two ounces of blood were transfused, this claim seems hardly acceptable. In the second case the patient died of hemorrhage in spite of the transfusion of 16 ounces of blood. Halsted's successful transfusion of his sister in 1881 has already been described.

Despite the fear of transfusion, interest in this subject remained high, and various types of apparatus and procedures were devised for the transference of blood from donor to recipient. Interest lagged in the 1890s when the intravenous infusion of physiological salt solution came into use. The simplicity of administering the saline solution and the absence of severe reactions made this procedure more acceptable than blood transfusion. In the Spanish-American War no blood transfusions were performed, but saline infusions were employed with relative frequency.

Why was it that the transfusion of blood was so successful in a few cases and so disastrous in others? This was the riddle that remained

311

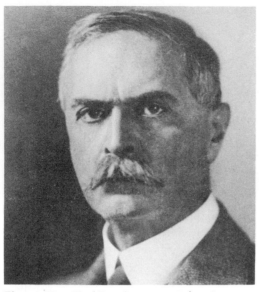

Figure 79. Karl Landsteiner. (From Corner, Geroge W.: A History of the Rockefeller Institute. New York, Rockefeller University Press, 1964.)

unanswered until 1900. Twenty-five years earlier, Leonhard Landois of Leipzig, Germany, had discovered that when animal serum is mixed with human blood, the human red blood cells disintegrate and liberate their hemoglobin. Landois reasoned that this might explain why animal blood is so injurious to human recipients, but it did not explain the failure with human donors. In 1900 an Englishman, Samuel G. Shattock, was the first to note that the blood serum of some individuals caused the red blood cells of other individuals to agglutinate (clump together). He attributed this phenomenon to disease. In the same year, Karl Landsteiner of Vienna examined the blood of all the workers in his laboratory and found by agglutination tests on their red blood cells that they could be divided into three groups. A fourth blood group was discovered by DeCastello and Sturli in 1902; and in 1909, Jansky of Prague defined and designated by letters the four main blood groups that we recognize today: A, B, AB, and O.

Landsteiner's discovery of the blood groups solved the riddle as to why some transfusions were successful while others were fatal or provoked such violent reactions as to make them unsafe. It now became apparent that to avoid such reactions it was necessary to transfuse an individual with blood that matched his own group.

After World War I the severe economic depression in Central Europe made research impossible for Landsteiner in his native Austria. He therefore accepted an invitation to join the staff of the Rockefeller Institute. He came to New York in 1922 and soon thereafter became an American citizen. In 1930, for his discovery of the blood groups, he received the Nobel Prize in medicine and became the first United States citizen to receive this award. (Carrel, who received the Nobel Prize in medicine in 1912, though he had been on the staff of the Rockefeller Institute since 1905, had not become a United States citizen).

After coming to the United States, Landsteiner periodically returned to his work on the blood groups. In 1927 he discovered the minor groups, designated M and N, which are of no importance in blood transfusion but are of significance for parental identification in establishment of paternity and in studies of racial differences. In 1940, working with A. S. Wiener, a Brooklyn physician, Landsteiner discovered the Rh factor, which is of such importance in obstetrical management. In addition to his work on the blood, Landsteiner also made monumental contributions to the science of immunochemistry and to the study of the mechanisms of allergy and the nature of antibody reactions.

Apart from the problems created by the different blood groups, other difficulties had to be solved before blood transfusion would become a fully practical procedure. One particularly troublesome matter had been the clotting of the donor's blood in the syringe or in the tubing through which the blood was injected. This difficulty was overcome when it was discovered that the addition of a citrate solution to the blood would prevent clotting. The use of citrated blood had two additional advantages: (1) the blood did not have to be used immediately but could be stored in a refrigerator for a few days and transported from one location to another; (2) blood could be accumulated in larger containers and injected steadily and with less haste.

Blood transfusion was first used extensively for the treatment of the wounded in World War I. During the latter part of the war it probably resulted in the saving of thousands of lives. It was not until 1917 that the citrate method of anticoagulation was sufficiently developed and standardized for large-scale use. Oswald Robertson, an American physician serving in the Canadian Army Medical Corps, did a great deal to improve the technique and to popularize the use of transfusions. Unfortunately, many soldiers died from loss of blood before they could be brought back to the area where the blood for transfusion was kept. Kenneth Walker recalls an effort that he made to carry blood to the front lines so that he could administer it where it was most needed. The policy then was to use Group O ("universal donor") blood so that it could be given without prior matching. Walker carried the blood into the front-line trenches in two bottles packed in ice in a large box slung from his neck by a leather strap. He says that this effort had an excellent effect upon the morale of the soldiers in the front line, "but it has to be confessed that the difficult conditions met with in the trenches prevented it from ever becoming a very effective method of treatment" (Walker, 1955).

After World War I civilian hospitals kept a roster of blood donors whose blood had been tested and whose blood groups were known. When a transfusion was needed or when a patient was about to undergo an operation that might require a blood transfusion, a donor of the appropriate blood group was called in. This manner of dealing with the situation was not always satisfactory; there were frequently difficulties in locating a donor and getting him to the hospital in time. Occasionally there was no donor of the proper group on the hospital roster. In order to avoid these difficulties and to have blood of the needed group always immediately available, Dr. Bernard Fantus, Professor of Pharmacology and Therapeutics at the Univer-

313

sity of Illinois College of Medicine, established in 1937 at the Cook County Hospital in Chicago the first blood bank. In the bank the blood was stored in a refrigerator in pint bottles to which an appropriate amount of citrate and glucose had been added to prevent coagulation and to enhance storage. Each bottle was labeled to show the date on which the blood was obtained, the blood group, and other important data. The blood bank principle was used extensively by the Army and Navy during World War II. The American National Red Cross collected 13 million bottles of blood between 1941 and 1945. Some of this blood was flown to the combat zones and was used for transfusions in the hospitals and in the field, but a considerable amount of the Red Cross blood was processed into dried blood plasma. The plasma was stored in lightweight packages, easy to handle and easy to transport; it was used for the treatment of shock and for other purposes after fluid had been added to it to make a clear solution.

It seems appropriate at this point to continue the transfusion story a little further. After the war many civilian hospitals organized their own blood banks. In 1947 the American Red Cross formulated a plan for the establishment of regional blood centers. The blood was collected by Red Cross teams in the cities and smaller communities. It was then stored in the center and was made available to hospitals in the region as needed. In time Red Cross Regional Blood Centers were established in every part of the United States. In 1962 there were 55 Red Cross Centers, and in addition there were 4400 hospital blood banks and 153 non-hospital blood banks. In that year the total amount of blood collected was between 5 and 6 million pints. By that time the method of preserving blood had been so improved that it could be kept in the banks for four weeks. Not all of the blood collected is used for transfusions of whole blood. Chemical and physical techniques have been developed for separating out various chemical fractions and cellular components for therapeutic use. These include plasma albumin, gammaglobulin, and antihemophilic plasma, and it is now possible to give transfusions consisting of red blood cells alone or white blood cells alone or platelets alone when these particular components are needed.

X-RAYS COME TO AMERICA The discovery of X-rays exemplifies the old dictum that chance favors the prepared mind. On November 8, 1895, Professor William Conrad Roentgen was working in his laboratory at the Physical Institute of the University of Wurzburg, Germany. He was experimenting with a Crookes tube, a bulblike glass structure from which air has been exhausted and into which positive and negative electrodes have been sealed. When a high-voltage electric current is passed through a Crookes tube the bulb displays a fluorescent glow. On this occasion Roentgen had covered the tube with a shield of heavy black cardboard. A piece of paper coated with barium platinocyanide lay on a nearby bench. While passing a current through the tube Roentgen noticed that a peculiar light appeared on the paper. No light could come from the tube, because the black shield that covered it was impervious to any known form of light.

314 Roentgen repeated this procedure several times and concluded that

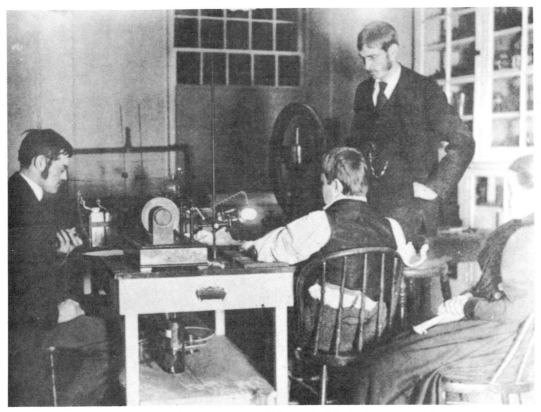

Figure 80. First diagnostic use of X-rays in North America, February 3, 1896, at Darmouth, Massachusetts. (From Brecher, Ruth, and Brecher, Edward: Rays—A History of Radiology in the United States and Canada. Baltimore, The Williams and Wilkins Co., 1969. Reproduced with permission.)

rays of some sort coming from the tube were passing through its covering and having a luminescent effect upon the paper. His penetrating grasp of the significance of this accidental observation led him to perform a number of additional experiments within the next few weeks, as a result of which he acquired much information about the unique physical properties of the new rays. He concluded that the light which he had observed on the coated paper had resulted from fluorescence caused by the rays. He found that a photographic plate was affected by the rays just as it was by ordinary light. He gave to these rays, which were destined to revolutionize medicine, the name *X-rays*. The first picture indicating what X-rays might mean for medicine was one showing the bones of Frau Roentgen's hand.

Roentgen announced his discovery in an article that was published in the last week of December, 1895. The news spread with extraordinary rapidity. Within a few weeks scientists in the United States were producing X-rays and carrying out experiments with them. Late in January Arthur W. Wright of the Department of Physics at Yale produced an X-ray picture of a dead rabbit that showed not only the bones of the rabbit but also the small round shadows of the shot with which it had been killed. On January 31, John Trowbridge of the Physics Laboratory at Harvard produced an X-ray picture of the human hand. On February 3, John Cox, Professor of Physics

315

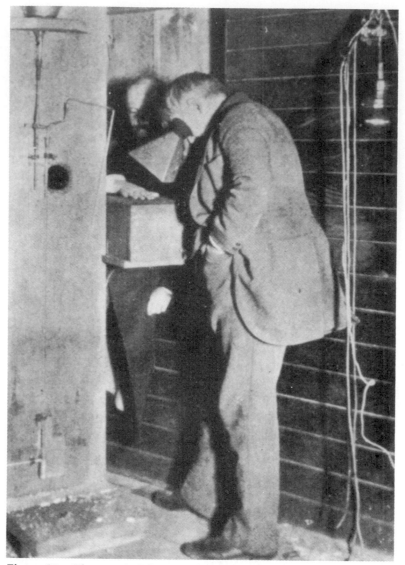

Figure 81. Thomas A. Edison examining hand through
fluoroscope, 1896. (From Brecher, Ruth, and Brecher, Edward:
Rays—A History of Radiology in the United States and Canada.
Baltimore, The Williams and Wilkins Co., 1969.)

at McGill University, was the first in North America to use X-rays successfully as an adjunct to surgery. He took pictures of a young man who had
been shot in the leg, which showed the damaged bones in the calf of the leg
and the bullet that had been responsible for the wound. The first American
physician to use X-rays successfully in his practice was a Chicago surgeon,
James Burry. On February 11, he employed a Crookes tube to localize and
remove some small buckshot from the hand of a patient.

Thomas A. Edison was among the prominent American figures to enter
the X-ray field at an early date. Concentrating as usual upon practical utility, Edison turned his attention to the development of a fluorescent screen
that would make it possible to observe moving objects in a subject or to set

a fracture while actually observing the damaged bone. By the end of March, 1896, Edison not only had developed a fluorescent screen but also had incorporated it in a practical apparatus that could be purchased by physicians.

Although many physicians and physicists were engaged in taking X-ray pictures in 1896, Dr. Francis Henry Williams of Boston deserves to be labeled America's first radiologist. Williams was peculiarly suited by both training and experience to pioneer in this field. He had graduated from the Massachusetts Institute of Technology before taking his medical degree and had a better understanding than most physicians of the technical problems involved in radiology. He was a member of the medical staff of the Boston City Hospital, and he utilized patients in that hospital for his early studies. He had the technical assistance of two members of the staff of the Massachusetts Institute of Technology, C. L. Norton and R. R. Lawrence, who designed more powerful X-ray equipment that took sharper pictures with a shorter exposure. The first X-ray picture published by Williams appeared in the Boston Medical and Surgical Journal for Febuary 20, 1896. On April 25, he gave a demonstration at the Massachusetts Institute of Technology, showing how X-rays could be used to detect enlargement of the heart. On May 2, 1896, he reported his early observations at a meeting of the Association of American Physicians and exhibited some of his work, including a dramatic picture of the bones of the foot taken through a heavy shoe. He also described the use of the fluoroscopic screen for studying diseases of the heart and lungs. A year later he reported to the same Association more extensive observations and noted that by the use of X-rays it was possible to detect pulmonary tuberculosis earlier than by other methods.

The first great American contribution in the field of radiology was made by Walter B. Cannon, who was then a Harvard medical student. Dur-

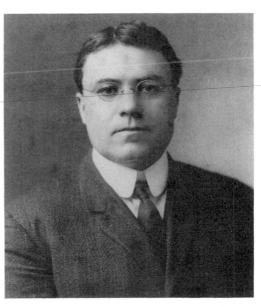

Figure 82. Walter B. Cannon. (National Library of Medicine, Bethesda, Maryland.)

ing his first year in medical school Cannon had worked in the physiological laboratory of Professor Henry I. Bowditch, who suggested that a way might be found to utilize X-rays to study the process of digestion. While traveling on a streetcar in Boston in December, 1896, Cannon heard two ladies across from him discussing with horror the fact that with the new X-rays a doctor could see right through you and could find out everything that was going on inside. During this discussion it occurred to Cannon that he might be able to visualize the activity of the intestines by feeding to an animal a substance that was opaque to X-rays. In his first experiment along these lines Cannon fed a button to a dog, and by using a fluoroscopic screen he was able to watch the button pass down the esophagus into the stomach. He soon found that he could visualize the stomach and intestines by giving the animal salts of heavy metals to swallow, either suspended in liquid or mixed with the animal's food. In this way he was able to observe the passage of food all the way from the mouth to the rectum. Cannon's first report of these studies appeared in 1898. Not only was his method of great value to the research worker but also it provided the foundation for the X-ray diagnosis of gastrointestinal abnormalities in man.

During his experiments Cannon had noted, while watching the movement of the intestine, that emotional reactions on the part of the animal, such as fear or rage, were followed by total cessation of all gastrointestinal movement. This led him to his lifelong and fruitful studies of the effect of the emotions and the autonomic nervous system upon the function of individual organs and of the body as a whole. In the course of these studies he evolved his concept of *homeostasis*—the manner in which the body maintains its steadiness and equilibrium when subjected to various stresses. Cannon became one of America's greatest scientists. He spent 50 years at the Harvard Medical School, most of the time as Professor of Physiology. Throughout these years he conducted his laboratory research in such a way as to provide a unique brand of stimulation to his students. Though in his early work he did not realize the dangers of exposure to X-rays, he was fortunate in that the apparatus which he used was partially shielded by lead sheets. Nevertheless, in later years he suffered considerably from X-ray dermatitis, the result of his exposure decades earlier.

It was not long after X-rays were discovered that some of their injurious effects came to light. One of the earliest reports came from Professor John Daniel of the Physics Laboratory at Vanderbilt University. In February, 1896, he attempted to take an X-ray picture of the head of one of his medical associates. To enhance the likelihood of success the tube was placed one-half inch from the subject's head, and the exposure was made for one full hour. Twenty-one days after this experiment the subject lost all of his hair in the area exposed to the X-rays. Soon after this, X-ray burns of the skin began to be reported. Most of these burns seemed at first to heal, and it was believed that the deleterious effects were only temporary and not serious. By the end of 1896 it was realized that some of the burns were slow in healing and could cause prolonged disability. It was also learned that burns could be prevented by shielding the X-ray tube or by protecting the skin with tin foil. It was only after longer experience that the more serious effects of overexposure to radiation became known.

318   After the danger of X-ray burns was well recognized, fewer cases were

reported. However, some people ignored the warnings and needlessly exposed themselves to X-rays without proper precautions. In 1904 it became apparent that overexposure not only could produce burns but also could induce the development of cancer. A glass blower who had made countless Crookes tubes in Edison's laboratory in 1896 had tested the output of each tube by placing one of his hands directly into the beam. He received severe burns, and his physician told him that if he did not give up this type of work it might be necessary to amputate both hands. He ignored this advice and continued to work through 1897 and 1898. Skin grafting was attempted without success, and finally it was noted that skin cancer was developing in the region of the burns. Both hands were amputated, but in spite of this the cancer spread by metastasis, and death occurred in 1904. Following this, other deaths from cancer were reported in X-ray workers. Among the victims were technicians and prominent physicians who had pioneered in radiology, quite innocent of the dangers to which their work exposed them. In 1939 an eminent Boston radiologist, Percy Brown, collected and published an account of these tragedies, entitled *American Martyrs to Science through the Roentgen Rays.* As a sad sequel to this account Dr. Brown himself died in 1950 of cancer resulting from exposure to X-rays.

The amateurish way in which the use of X-rays was introduced in three of America's leading medical institutions, the Massachusetts General Hospital, the Johns Hopkins Hospital, and the Mayo Clinic, seems worth recording. Roentgen's discovery aroused much excitement at the Massachusetts General Hospital, particularly among the house staff. Harvey Cushing, who was to become a famous surgeon, was then an intern on that house staff, and he was quick to perceive the various medical uses of X-rays. In a letter written to his mother on February 15, 1896, he said, "Everyone is much excited over the new photographic discovery. Professor Roentgen may have discovered something with his cathode rays which may revolutionize medical diagnosis. Imagine taking photographs of gall stones *in situ* — stones in the bladder — foreign bodies anywhere — fractures, etc., etc." (Fulton, 1946).

Early in 1896, Dr. John Collins Warren, who had been on a trip to Europe, brought back to the Massachusetts General Hospital a Crookes tube. In 1921 Cushing recalled what happened after Warren's return: "Dr. Warren had just brought back from Roentgen's laboratory a small tube about the size of a goose's egg and with it [Ernest A.] Codman and I ground out on the old static machine the first faint X-ray picture of the hand ever taken [at the Massachusetts General Hospital]" (Myers, 1929). Cushing, during the remaining six months of his stay in Boston, took an intense interest in X-rays and actually put up money to purchase "an X-ray machine," with the confident expectation that when the medical staff had learned to appreciate its usefulness he would be reimbursed. On May 10, he wrote to his mother, "It is great sport — very useful in the Out Patient to locate needles, etc. We could look through the chest readily this morning — count the ribs — see the heartbeat, the edge of the liver. It is positively uncanny" (Fulton, 1946).

The person who became involved most deeply in radiology at the Massachusetts General Hospital was Walter J. Dodd, who had begun his scientific career as janitor in a chemical laboratory at Harvard. In 1892 he was listed among the employees as *assistant apothecary.* Because of his interest and skill in photography he had also become the hospital's official pho-

319

tographer. He kept his equipment, developed his negatives, and made his prints in a small building on the hospital grounds known as the Kingsley Studio. As Cushing intimated in his letter of February 15, Roentgen rays were at first looked upon as a new photographic discovery. It was only natural, therefore, that Dodd should become involved, and from the first he played his part with intelligence and vigor. He began his work with the old static machine mentioned by Cushing and a crude X-ray tube. He solicited the cooperation of a Boston electric company in making a better tube, and he soon devised new sources of electric power. The Kingsley Studio was converted into an X-ray workroom, and here Dodd experimented with the various types of equipment and developed new technical procedures. Like many other pioneers in radiology before the dangers were recognized, Dodd developed X-ray burns and the more serious complications resulting therefrom. He died a martyr to his newfound profession (Brown, 1936).

It would seem that Cushing was not reimbursed, as he had hoped to be, for his purchase of the X-ray tube. At any rate he must have considered it to be his own, for when he moved from Boston to Baltimore in October, 1896, he carried the tube along with him. Within a short time of his arrival at the Johns Hopkins Hospital to take up his duties as Assistant Resident in Surgery, he discovered that the hospital which he had joined was not as far ahead in the field of X-rays as the hospital that he had left. In April, 1896, Osler had persuaded the Medical Board of the hospital to approve an order for an "X-ray apparatus," but apparently the apparatus had failed to materialize, for it was nowhere in evidence at the time of Cushing's arrival. It was young Cushing himself, just out of his internship, who with his own X-ray tube introduced the staff of the Hopkins Hospital to the new technique. In taking his pictures Cushing had the aid of a medical student who had to turn the crank of a static machine for 45 minutes to generate the current while Cushing exposed the photographic plate (Chesney, 1958). Cushing is said to have taken all the X-ray pictures at the Hopkins Hospital until October, 1897.

The use of X-rays at the Mayo Clinic came about in the following manner. Soon after Roentgen's discovery had been announced, Dr. J. Grosvenor Cross, a general practitioner in Rochester, Minnesota, became intrigued by the possible usefulness of X-rays in medical practice. In February, 1896, he obtained a Crookes tube and other equipment and after experimenting with it demonstrated its use at a meeting of the local medical society. About a week after the meeting a small boy who had swallowed a vest buckle was brought to the Mayo Clinic. The Mayo brothers asked Dr. Cross to use his X-ray machine to try to locate the buckle. The buckle was located in the esophagus, and knowing its precise location, Dr. Charles Mayo made an incision at the proper spot and removed the buckle. During the next several years Dr. Cross did a considerable amount of X-ray work for the Mayos, most of it to locate foreign bodies such as needles, bullets, and bits of glass or steel so that the surgeon could remove them more readily.

By the end of the first decade of the twentieth century, radiology was becoming recognized as a medical specialty, and X-rays were being used for therapy as well as for diagnosis. In the field of diagnosis the radiologists were improving their competence by checking their X-ray pictures and fluoroscopic findings against the findings at operation or at autopsy. At

320

about this same time the method for visualizing the intestinal tract that had been pioneered by Cannon began to be used in diagnostic radiology.

The therapeutic uses of X-rays began to be explored in Europe and in the United States at a very early date. The initial trials were directed at a great variety of diseases of the skin, where the results could be observed easily. There were many failures, many false reports of success, and many serious X-ray burns of the skin, but in time it became clear that exposure to X-rays would cure a relatively common skin cancer (epithelioma). One of the earliest successes in this field was reported by Dr. Wallace Johnson of the Georgetown University Medical School, who had begun his work in September, 1899, with the assistance of William H. Merrill, a medical student who had been placed in charge of the X-ray and photographic department of the dispensary. The therapeutic use of X-rays was hampered by the unpredictability of the amount of radiation emitted by the X-ray tubes then in use. The risk of X-ray burns often seemed to outweigh the potential benefits.

A great advance in radiology occurred when a new kind of X-ray tube was developed by William David Coolidge. Coolidge had begun some experiments with X-rays in 1896 at the Massachusetts Institute of Technology. At that time he succeeded only in acquiring a moderately severe X-ray burn. In 1905 Coolidge moved to the General Electric Company and began some experiments to improve the filaments in electric light bulbs. He finally succeeded in this work by using a filament of ductile tungsten, a discovery that was announced in May, 1910. Coolidge then began to investigate new uses for tungsten, and it occurred to him that its characteristics made it a suitable metal for use in X-ray tubes. In attempting to substitute tungsten for platinum in the so-called gas-tube then in use, he encountered a great many problems and ended up by inventing a tube based on entirely new principles. The old gas-tubes had a conventional cathode plus a hot filament to supply electrons, whereas the cathode in Coolidge's tube was itself the electron-emitting tungsten filament. In his application for a patent on this tube Coolidge specified that the electrons from the filament-cathode were to bombard the target and thus produce the X-rays directly. This was the essence of his new invention. Coolidge placed the tube in the hands of a radiologist, Lewis Gregory Cole of New York City, for testing. In December, 1913, Dr. Cole reported that the results with the new tube were excellent. The advantageous characteristics were greater accuracy of adjustment, stability, exact reproduction of results, flexibility, and high output. After this report Coolidge's tube, which was manufactured by the General Electric Company, was in great demand.

During World War I, owing to the need for X-rays in the treatment of the wounded, the Army training schools turned out additional radiologists and radiological technicians. As a result of the wide use of X-rays many more physicians became aware of the value of this diagnostic technique. When the war ended and these physicians returned to civilian practice, many of them decided to take training as radiological specialists. In 1913 there were only a few hundred radiologists and many of these also engaged in other medical activities. By 1931 the number of radiologists had increased to 1005, most of whom devoted full time to this specialty; by 1938 the number of radiologists had increased to 2191. One reason for this

321

increase was the greater number of technical procedures that had become available to radiologists.

CONTRAST
RADIOGRAPHY

Many of the new procedures depended upon the use of contrast radiography. In 1918 a young surgical resident, Walter E. Dandy, working in Halsted's Department of Surgery at Johns Hopkins, was searching for a method to improve the diagnosis and localization of brain tumors. Dandy thought that it might be possible to accomplish this by filling the ventricles of the brain, which normally contained fluid, with a substance that was opaque to X-rays. With this in view he carried out numerous experiments on animals, and although he could obtain some satisfactory X-ray pictures, he was unable to find an opaque substance that he thought would be safe to use in human subjects. At this point Dandy recalled the fact that bubbles of air in the intestinal tract stood out sharply as negative shadows in X-ray pictures. He remembered that Dr. Halsted had commented frequently on this phenomenon (Crowe, 1957). Dandy had also operated on a patient with a perforation of the intestine in which a bubble of air had accumulated beneath the diaphragm and had stood out sharply in the preoperative X-ray pictures. With these observations in mind Dandy decided to inject air into the ventricles of the brain. In the *Annals of Surgery* for July, 1918, he published an account of the first 20 patients in whom he had used air injections to visualize the brain. The results exceeded his expectations: whereas previously it had not been possible to achieve precise localization of tumors or other lesions in the brain, Dandy was able to localize such lesions in three of the first eight patients in whom he employed air injections. After its introduction and initial trials this technique became widely used by brain surgeons and neurologists for the diagnosis and localization of brain tumors and other lesions.

Working at the Mayo Clinic in 1921–22, Drs. Earl D. Osborne and Leonard G. Rowntree and their collaborators developed a different type of contrast radiography to visualize the kidneys. They found that when sodium iodide is injected into a vein it is rapidly extracted from the blood by the kidneys and is excreted by them in high concentration. They discovered that when X-ray pictures are taken of the kidney region while the sodium iodide is being concentrated and excreted, one could obtain a picture of the kidneys, ureters, and urinary bladder. This was due to the fact that the concentrated sodium iodide is opaque to X-rays. These results were reported in February, 1923. The method developed by the scientists at the Mayo Clinic soon became widely used for the diagnosis of abnormalities of the kidneys. The use of sodium iodide has since been superseded by the use of other chemicals that produce a better X-ray picture.

In the report of the kidney experiments in 1923 it was suggested that injections of sodium iodide might be used also for taking pictures of blood vessels to diagnose such abnormalities as aneurysms and arteriovenous anastomoses. Soon after this Dr. Barney Brooks of Washington University, St. Louis, injected a solution of sodium iodide into an artery in the leg of one of his patients and made X-ray pictures that showed the major vessels of the leg in beautiful detail. Visualization of arteries and veins and the

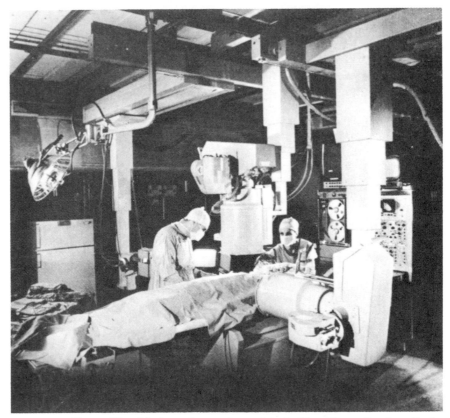

Figure 83. Modern cineangiographic facility. (From Brecher, Ruth, and Brecher, Edward: Rays—A History of Radiology in the United States and Canada. Baltimore, The Williams and Wilkins Co., 1969.)

chambers of the heart by injection of contrast media is now a standard procedure in diagnostic radiology.

Another breakthrough in radiology occurred in 1923 when Evarts Graham, Professor of Surgery at Washington University, St. Louis, asked one of his young residents, Warren H. Cole, to collaborate with him in trying to develop a contrast medium for visualization of the gall bladder. Graham was familiar with some previous work that provided hints as to how he might proceed. In 1909 Abel and Rowntree at Johns Hopkins had reported that a number of phenolphthalein compounds, including several containing iodine, are secreted by the liver into the bile. Rous and McMaster, in 1921, at the Rockefeller Institute, had shown that bile secreted by the liver enters the gall bladder and is there concentrated eight- to tenfold. Graham and Cole reasoned that a phenolphthalein compound containing iodine, which is opaque to X-rays, would be secreted in the bile and might be sufficiently concentrated in the gall bladder to make the latter visible in an X-ray picture. The early experiments to test this hypothesis were carried out on animals and initially were not very successful. The key to success was brought to light one day when the animal caretaker by chance gave the phenolphthalein to an animal that had not been fed. The gall bladder in this instance was clearly visible on the X-rays. From this point on, the

323

phenolphthalein compound was given to dogs in a fasting state with uniformly good results. After being fully tested in animals, the method was employed on a number of patients. In the first few patients the results were disappointing, but it was subsequently shown that all of these patients happened to have gall bladder disease. In other patients excellent visualization of the gall bladder was obtained, and the method, which became known as the *Graham test,* soon came into general use for the diagnosis of gall bladder disease and stones in the gall bladder.

RADIUM AND
X-RAY THERAPY

Prior to the 1920s there was little appreciation of the potentialities of X-ray therapy except for its successful use in the treatment of skin cancer and a few other superficial conditions. During this period of relatively little progress, advances were being made in the therapeutic use of another source of radiation, radium. The use of radium for the treatment of cancer was the subject of investigation in several European centers in the early years of the twentieth century. Work in this field lagged in the United States owing to the lack of adequate supplies of radium. In 1913 Howard A. Kelly, Professor of Gynecology at Johns Hopkins, acquired a supply of radium and began to use it for the treatment of patients in his small private hospital. In June, 1915, he and his associate, Curtis F. Burnam, reported their results in the treatment of 213 cases of carcinoma of the cervix and vagina treated between January, 1909, and December, 1914. The most favorable of these patients had been treated by surgery, and radium had been systematically used only for those treated in 1913 and 1914. With such a short period of follow-up it was difficult, in 1915, to assess the value of the radium therapy, but in some of those treated there had been at least a temporary regression of the carcinoma. Twenty-one years later, Burnam reviewed the cases that he and Kelly had treated with radium at the time of their 1915 report, and he said that he was impressed by two factors: (1) the number of severe injuries caused by the radium, and (2) the number of permanent cures.

In September, 1913, nine months after large-scale trials of radium therapy were begun at the Howard A. Kelly Hospital, the Cancer Commission of Harvard University secured one fifth of a gram of radium and inaugurated a therapeutic program at its new cancer center, the Collis P. Huntington Memorial Hospital of Boston. This program was directed by William Duane, a physicist whose interest in this field had been kindled by a visit to Pierre and Marie Curie, the discoverers of radium, in the late 1890s. From 1907 to 1912 he had conducted research at the Curie Radium Laboratory in Paris. In 1917 Duane and his co-worker, Robert B. Greenough, reported the results of the Huntington Hospital radium work up to that date. They had treated 642 patients with radium, and they stated that of these, 55 per cent had received definite benefit. As had been previously noted by Kelly, the results varied widely with the type of cancer treated. For example, cancer of the skin was apparently cured in 40 per cent, and only 12 per cent of the cases failed to obtain definite benefit. Good results were also secured with carcinoma of the cervix of the uterus, whereas cancer of the pharynx showed little or no benefit. In cases of recurrent cancer of the breast the

324

results were disappointing, and the authors believed that massive doses of therapeutic X-rays were preferable to radium in the treatment of this condition.

The Memorial Hospital in New York City, which specialized in the treatment of cancer and allied diseases, did not have an adequate supply of radium until the uranium deposits in Colorado were exploited in 1915. By 1916 the Memorial Hospital possessed one of the world's major supplies, more than 2.3 grams. A surgeon, Henry H. Janeway, had prepared himself to head Memorial's new Division of Radium Therapy by spending two years taking courses in physics at Columbia University. In 1915 he was joined by a brilliant young physicist, Gioacchino Failla. The early experience at the Memorial Hospital confirmed the findings in Baltimore and Boston, but greater attention was paid to the details of treatment, and ingenious methods were developed for measuring the amount of radiation so that the results of treatment could be related to the dosage. One of their conclusions was that the tissues of malignant tumors are more susceptible to radiation than are normal tissues.

While the therapeutic effect of radium was being evaluated, there had been new discoveries in radiation physics. In the course of his research at the Curie Laboratory, William Duane observed that radium emits a radioactive gas, which can be captured in a glass or metal container. This gas, first known as *radium emanation,* is now called *radon.* The emanation gas gradually deteriorates, and its useful life for radiation therapy is limited, but Duane found that if the gas is sealed in containers its radioactivity will last long enough to allow it to be used instead of radium for therapeutic purposes. Soon after his arrival at the Huntington Hospital in 1913 Duane set up there the first full-scale radium emanation plant, and one year later he helped to set up a similar plant at Memorial Hospital. Within a few years commercial concerns were producing emanation and offering it for sale. Emanation proved to have a number of advantages over radium; it is easy to handle; it can be obtained on short notice; it does not require long storage under special protective conditions; and it can be purchased at a relatively low price by doctors and hospitals that could not afford to buy radium. It also is useful in that the emanations from a small supply of radium can serve many people in widely separated areas.

The increasingly successful use of radium and its emanation during the years after 1913 tended to overshadow the therapeutic use of X-rays. However, about 1916 the Germans began to build transformers capable of delivering some 200,000 volts to an X-ray tube. Soon thereafter the General Electric Company combined a high-voltage transformer with a Coolidge tube to produce a special unit for X-ray therapy. One of the early problems in the use of this unit was that of measuring the dosage of X-rays delivered to the patient. By the end of the 1920s it had become possible to make this measurement with a relatively high degree of accuracy, by means of a chamber in which the amount of ionization produced by a beam of X-rays could be determined. In 1928, by international agreement, a unit (the *roentgen*) was established for the measurement of X-ray dosage.

As techniques improved and studies multiplied, it became apparent that results in X-ray therapy depended more upon the character of the tumor that was being radiated than upon the methods used or the dosage administered. It therefore became necessary to devote a long period of study to grading tumors according to their susceptibility to radiation. It was gradually learned, for example, that cancers of the cervix are not all alike in terms of malignancy. Further, it was learned that by examining the cells of the tumor under the microscope, their grade of malignancy could be roughly estimated. In general, it was found that tumors of low malignancy are relatively resistant to radiation, whereas more rapidly growing tumors seem to melt away when exposed to even modest doses of X-ray or radium.

15

Preventive
Medicine and
Public Health

*Bacteriology, by revealing the microorganisms concerned in those diseases which
are of the greatest racial and social importance to mankind, and by providing
methods for the study of their characters and behavior, transformed public health
from a blundering, empirical set of doctrines and practices to a science and laid
secure foundations for its further development along scientific lines.*

(William H. Welch, 1925)

The new scientific foundation for preventive medicine and public
health was created in the 1870s by the discoveries of Pasteur and Koch.
When it became known in the following two decades that some of the most
dreaded epidemic diseases were caused by micro-organisms, public health
officials found that they had something more substantial than the old
"miasmas" and "emanations" with which to grapple.

American physicians were slow to accept the "germ theory" of disease.
To them it was just another in the long line of theories that had come and
gone over the centuries and was perhaps even more fanciful than the
others. Most American scientists also lacked the cultural background that
would have enabled them to grasp the significance of this new concept of
disease. There were only a few to whom bacteria were a reality. Thomas J.
Burrill, in his course in botany at the University of Illinois, was the first to
introduce the study of bacteria, but he was more concerned with their biological than with their pathological significance. George M. Sternberg, who
taught himself bacteriology in the late 1870s, was the first American to investigate the relation of bacteria to disease and to gain some insight into

327

their importance for public health. William H. Welch was the first to teach medical bacteriology in the United States, not as a separate discipline but as part of his course in pathology. The first systematic course in bacteriology was offered by Victor C. Vaughan at the University of Michigan in 1889.

In spite of their late entry into the field of microbiological research, Americans were more adept than their European counterparts in the practical applications of the new science to the advancement of public health: they were the originators of the public health bacteriological laboratory.

PUBLIC HEALTH LABORATORIES
The earliest bacteriological laboratory was established by Joseph J. Kinyoun at the Staten Island Marine Hospital in 1887. A year later the first municipal public health laboratory was set up at Providence, Rhode Island. The primary purpose of this laboratory was the analysis of water and food, and it was utilized in the study of a typhoid fever outbreak of that year. Also in 1888, Victor C. Vaughan established the Michigan State Hygiene Laboratory, and George M. Sternberg opened the first privately endowed bacteriological laboratory, the Hoagland Laboratory in Brooklyn, which he used in the teaching of bacteriology at the Long Island Medical College.

It was at the New York City Bacteriological Laboratory, opened in 1892, that the new knowledge of bacteriology was first really applied in public health practice (Rosen, 1958). The laboratory was established principally through the efforts of the farsighted Hermann M. Biggs. Biggs had long been interested in the public health field; his A.B. thesis at Cornell University in 1882 was entitled "Sanitary Regulations and the Duty of the States in Regard to Public Health." Biggs completed his training at Bellevue Hospital just at the dawn of the bacteriological era and in 1885 was placed in charge of bacteriological work of the Carnegie Laboratory. Here he conducted a classic study of a major typhoid epidemic in Plymouth, Pennsylvania. Biggs then taught bacteriology at Bellevue Hospital and in 1888 became Consultant Pathologist of the New York City Health Department.

It was Biggs's interest in the bacteriological diagnosis of communicable diseases that led directly to the formation of the diagnostic laboratory. In 1892, New York City was faced with the threat of an epidemic of cholera that had appeared on ships from Hamburg, Germany. Biggs was appointed to an advisory committee on cholera, and when the Commissioner of Health, J. D. Bryant, established a Division of Bacteriology and Disinfection, he appointed Biggs chief inspector of this Division, which functioned in a small two-room diagnostic laboratory. The work carried on here was highly effective, for when seven ships carrying almost 100 cases of cholera entered New York Harbor in rapid succession, only 10 cases of cholera developed in residents of New York City, and there were no secondary cases (Smillie, 1955). After the cholera scare, the laboratory was not disbanded but began to employ bacteriological procedures for the control of diphtheria under the direction of William H. Park. Soon bacteriological studies were being made also on tuberculosis, dysentery, pneumonia, typhoid fever, and scarlet fever, and on the role of milk in the transmission of disease.

328

Establishment of public health laboratories by other local and state health departments followed rapidly after the example had been set by New York. In 1894, Henry P. Walcott, Health Commissioner of Massachusetts, organized a laboratory to produce diphtheria antitoxin, and in the following year a laboratory for the diagnosis and control of diphtheria was also established in Philadelphia. By 1914 all of the states except New Mexico and Wyoming had established public health laboratories in connection with their boards of health. These laboratories, to a great extent, took over the task of diagnosing communicable diseases and in order to control these diseases provided free vaccines and antitoxins to doctors in practice and to public health officers. Thus, the laboratories provided concrete evidence of the acceptance by government of the responsibility to protect the health of the people. At the same time their findings enabled public health administrators to deal more effectively with the control of epidemic diseases.

BOARDS OF HEALTH AND GOVERNMENT AGENCIES

The public health laboratory service was able to develop as rapidly as it did partially because most of the states had already organized state boards of health, which provided an institutional base for the establishment and growth of the laboratories. Louisiana established the first State Board of Health in 1855 in an effort to prevent further disasters from yellow fever. This Board was not very effective, as was indicated by Dr. Stanford Chaille, in addressing the Louisiana State Medical Society in 1879. "Louisiana," he said, "has legislated on *paper* a State Board of Health and Vital Statistics; but in reality we have no state, merely a city, board of health, organized under laws which nobody except politicians (and a designing or an ignorant class of these) can possibly approve" (Smillie, 1955). The second State Board of Health was established by the Massachusetts state legislature in 1869, just 19 years after Lemuel Shattuck, in his famous *Report of the Massachusetts Sanitary Commission,* had recommended that such a body be created.

Following the organization of the Massachusetts Board of Health, other states established similar boards in rapid succession during the 1870s and 1880s, the period in which the general principles of Pasteur and Koch were becoming better known. The organization of the various boards differed, but most included the following divisions: (1) registration of vital statistics, (2) general sanitation, (3) child hygiene, (4) prevention and control of communicable diseases, (5) laboratory service, and (6) social service, performed by public health nurses (Vedder, 1929). These boards provided an appropriate administrative mechanism for dealing with the community health problems of the state.

Action was also taken for interstate cooperation in the public health field. In 1878 a severe epidemic of yellow fever occurred in Louisiana that threatened the entire Mississippi Valley. The Louisiana State Board of Health proved inefficient in the handling of the outbreak, and a meeting was called by J. D. Plunket, President of the Tennessee State Board of Health, in order to form a "protective council." Representatives from five states attended in April, 1879, and organized the Sanitary Council of the

Mississippi Valley. The Council was highly successful in getting the Mississippi Valley states to act in unison on health matters of mutual interest. As a direct outgrowth of this Council, the Council of State Boards of Health of the United States was formed in 1884, an organization of all the states for consideration and regulation of public health affairs of interstate concern. In 1897, the Council changed its name to the Conference of State and Provincial Health Authorities of North America and included representatives not only from the state boards of health but also from Canada. Smillie stated in 1955 that "the Conference, which has remained in continuous existence since its formation . . . became *the most effective* single cohesive force in promotion of public health throughout the nation . . . it has maintained the integrity of state health services and has emphasized the primary responsibility of the state for the promotion of the health of its people" while working closely with the federal health services.

The federal government took almost no responsibility for public health during the first century except for the establishment of the Marine Hospital Service in 1798. The first Marine Hospital was built at Norfolk, Virginia, in 1800; and the second at Boston two years later. Subsequently, hospitals were built at other seaports as far west as San Francisco. In 1837 an Act of Congress provided for additional hospitals to serve seamen who were manning ships on inland waters.

The medical officers of the Marine Hospital Service were often the first to diagnose such diseases as cholera, yellow fever, and smallpox, which were being imported into the United States, and in the great cholera epidemics the Marine hospitals and their medical personnel were utilized for the treatment of those suffering from this disease.

The operation of the Marine hospitals was seriously hampered by the fact that their administration was entrusted to the United States Department of the Treasury, and the Director of each hospital was responsible to the local Collector of Customs. The Collectors handled all financial matters, including the deduction of 20 cents a month from each seaman's pay for the maintenance of the hospitals. (This was the first example in the United States of prepayment for hospital care.) Obviously, this system provided an opportunity for political abuse, corrupt practices, and misuse of federal funds.

The medical neglect and administrative incompetence became so flagrant that finally in 1870, at the urging of John Shaw Billings, the President approved an Act to reorganize the Marine Hospital Service. The Act provided for a supervising surgeon to direct all matters connected with the Service. Provision was made also for the disbursement of the funds furnished by the Act. John M. Woodworth was appointed by the President as the first Director of the Marine Hospital Service.

Woodworth proved to be an excellent choice, as he was highly successful in upgrading the administrative aspects of the Marine hospitals, patterning the organization along the lines of the Medical Department of the United States Army. He also agitated for federal control of port quarantine and was in large part responsible for the National Quarantine Act of 1878, which empowered the federal government to enforce port quarantine. However, no funds were appropriated for this purpose, and the Act stated that "there shall be no interference in any manner with any quarantine laws or regulations as they now exist or may hereafter be adopted under State laws." This made it clear that the doctrine of states' rights still handicapped the effective administration of nationwide public health activities.

The severe yellow fever epidemic in the Mississippi Valley in 1878 gave impetus to earlier agitation for a National Board of Health. In March, 1879, Congress passed an Act, sponsored by the American Public Health Association, which transferred from the Marine Hospital Service certain powers previously conferred upon it, including all maritime quarantine. The new Act created a National Board of Health consisting of seven physicians and representatives from the Army, the Navy, the Marine Hospital Service, and the Department of Justice. Fifty thousand dollars was appropriated to carry out the purposes of the Act. In June, 1879, Congress passed a second Act, giving the new Board wide quarantine powers and appropriating $500,000 for its quarantine work. This new Bill had a clause that proved to be a fatal weakness: it gave these quarantine powers for a period of four years only, and a re-enactment bill was necessary for continuation of the work.

The four-year history of the National Board of Health was a turbulent one. It had an unworkable administrative structure, and it became involved in states' rights controversies and personality conflicts. When an epidemic broke out in New Orleans in 1880, the members of the board tried to move too rapidly and made the fatal mistake of encroaching on the prerogatives of the individual states, whose representatives in Congress resented the federal centralization of power. While the controversy in New Orleans was raging, John Hamilton, the new Surgeon-General of the Marine Hospital Service, was doing his utmost to discredit the National Board. Hamilton's rise in the Service had been phenomenal; he had taken no part in the advancement of public health in the nation and had no knowledge or experience in the fields of quarantine, sanitation, and public health. However, he was distressed by the Marine Hospital Service's loss of power under the Act of 1879, and knowing that if Congress did not re-enact the Quarantine Law, the National Board would be powerless, Hamilton did his best to prevent re-enactment. He accused the members of the Board of misuse of funds, of extravagance and incompetence, and he insinuated that the funds of the Board had been used to corrupt local health officers. Hamilton was successful in blocking the Re-enactment Bill of 1883. The National Board of Health was given a grant of only $10,000 to continue its investigatory and advisory functions. In the Quarantine Act of 1890, Congress returned the responsibility for port quarantine to the Marine Hospital Service and, in addition, gave it power to control the interstate spread of certain infectious diseases, including plague, cholera, typhus fever, yellow fever, smallpox, and leprosy.

By 1902 it was felt that the name of the Marine Hospital Service no longer indicated the scope of its responsibilities, and its name was therefore changed to the Public Health and Marine Hospital Service. In was in this year, too, that the Hygienic Laboratory was established under an Act providing for the regulation of the interstate sale of viruses, serums, toxins, and similar products. Walter Wyman, who had succeeded Hamilton as Surgeon-General of the Marine Hospital Service in 1891, had invited Kinyoun in 1892 to move his laboratory from Staten Island to Washington, D.C. There Kinyoun was producing diphtheria antitoxin and carrying out a variety of useful activities; as a result his small research laboratory became

331

the nucleus around which the Hygienic Laboratory was formed. Next, the Service established a Biologics Control Division to test and to guarantee the safety and effectiveness of the various serums, vaccines, and related biological products that were being developed. Finally, in 1912 the present designation of the United States Public Health Service was adopted, the great emphasis now being upon public health affairs, but the Service continued to be responsible for the medical, hospital, and nursing care of sick and disabled sailors. The essential activities that were provided for in the Act of 1912 were as follows: (1) investigation and research, (2) improvement in methods of public health administration, (3) distribution of federal aid to state and local health departments, and (4) interstate control of sanitation and communicable diseases.

AMERICAN PUBLIC HEALTH ASSOCIATION
Although the promotion of health and the prevention of disease had clearly become responsibilities of government, the development of the public health and preventive medicine movements in the United States had, in many instances, been preceded and stimulated by the activities of independent, voluntary organizations such as the American Public Health Association. This Association was initiated by Stephen Smith of New York, a Commissioner of the Metropolitan Board of Health. In April, 1872, Smith called an informal meeting to consider the formation of a nationwide association of persons interested in the field of public health. The Association that resulted from this meeting established a policy of including in its membership not only physicians but also others professionally interested in public health. During the first seven years of the Association's existence, emphasis was placed on state health organization and a national health program. In 1875, for example, the following resolution was adopted (Ravenel, 1921):

> *That a committee consisting of a member of this Association from each state and territory of the Union . . . be appointed to petition Congress, at its next session, to institute a bureau of health, to be located at Washington City, with a branch at the seat of each state and territorial government. That this Association urge upon the governor and legislature of each and every state in the Union the importance of enacting laws creating state boards of health and providing adequately for sanitary administration.*

The Association was instrumental in motivating many states to establish state boards of health. Moreover, at its meeting in 1878, when the yellow fever epidemic was a paramount issue, a special committee was formed to draft the National Board of Health Law, which was finally passed by Congress in 1879. By that time the small group of men who had met in Stephen Smith's office in 1872 had grown to an organization consisting of almost 600 members. About 90 per cent of these were physicians, the remainder being civil engineers, educators, architects, and others not in the medical profession.

At about the same time that the American Public Health Association was founded, the American Medical Association established a section on "state medicine." Initially this section conducted a campaign to establish health departments in every state. At first the section had considerable weight and influence in the public affairs of the nation, but its influence waned with the growth of the American Public Health Association.

VOLUNTARY ORGANIZATIONS

The late nineteenth century also saw the development of a new type of voluntary health organization of which the first to have a major impact upon public health and health legislation was the National Tuberculosis Association. The founding of this association in 1904 and its broad and effective program have been described in an earlier chapter. In 1905, the voluntary concept began to spread to other fields. In that year the American Social Hygiene Association and the American Child Health Association were formed. Then came the National Committee for Mental Hygiene, in 1909, and the American Society for the Control of Cancer, in 1913, and many others were to follow.

PUBLIC HEALTH NURSING

Another major American institution, public health nursing, developed during the late nineteenth century out of voluntary organizations that depended for their support upon contributions and small service charges. In 1877 the *New York City Mission* began the employment of trained nurses for the purpose of giving bedside care to the sick poor in their homes. The idea gradually spread to other communities, and the first associations specifically designated as *Visiting Nurse Associations* were organized in Buffalo in 1885 and Philadelphia in 1886. A plan of public instruction was an integral part of the activities of these associations.

Through the efforts of Lillian D. Wald and Mary Brewster, The *Henry Street District Nursing Service* was opened in New York City in 1893. In 1902 Miss Wald loaned one of her nurses, Lina Rogers, to serve as a school nurse in the New York public school system. Within a short time Miss Rogers was appointed by the Health Department of that city as the first full-time trained school nurse in America. The successful outcome of this initial trial soon led to the employment of a group of nurses in the city schools. Soon thereafter nurses were employed to give instruction in infant hygiene and to visit the homes of patients with tuberculosis in order to instruct the family in the proper care of such patients. From 1905 on, public health nursing grew rapidly and soon was adopted as a community function by local health departments, school boards, state health departments, and eventually (1913) by the United States Public Health Service. Financial support for some of these services came from agencies such as the Rockefeller Foundation and the Milbank Fund. The National Organization for Public Health Nursing was founded in 1912.

By 1920, the organizations engaged in public health nursing numbered about 4000, employing approximately 11,000 nurses. Perhaps the most sig-

333

nificant factor in this phenomenal development was the rapid extension of state direction and control (Dock, 1921).

CONTROL OF DISEASE

The diseases against which public health measures were originally directed were those due to micro-organisms. Some of these diseases occurred in epidemics; others were endemic (habitually prevalent) in an area, as yellow fever was in Cuba before Walter Reed's discovery and as cholera is in India today. As more and more bacteria and other disease-producing organisms were discovered, people began to think that all diseases were caused by micro-organisms and that the one important job of the health official was to devise ways to protect the public from these living agents. Certainly some of the greatest triumphs of public health and preventive medicine have been in the realm of epidemic and other infectious diseases.

In the early years of the twentieth century it became evident that factors other than micro-organisms may cause disease and that some of these noninfectious diseases may be encountered in epidemic or endemic form. A classic example of a noninfectious endemic disease is pellagra. The U.S. Public Health Service became interested in this disease in 1914 because of its prevalence in the southern states and because knowledgeable people considered it to be infectious. One of the infectious-disease experts of the Public Health Service was therefore assigned the task of searching for the causative micro-organism. Fortunately, the expert chosen was Joseph Goldberger, who approached his task as a disciplined scientist and unprejudiced observer and, as described in Chapter 12, proved that pellagra is caused not by a micro-organism but by a dietary deficiency. It gradually became known that many serious diseases are caused by dietary deficiencies and that the detection and prevention of such diseases are within the province of public health. The provision of iodized table salt for the prevention of endemic goiter (introduced by David Marine in Ohio) and of vitamin D for the prevention of rickets are no less important public health measures than is the prevention of infectious diseases.

Many Americans have made discoveries or developed new procedures that are basic to public health practice. Some of these have been described in Chapter 12. Three examples of highly successful large-scale undertakings for the prevention of disease will be described in this chapter: (1) typhoid fever in the Spanish-American War; (2) prevention of disease during construction of the Panama Canal; and (3) the control of hookworm disease in the southern states.

TYPHOID FEVER: THE ARMY LEARNS A LESSON IN SANITATION

During the Spanish-American War the Army was less in need of surgeons than of sanitarians and physicians trained in modern diagnostic methods. Only 289 men were killed or mortally wounded in battle, whereas some 3700 died of disease. Of 107,973 soldiers encamped within the limits of the United States, 20,738 contracted typhoid fever. This disease alone accounted for 1580 deaths. Typhoid fever has a devastating effect upon an army because even when it does not result in death it produces a debilitating illness lasting several weeks and followed by a long period of convalescence. Its spread is due to poor sanitation, and as Samuel Eliot Morison has remarked, the American troops in this war "neglected even such principles of camp sanitation as were laid down in Deuteronomy" (Morison, 1965).

When the war began in April, 1898, the regular Army Medical Corps contained a number of first-class physicians, well trained and well informed; but the size of the Corps was small, even in relation to the small prewar Army. With the rapid expansion of the Army, many of the regular medical officers had to be assigned administrative duties, and the medical care of the troops was left largely to "contract surgeons" who had been appointed more for political than for professional reasons.

By 1898 a considerable amount of information about typhoid fever was available. It was known that (1) the disease is caused by a specific bacterium, the typhoid bacillus, discovered in 1880; (2) the disease is disseminated by contaminated drinking water and less commonly by personal contact with articles contaminated by the excreta of patients; (3) the disease can be positively diagnosed by post-mortem examination; (4) it can be diagnosed during life by a laboratory test (devised in 1896) on the patient's blood, the Widal test; and (5) malaria, the disease with which typhoid fever was then most often confused, can be diagnosed by microscopic examination of the blood for the malarial parasites. Lamentably, the contract surgeons in the camps had been educated in the old two-year medical schools and hence had no understanding of bacteriology and little or no knowledge of how to prevent the dissemination of the typhoid bacillus. They were too poorly trained in pathology to perform an autopsy; and if they were fortunate enough to have heard of the Widal test they had certainly had no experience in performing it. Few if any of them knew how to use a microscope or how to examine the blood for malarial parasites. The Army officials were by no means blameless; they had been overwhelmed by the magnitude of the problem; they were uncertain as to just what disease was causing all the deaths; and they had failed to provide the laboratory facilities required for the diagnosis of typhoid fever, malaria, and other diseases. In not a single Army camp was there a microscope!

Fortunately, the Surgeon-General of the Army, George M. Sternberg, was a physician of broad experience and an expert bacteriologist. In order to get a better understanding of the cause of the disease problems in the camps, General Sternberg, in August, 1898, appointed a three-member Commission to make a study of the situation. The Chairman of the Commission was Major Walter Reed, a highly competent regular Army medical officer. In 1890–91 Reed had taken Welch's course in pathology and bacteriology, during which he had carried out some special studies on the pathology of typhoid fever. In 1893 he became Professor of Bacteriology at the new Army Medical College, and while there, in 1896, he had conducted a study of an epidemic of malaria at Fort Myer, Virginia. He was therefore ideally qualified to head the Commission. The other members of the Commission were also carefully selected: Major Edward O. Shakespeare, who had made extensive studies on the epidemiology of cholera and typhoid fever, and Victor C. Vaughan, Dean of the University of Michigan Medical School and an expert in public hygiene and sanitation.

335

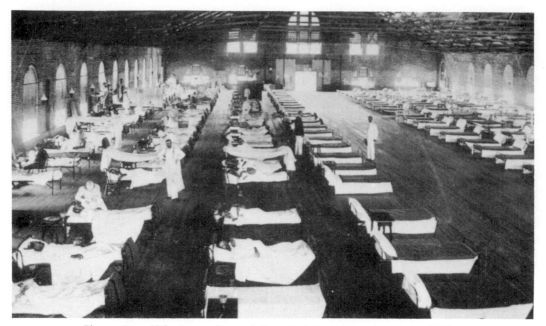

Figure 84. U.S. Army General Hospital, Fort Myer, Virginia, 1898.
(From Sternberg, Martha L.: George M. Sternberg, a Biography.
Chicago, American Medical Association, 1920.)

At the outset the Commission found in the camps hundreds of patients with what they believed was typhoid fever but who had been diagnosed as having malaria and were being treated as such. The camp physicians would not accept the views of the Commissioners, because they were convinced, purely on the basis of superficial observations, that the disease was either malaria or typhomalaria, a hypothetical disease entity (concocted during the Civil War) that was supposed to lie somewhere between malaria and typhoid fever. The Commissioners knew that they must obtain unassailable evidence to prove their point to the camp doctors. However, there were strong objections to performing autopsies, and there were no microscopes and none of the materials needed to perform Widal tests and malarial smears. The Commission therefore requested the Army to establish small, properly equipped diagnostic laboratories in each camp. General Sternberg promptly honored this request, and the new laboratories were set up and manned by the few people in the United States who knew how to use a microscope.

The Commission then asked to have 50 patients who had been diagnosed as having malaria or typhomalaria turned over to them for study. The laboratory tests on all 50 patients proved that they had typhoid fever rather than malaria. The camp doctors would not accept this conclusion, voicing their belief that the men who had performed the laboratory tests were creatures of the Commission and that they had merely reported results which they believed would please the Commissioners. In order to dispel any further doubts, the Commission asked to have another 150 cases of so-called malaria or typhomalaria selected. These patients were sent to leading hospitals in Baltimore, Philadelphia, New York, Boston, and Cleveland. In every instance the hospitals reported that the patients had typhoid fever. From

336

that time on no one questioned this diagnosis when it was backed up by the tests carried out in the camp laboratories.

Once it had been proved that the disease in question was typhoid fever, the Commission undertook an epidemiological study to determine how it got into the camps and how it spread once it had gotten there. How it got there was not always easy to determine, but in some instances it was shown that the outbreak of an epidemic was preceded by the arrival in the camp of soldiers from an area in which typhoid fever was prevalent. The manner in which the disease was spread was not hard to find: the hygiene and sanitation in the camps were appalling. Latrines were poorly constructed, and fecal matter was deposited carelessly and indiscriminately about the camps; in one camp, Vaughan remarked that he had never before seen so large an area of fecal-stained soil. There were clouds of flies, yet there was often no screening of mess halls and kitchens, and food was inadequately protected. The water supply was to blame in some instances, as when open sewers flowed into rivers close to the point from which the drinking water was obtained, or when water was dipped from springs by unwashed hands and transported in open barrels to the point where it was used. On the other hand, in a camp near Jacksonville, Florida, it was found that there were hundreds of cases of typhoid among the soldiers but very few cases in the city, though camp and city were supplied by the same water system. The dissemination in this camp was found to be due to other factors.

The camp hospital where typhoid patients were being treated was found in some instances to serve as a focus from which the disease spread. There were almost no nurses or orderlies, and every morning soldiers were detailed from the ranks to serve in the hospital for the day. Among other breaches of hygiene these men were observed to handle bedpans in an inexperienced manner, often soiling their hands as well as the bedding and floors. At noon and again at suppertime the hospital detail went to the regular mess hall, mostly without washing their hands, handling their own food and passing food to their comrades. Since different soldiers were detailed to hospital duty each day, the number thereby exposed either directly in the hospital or secondarily in the mess hall was considerable.

The Commission concluded from its investigations that the most important factor in the spread of typhoid in the camps was personal contact between a well soldier and a sick soldier, either his person, his clothing, his excreta, or articles that he had handled. However, the Commission recognized the role played by contaminated water or food and other factors mentioned above. The Commission also made an important new discovery: that the common housefly may serve as an agent to transmit typhoid bacilli from feces to food. In Vaughan's words, "We sprinkled lime over the contents of the latrines and soon we saw flies with feet whitened by the lime, walking over the food on the mess tables." The conclusion to be drawn from this astute observation was obvious (Vaughan, 1926).

As a result of the Commission's findings many new sanitary measures were taken in the camps. Latrines were better constructed and better protected, and their contents were covered periodically with disinfecting lime; careless disposal of human excreta was forbidden; water supplies were protected from contamination by sewage; mess halls were screened, and food was protected from flies; the practice of detailing soldiers for temporary duty in hospitals was discontinued; clothing and other articles that had been in contact with typhoid patients were either burned or disinfected. As a result of these measures the annual death rate among the troops fell from 879 per 100,000 in 1898 to 107 per 100,000 in 1899, and the incidence of the disease fell proportionately.

While the United States Army was having its problems with typhoid fever in the Spanish-American War, the British Army, at about the same time, was having similar problems in the Boer War (1899–1902). As a result of the high incidence of typhoid fever among British troops, Sir Almroth Wright decided to try to immunize the soldiers by injecting them with killed cultures of typhoid bacilli. Only soldiers who volunteered for the experiment received the vaccine. Due to unfortunate reports of a higher mortality among those who had been vaccinated, the British authorities, in 1903, prohibited further vaccination.

In 1908 the Surgeon-General of the United States Army, Robert M. O'Reilly, announced that he intended to make an investigation of methods to prevent typhoid. It is probable that Captain Frederick F. Russell, who had become interested in protective vaccination while working in Cole's laboratory at Johns Hopkins in 1906, was responsible for suggesting this investigation. At any rate, the Surgeon-General sent Captain Russell to Europe to inquire into the experience of the British and other workers in this field; he also appointed a Board of distinguished physicians, including Russell, to advise him on the matter. The advice of the Board was that "the practice of anti-typhoid vaccination is both useful and harmless and offers a practical means of diminishing the amount of typhoid fever in the Army."

In 1909 Russell began the gigantic experiment of vaccinating the United States Army against typhoid fever. In that year there were 173 cases of typhoid among the troops; by 1912 the number had been reduced to 9 cases. In 1911, when the United States Army was mobilizing along the Mexican border, antityphoid vaccination was made compulsory, and it continued to be compulsory for all United States troops through World War II. By 1915 the incidence of typhoid in the Army had been reduced to 3.24 cases per 100,000 troop-strength. Such a low rate was not achieved in the civilian population until 1935.

In the early years of World War I only the British Army had had anything approaching adequate antityphoid vaccination. In 1914 there were more than 45,000 cases of typhoid in the French Army. In 1915 the rate in the British Army was 4 per 1000, whereas in the Belgian Army it was 10 per 1000 and in the Italian Army, 18 per 1000. When the United States entered the war all troops were given typhoid vaccine, and the incidence of typhoid fever among them was negligible.

THE PANAMA CANAL: TRIUMPH OF SANITATION AND INSECT CONTROL

Had it not been for the work of Ronald Ross on the transmission of malaria, the work of the Typhoid Commission on the transmission of typhoid fever, and the work of the Yellow Fever Commission on the transmission of yellow fever, it probably would not have been possible to complete the construction of the Panama Canal.

The new American possessions in the Caribbean and the Pacific had emphasized the need for a shorter oceanic route between the east and the west coasts of the United States. During the Spanish-American War only one naval ship had been able to round Cape Horn to reinforce the Atlantic fleet. In this war, reinforcements had not been needed; but looking toward the future, more urgent circumstances could be foreseen. In 1900 President McKinley appointed a Commission to explore the feasibility of constructing a canal across Central America. After considering several possible routes the Commission reported strongly in favor of a route across the Isthmus of Panama. However, this area was known to be "a cesspool of disease" and had earned the title, *White Man's Grave*. It was described by a contemporary writer as a "damp, tropical jungle, intensely hot, swarming with mosquitoes, snakes, alligators, scorpions, and centipedes; the home, even as nature made it, of yellow fever, typhus, and dysentery." The author omitted to add that it was also the home of malaria.

In the late 1870s a French company had acquired the right to construct a canal through the Panamanian isthmus. Work on the project had started in 1881 under the supervision of Ferdinand de Lesseps, who had been responsible for the construction of the Suez Canal. The French effort was defeated not by engineering problems but by disease. In the single month of October, 1884, 654 members of the work force died of yellow fever. After the expenditure of $260 million and the sacrifice of hundreds of lives, construction was halted in 1889. When the United States made known its interest in the Isthmus of Panama, the French gladly offered to release their rights for $40 million. President Roosevelt was strongly in favor of the project, and after some rather questionable diplomatic maneuvers the United States agreed to pay the French $40 million for their rights and concluded a treaty with the new Republic of Panama to lease, *in perpetuity*, a "Canal Zone," for a down payment of $10 million plus $250,000 annual rent.

The construction of the Panama Canal, which began in 1904, was initially undertaken by civilian engineers on a private contract basis. The sanitation of the Canal Zone, however, was entrusted to the United States Army Medical Corps, which had had such a fine record in Cuba. Surgeon-General Sternberg selected Colonel William C. Gorgas as the sanitary officer for the Zone. Gorgas had been in charge of the work in Cuba that had brought an end to yellow fever in Havana, and he was experienced in sanitation and insect control. His first move was a vigorous attack on the mosquito population. His firm insistence on the enforcement of his anti-mosquito measures interfered with the freedom of action of some of his civilian superiors. Because of this, for several years, his orders were sometimes disregarded and occasionally countermanded. However, he had the staunch support of General Sternberg, who finally asked President Roosevelt to intervene and insist that Gorgas's sanitary orders be obeyed. The problems were lessened in 1907, when the construction of the Canal was taken out of the hands of civilian contractors and assigned to the engineers of the United States Army, with Colonel George W. Goethals in charge. In spite of the opposition that he encountered in the early years, Gorgas's sanitary measures and anti-mosquito campaign were highly successful. The last fatal case of yellow fever in the Canal Zone was reported in September, 1906. By the time the construction of the Canal was finished in 1914, the death rate from all

339

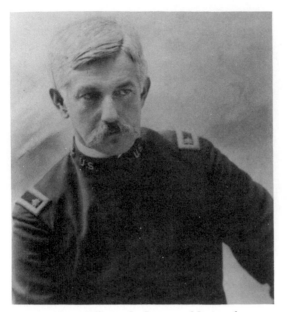

Figure 85. William C. Gorgas. (National Library of Medicine, Bethesda, Maryland.)

diseases in the Canal Zone was below that for any American city or state. In contrast to the experience of the French, American work on the Canal was never interrupted by disease.

HOOKWORM DISEASE   Hookworm disease is caused by the presence of the worm in the human intestinal tract. The tiny larvae of the worms hatch out of eggs in the soil, and when a person walks over the infected soil with bare feet, the larvae quickly penetrate the skin and find their way to a blood vessel, in which they are carried to the lungs, They then break through the air passages in the lungs, enter the sputum, and are swallowed with the sputum. In the intestines the larvae grow to adult worms about one-half inch in length. They cling to the inner coat of the intestine, where they live in colonies, usually of more than 1000 worms, feed on the blood of their host, copulate, and produce eggs. A single female worm lays 5000 to 10,000 eggs per day. The eggs become mixed with the feces, and if the feces are deposited on exposed soil or in a poorly constructed privy, as they may be in a primitive or unsanitary community, the eggs enter the soil, hatch into larvae, and burrow through the sole of the foot of a second unshod host. The symptoms produced by the hookworms while residing in the intestine are caused by the worms' avidity for human blood. As a result, anemia develops, the severity depending upon the number of worms in the intestine. Along with the anemia there are loss of vigor, increasing pallor, progressive weakness, and listlessness, and if the infestation persists, the individual may become short of breath and stuporous and may die. When a hookworm infestation is acquired during childhood it retards physical and mental development. A child may appear and act as though he were five to ten years younger than he actually is.

340

Though hookworm disease almost certainly has existed since prehistoric times, the worm was first discovered in the human intestine in an autopsy performed by Angelo Dubini in Italy in 1843. In the 1850s it was suggested for the first time that a severe form of anemia very common in Egypt was probably caused by hookworms. In 1878 two Italians, Grassi and Parona, discovered that hookworm infestation could be diagnosed by finding the eggs in human feces. The following year another Italian, Perroncito, made the important discovery that a severe and fatal anemia, which was prevalent among workers employed in the construction of the St. Gothard tunnel in Switzerland, was due to hookworm infestation.

As happened in the case of several other diseases, attention in this country was first focused on hookworm disease immediately after the Spanish-American War, when the United States Army had troops stationed on the island of Puerto Rico. In 1900, Captain Bailey K. Ashford of the Army Medical Corps reported that there were many cases of heavy hookworm infestation among the residents of the island and that this was associated with severe anemia and other symptoms. At about this same time Charles Wardell Stiles, a research zoologist of the United States Public Health Service, was making a study of parasitic worms, and he was the first to become cognizant of the prevalence of hookworm infestation in the southern states. Stiles was convinced that much of the chronic illness and retarded development observed among the people of the South at that time was due to hookworm disease resulting from poor sanitation.

In 1908, in connection with the work of President Theodore Roosevelt's Commission on Country Life, a conference was held for the purpose of hearing reports on the social, economic, and sanitary conditions of American farms. Stiles was among those attending the conference, and there he met Wallace Buttrick, Secretary of the (Rockefeller) General Education Board. Stiles took advantage of the opportunity to tell Buttrick about the devastating effect that hookworm disease was having upon the people of the South. He explained that the disease is both preventable and curable and that all that was needed to get rid of it was an intelligently organized campaign. He suggested that this might be an undertaking worthy of Mr. Rockefeller's support.

When he returned to New York, Buttrick told the hookworm story to Frederick T. Gates, Mr. Rockefeller's advisor. Gates was intrigued, but he was hesitant about taking any positive steps until he had verified Stiles's account of the situation. He asked Dr. Simon Flexner to make a study of the hookworm problem, and when Flexner reported that the disease was indeed widespread in the South and that he agreed with Stiles that it was both preventable and curable, Gates decided to present the matter to Mr. Rockefeller. The result was the creation of the Rockefeller Sanitary Commission, to which Mr. Rockefeller made a pledge of $1 million to be spent over a period of five years. Wickliffe Rose was appointed Director of the hookworm campaign, and Stiles served as scientific advisor (Fosdick, 1952; Penfield, 1967).

The campaign began with a survey to determine the incidence of the disease in the 11 southern states that were under study. It was quickly found that the disease was indeed rampant. In some of the rural schools the number of infected children ran as high as 90 per cent, and the overall incidence among a half million children examined between 1910 and 1914 was 39 per cent. The incidence was also high among adults; for example, 42 per cent in 300 college students and 32 per cent in three regiments of state militia. The survey also disclosed that most of the physicians of the affected areas were unaware of the problem and were unfamiliar with the methods for diagnosing and treating hookworm infestation.

While the facts on prevalence were being gathered, the battle against the disease was opened with a publicity campaign utilizing the newspapers, the schools, printed leaflets, and local boards of health to make the people aware of the extent and seriousness of the disease and of methods for prevention and treatment. The principal means of prevention were (1) the construction of sanitary privies to prevent the eggs in the feces from reaching exposed soil; and (2) the wearing of shoes to prevent the larvae from reaching the skin. For treatment, the medical organizations of the South cooperated with the Commission in establishing free outdoor clinics where the diagnosis could be made and appropriate medication started. Fortunately, a simple and effective remedy had been developed in Italy in the latter part of the nineteenth century. This treatment required only the administration of capsules of thymol and salts over a period of 18 hours.

The campaign against hookworm disease brought gratifying results very rapidly. The principal obstacle to success was ignorance and lack of interest on the part of some people. As a result not everyone took the necessary precautions against acquiring the infection, and not everyone who needed it received treatment. A report in 1940 by Keller, Leathers, and Densen indicated that in six of the southern states involved in the campaign, the incidence of hookworm infestation, which had been 36.6 per cent in 1910–14, had fallen to 11.2 per cent in 1930–38. The improvement in the morale, physical development, and sense of well-being of the people of the South was greater than these figures might seem to indicate.

PUBLIC HEALTH EDUCATION

University education in the field of public health and preventive medicine developed slowly in the United States. As early as 1850, Lemuel Shattuck, in his Report of the Massachusetts Sanitary Commission, recommended "that persons be specially educated in sanitary science, as preventive advisors as well as curative advisors. . . . Sanitary professorships should be established in all our colleges and medical schools, and filled by competent teachers. The science of preserving health and preventing disease should be taught as one of the most important sciences." At the first meeting of the American Public Health Association in 1872, Andrew White, President of Cornell University, contended that "fundamental instruction in Colleges, Universities and Medical Colleges should be provided in Physiology, Hygiene, and Sanitation."

Little heed was paid to such exhortations, however, and in 1881, J. M. Gregory, an educator, wrote that "the omission of hygiene as a subject for study in medical colleges is a serious defect in the education system." Although a number of textbooks on public health were available to medical students, Smillie states that hygiene, sanitation, preventive medicine, and

342

public health were taught only casually. "The subjects were assigned to one or more of the professors who were most interested in these fields, and a series of didactic lectures were given to apathetic and uninterested students. . . . The whole trend of the 19th Century was to limit the teaching of medical students to the intensely practical fields of diagnosis and treatment" (Smillie, 1955).

The year after his arrival in Baltimore, in 1885, W. H. Welch saw the need for better instruction in hygiene and preventive medicine, and he sent one of his graduate students, Alexander C. Abbott, to Europe to study under Koch in Berlin and under von Pettenkofer at the Hygienic Institute in Munich. Shortly after Abbott's return to Baltimore in 1889, he organized a miniature hygienic laboratory modeled on the Munich institute. But while Abbott was still in Europe, Victor C. Vaughan at the University of Michigan, early in 1889, had opened the first laboratory in America devoted to teaching and research in hygiene. A three-month course in bacteriology and related hygienic subjects was offered, at first only as an elective, but in 1890 courses in hygiene were provided in the regular curriculum for third- and fourth-year medical students. The little hygienic institute at Johns Hopkins was never fully launched, because Abbott was called to Philadelphia in 1890. There he served as assistant to John Shaw Billings, who had just organized a Laboratory of Hygiene at the University of Pennsylvania. Billings occupied the chair of Hygiene at that university until he was succeeded by Abbott in 1896. In the latter year Abbott also gave the first course of lectures in hygiene at the Johns Hopkins Medical School. The first School of Public Health and Preventive Medicine was organized at the Army Medical School in 1893 by Surgeon-General Sternberg. The University of Michigan, in 1910, was the first institution in the United States to award a specific degree in Public Health.

Even before the first laboratories and courses and professorships in hygiene and public health had been launched, two leading American educators had begun to urge that these subjects be raised to a higher level in the university faculties. The first of these educators was President Eliot of Harvard, who in his annual report for 1882–83 wrote (Cannon, 1934):

The University has no professorship of public health, or preventive medicine,—a modern subject of great importance which can be properly dealt with only through an endowed professorship, because the professor if properly devoted to his subject would be cut off from private practice. It would be a great service to humanity to divert even a tithe of the money annually given to charities of pauperizing tendency towards the promotion of medical teaching and research.

The following year, Eliot again drew attention to the desirability of a professorship of "Hygiene and Public Health." Year after year, Eliot continued to emphasize the importance of these subjects. At the dedication of the new buildings of the Harvard Medical School in 1906 (Cannon, 1934) he predicted that in the years ahead medicine would

deal more extensively than in the past with preventive medicine, or in other words, with the causes of disease as it attacks society, the community, or the state, rather than the individual. The object in view will be not only to arrest or modify a malady which has appeared in the body of the patient, but, as in the recent case of yellow

343

fever, to learn how the disease is communicated and how to prevent that communication.... The function of the nineteenth century physician will continue, ... but another sort of physician will be at work in the twentieth century preventing the access of epidemics, limiting them when they arrive, defending society from bad food and drink, and reducing to the lowest terms the manifold evils which result from the congestion of population.... And this work will be endless; for civilization involves constant changes in the environment of the human race; and it is on medical science that the race must depend for protecting it from the new dangers which accompany each novel environment.

In 1909, the year of Eliot's retirement, he finally got his wish. The professorship that he had proposed in 1883 became a reality with the appointment of Milton J. Rosenau as Professor of Preventive Medicine and Hygiene. In 1913 Rosenau joined forces with W. T. Sedgwick, who since 1883 had given a course at the Massachusetts Institute of Technology in what today would be called "sanitary engineering." Their joint venture was named *The Harvard Medical School and Massachusetts Institute of Technology School of Public Health.* This school functioned effectively until 1922, when it was discontinued because of a court ruling that the granting of a joint degree was not permitted under the charters of the two schools. Following this, each institution continued its own separate School of Public Health.

The second educator to emphasize the importance of hygiene and public health was William H. Welch. In 1884 when he was studying in Germany, Welch wrote to President Gilman of Johns Hopkins: "I have long been particularly impressed with the hygienic institute which is the pride of the Medical School in Munich. I hope we may have a similar institute in Baltimore" (Flexner and Flexner, 1941). Welch felt that the essential feature would be an institute "which would not only train health officers but would react upon the medical school of the university where it was placed and contribute to the training of physicians going into general practice."

Like Eliot, Welch never missed an opportunity to set forth his views on the importance of hygiene and preventive medicine in the education of a physician. In 1899 he said, "The development of laboratories connected with Boards of Health is one which is peculiarly American. Their greatest usefulness has been their assistance to physicians in making diagnoses of such diseases as tuberculosis, typhoid fever, malaria and diphtheria, and the work they have done in furthering the treatment of diphtheria by antitoxin has been particularly valuable." However, Welch was not at all satisfied with this accomplishment alone. He still pointed out vigorously that such laboratories of hygiene should also be established in universities, since they were greatly needed to train scientific hygienic workers and to make new discoveries, which the state laboratories could then practically apply. It was his regret at this time that only a few such laboratories connected with medical colleges and universities were in existence in this country.

Welch was not only interested in giving hygiene and public health a more important place in the faculty; from time to time he harked back to his view, first expressed in 1884, that a separate Hygienic Institute, similar to the one in Munich, was desirable. By 1914 other influences were converging to support this view. Wickliffe Rose, in his efforts to organize the hookworm campaign in the southern states and in his planning to develop similar campaigns in Brazil and other countries, had come face to face with the lack of trained public health workers. He discussed with Gates, Buttrick, Abraham Flexner, and other Rockefeller officials the desirability of developing a program to train workers in this field; and he outlined a plan for creating an Institute of Hygiene in connection with an existing university. At about the same time (1914), Hermann M. Biggs, who had become a very influential figure in public health circles and who had just been appointed Health Commissioner of New York State, drew attention to the fact that there were 1200 health officers in his state who had been very indifferently trained in the principles that they were expected to apply. He stated that it would be desirable to have a one- or two-year course designed specifically for the education of public health workers.

In October, 1914, a conference on training for public health was held at the office of the General Education Board in New York. The discussion at this meeting established substantial agreement on the following points: (1) that a fundamental need in the public health service of this country at the present time is for men adequately trained for the work; (2) that a distinct contribution toward meeting this need could be made by establishing at some convenient place a School of Public Health of high standard; (3) that such an institution, while maintaining its separate identity, should in the interest of both economy and efficiency be closely affiliated with a university and its medical school; and (4) that the nucleus of this School of Public Health should be an Institute of Hygiene (Welch and Rose, 1920).

At the conclusion of the meeting, Rose and Welch, both of whom had participated in the discussion, were asked to formulate a plan for an Institute of Hygiene. The plan that they prepared was presented to the General Education Board in May, 1915, and to the Trustees of the Rockefeller Foundation in January, 1916. It recommended the creation of a separate Institute of Hygiene and Public Health within an established university and outlined the educational program that would be provided by the proposed institute. The concluding paragraph of the report was as follows:

> *The benefits to be expected from the establishment of such an institute as that proposed are not to be measured solely by the number of students trained within its walls. The institute can supply only a relatively small number of those who desire to enter upon public health service. The far-reaching influence of the institute should be felt in the advancement of the science and the improvement of the practice of public health, in establishing higher standards and better methods of professional education in this field, in stimulating the foundation of similar institutes in other parts of the country, in supplying teachers and in cooperating with schools of a simpler character designed for briefer technical training which should be established in each state in connection jointly with boards of health and medical schools.*

When it became known in educational circles that the General Education Board, with Abraham Flexner at the helm, was considering making a grant to the Johns Hopkins University for the establishment of an Institute of Hygiene and Public Health, Mr. Eliot, no longer President of Harvard but still concerned about public health education, was disturbed and wrote a letter to Abraham Flexner on February 1, 1916, in which he said (Flexner and Flexner, 1941):

> The more I consider the project of placing the proposed Institute of Hygiene at Baltimore, the less suitable and expedient I find it. . . . In comparison with either Boston or New York, it [Baltimore] conspicuously lacks public spirit and beneficent community action. The personality and career of Dr. Welch are the sole argument for putting the Institute in Baltimore—and he is almost sixty-six years old, and will have no similar successor. . . . My life-long interest in the great problems of public health and sanitation will account in your mind for this frank statement.

According to the Flexners, "Abraham Flexner replied that the argument for locating the school in Baltimore was based not on Welch alone, but also on the medical school, and he ventured to prophesy that the medical school would endure after Welch's days were over. However, Eliot was not appeased; he wrote that the Hopkins school was 'one man's work in a new and small university made comparatively independent of community action by large bequests from one benefactor.' "

Regardless of Eliot's protest, the Rockefeller Foundation proceeded with its plan to locate the proposed Institute in Baltimore. A Committee appointed to study the matter, deciding that the success of such an undertaking would depend largely on who was chosen as its Director, recommended that Welch be asked to retire from his other duties at Hopkins to accept this new responsibility. Welch, after some deliberation, accepted the directorship, and the Rockefeller Foundation appropriated $267,000 to found the institution that became known as the Johns Hopkins School of Hygiene and Public Health. The School was opened in October, 1918, and in its early years was supported by annual grants from the Rockefeller Foundation. In 1922 the Foundation awarded it an endowment fund of $6 million.

By the time the School's new and handsomely equipped building, located across the street from the Medical School, was opened in 1925, Welch had selected a distinguished faculty in a variety of disciplines related to sanitation, preventive medicine, and public health. Courses were offered in physiology, epidemiology, bacteriology, immunology, virology, vital statistics, chemistry, and nutrition including vitamins and other accessory food factors. These studies led to the degree of Doctor of Public Health or Doctor of Science in Hygiene, or to a certificate in public health.

According to F. F. Russell (Flexner and Flexner, 1941), Professor of Preventive Medicine and Epidemiology at Harvard, the Hopkins School of Hygiene and Public Health

> marked the turning point in public health education not only in this country but throughout the world. As everyone knows the early efforts of von Pettenkofer were for a time overshadowed by the advent of the bacteriologists, and education in public health became, as a result of this, the education of the health officer in the control of infectious diseases, to the almost complete exclusion of all other aspects of public health. In Britain and on the continent and here at the University of Pennsylvania under Abbott, and at the Massachusetts Institute of Technology under Sedgwick the main subject was bacteriology. Dr. Welch appreciated the one-sidedness of public health education and went back to von Pettenkofer and introduced into the new Hopkins curriculum all the disciplines which had any bearing

on hygiene, statistics, nutrition, administration, parasitology and physiology, and he provided a faculty that was competent in all these fields, in contrast with the institutions of hygiene of Germany and Great Britain, where the education in public health was under the charge of the professor of bacteriology of the medical school. Of the new departments, that dealing with vital statistics was perhaps the most important, and [Raymond] Pearl developed this field in such a way that it has influenced all the departments. . . . The entire personnel of our public health services is now being built up with men who have graduated from the new schools, and the day of the self-educated health officer has already passed. While it is too early to say that the new schools have eliminated politics from public health, it is fair to say that political appointments are now the exception rather than the rule. The papers presented at public health officers' meetings have radically changed; formerly the best dealt with methods of administration; at present more and more papers deal with the scientific basis on which administrative practices can be made more effective. Gradually a better class of men is being attracted to careers in public health. . . . This change in the whole question of public health is, I believe, due to Dr. Welch, and he foresaw the entire development when he planned the Hopkins, which in turn influenced other schools.

As indicated in Professor Russell's comments, it did not take long for other universities to follow the example set by Welch. The Harvard School of Public Health, which would have afforded great satisfaction to Eliot, was founded in 1922 and has had a very distinguished career.

VITAL STATISTICS

The word "statistics" came into the English language at about the time of the Revolutionary War, to signify that branch of political inquiry concerned with the collection and classification of facts bearing on the condition of a state. *Vital statistics,* comprising numerical records of marriages, births, sickness, and deaths, provide the data needed for the study of the growth and health of a community. These data are of value from many points of view, but they are absolutely essential to guide the work of public health officials.

Death rates, which are perhaps the most important vital statistic from the point of view of public health, are usually expressed as the number of deaths per 100,000 population per year. To determine the total death rate or the death rate for any particular disease it is therefore necessary to know not only the number of deaths but also the size of the population within which those deaths occurred; the number of deaths is the *numerator,* and the size of the population is the *denominator* of the death-rate fraction. The numerical data for the denominator of this fraction began to be gathered in the United States when the first census of the population was taken in 1790. Although the census has been recorded every 10 years since that time, the data required for the numerator of the fraction were never accurately recorded on a national scale during the first century. In the census of 1850, the census-takers were instructed to record the number of deaths that had occurred in each household during the last year of the census period. This procedure was repeated in 1860 and 1870. Theoretically, the data obtained in these three censuses should have made it possible to calculate death rates for the nation and for each state. However, a critical study of the data disclosed that they were altogether untrustworthy. Some of the larger cities had been keeping accurate records of all deaths within their jurisdictions, and when these figures were compared with those of the census-takers it was found that the latter were sometimes as much as 40 per cent below the actual number.

When the census of 1880 came around, John Shaw Billings, who was the instigator of so many other important advances in medicine, decided that he would try his hand at improving the compilation of death statistics. He prepared a supplement to the census report, which was based on a study that he had made of the accuracy and completeness of the mortality records kept by many cities and a few states. For his supplement he selected the records that he found to be most trustworthy. The records included were those of two states, Massachusetts and New Jersey, the District of Columbia, and 19 cities from other states. Thus, a reasonably accurate numerator was provided for calculating the death rate in a population of about 4 million. This was only about 17 per cent of the total population of the nation, and just how applicable the figures were to the nation as a whole is questionable, since they came largely from urban populations at a time when 85 per cent of the population was rural. Nevertheless, the figures were far more accurate than any which had previously been available, and the sample was large enough to permit limited conclusions regarding death rates. The area from which Billings derived his data became known as the *death registration area.*

During the next two decades, in a number of lectures and papers, and with constant support from the American Public Health Association, Billings attracted attention to the value of vital statistics in public health work, and he urged the various states to improve their methods of collecting data so that they could be included in the registration area. In this effort he was joined by a number of others who understood and approved of his objectives.

The annual compilation of mortality statistics in their present form began in the United States in 1900. In that year the registraton area included 10 states and many cities in other states. Only one "western" state, Michigan, was in the area. No state with a large black population was admitted to the registration area until 1906, when Maryland was added. By 1920 all except 14 states were included, and by 1933 the area included all of the 48 states then in the Union (Cassedy, 1965).

A great advance in the registration of deaths occurred about 1900, when a standard death certificate was devised. This certificate came into general use in the registration area in 1915. Physicians were required to report every death and the cause of death on the standard form. The reporting of births on a standard birth certificate began in the registration area in 1915.

The gross death rate has little significance to the public health official. It is only when the cause of death is recorded and tabulated that the health officer has information on which he can take action. The recording of deaths according to cause has always presented problems. These problems were insuperable in the first century, when Benjamin Rush and his followers believed that almost all deaths were due to a single cause and when the methods of diagnosis were so inadequate. In the second century, the dif-

348

ferentiation of one disease from another has become much more precise, but there are still more than a few cases in which the attending physician has to make an educated guess when he enters the cause of death on the certificate. However, the real difficulty in the beginning of the second century was to devise a practical, comprehensive, uniform nomenclature of the causes of death, which could be understood and applied by physicians everywhere.

When Billings began collecting information on death rates, the nomenclature that was most widely used for death registration was a list of the causes of death devised by William Farr, Registrar-General of England. New developments in medicine made Farr's list obsolete before 1900, and shortly

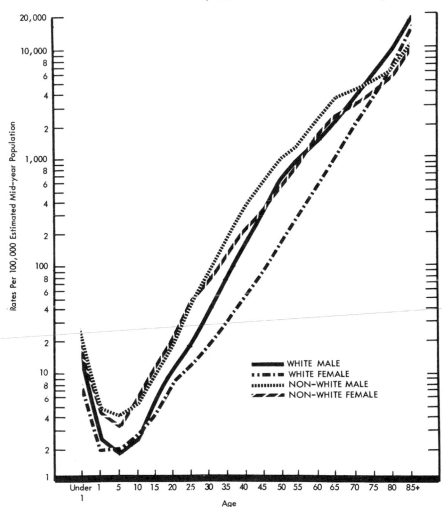

DEATH RATES FROM MAJOR CARDIOVASCULAR RENAL DISEASES
BY FIVE YEAR AGE GROUPS, COLOR AND SEX - UNITED STATES, 1962

Figure 86. Death rates from major cardiovascular diseases—United States, 1962. (President's Commission on Heart Disease, Cancer and Stroke. Vol. II. Washington, D.C., Government Printing Office, February, 1965.)

after that year American registrars substituted for it the new *International List of Causes of Death* prepared by a Frenchman, Jacques Bertillon. The Bertillon system of nomenclature took into account the more modern methods of diagnosis, including the precise identification of infectious diseases by bacteriological methods. The International List has been kept up to date; it had its fourth decennial revision in 1939, and other revisions have been published since then. Another classification that has been used extensively in the United States is the *American Standard Nomenclature,* which was first published in 1931. The responsibility for revisions of this system was assumed by the American Medical Association. At present the cause of death recorded on the death certificate by the attending physician is translated into a uniform language according to the *International Statistical Classification of Diseases, Injuries and Causes of Death,* prepared under the sponsorship of the World Health Organization of the United Nations. The data are sorted, classified, and tabulated at the National Center for Health Statistics of the United States Public Health Service in Washington, D.C. (Peery, 1975).

Maintenance of accurate vital statistics has been more difficult in the United States than in some of the older, more stable European countries because of the varying tides of immigration. In addition, there have been great movements of the population from the relatively settled East to the open spaces of the West and from the country into the cities and more recently from the cities to the suburbs. These movements of the population have made the denominator in the death-rate fraction almost as variable and unpredictable as the numerator. In order to obtain a reasonably accurate denominator for the annual tabulation of death rates, the Census Bureau has had to provide estimates of the size of the population for the years between the decennial census years.

Another factor affecting the significance of death rates has been the rise in the average age of the population. As effective methods have been developed to reduce infant mortality and to prevent or cure the infectious diseases, which killed so many children and young adults in the nineteenth century, the proportion of the population surviving beyond the sixth decade of life has increased dramatically. While the deaths from infectious diseases have declined, some of them almost to the vanishing point, those from the diseases of the elderly—cancer, heart disease, stroke, and so forth—have risen proportionately. Deaths from these diseases have increased chiefly because there are more old people (see Table 3). Indeed, if an adjustment is made for age, there is evidence that the death rate from cardiovascular disease has actually declined among females and has not risen in the male population (see Figure 87).

The activities of state and national health services are guided not only by surveillance of the causes of death but also by keeping close track of the actual incidence of various diseases. If a rise in incidence of an infectious disease is detected early enough, effective preventive measures (such as isolation of patients, administration of vaccines, and extermination of animal hosts and insect vectors) can be taken. In England, reporting of "dangerous infectious diseases" began on an informal basis in the mid-nineteenth century and was made compulsory by an Act of Parliament in 1889. Reporting of diseases in the United States was started by individual

TABLE 3. PROPORTION OF POPULATION OVER 64 YEARS OF AGE

Year	Per Cent Over 64
1850	2.5
1900	4.1
1940	6.9
1950	8.2
1965	9.4
1972	10.0

states, and it is still governed by state laws. The Massachusetts State Board of Health, in 1874, inaugurated a system for the voluntary reporting of prevalent infectious diseases and obtained the cooperation of more than a hundred physicians in submitting weekly reports. Two years later a similar voluntary system was instituted in Michigan, in which the physicians submitted their reports on postcards provided for the purpose. Michigan was

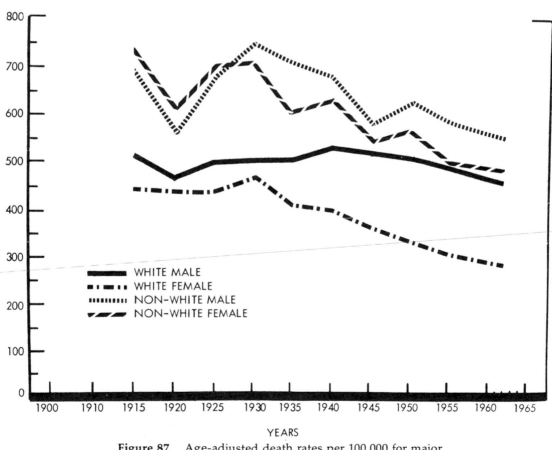

Figure 87.   Age-adjusted death rates per 100,000 for major cardiovascular diseases, United States, 1900–1962. (President's Commission on Heart Disease, Cancer and Stroke. Vol. II. Washington, D.C., Government Printing Office, February, 1965.)

351

also the first state (1883) to make obligatory the reporting of contagious diseases to the public health officials, but oddly enough it was the owner of the house where the disease occurred rather than the attending physician who was responsible for submitting the report. The following year Massachusetts passed a similar law, but this time it was the physician rather than the householder who had to notify the health officer. By the 1940s, each state had a long list of diseases on which physicians and hospitals were required to report.

16

Federal Government and Medicine

The year 1940 marked the beginning of a new era in the relations of the federal government and science. So far as a line can be drawn across the continuous path of history this date separates the first century and a half of American experience in the field from what has come after. As the scale of operations changed completely, science moved dramatically to the center of the stage. By the time the bombs fell on Hiroshima and Nagasaki, the entire country was aware that science was a political, economic and social force of the first magnitude.

(A. Hunter Dupree, 1957)

Except for research conducted by the regular governmental departments, such as the Army, the Navy, the Department of Agriculture, and the Public Health Service, the federal government showed little interest in providing funds specifically for medical research prior to World War I. During the war, the medical affairs of the armed forces were carried out under the general supervision of the Medical Division of the Council of National Defense, which had been created by President Wilson in 1916. One of the major wartime problems with which the Medical Division had to grapple was that of venereal disease in the Army camps, and it was on the recommendation of this Division that the first substantial federal appropriation specifically designated for research was made, under the Chamberlain-Kahn Act of 1918 for the study of venereal disease control.

During the period after World War I the government was involved to a modest extent in the support of research. It was not until the establishment of the National Institute of Health (NIH) in 1930 that the groundwork was laid for the ultimate role of the government in this area.

The National Institute of Health grew out of the Hygienic Laboratory,

353

the origin of which was described in an earlier chapter. This Laboratory gained official recognition in 1901 when Congress appropriated $35,000 for a building to house it. Its functions at that time involved chiefly practical matters: foreign and interstate quarantine; medical inspection of immigrants; and the acquisition of up-to-date information on the causes, sources, mode of spread, diagnosis, and prevention of major communicable diseases. To coordinate the activities of the Hygienic Laboratory with other activities of the Public Health Service (PHS), a Division of Scientific Research was created in 1901, and the Laboratory was operated as a unit of this Division.

The initial work of the Hygienic Laboratory was concerned almost exclusively with microbiology and communicable diseases, but its research moved into a new area in 1910, when the Public Health Service turned its attention to cancer. In 1922 the Division of Scientific Research sponsored a small laboratory at the Harvard Medical School for the study of malignant disease. Only a modest amount of money was allocated for cancer research: the combined expenditures for this purpose at the Hygienic Laboratory and at Harvard amounted to no more than $11,000 in 1922, and it was projected that it would not exceed $25,000 per year in the future. Emphasis on the study of chronic noncommunicable diseases continued to increase. By 1930 the Public Health Service was becoming involved in the study of heart disease and the biochemical and endocrinological aspects of mental disease.

In the late 1920s two United States senators, Matthew Neely and Joseph Ransdell, began to agitate in the Congress for appropriation of funds for the support of cancer research. The interest of the public in this subject and in research in general was aroused by some excellent science-writing in the magazines and news media. Increased public awareness and support led to the passage, in 1930, of the Ransdell Act "to establish and operate a National Institute of Health, create a system of fellowships in said Institute, and to authorize the government to accept donations for use in ascertaining the cause, prevention and cure of disease affecting human beings, and for other purposes." The act also provided $750,000 for the erection of additional buildings to house the Public Health Service. The major share of credit for the passage of the Ransdell Act should go to Lewis Thompson, then Assistant Surgeon-General of the U.S. Public Health Service, who became the first Director of the National Institute. Thompson was also responsible for obtaining a gift of land to the government from Mr. and Mrs. Luke I. Wilson — 82 acres in Bethesda, Maryland, adjoining the District of Columbia. The National Institute of Health was built on this land.

Additional expenditures for investigation of disease and problems of sanitation were authorized by Congress in the Social Security Act of 1935. Two years later, following a widely publicized crusade for the "conquest of cancer" in which the members of Congress were deluged with letters, a Bill was enacted to establish a National Cancer Institute, and $700,000 was appropriated for this purpose. A building for the Institute was constructed on the Bethesda property.

The National Cancer Institute was authorized to conduct and foster studies and research relating to the cause, prevention, and methods of diagnosis and treatment of cancer; to promote the coordination of cancer research; to provide fellowships at the Institute as well as at other institutions; to secure counsel and advice from cancer experts in the United States and abroad; and to cooperate with state health agencies in the prevention, control, and eradication of cancer. Dr. Carl Voegtlin, who was mentioned in an earlier chapter as head of the Chemical Division of Barker's Medical Clinic at Johns Hopkins, was made Director, and a staff of some 30 scientists was secured representing basic approaches to cancer research in such fields as biophysics, biochemistry, biology, bacteriology, pharmacology, and statistics.

In spite of opposition from the Public Health Service, an Advisory Council on Cancer was created and was given authority to review all research proposals and to certify them for approval prior to funding by the Surgeon-General. Thus was born an important principle: peer review and certification prior to allocation of government funds for medical research.

In order to stimulate outside research, the Institute considered 137 applications for grants-in-aid between 1938 and 1940 and awarded 33 grants involving a total of $220,000. Here was the first concrete evidence that federal funds would provide a new order of magnitude of financial support for research.

Other important developments were establishment of the Walter Reed Hospital with its Institute for Medical Research as the principal Army Medical Center and the Naval Hospital with its Institute of Medical Research. Another Washington-based center of government research was developed at St. Elizabeth's Hospital under the auspices of the Department of Interior, an institution which since the Civil War days had treated mentally ill patients from the military services. Here the first American studies of the use of malaria in the treatment of syphilis of the central nervous system were carried out.

By 1937 more than 120 government agencies were involved to some degree in research of some type. Total federal research expenses for that year reached a high of $124 million. In comparison to the situation in universities, where the ratio of research to total expenditures was as high as 25 per cent, that in governmental activities was only 1.4 per cent, and only two thirds of federal funds were allocated to the natural sciences and technology, including medicine.

In 1947 the national expenditure for medical research totaled $87 million, of which the federal share was $27 million, or 31 per cent. The National Institute of Health that year expended $8.3 million, or 10 per cent of the national total and 30 per cent of the federal share. This was no more than a fraction of what the expenditures would be in subsequent years.

The transformation of the role of the federal government in national affairs that took place in the 1930s was a major event. For the first time in its history, the government reached out directly in a time of peace to involve itself in the social and economic security of the people of the nation in a massive way. This shift of governmental action set the scene for the great events of the future.

In the period just preceding World War II there was concern over the decline in private foundation aid to research and a growing demand for coordination of research on a larger scale and with more government support. However, few steps were taken in this direction until the advent of the national emergency of 1941. In fact, as Shryock (1945) points out: "The manner

355

in which the federal government turned to scientists in the successive emergencies of 1861, 1917, and 1941 provides a very good measure of the growing recognition that even national survival might turn on the adequacy of research." Prior to World War II, the mechanism for coordinating different federal agencies working in the health field presented a vexing problem. In 1939 the Public Health Service and the Food and Drug Administration were placed in the Federal Security Agency, which later was incorporated into the Department of Health, Education and Welfare.

World War II brought many changes. The several military services and the PHS were unable to agree on a coordinated approach to military medical problems. In 1941 the Office of Scientific Research and Development was created by order of President Roosevelt and placed under the direction of Vannevar Bush, President of the Carnegie Institution. Alfred Newton Richards, who was then Vice-President for Medical Affairs of the University of Pennsylvania, was appointed Chairman of the Committee on Medical Research. The CMR had the job of "mobilizing the medical and scientific personnel of the nation; recommending contracts to be entered into with Universities, Hospitals and other agencies conducting medical research activities; and submitting recommendations with respect to medical problems related to the national defense." Committees and panels to review the needs in many fields were set up, which ultimately led to 593 contracts with 135 universities, hospitals, research institutions, and industrial firms. The activities of the CMR utilized the services of approximately 17,000 doctors of medicine and 38,000 scientists and technologists. Between 1941 and 1947, $25 million was spent through the six CMR divisions. "Never before," Dr. Richards said, "has there been so great a coordination of medical scientific labor." The Congress was impressed and attributed "the magnificent progress" in medical research to "adequate financing, coordination and team work." The success of this enterprise gave the impression that adequate financing could speed up the conquest of disease.

Throughout the war period the study of chronic and degenerative diseases was necessarily put aside. However, there was an increase in the magnitude of research in certain fundamental areas which had great value for the peacetime population. Advances were made in all the major divisions into which the CMR organized its work. In aviation medicine the chief advances related to overcoming some of the hazards of high-altitude and high-speed flying. In surgery progress was made in the prevention of infection in wounds and burns, the use of penicillin and the sulfonamides, and development of a new type of suture material. An outstanding contribution was the successful separation of blood derivatives by E. J. Cohn's group at Harvard. The protein fractions that they isolated proved invaluable for the prevention and treatment of shock, control of hemorrhage, and the prevention of certain infectious diseases by the use of one of the fractions, gammaglobulin. In chemistry the most spectacular gain was the development of effective insecticides and rodenticides. But the outstanding achievement of the whole program was the development of penicillin. For this the Committee entered into contracts with the Bradley Polytechnic Institute at Peoria, Illinois, to support studies conducted by Robert Coghill of the Northern Regional Research Laboratories.

356   It was necessary to sort out the strains of the fungus *Penicillium* adapt-

able to large-scale production of the active principle, to find suitable conditions of growth, and to seek better methods of extraction and purification. The information obtained by Dr. Coghill was promptly transmitted to commercial firms already working on the problem. Production was stepped up from one-liter bottles to 15,000-gallon tanks. The development of penicillin affords a striking illustration of the effectiveness of a well-financed and coordinated approach to the practical application of a basic medical discovery. No private, uncoordinated effort could have secured such results in a comparable period of time, as evidenced by the slow progress in the development of this drug after its discovery by Fleming in 1928.

The nation was impressed by these accomplishments which generated great expectations for scientific research as a way to solve national problems. Thus, as a result of the development of penicillin and the atomic bomb, the public was ready to give generous support to science and particularly to medical research.

In 1943 the Surgeon-General of the Public Health Service, Dr. Thomas Parran, appointed a Committee to make recommendations for the reorganization of the PHS. These recommendations ultimately led to a legislative proposal to revise and consolidate all of the laws under which the PHS operated. This proposal resulted in the adoption of the Public Health Service Act of 1944. The Act gave the Service authority to "pay for research to be performed by laboratories, hospitals, universities and other public or private institutions." The Service was authorized to support such research through grants rather than through contracts, and it was given specific authority to award grants to individuals.

At about the same time, President Roosevelt requested Vannevar Bush, Director of the Office of Scientific Research and Development, to recommend measures for utilizing the wartime experience to develop a postwar research program that would be useful to the public and would enable the federal government to aid research in public and private institutions. While Bush was preparing his recommendations, the American Association for the Advancement of Science, in September, 1944, took a strong stand in favor of a national research establishment equivalent in rank and authority to the legislative, executive, and judiciary branches of the federal government.

Bush's report, which was submitted to President Truman in 1945, recommended that Congress establish a National Research Foundation as an independent entity, which would ensure a coordinated approach to all the nation's research needs and would simultaneously prevent government interference in the conduct of research in the private sector. Bush's recommendations were not implemented, however, because the spokesman for the Public Health Service, Rolla E. Dyer, Director of the National Institute of Health, pointed out that the PHS already had "all of the authority in reference to health and medical research that was contemplated for the proposed National Science Foundation." The PHS was obviously anxious not to have its authority undermined by a new foundation, and it would appear that this objective also had prompted a letter which Dyer had written to A. N. Richards in 1944, suggesting that the contracts awarded by the Committee on Medical Research be continued after the war by transferring them to the PHS. This transfer of contracts did indeed take place; those in the

357

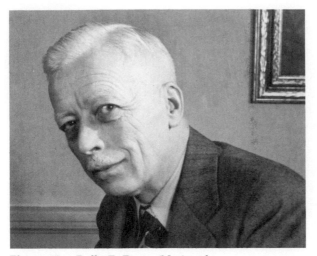

Figure 88. Rolla E. Dyer. (National
Library of Medicine, Bethesda,
Maryland.)

biomedical area were transferred to the National Institute of Health and
those in the physical sciences to the Office of Naval Research. These
transfers to government agencies rather than to an independent science
foundation set a precedent that had far-reaching consequences in the
provision of federal support for research conducted in universities.

As a result of its new statutory authority and its new contracts, the PHS
needed more manpower and a bigger administrative budget. In 1946 the
Congress appropriated for the National Institute of Health almost $8 mil-
lion—more than a tenfold increase over its annual funding at the start of the
war. Thus, whatever course the government ultimately chose for its peacetime mechanism of research support, the NIH would inevitably play an important role.

These events came at a very propitious time. The biomedical sciences
had developed rapidly during the first four decades of the second century.
American contributions to this development had been impressive. These
advances could now be coupled with the new technical and research capability. The war effort brought much of this magnificent potential into focus.
When the war ended, American medical science was ready for major expansion. It was soon realized, however, that medical science could not attain
its objectives without public support. To gain such support the relevance to
public needs and expectations would have to be clearly delineated, as was
emphasized later by James A. Shannon, who became Director of the NIH in
the postwar era.

An important event influencing the growth of government support for
medical research was the appearance on the scene of Mrs. Albert D. Lasker,
wife of a prominent and wealthy citizen who had been Chairman of the
Shipping Board during World War I. Mrs. Lasker had for some time worked
with voluntary organizations and had been responsible for a streamlining
of the American Cancer Society. She was aware of the National Health Survey of 1936, which emphasized the poor state of health of the American

people. This seemed to be confirmed by the fact that of 14 million men examined for military service prior to June, 1944, no less than 4 million had been rejected as mentally or physically unfit. Her experience with private health-oriented organizations had convinced her that the private sector alone could never fill the total needs in the fight against disease. Mrs. Lasker, as a result of her background, had the capacity to "think big," and she also had the conviction that something could and should be done.

Mrs. Lasker had a friend, Mrs. Daniel (Florence) Mahoney, who had had experience in campaigning for improvement of health programs; and she had the power, through her family's newspaper connections, to help on the political front in the battle for expanded medical research support. Both ladies knew that Senator Claude Pepper was running for re-election in the spring of 1944. They supported him in his campaign, Lasker with money, Mahoney with editorial endorsement. Consequently, they were in a position to ask the senator, in the important 1944 hearings of his special Subcommittee on Wartime Health and Education, to give emphasis to the future of medical research. Thus, as emphasized by Strickland (1972), there appeared on the scene important lay reinforcements for the political battle to secure better support of medical research and education as well as better legislation for health care.

When Senator Pepper's hearings opened in December, 1944, the committee heard from 16 witnesses, half from the federal government and at least half of the others called at the suggestion of Mrs. Lasker. These witnesses testified that the existing sources of funds for peacetime medical research were inadequate. It was recommended that any new funds should be distributed equitably according to the importance of the medical problems. Senator Pepper supported this view and stated that "the volume of research which is carried out in the medical field should in my opinion not be limited by the lack of money."

The next big problem was the choice of a mechanism for the distribu-

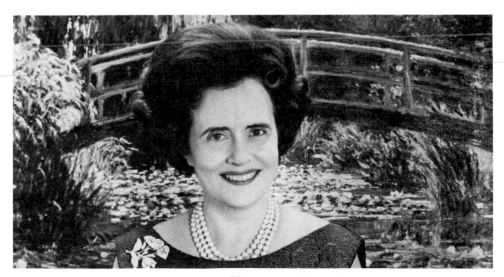

Figure 89. Mrs. Albert D. Lasker.

tion of the federal monies voted for medical research. Although the Public Health Service already had the statutory authority, the lay group was not convinced that the PHS had the vision to do the job successfully. At this critical point Leonard Scheele became Surgeon-General of the USPHS, and Mrs. Lasker quickly developed confidence in him and thus in the Public Health Service as the best sponsor for the government research program.

Up to this time the *American Society for the Control of Cancer* had been spending its efforts and funds on every aspect of malignant disease except research into its causes. In 1945 Mrs. Lasker began a special fund-raising effort for the Society with the promise that at least one quarter of the funds thus raised would be spent on research. Impressed by his wife's success, Albert Lasker joined the effort and got help from many important friends in business and industry. This group raised $4 million for the Cancer Society in 1945 in contrast to the $780,000 that had been raised the previous year. In 1946 the Lasker group raised $10 million, and the new Board of Directors, of which Mary Lasker was a member, changed the name of the organization to the *American Cancer Society* (Strickland, 1972).

As public demand increased for more and more government money for cancer research, the Public Health Service adopted a conservative attitude. This led Senator Neely to seek other avenues for administrative management under the provisions of the Neely Cancer Bill, which was backed by the Lasker forces. The PHS realized that not just money but also control over a new cancer effort was about to elude them. Scheele told Congress that while the Institute probably would not use all of the additional dollars the very next year, NIH hoped that Congress would authorize a higher appropriations ceiling so that as soon as the Cancer Institute built up its capacity to put the extra money to good use, it would be available. This satisfied Neely, but from then on the PHS knew that it had to think in terms of larger commitments in order to stay alive.

In 1945 Congressman Percy Priest introduced a Bill that would establish a Mental Health Division within the PHS and provide funds for the training of psychiatrists. Mrs. Lasker, though she favored the Bill, was then too involved in other matters to give it her personal attention (Strickland, 1972). Therefore, she suggested to the National Committee for Mental Hygiene that they employ a lobbyist. Mrs. Lasker put up the money, and Mr. Lynn Adams was hired. Within a year after its introduction, the National Mental Health Act was adopted (1946)—another legislative landmark and one that proved the effectiveness of a full-time paid lobbyist.

President Truman in October, 1946, asked his Scientific Research Board to examine the entire scientific program of the federal government. The report, known as the Steelman Report, stated that "the conquest of disease like the conquest of hunger is of primary concern to the people." The Board felt that "two major steps are needed promptly to assist in overcoming those barriers to realizing recent gains in medical science and to further progress. These were: (1) provision of substantial additional funds for training and research at the earliest possible moment; (2) formulation of a national policy on medical research."

Though deeply involved in medical research and public health services, the federal government in 1946 had not yet entered the field of medical care. Its only significant involvement in the delivery of personal health services was in the Marine hospitals and the hospitals and other medical facilities of the Veterans' Administration. The American Medical Association had strongly rejected every effort by government to enter the area of civilian medical care and had denounced President Roosevelt's flirtation with a national health program. As the 1876–1946 period was coming to an end, another battle between organized medicine and a liberal president was shaping up, for President Truman was preparing to follow the lead of his predecessor by submitting a new plan for a national system of health insurance.

17

American Medical Association

Resolved,*That the American Medical Association declares its opposition to the institution of any plan embodying the system of compulsory contributory insurance against illness, or any other plan of compulsory insurance which provides for medical service to be rendered contributors or their dependents, provided, controlled or regulated by any state or the Federal government.*

(Resolution of House of Delegates of the AMA, April, 1920)

In 1900 the American Medical Association (AMA) was still an ineffective organization, and it could not claim to lead or even to represent the medical profession. In the 45 states, 4 territories, and the District of Columbia, the AMA had a total of 8400 members, and of these, only 4332 subscribed to the *Journal* of the AMA. The ratio of members to the total number of medical practitioners varied: it was 1:4 in Colorado, 1:9 in Pennsylvania, 1:10 in Illinois, 1:13 in California, 1:19 in Massachusetts, 1:28 in New York, and 1:40 in Texas. With the reforms in the organization and leadership of the AMA that took place during the first decade of the twentieth century there was an extraordinary increase in the number of members. The membership in 1910 was 70,146, and by 1920 it had increased to 83,338, of whom 74,372 received the Journal. The percentage of the entire profession that held membership in 1920 varied from a low of 51.5 in the southwest central states to a high of 64.2 in the New England states. At this point the AMA could reasonably claim to be the voice of American medicine, though a significant segment of the profession was not included in its ranks.

During its first 50 years the AMA, in its weak way, championed a number of worthy and important causes, but it exerted almost no influence on legislation at either the state or national level. Its efforts to bring about a uniform nomenclature of diseases failed; its attempts to get the states to gather and record vital statistics were only partially successful—nine states in 1900 met the requirements of the census bureau for classification as "registration states." With the assistance of the American Public Health Association and aided by the anxiety created by the yellow fever epidemic of 1878, Congress was prevailed upon to establish a National Board of Health, but this victory was short-lived, since Congress, in effect, abolished the Board in 1883 through failure to appropriate funds for its support. However, toward the end of the nineteenth century, progress was at last being made in medical education and medical licensure; these were objectives toward which the AMA had striven since its creation.

The first major step in the reformation of the American Medical Association was taken in 1899 when it created a permanent *Committee on National Legislation* to represent the Association before Congress. The following year a *Special Committee on Reorganization* was appointed, composed of Joseph N. McCormack of Kentucky, P. Maxwell Foshay of Cleveland, and George H. Simmons of Chicago. At the annual meeting in 1901 the Special Committee presented proposals for a complete reform in the constitutional structure of the Association. It was recommended that the membership of the AMA be made up of all members of local medical societies affiliated with state societies. It would only be necessary for an applicant for membership to present a certificate of good standing in his local society and to pay the annual dues. The proposed new constitution made provision for a legislative body to be known as the House of Delegates and made up of representatives from state, rather than local, medical societies. In addition to the state representatives, provision was made for representation of the Army, Navy, and Marine Hospital Service, and also of the specialist sections of the Association. The basis of representation from the state and territorial societies was 1 delegate to every 500 members or fraction thereof. The membership of the House of Delegates was limited to 150. To stay within this limit, the constitution provided that as the membership of the state societies increased, the ratio of physicians to delegates would rise. A reapportionment of delegates was to be made every three years.

The Special Committee realized that the strength of the AMA would depend upon the strength of the county and state medical societies, and they urged the state societies to become incorporated and to accept as members all physicians who held membership in a county society. Following its own internal reorganization and the drafting of a Model Constitution for state societies, the Association launched a drive to strengthen existing local societies and to start new societies where none existed.

The organizational work fell largely to Dr. Joseph N. McCormack, who before undertaking this job had won the commendations of the public and the medical profession in his home state, Kentucky, where he had successfully agitated for the adoption of new public health laws and for enforcement of licensing statutes. McCormack persuaded the state societies to adopt the Model Constitution, and he assisted them in strengthening their organization. He stressed the advantages that better organization offered not only to the profession but also to the public. "No great reform," he said, "is possible without high ideals, and our ideal is a society in every county, in every state, containing as many as three or four medical men, embracing in its membership every reputable physician in the country and existing solely for improvement and helpfulness in everything related to the prosperity and well being, not only of every member of the profession as a whole, but of every citizen of this jurisdiction." In his organizational work McCormack also stressed the need for continuing education for physicians, and he urged the state and local societies to play a leading role in this field by encouraging publications, lectureships, and university extension courses to keep physicians abreast of new developments.

As a result of McCormack's organizing campaign, which extended into every portion of every state and territory, there was a phenomenal growth in the number of local medical societies and in their membership and in the membership of the AMA. By the time the campaign ended in 1911, more than 200 medical societies had established postgraduate training courses, and many state societies were publishing their own medical journals.

During the decade of reform, the AMA had some strong and distinguished leaders. Its presidents included William J. Mayo in 1905, William C. Gorgas in 1908, and William H. Welch in 1909. George H. Simmons, a wise and able physician, was Secretary of the Association and the Editor of its *Journal*. In his presidential address in 1910 Dr. Welch said that Simmons "has done more than anyone else to determine and further the policies of the Association and to place it in its present high position of influence and usefulness." It was during this same decade that the Association decided to establish its permanent headquarters in Chicago.

As part of its reform movement, the AMA began in 1904 to concentrate attention upon medical education. In that year the Council on Medical Education was established. This body, as described previously, played an important role in educational reform.

In its effort to gain greater political effectiveness, the AMA tried to persuade its members that some of them should run for political office. It was pointed out that 12 of the 13 original states had sent at least one physician to the Congress when it was first assembled. In 1900, with 45 states in the Union, there were only one physician in the Senate and five physicians in the House of Representatives. The one physician in the Senate, Jacob H. Gallinger of New Hampshire, though he possessed an M.D. degree, was in fact an old fashioned homeopath, and he created problems for the future of medical research by sponsoring in the Senate an Antivivisection Bill. The passage of the Bill was defeated largely through efforts organized by W. H. Welch. According to the Flexners, Dr. Welch "dropped all other activities and during the winter of 1897–98 changed himself into a political lobbyist." The following year Gallinger presented his Bill again. At the committee hearings on this occasion Welch appeared with a number of distinguished individuals, and their evidence was so overwhelmingly in favor of vivisection that Gallinger withdrew his Bill before it could be put to a vote.

The AMA did not succeed in its campaign to get more doctors into Congress. On the other hand, it found that its new organizational structure, sprouting from the grassroots of the local and state medical societies, gave it unexpected political strength. The AMA could get its message to its widely scattered members, who in turn could effectively pressure their representatives in the state legislature or in the national Congress. In 1905 the AMA's Committee on Medical Legislation prepared a list of local political leaders in all recognized and organized political parties; this list included the names of over 11,000 politicians. In 1907 the AMA made another move that was of political importance: it published its *Directory of Physicians*. Not only did the new Directory enhance the prestige of the Association but also it served the purposes of the Association by listing licensed practitioners but failing to list those who were unlicensed. In the year in which the Directory was published, the House of Delegates established the *Bureau of Medical Legislation,* which was given a permanent staff and took an active part in politics from that year onward.

The AMA's greatest political victory in the decade of reform occurred before the Bureau of Medical Legislation was established, with the passage of the *Pure Food and Drugs Act* of 1906. The *Journal* of the AMA and several of the Association's committees had joined in the battle for the passage of this Act, and for the first time the grassroots mechanism had been employed to influence the votes of some members of Congress.

The AMA's efforts to bring about the creation of a National Department of Public Health, which had started in the nineteenth century, were continued in the first decade of the twentieth century. In 1902, with the official blessing of the AMA, Congress passed a bill changing the name of the Marine Hospital Service to the *United States Public Health and Marine Hospital Service*. The powers granted to this newly named service were very limited, and in 1906, after the passage of the Food and Drugs legislation, the AMA began again to agitate for a federal Department of Health headed by a Secretary at cabinet level. The creation of such a Department was opposed by President Roosevelt and by his successor, President Taft. It was also opposed by certain medical sects, which claimed that the Bill would create a centralized bureaucratic system in place of the "democracy of our fathers" and would result in an enormous and ever increasing tax burden. In this excursion into politics the AMA failed to achieve its objective.

COUNCIL ON PHARMACY AND CHEMISTRY Another important event during the decade of reform was the creation (1905) by the AMA of a *Council on Pharmacy and Chemistry*. It was expected that this Council would concern itself with the usefulness and advertising claims of "ethical" drugs. It was then believed that the proposed Food and Drugs Law would dispose of the "unethical drugs." But the Food and Drugs Act of 1906, as finally adopted, failed to embody those provisions which the AMA considered most important for the control of the drug industry. When it became apparent that the provisions of a feeble Act would be even more feebly enforced, the Council on Pharmacy and Chemistry decided to turn its attention to the flourishing trade in *nostrums* (patent medicines). The anti-nostrum campaign was bitterly contested every step along the way by the manufacturers of proprietary medicines. Most of the nostrums had won their popularity as a result of (1) false advertising claims, (2) naive or fabricated testimonials, or (3) the high alcoholic content of the nostrum, which enabled those who lived among the rabid teetotalers of the era to drink their toddy disguised as medicine.

The principal instruments used by the council in its campaign were (1) the Chemistry Laboratory of the AMA, established in 1906, where analyses of the nostrums under scrutiny were performed, and (2) a series of publications, which informed physicians and the reading public about the composition of patent medicines and the validity of their advertising claims. From the point of view of physicians the most effective publication was the annual volume, *New and Nonofficial Remedies.* This book was widely used by physicians in prescribing drugs; it contained carefully documented information about the composition and physiological activity of many pharmaceutical products. To be listed in *New and Nonofficial Remedies,* a drug had to comply with specified rules: its chemical composition must be disclosed; tests for determining the identity and purity of the drug must be provided; if advertised to the public there must be no directions for self-medication; the name of the drug must not be misleading; there must be no false or misleading claims; the usefulness of the product must have been established.

These rules induced many drug manufacturers to raise their standards of production and advertising, for when a manufacturer wished to persuade physicians to prescribe his product, no advertisement was as effective as listing in *New and Nonofficial Remedies.*

The Council succeeded in inducing publishers of medical journals, magazines, and newspapers to reject advertisements for drugs that made false or exaggerated claims, and it provided lists of products that fell into this category. In this part of its campaign the Council received great assistance from Samuel Hopkins Adams, author of a series of 12 articles which appeared in *Collier's* Magazine, in 1905 and 1906, entitled "The Great American Fraud." Adams had investigated the subject with unusual thoroughness, and his denunciations of quackery and nostrums were written with force and conviction. The AMA had Adams's articles printed in booklet form, and between 1906 and 1911 it distributed 150,000 copies to libraries and individuals throughout the nation.

The Council also kept an eye on the cost of drugs and made it known when a product was sold at an unjustifiably high price. In this regard it was particularly critical of the Bayer Company, a German firm that was the original producer of *Aspirin.* This drug is a relatively simple and easily manufactured chemical, acetylsalicylic acid. The exaggerated advertising claims for "Aspirin-Bayer" led the Council to eliminate it from *New and Nonofficial Remedies.* In 1917 the AMA also tried to prevent the Bayer Company from renewing its patent on aspirin, which had given the company a monopoly on the manufacture and sale of acetylsalicylic acid in the United States. The AMA stated that

> . . . *practically no other country in the world, not even the original home of the preparation [Germany], would grant a patent on acetylsalicylic acid, the product, or on the process for making that product. The United States granted both! As a result, for seventeen years it has been impossible in this country for anybody except the Bayer Company to manufacture or sell acetylsalicylic acid, either under its chemical name or any other name.*

The *Journal* of the AMA publicized the fact that in European countries that had refused to grant a patent on aspirin, acetylsalicylic acid sold for 4 to 6 cents an ounce, whereas in the United States, where the company was

367

protected by its patent, the price was 43 cents an ounce. Partly as a result of the AMA diclosures the Bayer patent was not renewed in 1917, but the company retained, for several additional years, its Aspirin trademark. Therefore, acetylsalicylic acid still could not be sold as "aspirin," the name best known to the public. During the years that aspirin was protected by the trademark, the AMA urged physicians to save their patients unnecessary expense by specifying "acetylsalicylic acid" rather than "aspirin" in their prescriptions. In this action the AMA took a stand in favor of prescribing a drug by its *generic* (chemical) name, rather than by its *proprietary* name. Adherence to this principle is still the subject of debate.

The anti-nostrum campaign did not succeed in driving all patent medicines out of the drugstores (Burrow, 1963):

Nevertheless, the Association viewed with considerable satisfaction the accomplishments of a decade and a half of leadership in the proprietary fight. It had largely driven the nostrum from medical journals and had raised the standard of medical advertising to a position probably unsurpassed in Europe. A decided improvement appeared in the type of claims that proprietary concerns made for their products, and the growing number of states that had enacted a uniform law controlling advertising was also encouraging. The thousands of letters that it received from laymen showed rising interest in national health problems, as well as public recognition of the Association's service, and even abroad its struggle had not been ignored.

COMPULSORY HEALTH INSURANCE

In the first two decades of the twentieth century, the AMA had become a formidable organization. Its internal structure, with its democratically chosen House of Delegates and its Committees, Councils, and Bureaus, provided an effective mechanism for dealing with a variety of medical problems. Its well-respected Committee on Legislation and its grassroots machinery for influencing those who were making and administering the laws gave it a degree of power that no politician could afford to ignore. Its *Journal,* edited by George Simmons, was read not only by physicians but also by news editors and feature writers, who helped to shape public opinion.

The AMA in that period was no stand-pat organization; it had a progressive, forward-looking program. To be sure, it was concerned for the welfare of the medical profession, but it was no less mindful of the welfare of the public. The public would receive the greatest benefit from the Food and Drugs Act and the anti-nostrum campaign; from the elimination of poor medical schools; from the creation of a federal Department of Health; from the establishment of the Children's Bureau (1912); from stricter licensing laws; and from educational programs to keep practicing doctors abreast of the newest and best methods of treatment. The AMA and its *Journal* had fought for the adoption of all these measures. Since some of its undertakings were directed against vested interests and were opposed by reactionary politicians, the Association gained the goodwill of the reformers and the liberal press. However, between 1915 and 1925 the AMA gradually changed (at least, in the eyes of the reformers) from an organization with a positive, progressive program, to an organization with a negative, stand-pat program. The issue that brought about this change was that of compulsory health insurance or, to use the terms popularized by the AMA, "socialized medicine," or "state medicine."

James G. Burrow, in his book, *AMA—Voice of American Medicine,* has given a balanced, well-documented account of the struggle over compulsory health insurance. The following much abbreviated description has made liberal use of the material presented by Burrow.

Compulsory health insurance got its start in Germany in 1883. It entered English-speaking territory in 1911, when it was adopted in modified form in Britain. In the United States, workmen's compensation laws had been enacted by many states (41 states by 1920), but these laws applied only to disabilities arising in the course of employment. There was no other form of legally required health insurance. In 1907 the *Association for Labor Legislation* began to agitate for a broad program of social legislation including sickness insurance. The original proposal was for voluntary insurance subsidized by the states. In 1911, Louis D. Brandeis, a prominent pro-labor and social-justice lawyer (later a justice of the Supreme Court), in addressing the *National Conference on Charities and Correction,* strongly advocated a national program of social insurance. Through the influence of Brandeis and others, the Progressive party, in 1912, was persuaded to include in its platform a plank advocating compulsory health insurance; this was the first time that a major political party had taken such a step. When the Progressive party lost the election by a wide margin, there was little encouragement for others to follow its example.

The Association for Labor Legislation announced in 1915 that it was preparing a *Standard Bill,* which it intended to introduce into state legislatures in 1916. This Bill called for social legislation, including compulsory health insurance, for employed persons earning $1200 or less and for other employees who wished to subscribe. The insurance provided hospitalization with necessary medical, surgical, and nursing care and cash payments equal to two thirds of the employee's wages for up to 26 weeks of illness. There was also provision for maternity benefits and an allowance of up to $50 for medicines, appliances, and other associated needs. There was to be free choice of physicians from a panel made up of those willing to serve and approved by the state.

The Standard Bill was supported by the *American Sociological Society,* the *American Economic Association,* and the *American Statistical Association.* It was endorsed by Governor Hiram W. Johnson of California and Governor Samuel W. McCall of Massachusetts, by a number of physicians and public health officials, and, significantly, by the Medical Society of the State of New York. Although some labor leaders endorsed the Bill, it was opposed by the powerful President of the American Federation of Labor, Samuel Gompers.

Up to this time the AMA had taken no official position on compulsory insurance, and the *Journal* stated that it hoped that "lack of cooperation" between physicians and legislators could be avoided; it merely urged physicians to examine the Standard Bill and to submit any criticism or suggestions to the Association for Labor Legislation. To deal with the problem in greater depth the AMA early in 1916 appointed a *Committee on Social Insurance,* with Isaac M. Rubinow as Secretary. After preliminary study this Committee expressed a generally favorable attitude toward compulsory health insurance as it existed in Britain.

In the summer of 1916, reporting on the introduction of compulsory health insurance bills in the New York and Massachusetts legislatures, the *Journal* stated that the bills had been drafted by the Association for Labor Legislation *with the aid of the AMA's Committee on Social Insurance;* and the *Journal* added, "Much of the best informed opinion of this country is in favor of these proposals. . . . The introduction of these bills marks the inauguration of a great movement which ought to result in an improvement in the health of the industrial population and improve the conditions for medical service among wage earners."

By late 1916 social insurance bills had been introduced into other legislatures, and Congress was holding hearings on social legislation including health insurance. In January, 1917, the *Journal* again made favorable editorial comments about social insurance, pointing out that among the large industrial nations, the United States was practically the only one that had failed to adopt compulsory health insurance laws. The report of the Social Insurance Committee, presented to the House of Delegates in June, 1917, took a position in favor of compulsory insurance, noting that it had operated with a considerable degree of success in Europe. However, the Committee suggested that a compulsory scheme should (1) make provision for free choice of physician; (2) pay for physicians' services according to the amount of work required rather than on a flat salary basis; (3) provide for adequate representation of the medical profession on the administrative body exercising control over the program; and (4) prevent administrative supervisors from interfering with the physician's function in caring for the patient. Though the House of Delegates endorsed these specific reservations, it took no action for or against compulsory health insurance.

During 1917 the *Journal,* which up to that time had commented favorably on social insurance, began to swing toward opposition. In 1920, Malcom L. Harris, a new member of the Committee on Social Insurance, contributed two articles to the *Journal* severely criticizing socialized medicine; and following Harris's lead, the House of Delegates, at a meeting in August, 1920, adopted for the first time a resolution opposing compulsory health insurance "or any other plan of compulsory insurance which provides for medical service to be rendered contributors or their dependents, provided, controlled or regulated by any state or the Federal government." Having taken such a firm stand on this controversial issue, the AMA sought to justify its position at home and abroad by inviting Alfred Cox, the Secretary of the British Medical Association, to submit an authoritative account of the British compulsory health system for publication in the *Journal.* Prior to extending this invitation to Cox the authorities of the AMA had been misled into believing that the account would be an unfavorable one. It was quite the reverse: Cox maintained that whether one considered the matter from the point of view of the medical profession or the public, the British system had been a success. Though disappointed by Cox's report, the AMA did not modify its opposition to compulsory health insurance.

Federal legislation during the next several years convinced the AMA that the government was in the process of embracing socialized medicine,

370

piecemeal. The *Sheppard-Towner Act* of 1921 provided federal funds to states for infancy and maternity welfare programs; and the *World War Veterans Act* of 1924 provided hospitalization and other health benefits for veterans with non–service-connected, as well as service-connected, disabilities and illnesses. Though these acts had strong public support, the AMA viewed them as an attempt by government to pre-empt the medical care of a large segment of the population.

After 1920 the tone of the *Journal's* opposition to socialized medicine seemed to rise to a higher pitch. This was due, at least in part, to the presence of Morris Fishbein on the editorial staff. Fishbein graduated from the University of Chicago in 1910 and received his M.D. degree from Rush Medical College in 1912, and one year later he became Assistant Editor of the *Journal*. Within a few years he had proved himself to be an able and effective writer, and when George Simmons retired as Editor in 1924, Fishbein was chosen to succeed him. For the next 25 years Fishbein energetically devoted his talents as a writer and speaker to what he considered to be the best interests of the medical profession. He was not the sort of editor to take an equivocal position on an important issue. His stand on compulsory health insurance was one of uncompromising and bitter opposition; it was, he seemed to believe, a scheme of the communists, unworthy of adoption by a democratic people. These views were evidently shared by Olin West, who had become General Manager of the AMA in the same year that Fishbein had become Editor of the *Journal*. Moreover, the speeches made by the Trustees of the AMA and at the meetings of the House of Delegates made it clear that Fishbein's editorial utterances did not lack support. The position of the AMA had hardened.

In the 1920s and 1930s the AMA encountered other issues on which it took a negative stand. It opposed group medical practice: "May it not be one more step," said the *Journal* in 1921, "toward the complete elimination of the medical practitioner—of the family adviser—of him who heretofore has reflected to the public the altruistic motives of the medical profession? Does it mean that the family physician is being replaced by a corporation?" There was also the problem of "contract practice"—physicians hired by industrial and other organizations to provide medical care for particular groups of individuals. There was no objection to salaried physicians in the Army, Navy, or Public Health Service, but when a civilian physician worked for a salary that was less than he might have earned on a fee-for-service basis, he was considered by the AMA to be unethical.

In spite of the AMA's opposition, group practice and contract practice continued to spread, and until the end of the Hoover administration in 1933 there was an almost constant but unsuccessful battle with Congress to effect a change in the law governing the medical care of veterans. In the early 1930s other influences were affecting medical practice: (1) The severe depression was making it difficult for patients to pay for their medical care on a fee-for-service basis, and more physicians, in order to gain economic security, were turning to group and contract practice. The depression also gave impetus to the development of prepayment plans such as Blue Cross or even to a more comprehensive type of sickness insurance such as was being offered by some of the group practice clinics. (2) The advances in surgery and the many technical improvements in methods of diagnosis and

371

treatment were tending to make the hospital, rather than the doctor's office, the core of medical practice.

As in the case of other developments that ruffled the traditional economics of medical practice, the AMA voiced its opposition to the spread of prepayment schemes. In 1932, the *Journal* ran a series of articles about prepayment plans, which by focusing attention on the more disreputable types, placed the whole development in an unfavorable light. However, the effects of the depression could not be ignored, and to deal with the economic situation in a more positive and thorough manner the House of Delegates established a *Bureau of Medical Economics.*

In the same year, 1932, the final report of the *Committee on the Costs of Medical Care* appeared. This report had been five years in preparation by a Committee of some 45 members, most of whom had medical degrees, with a scattering of economists and representatives of the general public. The report directed attention to the maldistribution of physicians and hospitals and the poor medical care received by families of limited means. The Committee's recommendations for improvements in medical care contained the very proposals against which the AMA had been campaigning: (1) group practice centered in hospitals; (2) planning, evaluation, and coordination of medical services by state and local government; and (3) payment for the costs of medical care "through the use of insurance, through the use of taxation, or through the use of both these methods."

Fishbein lost no time in castigating the Committee's report. He accused the Committee of bias in favor of health insurance schemes: "So definite was the trend in the committee's studies in this direction that one must review the expenditure of almost a million dollars by the committee and its final report with mingled amusement and regret." In addition to detecting bias in the report, Fishbein found that it contained enough evidence of "socialistic leanings" to discredit it.

By the time President Roosevelt and his New Deal came into power in 1933, the AMA had established its position in strong opposition to both compulsory and voluntary health insurance, and its reaction to the report of the Committee on the Costs of Medical Care had indicated that it was opposed to any material change in the existing system of health services.

During the first year or two of the New Deal, the AMA cooperated with the program of Emergency Legislation, including the employment by the government of physicians to render medical care to needy citizens. However, conflicts began to develop as the administration was formulating its plan of social security legislation. The influence of the AMA was probably crucial in keeping compulsory health insurance out of the social security measures that the President presented to Congress in 1935. But this was not the AMA's only worry. There was the Wagner-Doughton-Lewis Bill, which had been introduced into the Congress early in 1935. The principal defect in this Bill, in the view of the AMA, was that it placed the medical services that it proposed to provide under the direction of a lay board of the Department of Labor. Then there was the Epstein Bill, which called for an undisguised program of compulsory health insurance. This Bill never came close to adoption by Congress, but it was introduced into several state legislatures, and though it was not enacted by any of them, it was a source of great anxiety to the AMA.

During the first Roosevelt administration, the AMA was embarrassed by several developments that raised doubts as to its leadership of the medical profession. In 1933, the Michigan State Medical Society joined with the American College of Dentistry in financing an independent survey of the British national health system. The report of this survey provided overwhelming evidence from prominent physicians and others that the system was effective and widely approved. Moreover, the survey disclosed that the London correspondent of the AMA, who for years had been feeding the *Journal* unfavorable accounts of the British system, was neither in regular medical practice nor a member of the British Medical Association. Even worse than the embarrassment occasioned by this report was the action by the California State Medical Society, in 1935, when it submitted to the state legislature a Bill that made provision for both voluntary and compulsory health insurance. The Bill failed of enactment, but the fact that a state medical society would take action so far out of line with AMA policy was a source of great concern.

When Roosevelt was elected for a second term in 1936, the AMA foresaw that the dreaded compulsory health insurance might be incorporated in a new proposal for social legislation. To gain more solid backing from the medical profession and to explain its position to the public, the AMA started an educational campaign through its own publications and through news releases to the press. The effect of the propaganda was mixed; as Burrow (1963) describes it, "The Association's attack upon threatened political innovations appears to have made a greater impression on the medical profession than on the public. Its alarmist literature kindled an evangelistic fire among some physicians who were shaken by the government's alleged attack on human liberties."

On a more positive note, and with the hope of weakening the case for compulsory health insurance, the AMA encouraged county medical societies to develop local medical service bureaus, in which physicians would share the burden of caring for the indigent and the medically indigent (those who could pay the basic costs of living but could not pay medical bills). The success of many of these bureaus served not only to blunt the agitation for compulsory health insurance but also to enhance the public image of the medical profession. A similar system of service bureaus was organized on a statewide basis by some of the state medical societies. In 1940, 14 statewide programs were being developed, but by then the needs were changing as the depression gave way to the high employment of the war period.

In the meantime, the *National Health Survey* of 1935–36 (see Chapter 10) had again drawn attention to the deficiencies in the medical care of poor families, and the *National Health Conference* of 1938 had addressed these issues. Following the Conference, President Roosevelt had signified his intention of including medical provisions in a revised system of social security. The administration's new health program was introduced into Congress by Senator Wagner of New York early in 1939. The AMA protested that it had not been consulted in the preparation of the Wagner Bill, and it stoutly opposed some of its most important provisions. The Bill provided federal aid to those states which agreed to develop acceptable health service programs, and though the AMA's chief concern was that this measure would

373

lead to compulsory health insurance, its arguments against the Bill placed greater stress on the "extravagantly high cost" of the proposals and the lack of any need for a program of this type.

Actually, the Wagner Bill of 1939 was relatively innocuous compared with the Bill introduced by Senator Wagner in 1943, with Senator Murray of Montana and Representative Dingell of Michigan as co-authors. The so-called Wagner-Murray-Dingell Bill proposed a great extension of the social security system. It provided increases in unemployment compensation and in old age and survivors' benefits. It also made provision for disability insurance and a uniform public assistance program. However, most alarming, in the eyes of the AMA, was its provision for a federal system of compulsory medical and hospitalization insurance, which included everything except the cost of drugs, dentistry, and home nursing care.

Between the introduction of this bill and the end of the World War II the AMA utilized all the resources at its command to convince the public and any doubting members of the medical profession of the dangers of compulsory health insurance. Its campaign was successful in that the Wagner-Murray-Dingell Bill was not adopted. However, this was not the end of the struggle: after the war the same problem had to be faced again.

In its endless campaign to defeat compulsory health insurance, the AMA found it expedient to play down its objections to voluntary health insurance. In the period from 1933 to 1941, as Burrow puts it, "its attitude [toward voluntary insurance] evolved from pronounced hostility to suspicious friendliness."

OTHER ACTIVITIES

While waging its war against compulsory health insurance the AMA did not overlook its other responsibilities. It continued its fight against quackery and nostrums and exposed a variety of fake cancer-cures, obesity-cures, arthritis-cures, and so forth. When the Wagner Bill of 1939 was being considered, the AMA reiterated its almost forgotten plea for a federal Department of Health headed by a Secretary of cabinet rank. The campaign for a stronger Food and Drugs Law continued through the 1920s and 1930s without notable success until 1937, when a tragic incident, followed by a public outcry, forced the hand of Congress. The incident involved a product called "Elixir Sulfanilamide," made by a drug manufacturer in Tennessee. The elixir consisted of sulfanilamide dissolved in diethylene glycol. Though sulfanilamide itself was a useful and highly effective drug, when mixed with diethylene glycol it became a deadly poison. At least 73 deaths resulted from the use of Elixir Sulfanilamide, and it was obvious that the product had not been adequately tested for toxicity before being placed on the market. In commenting on what had happened, the *Journal* remarked that the weak law for the control of drugs had placed the Food and Drugs Administration in the role of "a hunter pursuing a tiger with a fly swatter." As a result of this tragic incident Congress adopted the much stronger *Food, Drug and Cosmetic Act* of 1938.

18

Medical Licensure and Medical Literature

The knowledge a man can use is the only knowledge which has life and growth in it and converts itself into practical power. The rest . . . dries like raindrops off the stones.

(William Osler)

MEDICAL LICENSURE The attempts that were made during the first century to create effective state licensing boards failed because the profession and the public had chosen not to recognize the authority of such bodies. In the 1870s, however, various state legislatures began to take renewed interest in protecting the public from incompetent practitioners. Texas, in 1873, was the first state to adopt a modern medical practice law, and the following year the Kentucky legislature authorized the governor to organize a system of medical licensure; other states, in rapid succession, took similar action during the period 1875 to 1900.

An interesting and important influence during these years was exerted by the Illinois Board of Health, which was founded in 1877. This Board possessed no licensing powers, but it was authorized to keep a statewide register of recognized physicians. As part of its responsibility in preparing this register, the Board made a survey of all medical colleges in the United States and Canada. The list designated those colleges that the Board considered to be "in good standing." This was the first effort by an official body to categorize medical educational institutions as either good or bad; it served as a prelude to the rating system instituted some 25 years later by the American Medical Association. The first list was published by the Illinois Board in 1880, and it was revised five times between 1883 and 1889. The criteria used for determining whether a school was in good standing were essentially the same as those subsequently adopted by the Association of American Medical Colleges. In 1889 the Board's analysis included 179 regular schools (of which 16 were in Canada), 26 homeopathic, 26 eclectic, 13 other sects, and 13 indicted as "fraudulent" (Shryock, 1967). Shryock believes that the reports of the Illinois Board of Health may have exerted a more favorable influence upon medical education during the 1880s than did reforms in any particular college.

One of the problems with which all of the state boards had to contend was that of the licensing of the medical sects. This was important because relatively large segments of the public were dependent upon the sects for medical care. For example, in Philadelphia in 1881, of the 1480 physicians engaged in practice, 237 were homeopaths (Shryock, 1967). Some of the states solved this problem by creating separate boards for licensing: (1) regular physicians, (2) homeopaths, and (3) eclectic physicians. But before 1880, both the Michigan and the Louisiana state medical societies had agreed to establish joint licensing boards with the homeopaths, and in 1884 Massachusetts established a single licensing system to include regular physicians, homeopaths, and eclectics.

The problem of licensing the homeopaths and the eclectics, which aroused so much controversy in the 1880s and 1890s, was eventually solved during the first quarter of the twentieth century, when both of these sects gave up their narrowly based systems and merged with the regular profession. Osler was one of the few regular physicians who foresaw at an early date the direction in which sectarian affairs was moving. When he expressed the following views in 1889, they were considered to be almost reprehensively radical:

> . . . in the eyes of the law we all [the regular profession and the sects] stand equal, and if we wish legislation for the protection of the public we have got to ask for it together, not singly. I know that this is gall and wormwood to many — at the bitterness of it the gorge rises; but it is a question which has to be met fairly and squarely. When we think of the nine or ten subjects which we have in common, we may surely, in the interest of the public, bury animosities, and agree to differ on the question of therapeutics.

The establishment of state licensing boards proceeded at such a pace during the 1880s and 1890s that by 1898, according to Shryock (1967)

> only the Alaska Territory had no regulations whatever. In Michigan and five states west of the Mississippi the registration of any diploma entitled a man to practice, and eleven states still accepted either approved diplomas or examinations. But there were already 22 states which required both diplomas and state examinations — the program of the future.

In 1891 the state licensing bodies formed their own organization, the *National Confederation of State Medical Examining and Licensing Boards*. This Confederation worked closely with the Association of American Medical Colleges and the Council on Medical Education of the American Medical Association.

376

One of the most complicated problems in the early years of state licensing was that of achieving an acceptable basis for reciprocal licensure so that a physician could move from a state in which he was licensed into another state, and practice there, without having to go through another round of examinations. To cope with this problem the *American Confederation of Reciprocating Examining and Licensing Medical Boards* was formed. This body succeeded in bringing about a degree of uniformity in state licensing laws that made reciprocation of licensure less difficult. Whereas the mission of this Confederation was to deal specifically with reciprocation, the *National Confederation of State Medical Examining and Licensing Boards* concerned itself with improving the standards of medical education: preliminary requirements, graded curriculum, length of course, facilities, and other factors. In 1913 the two confederations merged to form a new organization, which happily had a shorter name, *Federation of State Medical Boards*.

The animator of the Federation for many years was Walter L. Bierring, who in 1915 became its Secretary and the Editor of its monthly publication, the *Federation Bulletin*. Bierring was born in Iowa of Danish parents, and he received his M.D. degree from the State University of Iowa in 1892. He then spent two years in Europe, where he studied at Heidelberg and Vienna and had a stimulating experience in Paris working at the Pasteur Institute with Pasteur, Metchnikoff, and Roux. After returning to the United States he became, successively, Professor of Pathology and Bacteriology and Professor of the Theory and Practice of Medicine at the State University of Iowa. He also served for three years as Professor of Medicine at Drake University. Bierring therefore brought to the Federation a cultural, scientific, and educational background that equipped him admirably for his duties. He also possessed tact and statesmanship, which enabled him to develop excellent working relations with state boards of medical examiners, the Council on Medical Education of the AMA, the Association of American Medical Colleges, and other organizations concerned with medical education and licensure. It was largely through Bierring's influence that the Federation became a potent force for the betterment of medical education and practice (Derbyshire, 1969).

Another important body that came into being at about the same time as the Federation was the *National Board of Medical Examiners*. From the earliest days of the AMA there had been occasional talk about the desirability of having a national system of medical licensure. In 1902 the *Journal* of the AMA suggested in an editorial that the President appoint a National Board of Medical Examiners for physicians seeking government positions; and the hope was expressed that those accredited by the Board might be accepted without further examination for state licenses. This editorial was prompted in part by the great difficulty that was then being encountered in achieving reciprocal licensure among states. When a proposal for a voluntary National Board was submitted to the House of Delegates of the AMA it became apparent that states which objected to honoring the licenses of other states were no more inclined to accept certification by a national body.

Another proposal for a voluntary National Board appeared in 1906 in the *Journal* of the AMA. This attracted little support. Then in 1910 came Flexner's report on medical education, which sharply criticized the state boards for their lack of success in limiting the practice of medicine to qualified physicians. Flexner's chapter on the state boards ended with a concise summary of the licensing situation as of that date and a rather muted hope for a national examining body (Flexner, 1910):

> *Despite imperfect and discordant laws and inadequate resources, the state board has abundantly justified itself. It is indeed hardly more than quarter of a century old; yet, in summing up the forces that have within that period made for improved conditions, the state boards must be prominently mentioned. Their role is likely to be increasingly important. They have developed considerable* esprit de corps. *Their power of combined action on broad lines has distinctly increased even in the last few years. Reciprocity between states whose laws are measurably concordant and whose ideals are taking similar shape tends to demonstrate the fundamental sameness of the problems requiring solution. Out of these first cooperative efforts, a model law will emerge; federated action may become possible. Perhaps the entire country may some day be covered by a national organization engaged in protecting the public health against the formidable combination made by ignorance, incompetency, commercialism, and disease.*

In 1914, another editorial in the *Journal* of the AMA urged the creation of a National Examining Board, and a year later Dr. William L. Rodman, in his presidential address before the American Medical Association, announced that a National Board of Medical Examiners had been founded. The House of Delegates took cognizance of Rodman's announcement and referred the matter to the Council on Medical Education, which gave the National Board its unanimous approval.

The membership of the original Board was such as to attract immediate attention. The representatives of the federal medical services were as follows: Surgeon-General Gorgas and L. A. LaGarde of the Army, Rear Admiral Braisted and E. P. Stitt of the Navy, and Surgeon-General Blue and W. C. Rucker of the Public Health Service. The Federation of State Medical Boards was represented by Herbert Holden; the Association of American Medical Colleges by Isador Dyer; the American College of Surgeons by E. W. Andrews; the Mayo Foundation by Louis B. Wilson; and the AMA by V. C. Vaughan and W. L. Rodman. In addition, there were three members-at-large, H. D. Arnold, Austin Flint, and Henry Sewell. Dr. Rodman, the founder of the Board, died in 1916, and his place was taken by Walter Bierring. At the same time Rodman's son, J. Stewart Rodman, succeeded his father as the Board's Secretary.

Eight states endorsed almost immediately the certificate of the National Board, and the Board thus gained legitimacy as an accredited medical examining body. The first examinations were held in Washington, D.C., in 1916. Thirty-two candidates had applied for the examinations, but the Board found only half of these to have acceptable qualifications. Ten candidates took the examinations, and only five of them passed. Between 1916 and 1921 there were 498 applicants, of whom 427 were found to be qualified; 325 took the examinations, 269 passed. During this period the number of applications was probably limited by World War I.

After the war the number of applicants increased. In 1921 the Board acquired legal status by being incorporated and gained financial support from the Carnegie Foundation.

In 1922 the National Board examinations were divided into three parts:

Part I, a written examination on preclinical subjects to be taken after the first two years in medical school; *Part II*, a written examination on clinical subjects at the end of the fourth year; and *Part III*, an oral examination on both clinical and laboratory subjects after the completion of an internship. The superior quality of the examinations, the recognized stature of the examiners, and the elimination as far as possible of personal bias in the rating of candidates, all served to enhance the prestige of the Board, and gradually young doctors came to view the possession of a National Board certificate as an honor. Since the medical schools were informed about the marks achieved by their students, the examinations served to reorient and upgrade the educational programs in some of the weaker schools.

By 1940 the number of candidates taking the National Board examinations had increased to about 1400 a year, or about one quarter of all medical school graduates. By that time all except five states were accepting the National Board certificate as qualification for licensure without state Board examinations. The National Board cannot, itself, issue licenses; its legal status is that of a corporation authorized to examine and grade those medical students and medical graduates who apply to be examined; its strength lies in its high professional standards and its lack of involvement in state and national politics.

Other medical examining boards of national scope are the specialty boards, whose members are chosen by the relevant specialist association. These boards are designed to examine candidates who apply for certification as specialists. The first specialty board to be established was the American Board of Ophthalmology, which began to accredit ophthalmologists before World War I. Since then many similar boards have been created; at first, in broad specialties such as medicine, surgery, and pediatrics and later, in specialties of narrower range, such as heart surgery, gastroenterology, and cardiology.

Accreditation by a specialty board has no legal basis, but from many points of view it is an asset to its possessor. Many state and voluntary agencies that refer patients for medical consultations or surgical operations are required to make their referrals only to those who have the correct specialty accreditation. More and more hospitals are restricting privileges in a specialty field to possessors of the certificate of a specialty board. Even in the courts, a surgeon who has performed an operation usually performed by a specialist is at a great disadvantage in a malpractice suit if he does not have accreditation in that particular specialty. In other words, the specialty boards have come to be recognized as quasi-official examining and accrediting bodies.

MEDICAL LITERATURE

The *Journal of Morphology* was the first American scientific periodical dealing with a field related to medicine. This journal was founded in 1888 under the editorship of the zoologist Charles O. Whitman. When it was launched, Whitman had just accepted a position as Professor of Zoology on the original faculty of Clark University in Worcester, Massachusetts. This small university had been organized by G. Stanley Hall, who from 1881 to 1888 was Professor of Psychology at Johns Hopkins. The original Clark Uni-

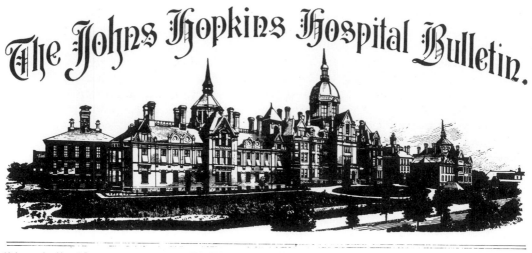

Volume I.—No. 1.] BALTIMORE, DECEMBER, 1889. [Price, 15 Cents.

MEDICAL INSTRUCTION IN THE JOHNS HOPKINS HOSPITAL.

During the year 1889–90, instruction will be given at the Johns Hopkins Hospital in Pathology and Bacteriology, Medicine, Surgery, Gynaecology, and Hygiene, by lectures, demonstrations, laboratory courses, bed-side teaching and general clinics in the laboratories, wards, dispensary, amphitheatre and private operating rooms.

1. PATHOLOGY AND BACTERIOLOGY.

PATHOLOGY.

The instruction in Pathology is under the charge of Dr. W. H. Welch, Professor of Pathology, Johns Hopkins University, and of Dr. W. T. Councilman, Associate in Pathology and Associate Professor of Anatomy, Johns Hopkins University. It is conducted in the Pathological Laboratory, which is one of the buildings of the Johns Hopkins Hospital, especially constructed for pathological work. Here are to be found an autopsy theatre, rooms for bacteriological and special research, rooms for pathological histology, experimental pathology and photography and a museum.

Courses of instruction in Pathological Histology are continued throughout the academic year. In connection with the course in Pathological Histology fresh pathological specimens are demonstrated and also studied microscopically, especially by the aid of frozen sections. Instruction is also given in the methods of making post-mortem examinations and of recording the same.

Much attention is given to the collection and study of material in Comparative Pathology.

The resources of the laboratory are open to those who are fitted to engage in special investigations in any department of pathology.

In addition to regular practical courses in the laboratory extending throughout the academic year, special courses of lectures on pathological subjects will be given during the months of January and February, 1890. Professor Welch at this time will lecture once a week upon the Pathology of Diseases of the Heart and Blood Vessels. The subjects of fatty heart, fibrous myocarditis, diseases of the coronary arteries of the heart, thrombosis, embolism, infarction, and endarteritis, will be considered.

Professor Councilman will lecture upon Inflammation. The modern doctrines of inflammation, the origin of pus, the behavior of fixed cells in inflammation, the relation of bacteria to inflammation, are among the subjects to be considered. The lectures will be illustrated by gross and microscopical specimens.

BACTERIOLOGY.

The instruction in Bacteriology is under the charge of Professor W. H. Welch and of Dr. A. C. Abbott, Assistant in Bacteriology and Hygiene.

The rooms for bacteriological work are in the Pathological Laboratory. They are supplied with all of the apparatus required by modern bacteriological methods, such as those employed in the Hygienic Institute in Berlin. The laboratory has a full set of cultures of pathogenic micro-organisms, and of others useful for study and teaching.

Opportunities for studying bacteriology are available for students during the entire academic year, the laboratory being open on week days from nine o'clock in the morning until six in the evening. As much time can be given to the work as the student has at his disposal.

In the bacteriological course the student becomes familiar with the preparation of the various culture media, with the principles and methods of sterilization, and with the morphological and biological characters of the micro-organisms which belong to this

Figure 90. Title page of the Johns Hopkins Hospital Bulletin, 1889.

versity faculty was "one of the most remarkable faculties of young men ever brought together in this country" (Sabin, 1934). This characterization applies particularly to those chosen in the scientific disciplines: among them were such stars as Albert A. Michelson in Physics, Whitman and Frank Lilly in Zoology, Franz Boas in Anthropology, Henry H. Donaldson in Neurology, and Franklin P. Mall and James P. McMurrich in Anatomy. With the support given by this group, the *Journal of Morphology* flourished. Though Whitman moved to the University of Chicago in 1892, he continued to edit the *Journal* until 1910.

When the Johns Hopkins Hospital opened in 1889, the hospital Trustees authorized and provided funds for two medical publications. One, the *Johns Hopkins Hospital Bulletin,* was to be a monthly publication, and it was expected that it would serve as a news bulletin for the hospital. The second, the *Johns Hopkins Hospital Reports,* was to serve as the vehicle for the publication of the scientific work performed at the hospital and medical school. With the passage of time, however, more and more relatively short articles dealing with original work carried out at the two institutions made their appearance in the *Bulletin,* which has been published continuously since its founding, though it has recently adopted a new name, *The Johns Hopkins Medical Journal.* The *Reports,* which appeared at irregular intervals, filled a need for a publication that would carry longer articles and monographs. It was planned that the first volume of the *Reports* would be edited by Welch and would be devoted to articles reporting work carried on in his laboratory and that the second volume would be edited by Osler and would be devoted to the clinical work conducted at the hospital. As it turned out, Volume II appeared in 1890, but Volume I, owing to the slow and meticulous manner in which it was edited by Welch, did not appear until 1897.

In the meantime Welch had become aware of the need for a scientific journal devoted to reports of medical research carried on not only at Johns Hopkins but also at other institutions, where the amount of research was steadily increasing. With this in view and with enthusiastic support from President Gilman, who agreed that the Hopkins University would contribute $1000 annually, Welch founded the *Journal of Experimental Medicine* and became its Editor. This was the first regularly published American periodical devoted to medical science. Welch immediately set to work writing letters to medical research workers all over the country, encouraging them to submit papers for the new journal, of which the first number appeared in 1896. In commenting on Welch's editorship, the Flexners have stated: "Welch's greatest difficulty as an editor arose less from outside engagements than from his own temperament, which demanded scrupulous attention to detail, but would not allow him to accept assistance in this time-consuming work. He rarely consulted the associate editors, and, shunning secretaries, wrote all the voluminous correspondence in his own hand" (Flexner and Flexner, 1966). Contrary to expectations, the editor gradually was overwhelmed by the number of papers submitted for publication. The editorship became such a burden that Welch after several years began to look around for someone to take over the job.

In 1901 Welch heard that Harold Ernst, Professor of Bacteriology at Harvard, was planning to start a new periodical. In 1896 Ernst had founded the *Boston Society of Medical Sciences,* and he had been editing its proceedings, which were published in a small pamphlet. He now had in mind the publication of a national journal as the official organ of the newly organized *American Association of Pathologists and Bacteriologists.* Welch tried to persuade Ernst to give up this project and offered to turn over to him the editorship of the *Journal of Experimental Medicine.* When President Gilman heard about this offer, he told Welch that he had no right to take such a step

381

without first obtaining the consent of the university, which was financing the *Journal* in part. As a result Welch withdrew his offer, and Ernst proceeded with his original plan. The first issue of the new periodical, the *Journal of Medical Research,* appeared in July, 1901. Finally in 1903 President Gilman agreed to let Welch turn over the *Journal of Experimental Medicine* to Rockefeller Institute, and Simon Flexner and Eugene Opie became its editors.

While Welch was struggling with the *Journal of Experimental Medicine,* a new scientific publication appeared in 1898: *The American Journal of Physiology,* sponsored by the *American Physiological Society* and edited by Henry P. Bowditch, Professor of Physiology at Harvard. Then in the early years of the twentieth century, other scientific periodicals of national scope appeared in rapid succession: *American Journal of Anatomy,* in 1901; *Journal of Experimental Biology and Medicine,* in 1903; *Journal of Infectious Diseases,* in 1904; *Journal of Experimental Zoology,* in 1904; *Journal of Biological Chemistry,* in 1905; *Journal of Pharmacology and Experimental Therapeutics,* in 1909; *Biochemical Bulletin,* in 1912. These publications are indicative of the speed with which biomedical research was spreading through the United States. When the *Journal of Experimental Medicine* was founded in 1896, it stood alone as a vehicle for reports on basic medical research, but within two decades it was only one of a growing family of such periodicals.

In addition to the strictly scientific journals, well-edited clinical journals of excellent quality were appearing in increasing numbers. For example, the American Medical Association established several good clinical journals, such as the *Archives of Internal Medicine* (1908). Two journals established in the first century, *The American Journal of the Medical Sciences* and *The New England Journal of Medicine,* along with the *Journal of the American Medical Association,* established in 1883, carried clinical and scientific articles of broad medical interest together with reviews of books and articles published in America and foreign countries. First-class textbooks, monographs, and treatises on both clinical subjects and the basic medical sciences also began to appear in increasing numbers.

John Shaw Billings's two projects, the *Index Catalogue of the Surgeon-General's Library* and the *Index Medicus,* served to make the increasing volume of medical publications more accessible and more useful. The *Index Medicus,* which was published monthly, contained a listing of the world medical literature in alphabetical sequence both by author and by subject. The first series of the *Index* (1879–1899) was edited by Billings and Robert Fletcher. After a lapse, the second series began in 1903 under the auspices of the Carnegie Institution of Washington, with Fletcher as Editor-in-Chief. The value of the *Index* has been attested by its worldwide list of subscribers; no medical school, medical library, hospital, or research institution either in this country or abroad can afford to be without it.

PART THREE

Period of
Explosive
Growth–1946-1976

19

The
National Scene

As American civilization became increasingly permeated by its technology, it lay increasingly at the mercy of the internal logic of advancing knowledge. Science and technology had a momentum of their own: each next step was commanded by its predecessor. To fail to take that next step was to waste all the earlier efforts. Once the nation had embarked on the brightly illuminated path of science, it had somehow ventured into a world of mystery where the direction and the speed would be dictated by the instruments that cut the path and by the vehicles that carried man ahead. The autonomy of science, the freedom of the scientist to go where knowledge and discovery led him, spelled the unfreedom of the society to choose its way for other reasons. People felt they might conceivably slow the pace of change — but they wondered whether they were in a position to stop it.

(Daniel J. Boorstin, 1973)

In the years 1946 to 1976 the world was seething with social unrest and political struggle. The Communist form of government, which before World War II had prevailed in the U.S.S.R. only, spread to other countries during the latter part of the war, and by 1950 China and the nations of eastern Europe and the northern Balkans all had Communist governments. During the same period the great colonial empires of Britain, France, and Holland were falling apart, and the overseas possessions of other European nations were agitating for independence. For the 25 years that followed, the dominating factor in world politics was the "cold war," in which the United States and the Soviet Union were the leading antagonists.

Through these years of turmoil and threats of a nuclear war, science and technology advanced at a pace never before imagined and with an autonomy oblivious to the stresses of the sociopolitical environment. The atom was broken down into ever smaller particles; fission bombs were superseded by fusion bombs; nuclear power plants were constructed; computers performed mathematical feats with steadily increasing speed and

385

precision; rockets of fantastic power sent men first into space and then to the moon; transistors replaced vacuum tubes; jet power succeeded propeller power; insecticides and hybrid grains increased agricultural production. Medical science and technology also moved forward with a momentum of their own: the secrets of genetics were unraveled; the science of immunology had to be completely revised in the light of new discoveries; the chemistry of neural activity was revealed; enzymes controlling blood pressure and regulating many other bodily functions were discovered; new viruses were brought to light; new protective vaccines were developed; ways were found to transplant organs from cadavers to living subjects; artificial kidneys, heart-lung machines, and cardiac pacemakers were devised to carry on the function of vital organs; the heart could be opened for repair of congenital defects and malfunctioning valves, and plugged coronary arteries could be bypassed; successful methods were developed for the treatment of some forms of cancer; new antibiotics were extracted from a host of soil micro-organisms, and many effective drugs were discovered or synthesized; hearing aids were improved, and operations were performed under a microscope for the relief of deafness.

The research that led to many of the major advances in medical science and medical therapy took place in laboratories in the United States, and it would not have been possible without generous financial support, principally from the federal government but also from foundations and individuals. Congress provided massive funding for medical research through the mechanism of the National Institutes of Health. Some of these funds were used to support the work being conducted in the laboratories of the NIH, but much of the money was parceled out in the form of research and training grants for institutions throughout the country.

While research was in the ascendancy, medical education went through a period of relative neglect. There was almost no increase in the number of students graduating from the medical schools while the population was increasing by the tens of millions, and in the 1950s the country was faced by a serious shortage of physicians. Part of the shortage was made up by a large and long-continued influx of foreign medical graduates. Between 1955 and 1975 the number of medical schools in operation increased from 82 to 116, and the number of students graduating each year doubled. To bring this change about a huge financial outlay was required, and a large number of basic scientists and clinicians had to be recruited for the expanded faculties.

Medical practice during 1946 to 1976 underwent many changes made necessary by the expansion of knowledge and improvement in equipment. Hospitals more than ever became the center of practice for the proliferating number of specialists; and all types of physicians and surgeons were dependent upon the facilities and services of a hospital for the care of their seriously ill patients. Medical practice was also faced by special problems presented by the increasing proportion of old people and the increasing number of nursing homes provided for their care. The practitioner also had to devote professional time to continuing education and to serving on various hospital and medical society committees, utilization review boards, and Professional Standards Review Organizations (PSROs). Blue Shield, commercial health insurance, and the federal and state programs for the care of the elderly and the indigent burdened the practitioner with a heavy

386

load of paper work but at the same time paid fees that he might otherwise not have collected. Many busy physicians would have been happy to forego the fees in order to rid themselves of the paper work.

The aspects of medical care that were of the greatest concern to the public and their elected representatives were the staggering increase in cost and the decrease in the number of family doctors. People harked back to the "good old days" when hospitals were unnecessary and when a family doctor, carrying all of his diagnostic equipment and medicine in a little black bag, would make house calls for three or four dollars a visit. That pleasant dream was really not so pleasant if one had to have with it all the serious illnesses and infirmities that the old family doctor could not treat.

The public image of the physician suffered during this 30-year period. News stories focused attention on the unethical doctors who grew rich on Medicaid fees and the shoddy practitioners whose careless misdeeds drove the cost of malpractice insurance to intolerable levels. The American Medical Association, which was looked upon as the spokesman for the doctor, did little to improve the physician's image. In spite of its many fine services for the public and for the profession, the Association gained a reputation as a negative advocate, opposed to change and overly concerned about the physician's income. The Association took some unfortunate stands which circumstances forced it to abandon: opposition to voluntary health insurance, denial of a shortage of physicians, and opposition to government support of medical education.

The public and the legislators were particularly concerned about the health of the poor. This was indeed a matter for concern, but the health of the poor suffered more from socioeconomic factors—poor housing, inadequate fuel, inadequate and poorly balanced diet, and the depressing effect of unemployment—than from the factors usually causing disease among those with a higher standard of living. The poor unquestionably did not receive the same quality of care as did their more fortunate neighbors, and it was therefore surprising to note that the death rate per 1000 population in New York City, with its large population of blacks, Puerto Ricans, and other poor minority groups, had fallen over the years and in 1975 reached its lowest level, 9.6, only slightly higher than the national death rate of 9.2 (*New York Times,* January 1, 1976).

| PLAN OF PRESENTATION FOR PART III | In dealing with this period of fantastic change, we shall present briefly the international and domestic developments that provided the setting in which medicine moved forward. This will be |

followed by separate chapters dealing with medical education, and the role of government in medicine. Medical research, which was treated in a single chapter in Parts I and II, will be broken down into a series of chapters in Part III. It would be impossible in a volume of this size to give an adequate account of the tremendous progress that has been made by research and development in almost every aspect of medine. We have chosen instead to

387

concentrate attention on several areas·in which the developments of the past 30 years have made major contributions to both medical science and medical practice. In presenting each of these subjects we shall carry the story back into the pre-1946 period to the extent necessary to set the stage for the post-1946 developments. Finally we shall consider the effect of these various factors on the practice of medicine.

FOREIGN AFFAIRS

The hope of a lasting peace after World War II proved to be an illusion. The high-sounding resolutions with which the United Nations had been established had a very limited effect in restraining national ambitions. Throughout the years 1946 to 1975 the Soviet Union and the United States were engaged in a "cold war," which failed to become a hot war largely because of bilateral fear of a nuclear holocaust. Nevertheless, limited hot wars in which one or the other or both of the great powers were involved were waged in the Middle East, Africa, India, China, Korea, and Southeast Asia.

The cold war began when President Truman, alarmed by the spread of communism in eastern Europe and the Balkan States, offered aid to any nation which would resist Communist infiltration. At the same time the Marshall Plan was instituted to provide funds for the reconstruction of the war-torn countries of Europe. In 1949 the North Atlantic Treaty Organization (NATO) was established as a defensive alliance against the Communist bloc. General Eisenhower was made Supreme Commander of the combined NATO military forces, with headquarters in Europe. A year later, on the other side of the world, the United States, backed by the United Nations, sent troops to the Korean Peninsula to prevent the Communists of North Korea from taking over the entire peninsula. The United Nations forces, under the energetic leadership of General Douglas MacArthur, not only drove the Communists out of South Korea but also continued their march northward to the Chinese border. At that point the Chinese sent an army of 200,000 men to the aid of their Communist friends, and the Korean War ended without victory for either side. While the Korean War was in progress, the Truman administration also took the first step down that thorny trail in Southeast Asia by providing funds and sending a military mission to Vietnam to aid the French, who were waging a losing battle against the Communist Viet Minh.

During Truman's second term as President, the Russians exploded their first atomic bomb, and by the time of President Eisenhower's inauguration they were known to have a stockpile of bombs ready for use. Shortly after Eisenhower moved into the White House, the Soviet dictator, Joseph Stalin, died. The American Secretary of State, John Foster Dulles, was determined that Stalin's successor should have no misconceptions about the American position; he announced that the United States would meet Soviet aggression with "massive retaliation" with nuclear weapons, striking back, "at places and with means of our own choosing." Dulles also insisted that Vietnam must not be allowed to fall to the Communists, and by the end of Eisenhower's first term the United States was paying four fifths of the cost of the fight against the Viet Minh.

On October 4, 1957, the Russians startled the world by sending their *Sputnik* satellite into orbit. Prior to the surprise flight of *Sputnik*, the United States armed services had been experimenting with rocketry for military uses. This work had gone forward at a rather leisurely pace. Although the Soviets had mastered the production of atomic bombs, this feat was reputed to have been accomplished merely by stealing American secrets. No one seriously believed that Russian technology could rival that of the United States. The flight of *Sputnik* put an abrupt end to that type of complacency. To prove that *Sputnik I* had been no accident, less than a month later the Russians sent *Sputnik II* into orbit, this time carrying the first space traveler, a dog whose heartbeat and other vital signs were monitored as the vehicle circled the globe.

When *Sputnik I* rose into orbit, the American effort to launch a satellite was thrown into high gear. It was well known in military circles that rockets that propel spacecraft into orbit could serve to launch intercontinental missiles with atomic warheads. In July, 1958, Congress established the National Aeronautics and Space Administration (NASA), an independent agency, to coordinate all developments in space technology and to conduct nonmilitary space science programs. The creation of NASA did much to speed the progress of the American space program and to keep it directed toward well-defined goals.

In December, 1958, the U.S. Air Force successfully launched a four-ton monster from Cape Canaveral. During the next three years many satellites carrying a variety of sophisticated equipment were sent into orbit by both Russia and the United States. People began to speculate whether the Russians or the Americans would be the first to send a man orbiting around the earth.

On April 12, 1961, the Russians sent Major Y. A. Gagarin on a single orbit around the earth and brought him back safely to his homeland. The following August, a second Russian spaceman circled the earth 17 times. It was not until February of the following year (1962) that Colonel John H. Glenn, Jr., was blasted off the pad at Cape Canaveral and orbited the earth three times, the first American to circle the globe. Although the United States was about a year behind the Russians in space exploration, Glenn's flight had great propaganda value. The Russian flights had been kept from public view and were shrouded in mystery, but the whole American exploit, from blast-off to landing, was carried out in full view of news reporters, photographers, and television and moving-picture cameramen. People the world over had an opportunity to behold at close range the precision, the technical perfection, and the personal courage with which this feat was accomplished.

The race in space technology was going on throughout most of President Eisenhower's eight years in office. When the race began with our side apparently far behind, there was a frantic search for an explanation. It was held that our educational system was at fault, that our training of scientists was less thorough than that of the Russians, and that we were not training enough scientists. Some of these charges had a beneficial effect upon medical research by encouraging public support for all types of scientific endeavor.

After Nikita S. Khrushchev assumed leadership of the Soviet government, he and Eisenhower met for a "Summit Conference" in July, 1955. Khrushchev seemed a more open and cooperative person than Stalin had been. The two leaders agreed that an atomic war would be a disaster for both sides, and Khrushchev's attitude raised hopes of a lull in the cold war. These hopes were reinforced in February, 1956, when Khrushchev called for "peaceful coexistence between East and West" and made it known that he disapproved of Stalin's "needless brutalities." When a second Summit Conference was scheduled for May 15, 1960, it was believed that this meeting might further improve Soviet-American relations. Unfortunately, shortly before the date of this conference a United States reconnaissance (U-2) plane was shot down over Russia. The pilot, who landed safely by parachute, confessed that he was a United States spy. When the Summit Conference was convened, Khrushchev demanded that the President apologize for the U-2 incident, and when Eisenhower refused, Khrushchev broke up the meeting and left for home.

A few days before President Kennedy was inaugurated in 1961, the United States broke off diplomatic relations with Cuba, where Fidel Castro had established a Communist government. Castro had signed five-year trade agreements with the Soviet Union and Communist China and had seized 850 million dollars' worth of United States property. In retaliation, the United States, which had been Cuba's largest customer for sugar, refused to import any more of this commodity. In an address to the United Nations Castro characterized the United States refusal to purchase sugar as "economic aggression."

In April, 1961, with President Kennedy's approval and with military assistance from the United States, a group of Cubans who had left their country to escape Castro attempted to invade Cuba, in the hope of overthrowing the Castro government. This ill-conceived and ill-planned expedition, the Bay of Pigs fiasco, was quickly defeated, much to the embarrassment of the Kennedy administration.

The Russians took advantage of the change in American administrations to create trouble in Germany. They threatened to give Communist East Germany control over West Berlin and the air supply routes into the city. In June, 1961, President Kennedy had a two-day conference with Khrushchev in Vienna, at which the Berlin situation was discussed. Nothing was settled, but it was made known that the United States would strongly oppose any effort of the Communists to take over West Berlin. Seeing that they could not make the Americans back down, the Russians settled the matter by sealing the border between East Berlin and West Berlin. This was done to prevent the steady flow of East Germans to the West, which had been a source of concern to the Communists for several years.

In August, 1961, President Kennedy presented to Congress a program aimed at putting explorers on the moon before 1970. Although the President estimated that this program would cost several billion dollars, it was approved wholeheartedly by Congress.

Cuba again became the focus of the cold war in late 1962, when President Kennedy successfully demanded that the Russians dismantle their missile bases and remove the offensive weapons that they had been setting up to give Castro greater strength in his dealings with the United States.

During the Kennedy administration the friendship of the Communist partners Russia and China began to show signs of tension. Khrushchev's call for peaceful coexistence between East and West had not pleased the hard-line Chinese, and they accused the Soviet leader and his followers of deviating from basic Communist doctrine. To the President and his Secretary of State, Dean Rusk, the theme of peaceful coexistence seemed worthy of further emphasis, since not only would it advance the prospect of peace but also it might widen the gap between the major Communist powers. In June, 1963, President Kennedy delivered a public address in which, after referring to the differences between Russia and the United States, he went on to say "Let us not be blind to our differences, but let us also direct attention to our common interests and the means by which these differences can be resolved. And if we cannot end our differences, at least we can make the world safe for diversity." The overriding common interest was, of course, the desire to avoid a nuclear war, and the first significant step toward the realization of this desire occurred on August 5, 1963, when, at a ceremony in the Kremlin, Russia, Great Britain, and the United States signed a nuclear test-ban treaty in which it was agreed not to hold any further open-air or underwater tests of nuclear explosives.

In the autumn of 1963, President Kennedy began to look forward to the political campaign of the following year. He flew to Texas in November to make some speeches, and on November 22 while riding in a motorcade through the streets of Dallas he was assassinated.

Immediately after the assassination, Vice-President Lyndon Baines Johnson was sworn in as President. Johnson had served continuously as a member of Congress, first as a representative and then as a senator, from 1937 until his election as Vice-President. He had risen to the position of majority leader of the Senate, where he was admired by his colleagues for his skill in legislative tactics.

The Johnson administration and the rest of the world were caught by surprise when it was announced from Moscow that Khrushchev had been removed from office and that Aleksei N. Kosygin had been named Premier and Leonid I. Brezhnev, First Secretary of the Party. Just how this switch would affect relations with the Soviet Union was a puzzle.

The American involvement in Vietnam plagued Johnson throughout his presidency; his dogged insistence on pushing the war to a victorious conclusion transformed a popular president into an object of vilification and hatred; and though his obstinate stand had many staunch supporters, their numbers gradually diminished, and in the end his position was so weakened that he decided to withdraw from politics. Johnson's tragedy was heightened by the fact that during the Eisenhower administration he had taken a strong stand against involvement in Vietnam.

Affairs in South Vietnam were in a fluid state when Johnson became President. The Vietnamese government was virtually leaderless, and many Americans had lost faith in its ability to wage a successful war. At first the President was cautious about committing the United States to all-out military aid to a faltering regime, but his hesitation came to an end in August, 1964, when North Vietnamese PT boats attacked two U.S. destroyers in the

391

Gulf of Tonkin off the coast of Vietnam. The President took advantage of this incident to secure from Congress the "Tonkin Resolution," which authorized him to take "all necessary measures" to prevent future aggression against the forces of the United States. With this resolution behind him, when the Viet Cong attacked an American camp in February, 1965, killing 8 American soldiers and wounding more than 100 others, Johnson promptly ordered carrier-based air strikes against North Vietnam. Although the President claimed that the bombing missions were carried out only in retaliation for the attack on the American camp and insisted that "we seek no wider war," the air strikes continued, and about a month later the first United States combat units, two battalions of Marines, landed in Vietnam.

From the first landing of U.S. combat units onward, the war was escalated and intensified: the North Vietnamese sent more and more troops to support the Viet Cong; the United States sent regiments and divisions and planes and gradually took over from the South Vietnamese full control of the fighting. By the end of Johnson's term as President the total United States forces in the Vietnam area exceeded half a million, and more than 30,000 Americans had been killed and another 100,000 wounded.

In Johnson's last year as President the country was sharply divided between those who felt humiliation at the perplexing failure of the American forces in a war against a second-rate Communist nation and those who wanted out, shame or no shame. There were antiwar speeches, antiwar marches, and antiwar riots; draft cards were burned individually and *en masse,* the American flag was desecrated, and bombs were exploded in protest against the war. The younger generation made up the greater part of the antiwar demonstrators, and this was no more than natural: their education had been disrupted, their early careers had been blighted, and many of them had been dragged halfway round the world possibly to be maimed or killed in a war which to them had no validity. For those who took no stock in the Communist menace or the domino theory, the validity was indeed hard to find.

Before he went out of office President Johnson evidently had decided that there was little prospect of victory in the Vietnam War. He authorized the opening of peace negotiations between the United States and North Vietnam, and these negotiations began in Paris in May, 1968.

The first year of the Nixon administration was full of excitement and hope. In July, 1969, an Apollo aircraft, the eleventh in its line, landed two Americans on the moon, and this amazing feat was repeated by *Apollo 12* in November. Thanks to television, almost every American as well as people in many other parts of the world had an opportunity to experience the excitement of the moon landings. The bleak moonscape was displayed vividly, and above the mountains of the moon, 240,000 miles away, lay the tiny globe of mother earth. In the elevation of spirit stimulated by the moon landings the prospect of nuclear warfare seemed to fade into the background. Even among the atomic experts there was new hope: at preliminary meetings of Russian and United States representatives it had been agreed in December to open Strategic Arms Limitation Talks (SALT) in April, 1970.

Nixon, under constant pressure from increasingly formidable antiwar forces, did not long delay in reaching a decision to get out of Vietnam as soon as this could be done "with honor." After a major antiwar rally in October, 1969, he addressed the nation on television and made it known that South Vietnamese forces were being trained and equipped to replace United States troops and to take over a larger share of the fighting.

United States troops were gradually withdrawn from Vietnam in the latter part of 1969 and early 1970, and the President announced that 150,000 soldiers would be brought home during the ensuing year.

During this period United States space exploits continued to be spectacular. After a near disaster with *Apollo 13,* which failed to complete its mission to the moon in 1970, *Apollo 14* and *Apollo 15* made successful moon landings, the latter for a 66-hour exploration of the lunar surface.

During 1971 the Nixon administration made an about-face in its policy toward the major Communist powers. Henry A. Kissinger, the President's advisor on national security affairs, made secret visits to Peking in July and October to make arrangements for a presidential visit to Communist China. In September the President announced that the United States would no longer oppose the admission of the Peking regime to the United Nations, and China was admitted shortly thereafter. In October it was announced that the President planned to visit both Peking and Moscow in 1972. These visits were made as scheduled, China in February and Russia in May.

In August, 1972, it was announced that the American force in Vietnam, which had exceeded 500,000 when Nixon took office, would be down to about 25,000 by the end of the year. Then 10 days before the November election, the North Vietnamese announced that an agreement had been reached to end the hostilities in Vietnam. This turned out to be a premature announcement, but it certainly did Nixon a political favor.

During the election campaign, with everything going for him, Nixon maintained a low profile; he held few press conferences and made few speeches. His Democratic opponent, Senator George S. McGovern of South Dakota, based his campaign for the presidency on opposition to Nixon's Vietnam policy, but when election day arrived such impressive progress had been made toward bringing the war to an end that the President's Vietnam policy had become a political asset. Nixon won the election by a landslide, McGovern receiving only 37.5 per cent of the votes.

Prior to the election almost no serious attention was given to what turned out to be the most important event of the campaign. On June 17, five burglars wearing rubber gloves and carrying wiretapping devices were caught by police in the headquarters of the Democratic National Committee in the Watergate Apartment and Office Complex. The scandalous nature of this undertaking began to come to light when the robbers went on trial early in 1973. From then on an extraordinary sequence of events gradually unfolded, involving one after another of the President's staff and those who ran his election campaign. Finally the President himself was so deeply implicated in the obstruction of justice that impeachment proceedings were started against him, and on August 9, 1974, he resigned.

Nixon's last year in office was spent under the blackening cloud of Watergate, which cast its shadow over all other happenings. But in the shadows there had been other important events. Retired Ambassador David K. E. Bruce was sent to Peking to head the United States liaison office in China. Brezhnev and Nixon signed four treaties involving agriculture, oceanography, cultural exchanges, and transportation, and the two leaders joined in a pledge to work for nuclear arms control. American prisoners of war were released by the North Vietnamese. The South Vietnamese Army, trained, equipped, and supplied by the United States, appeared at least temporarily to be holding its own against continual pressure from the Communists.

One event that could not be obscured by Watergate occurred in the Middle East. The Arab countries, reacting strongly to United States support of Israel in the October war of 1973, shut off oil supplies to the United States. This led to alarming shortages and rapid increases in the price of gasoline, fuel oil, and other petroleum products. Efforts were made to persuade the Arabs to lift the embargo, but they were obviously pleased to have the United States at a disadvantage, and it was March, 1974, before they agreed to resume shipments of oil. However, they did not agree to roll back the high prices that had been put into effect when the embargo was established. The high oil prices had a far-reaching effect upon the economy of every industrial nation, and the oil situation was one of the most difficult with which President Ford had to deal when he took office.

About a year before President Nixon's resignation, Vice-President Agnew was forced to resign as a result of an entirely unrelated scandal arising from his alleged acceptance of bribes and his indictment for income tax evasion. Following Agnew's resignation, President Nixon nominated Representative Gerald R. Ford of Michigan for the vice-presidency, and this nomination was confirmed by Congress. Thus when Nixon resigned the following August, the nation for the first time had a president who had not been elected to office.

Ford's entry into the White House was greeted by an almost universal sense of relief. His accessibility, openness, forthrightness, and lack of complexity were welcomed by everyone. However, about a month after he took office his popularity went into a sharp decline when he announced that he was issuing a presidential pardon to Nixon for all federal crimes that he might have committed as Chief Executive.

In foreign affairs Ford's Secretary of State, Henry A. Kissinger, played a prominent role. His widely publicized "shuttle diplomacy" between Israel and its Arab neighbors finally succeeded in achieving at least a temporary stabilization in that area. The President's most difficult foreign affairs problem was in Southeast Asia. In spite of the cease-fire agreement which had been signed in Paris in 1973, the war in Vietnam went on about as before, except that all American combat units had been withdrawn. Congress, unhappy about lending further support to what appeared to be a lost cause, reduced the appropriations for South Vietnam for fiscal 1975 from the requested $1.45 billion to $700 million. The Communist forces stepped up their military pressure in 1975, and as the South Vietnamese Army fell back, leaving much valuable equipment behind, it became evident that they were no match for the enemy. The final collapse of the Saigon regime came with calamitous speed. United States officials, civilians, and military personnel still in Saigon had barely time enough to make a scrambling, undignified exit by ship, plane, and helicopter before the Communists occupied the city. Thousands of South Vietnamese also fled to American territory, thus presenting to the United States government the difficult task of finding homes for a large number of refugees who knew little or nothing about our language or customs.

DOMESTIC AFFAIRS President Truman's domestic program, which was known as the *Fair Deal,* included (1) an expanded social security system, (2) government aid for scientific research, and (3) a permanent Fair Employment Practices Commission (FEPC) to protect minority rights. In a message to Congress in November, 1945, Truman made a number of proposals which, he said, were designed to "reach the health objectives of our economic Bill of Rights." These proposals, which included a plan for prepayment of medical costs "through expansion of our existing compulsory social insurance program," revived the old battle with the American Medical Association. Truman's program also aroused the opposition of other groups, and in the election of 1946 the Republicans gained control of Congress and blocked most of the Fair Deal domestic measures. Congress also passed, over Truman's veto, the Labor-Management Relations Act (the Taft-Hartley Act).

No action on the part of President Eisenhower had a more far-reaching national effect than his appointment in 1953 of Earl Warren as Chief Justice of the Supreme Court. In May, 1954, the Supreme Court, under the leadership of Warren, ruled unanimously that segregation of the races in public schools is unconstitutional. This decision overturned a ruling of the Supreme Court in 1896 that Negroes could be taught in "separate but equal" schools. The new decision held that "separate educational facilities are inherently unequal." Realizing that it would take time to effect such a radical change in the educational system of the southern states, the Court set no deadline for obeying the ruling. In May, 1955, the Court directed the states to end racial segregation "with all deliberate speed" but still set no deadline for compliance. In November, 1955, the Supreme Court, again by unanimous decision, banned racial segregation in public parks, playgrounds, and golf courses. In 1956, undeterred by heavy criticism of its desegregation decision, the Court extended its ban on segregation to tax-supported colleges and universities, and it ruled that segregation on buses and trains was unconstitutional.

Other important national events that occurred during Eisenhower's presidency include: the admission of Alaska and Hawaii to the Union as the forty-ninth and fiftieth states, respectively; the adoption of an Education Act, spurred by the Russian achievements in space technology, which provided millions of dollars for student loans and for the support of teaching in sciences and languages.

An additional matter of national concern was President Eisenhower's health. In September, 1955, he suffered a moderately severe myocardial infarction, which kept him away from his desk for about three months. He had been back at work for only six months when he had to undergo an emergency intestinal resection for regional ileitis. This was only a short time before the presidential election of 1956, but in spite of his precarious health Eisenhower and his running mate, Richard M. Nixon, won the election by a larger majority than they had obtained in 1952. Eisenhower's health was threatened again in November, 1957, when he had a mild stroke which affected his speech for a short time. He made a good recovery from this episode and had no further serious illness until his retirement in 1961.

On the domestic front, President Kennedy was occupied largely with civil rights problems and the national economy. It was apparent that in many areas of the South the desegregation of schools and colleges was not going to be accepted without a struggle. There were bloody riots in several communities, and when an unruly crowd in Oxford, Mississippi, prevented a young black student from entering the state university, President Kennedy ordered federal troops to Oxford to insure safe registration and attendance of black students at that school. With regard to the economy, Kennedy was worried about the poor balance of trade with foreign countries and the shrinkage of the United States gold reserve. In 1962 the gold reserve reached its lowest level since 1939. In explanation of the poor balance of trade the President emphasized that during the period of reconstruction in the countries that had been so heavily damaged during the war, new and efficient factories had been built. With new industrial plants and lower wages, the foreign countries were getting an increasing share of international trade. President Kennedy was evidently too distracted by foreign affairs to give much emphasis to the social legislation which he was known to favor. With regard to health matters, he asked Congress to adopt a Medicare Bill, but he exerted no great pressure to have this Bill accepted, and it did not get very far in Congress.

President Johnson, with his background of long experience and leadership in the Congress, quickly displayed his political adroitness and his mastery of the legislative machinery by gaining passage of a number of important pieces of legislation which Kennedy had proposed without effect. Within a few months Congress had approved the allocation of $1.2 billion for college construction and had adopted a mass transit bill and legislation to protect wilderness areas. Though Johnson was the first resident of a southern state to occupy the White House in almost a century, he used his influence to force through a reluctant Congress the Civil Rights Act of 1964, which prohibited discrimination in places of public accommodation; strengthened voting rights statutes; created an Equal Opportunity Commission to deal with job discrimination; empowered federal agencies to withhold funds from programs that discriminated against blacks; and authorized the Attorney General to take legal action to speed up desegregation in schools and colleges. Congress also passed the Equal Opportunity Act of 1964 and various other measures to fight poverty and to provide better educational opportunities for children of poor families.

The Eighty-ninth Congress, which held its sessions during the first two years of Johnson's second term, produced more social legislation than any Congress since the New Deal. Martin Luther King was then at the peak of his influence, and his demonstrations and marches were largely responsible for the passage of the Voting Rights Act of 1965 and other civil rights legislation. Congress also adopted bills for rent subsidies, for economic support for the depressed Appalachian area, for demonstration cities, for the creation of small urban parks, for federal aid to the arts, for highway beautification, and for aid to elementary education.

396   In the medical field, under urging from President Johnson, the over-

whelmingly Democratic Congress adopted the Medicare Act, which was signed into law on June 30, 1965. The Act provided funds under the Social Security Law for the health care of all citizens (and aliens with more than five years' residence in the United States) 65 years of age and older. This type of legislation, which had been proposed successively by Presidents Roosevelt, Truman, and Kennedy, had been strongly opposed by the American Medical Association and had never gotten beyond congressional committee hearings until 1964, when both houses of Congress approved Medicare bills. However, the bills of the House and the Senate differed, and before the differences could be reconciled, Congress adjourned and the bills died. Seeing that the passage of some type of Act for the medical care of the elderly was inevitable, and in an effort to gain what it considered to be preferable legislation, the AMA sponsored an "Eldercare" Bill. This Bill would have placed responsibility for the administration of the program on the states rather than on the federal Social Security Agency and would have been funded through federal grants-in-aid to the states. This proposal was rejected in committee and never reached the floor of the House.

As a companion piece to the Medicare legislation, Congress also approved a Medicaid program, which provided grants-in-aid to the states for the health care of needy persons under the age of 65. In addition, the Eighty-ninth Congress approved increases in the appropriations for hospital construction (Hill-Burton Program) and for the National Institutes of Health; it also approved two new and important medical programs: (1) President Johnson's proposal for a "Heart, Cancer and Stroke Program" (Public Law 89–239), which was given the name *Regional Medical Program* (RMP), and (2) a Comprehensive Health Planning Act (CHP) (Public Law 89–749). The administration of both of these new programs was placed in the hands of the Department of Health, Education and Welfare.

Among President Nixon's most urgent domestic problems was inflation, which during the Johnson administration had been rising at a rate of almost 10 per cent per year. During his first year in office Nixon tried to deal with this problem by persuading business and labor leaders to show "a sense of responsibility" in their decisions regarding wages and prices. This policy was ineffective, and as inflation continued to mount and more and more people began to raise their voices in protest, the President ordered a 90-day wage-price freeze in the summer of 1971. When the freeze expired in November, a *Phase 2* economic program was instituted, which limited wage increases to 5.5 per cent per year and price increases to 2.5 per cent. It was obvious that an important inflationary factor at that time was the high level of government expenditures due in large part to the war in Vietnam. Additional factors which troubled the Nixon administration and almost everyone in the country were the increase in violent crime and the widespread use of drugs, particularly by school and college students.

In domestic affairs President Ford had to deal with soaring inflation, rising prices, a business recession, and widespread unemployment. Efforts to bring these matters under control had met with no success by the end of 1975, although there was some indication of an improvement in the recession. All attempts to persuade the oil-producing nations to lower the price of oil were futile.

In health affairs President Ford showed no inclination to swim against

397

the tide of federal involvement, which had been rising steadily during the preceding administrations. The Nixon administration had made an effort to stem the tide by reducing the budget or actually withholding money appropriated by Congress for the Hill-Burton Program, the National Institutes of Health, the Regional Medical Program (RMP), and the Comprehensive Health Planning Program (CHP). Some of Nixon's actions were reversed by the courts, but many of them remained in force and gave rise to loud objections on the part of medical educators and medical scientists. President Ford, though he vetoed many other acts of Congress, affixed his signature to the *National Health Planning and Resources Development Act of 1974,* under which Hill-Burton, RMP, CHP, and other federal health programs were to be combined under the Department of Health, Education and Welfare and administered regionally by health systems agencies. The success of this ambitious federal program will depend upon the amount of money that Congress is willing to appropriate for its support. It was generally believed in 1975 that the next major move on the part of the federal government would be the adoption of a Compulsory National Health Insurance Plan financed in part by contributions on behalf of those insured and in part by taxation.

20

Medical Education

The student—the doctor—will need his basic sciences throughout his career. They are the life-blood of his practice. When he leaves the medical school for the hospital, it is only to return to the former, often to add to his knowledge. He will be going back and forth between the two until he graduates, and, we will hope, frequently thereafter. If he does not do this, his professional life becomes static.

(James Howard Means, 1953)

EFFECT OF MILITARY REQUIREMENTS
From 1940 until the closing phases of the war in Vietnam, medical education was affected to a variable degree by the need for doctors in the military services. About a year before the United States entered World War II, Congress adopted the Selective Training and Service Act, under which men of the ages 21 to 36 years who were physically and mentally sound could be drafted into the armed forces for a period of one year. The AMA was opposed to the idea of a "doctor draft." When the Selective Service law was adopted, the Association organized the Committee on Medical Preparedness, which undertook the enormous task of canvassing 184,000 physicians to determine their qualifications, readiness, and suitability for service. Under urging from the AMA, President Roosevelt in 1942 established the Procurement and Assignment Service for Physicians, Dentists and Veterinarians for the purpose of effecting orderly recruitment and proper assignment of these professionals.

After the attack on Pearl Harbor in December, 1941, all men aged 18 to 45 years were required to register for the draft, and the term of service was lengthened to the duration of the war. Deferments from military duty were granted to those who were employed in occupations essential to the war effort (workers in shipyards, munitions factories, and the like). Some physicians came under this heading; for example, those who were providing the only medical service for a community and those who held indispensable positions in medical schools and hospitals. Actually, the draft

399

created no real problems for physicians. Large numbers of doctors volunteered for military service, and the real difficulty was to decide how to distribute the limited supply so as to meet both civilian and military needs. It was those desiring to become physicians who were most seriously affected by the military situation. Under the Selective Service law premedical and medical students were as vulnerable as any other men of the same age.

When it became obvious that something had to be done to assure a continuing supply of physicians, the government agreed to grant commissions in the Army or Navy to physically fit students in the junior and senior classes of the medical schools and to postpone their call to active duty until they had completed a one-year internship. Later this arrangement was extended to apply to students in the freshman and sophomore classes. Furthermore, to provide a flow of students into the medical schools, the government in 1943 instituted a recruitment plan for medical training. Under this plan the Army Specialized Training Program (ASTP) supplied 55 per cent of the students for the freshman classes; the Navy V-12 Program, 25 per cent; the remaining 20 per cent being drawn from the civilian population. The medical schools, many of them in a precarious financial position, welcomed this arrangement, since the government not only supplied 80 per cent of the students but also paid the educational expenses for those who were selected.

When many of the young medical teachers left to join the armed forces, the medical schools had to operate with greatly reduced faculties. The shortage of teachers was aggravated by the condensation of the medical curriculum, which was introduced in order to speed up the production of doctors. The long summer vacations of the prewar years were abolished, shortening the period of study for the medical degree from the usual four years to three years or even less. Moreover, the enrollment of students in the first-year classes was increased, usually five to fifteen per cent. The schools also agreed to admit students for the duration of the emergency after only two years of college work.

POSTWAR FINANCIAL PROBLEMS

After the war it took several years for the medical schools to get back to normal operating schedules. During this period the financial predicament of the schools worsened as a result of inflation and a shrinkage in capital funds and philanthropic gifts. For a time it appeared that several schools might have to close their doors. Though the AMA recognized the seriousness of this situation, it stoutly opposed any direct financial support of medical education by the federal government. To explore other alternatives for raising funds, the AMA joined with the Association of American Medical Colleges (AAMC) in 1947 in sponsoring a meeting with leaders of industry, business, education, and philanthropic organizations. The result of this meeting was the formation of the National Fund for Medical Education, which was to solicit funds from individuals, business firms, and foundations. The National Fund had just started its fund-raising efforts when Senator Claude Pepper of Florida succeeded in getting a bill through the Senate to provide financial aid to the medical schools. This Bill could not become law until a companion Bill had been adopted by the House of Representatives. The House Bill, which was very similar to the Pepper Bill, offered federal support to the medical schools in the form of $500 per student based on the regular enrollment of each school; and, in order to encourage schools to enlarge their student bodies, $1000 for each student over and above the customary enrollment. The bill also called for an annual appropriation of $5 million for construction and expansion of medical schools. For several reasons the AMA opposed this bill: (1) its old fear that direct government financial support would lead to government control; (2) it objected to the provision of financial support for osteopathic as well as orthodox schools; and (3) it opposed giving the National Council on Education for Health Professions power to interfere in the administration of those medical schools which received financial aid under the bill. Largely as a result of the AMA's opposition the House Bill died in committee, and Senator Pepper's Bill came to a similar end because of the failure of the House to act.

In 1948 President Truman signed a new peacetime Selective Service Act, which required men 19 to 21 years of age to serve 21 months of active duty with one of the military services. When the Korean crisis erupted in 1950, Congress amended the Act of 1948 to permit the President to call up all reserves in the armed forces, with or without their consent. The amended law also required a special registration of all doctors, dentists, veterinarians, and allied specialists under the age of 50 years. The regulations allowed local Selective Service Boards to grant draft deferments to medical students and to those who had been accepted for admission to a medical school. Arrangements were also made (under the Berry Plan) to allow selected individuals to complete residency training in a specialty needed by one of the services, provided the individual would agree to go on active duty for two years after completion of the residency.

EDUCATIONAL COSTS AND PATTERNS

In 1951–52, at the time of the survey made by President Truman's *Commission on the Health Needs of the Nation,* there were in the United States 79 medical schools, of which 7 were two-year schools teaching only the basic medical sciences. The total undergraduate medical school enrollment was 27,076, and the operating expenses of all 79 schools for the academic year 1951–52 was $110 million. The income to offset these expenses came from the following sources: tuition and fees, $16.3 million; special training grants, $5.1 million; grants from outside agencies for research, $33.8 million; and the remainder from endowment income, university funds, state appropriations, and other sources (Report of the President's Commission on Health Needs of the Nation, vol. IV, p. 224, 1952).

The standard prerequisite for admission to a medical school at that time was a bachelor's degree or at least three years of college in a program that provided the essential premedical sciences. Many colleges and universities offered special "premedical courses." Some medical schools would admit well-qualified students at the end of three years' college work, with

401

the understanding that the bachelor's degree would be awarded after the satisfactory completion of the first year in medical school. These combined courses, saving a year on the way to the medical degree, were offered usually when the student took his undergraduate college course and his medical studies in the same university.

Prior to World War II, a number of young physicians still were going into practice immediately after receiving their M.D. degree. The degree and the successful completion of a State Board or National Board examination were all that were required for licensure in many states, though some states required an internship as well. After the war, very few students were willing to embark on practice without an internship, and with each passing year more and more of them went on for residency training in medicine or surgery or one of the specialties. By the late 1950s, almost all graduates were taking residencies in order to qualify for certification in a specialty; even family doctors and general practitioners began to find it desirable to spend at least one or two years as a resident before beginning practice, and before the end of the 1960s family practice itself had been recognized as a specialty.

INCREASE IN APPLICATIONS FOR ADMISSION TO MEDICAL SCHOOLS

Another change occurring after World War II was a sharp increase in the number of applications for admission to medical schools. This was due, in large part, to the "G.I. Bill," which provided educational funds for veterans. In 1949 and again in 1950 almost 25,000 students applied for admission to medical schools, though the schools in those years were able to admit only about 7000 first-year students. Prior to the war a few of the top-flight schools had more well-qualified applicants than they could accept, but most students who had taken the proper courses and had obtained average grades in their college work could gain admission to some medical school. After the flood of applications due to the G.I. Bill had subsided, the number of applicants fell back to a level about three thousand higher than it had been before the war (Table 4). In the late 1950s the medical schools were able to accept only about half of those who applied for admission.

While the medical schools, during the postwar years, were turning away large numbers of applicants, there was evidence of a growing shortage of medical practitioners. In 1905, 160 medical schools awarded the M.D. degree to 5606 students. In 1920, after the Flexner Report and the Council on Medical Education of the AMA had induced about half the schools to close, the number of students graduating fell to 3047. After that the number graduating each year slowly rose, and in 1935 the 77 schools then in existence graduated 5101 students. The number graduating each year then remained at approximately the same level for 15 years. In 1950, 79 schools turned out 5553 graduates. During this 15-year period the population had increased from about 127 million to about 151 million. Thus the annual number of graduates per million population had fallen from 40.7 in 1935 to 36.8 in 1950. The effect of the reduced number of graduates was aggravated by a number of other factors: more graduates were remaining in academic

TABLE 4.   MEDICAL STUDENT DATA*

Academic Year	No. of Schools	No. Applying for Admission†	No. of 1st-Year Students	Total Enrollment	Number Graduating
1929–30	76	13,655	6457	21,597	4565
1939–40	77	11,800	5794	21,271	5097
1949–50	79	24,434	7042	25,103	5553
1955–56	82	14,937	7687	28,639	6845
1959–60	85	14,952	8173	30,084	7081
1964–65	88	19,168	8856	32,428	7409
1966–67	89	18,250	8964	33,423	7743
1968–69	99	21,118	9863	35,833	8059
1969–70	101	24,465	10,433	37,669	8367
1970–71	103	24,987	11,348	30,487	8974
1971–72	108	29,172	12,361	43,650	9551
1972–73	112	36,135	13,677	47,546	10,391
1973–74	114	40,506	14,159	50,886	11,613
1974–75	114	42,624	14,763	54,074	12,714
1975–76	116				

*Basic data from Lambson (1975), with additions from other sources.
†The number of applications per applicant was 3.9 in 1959–60, 5.5 in 1969–70, and 8.5 in 1974–75.

medicine, medical research, public health, and industrial medicine; and a steadily increasing proportion were choosing specialty practice rather than general practice. These trends were to continue, and the result was a steady decline in the number of physicians engaged in the primary care of patients. By the 1950s those who had gone to medical school prior to 1920, when general practice was the objective of most students, were rapidly dying off or retiring, and many communities that had two or three general practitioners in 1940 found themselves without even one physician 25 years later.

THE SUPPLY OF PHYSICIANS   For years the AMA tried to insist that there was no doctor shortage. Its argument was based on statistical data produced by its Bureau of Medical Economic Research under the direction of Frank G. Dickinson, who pointed out that the number of physicians per 100,000 population, which was only 131 in 1938, had risen to 136 in 1949 and that the improvement in medical facilities and equipment made it possible for a smaller number of physicians to take care of a larger number of patients. Dickinson maintained that the lack of physicians in some areas was due to maldistribution rather than to a true shortage.

In spite of AMA denials, the country began to awaken to the seriousness of the doctor shortage in the late 1940s. One of the problems was that between 1925 and 1950, while the population was increasing from about 115 million to 151 million, only six new medical schools were established. In 1949, 18 states had no medical school, and 15 schools rejected all out-of-state applicants.

403

FOREIGN MEDICAL GRADUATES

The rise in the physician-to-population ratio to which Dickinson had called attention was due in part to the licensing of foreign medical graduates. Before and during the war, many physicians, some of them trained in the best German schools, had come to the United States to escape the persecutions of the Fascist dictators. Most of these foreign medical graduates (FMGs) sought licenses to practice in one or another of the states. Foreseeing that the licensing of foreign physicians was going to present a problem in the United States, the Council on Medical Education and Hospitals of the AMA, assisted by the Association of American Medical Colleges and an Advisory Council representing a number of private and governmental agencies, began immediately after World War II to collect information about foreign medical schools in order to assess their educational standards. By 1950 a list had been compiled that included 44 medical schools in eight countries whose programs were close enough to American standards to make their graduates qualified for licensing in the United States. Nevertheless, state laws and the attitude of many state boards made it difficult for a graduate of these better schools to obtain a license. Twenty-two states refused to recognize foreign medical degrees, and no state allowed an immigrant physician to become licensed without examination. Twenty states required full citizenship, and an additional eight required at least first papers for citizenship. Some states also required an internship or even a longer period of postgraduate training. New York was one of the more lenient states in its attitude toward foreign medical graduates, but between 1942 and 1946 only 2878 of 4975 foreign physicians who took the New York licensing examination passed. The failure rate for this group was 42 per cent, while the failure rate for graduates of New York State schools during this same period was only 6.6 per cent. Although the Council on Medical Education had performed a valuable service in listing acceptable foreign medical schools, the AMA made almost no effort to induce the states to modify their licensing laws, and some of the state medical societies were actually opposed to making any modifications in the law that would make it easier for foreign graduates to obtain a license.

In spite of the difficulties in obtaining a license, foreign medical graduates came to the United States in ever-increasing numbers. They could enter the country either on a permanent visa as immigrants or on a temporary visa as visiting scholars. Some of those who entered on a temporary basis were able later to change their status to that of immigrant. Many of those who entered on a temporary visa were bona fide students seeking several years of postgraduate medical education before returning home to practice medicine. Those who planned to stay as immigrants found that the best way to obtain an American license was to serve an internship and several years of residency training in an American hospital before taking the licensing examinations.

Since World War II the number of approved internships and residencies has more than doubled, and many of these positions have not been filled. Hospitals with the less desirable teaching programs have found it difficult to fill their positions with graduates of American schools, and they have therefore been happy to accept FMGs. It can be seen from Table 5 that the approved internships and residencies have been filled by an increasing

TABLE 5. NUMBER OF GRADUATES OF U.S. AND FOREIGN
SCHOOLS LICENSED TO PRACTICE IN U.S.*

| Year of Licensing | Number Licensed | | Physicians in U.S. | |
	Graduates of U.S. Schools	Graduates of Foreign Schools	U.S. Graduates	Foreign Graduates
1962	6648	1357		
1963	6832	1451	245,550	30,925
1964	6605	1306		
1965	7619	1528		
1966	7217	1634		
1967	7267	2157		
1968	7581	2185		
1969	7671	2307	271,390	53,552
1970	8016	3016	276,811	57,217
1971	7943	4314	282,609	62,214
1972	7815	6661	288,525	68,009

*Modified from Crispell (1974).

proportion of foreign graduates. According to Dublin (1974), since 1962, 43,000 foreign graduates have entered the United States as immigrants or have converted from temporary visitor to permanent resident by securing an immigrant visa, and during these same years under the exchange visitor program "over 55,000 FMGs, largely from developing countries, have made their initial contact with American medical practice and American medical institutions." Table 5 also shows the steady increase in the number of FMGs licensed each year. FMGs received 46 per cent of the licenses issued in 1972, and in that year 19 per cent of the physicians in the United States had received their medical degrees abroad. In addition to the FMGs who are licensed to practice or who are serving as interns and residents in United States hospitals, there is a large group (estimated at about 10,000 by Dublin in 1974) who have not been able to meet the qualifications for licensure and therefore cannot practice independently. They nevertheless hold jobs in state chronic-disease and mental institutions, where the law allows them to care for patients under qualified professional supervision.

Many of the foreign graduates entering the United States are poorly qualified and have been unable to pass licensing examinations. On the other hand, a considerable number have obtained important teaching and research positions and have risen to distinction. In 1972, Checker, Fribush and Larson examined the records of 22,611 faculty members with M.D. degrees, and found that 4165 were graduates of foreign medical schools. They noted, however, that one third of the foreign-educated faculty did not have patient-care responsibilities. In the early years of the flood of FMGs it was hoped that they would become family practitioners and settle in some of the areas where doctors were most urgently needed. This has turned out not to be the case. Foreign graduates tend to settle in the same densely populated areas as United States graduates, and in 1973 (Sprague, 1974b) only 11.9 per cent of FMGs were engaged in general practice whereas 18.6 per cent of United States graduates were so engaged.

405

To help regulate the flow of FMGs, the Educational Council for Foreign Medical Graduates (ECFMG) was established in 1958 "for the primary purpose of determining on an individual basis, whether a graduate of a medical school outside of the United States or Canada could be considered sufficiently well-qualified to serve as intern or resident in an American hospital." The ECFMG examination is a test of medical knowledge based on questions taken from Part II of the National Board examinations and of basic knowledge of the English language. The average passing rate of FMGs on a single ECFMG examination is 39 per cent (Weiss et al., 1974a). A foreign graduate must pass the ECFMG examination in order to obtain an approved internship or residency in an American hospital. The foreign countries contributing the greatest number of physicians to United States graduate medical programs in 1972 were as follows: India, 3229, the Philippine Islands, 2440, and Korea, 1171.

Because of the difficulty in getting into an American school, an increasing number of United States citizens have been going abroad to obtain a medical education. It was estimated in 1974 that approximately 5000 Americans were attending foreign medical schools. Since most of these individuals had been rejected for admission to American schools, they were in general not the best students, and in addition most of them had a serious language problem in the foreign schools. It is not surprising, therefore, that American graduates of foreign schools have done less well in the ECFMG examinations than have foreign citizens. For example, in the January, 1974, examinations of 18,765 candidates, including the Americans, 40.7 per cent passed, but only 35.7 per cent of the Americans passed. In that year, 663 American citizens graduating from foreign schools took the examination.

In 1970 a plan was developed to give American students who were doing unusually well in their foreign medical schools an opportunity to transfer back to American schools with advanced standing. This program became known as COTRANS (Coordinated Transfer Application System). United States citizens in foreign schools who apply for transfer are given a Part I National Board examination, and if they pass a place is sought for them in an American school. In five years (1970–74), 826 students obtained transfers under the COTRANS program; 611 of them were admitted to the third-year class (Dubé, 1975a and b).

In recent years there has been a mounting wave of protest against the admission of such large numbers of foreign graduates into the American health care system. We shall not attempt to enumerate all of the many valid objections. One of the most important is that during the past two or three decades thousands of foreign physicians have been allowed, even encouraged, to take up permanent residence in the United States, thus depriving many developing countries of a valuable and irreplaceable asset. Another important objection is that a large number of these FMGs, both licensed and unlicensed, are providing a very inferior form of medical care for American citizens. Differences in cultural background add to the difficulties of the FMG. In the course of a hearing before a congressional committee, Congressman William R. Roy, himself a physician, put the matter very succinctly: "May I suggest to you as a physician that it is extremely difficult to deal with the patient population unless you know something of their background, something of their culture, something of their mores, and that foreign physicians almost without exception fall short in this area." (Quoted from Weiss et al., 1974b). (For additional recent comments on the FMG problem, see Crispell, 1974; Mason, 1974; Ronaghy, 1974; Sprague, 1974b; two articles by Weiss and others, 1974a and b; Margulies and others, 1968.)

The growing shortage of physicians during the postwar era was the factor that made it easy for foreigners to gain admission to the American health care system.

NEW SCHOOLS OF MEDICINE During the period 1940–1950 only two new medical schools were established, and two other schools, Bowman Gray in North Carolina and the University of Utah in Salt Lake City, which formerly had offered only the first two years of medical school, extended their programs to four years and began to award M.D. degrees. These developments brought about an increase of about 500 medical graduates each year. The AMA, which at that time maintained that there was no doctor shortage, showed no enthusiasm for the development of new schools. However, in the 1950s there began to be evidence of a change in the position of the AMA. In 1951 the House of Delegates made it known that they would support a policy of federal grants to medical schools, provided the funds were given for construction, equipment, or renovation and provided they were controlled and allocated in the same manner as the Hill-Burton grants. The AMA also showed its concern by establishing the American Medical Educational Foundation, through which it hoped to raise funds for the medical schools from private sources. The Foundation fell far short of its goal of raising $2 million in 1951 and $5 million in 1952; nevertheless, it was able to provide some much needed unrestricted funds to the medical schools.

Between 1950 and 1965, nine new medical schools were established, and some of the older schools had increased the size of their classes. The number of medical students graduating in 1965 was about 2000 more than in 1950 (See Table 5). However, by this time it had become apparent that in spite of the increase in the number of graduates of American schools and the flood of graduates of foreign schools, the shortage of physicians had reached a critical level to which the only satisfactory solution would be a considerable increase in the output of the American schools.

During the 1960s, plans were being developed for a substantial number of new schools in various parts of the country; but after planning has begun, it takes five to ten years or even longer before a new school is ready to accept its first students. During the interval, the plans have to be completed, facilities have to be constructed and equipped, and a faculty has to be assembled. Another four years elapses before the first students are graduated, and then the graduates spend usually three to five years in clinical training before they are ready to become practitioners. Thus, from the initial planning phase, 15 to 20 years elapse before the graduates of a new school begin to enter practice.

The first significant though modest federal aid for expansion of the medical schools came with the Health Education Assistance Act of 1963, and the first applications for funds for construction under this Act were submit-

407

ted in 1965. Between 1966 and 1973 (see Table 4), 26 new medical schools opened and were admitting students. Six of the 114 schools operating in 1973 were two-year schools, teaching only the basic medical sciences. However, three of these schools were in the process of changing to a four-year curriculum leading to the M.D. degree. When the academic year 1973–74 opened, 10 of the most recently established schools had yet to graduate a student. In other words, 13 schools (of the total of 114), which had not awarded an M.D. prior to 1974, would be contributing to the pool of medical graduates by 1978. Moreover, 16 additional medical schools were in various stages of planning and implementation in 1974, and it was expected that at least 5 of these schools would be opened by 1980. The number of students enrolled in the medical schools increased from 23,216 in 1945–46 to 47,546 in 1972–73, and the number graduating at the end of each of these years rose from 5826 to 10,391. It is estimated that when all of the 114 schools are operating at full capacity, the number graduating each year will exceed 14,000, and if the schools that were being planned in 1975 proceed to the stage of operation, the number graduating each year may reach 17,000 to 18,000 by the end of the twentieth century. In the mid-1970s some of those concerned with the problems of medical education were beginning to wonder whether we were not building too many medical schools (Kerr, 1975).

An important element in the increased enrollment of medical students during the 1970s was a marked rise in the number of women admitted to the schools. In 1970–71 women made up 11 per cent of the first-year class; this figure has risen to 22 per cent in 1974–75. There was also an increase in the enrollment of black students; from 3.8 per cent in 1970–71 to 6.5 per cent in 1974–75.

In commenting recently (1973) on the change in the composition of the student body, Dr. David E. Rogers, President of the Robert Wood Johnson Foundation and former Dean of the Johns Hopkins School of Medicine had this to say:

> ... *until quite recently, our backgrounds and those of our medical students were disturbingly similar. We and they came from upper and middle class backgrounds. We and they were white, male, raised on the work ethic, and placed high values on science. We were, and are, a group concerned with academic achievement, competition, intellectual rigor, research, and the ability to grasp abstract concepts. I do not decry these values—they are certainly mine. However, in so doing, we have excluded many who possess other kinds of skills now clearly needed to deal effectively with many problems in health that need physician input. As my colleague, Walsh McDermott, has put it, "We've designed a system to train nothing but pitchers—no shortstops, no outfielders, no catchers," and that does not make a balanced ball club that can field promptly or smoothly the complex issues of health and medical care today.*

> *Recently, and with prodding, we have begun to admit an increasing number of minority students and women—both long overdue. These individuals often have outlooks and aspirations quite at variance with those that I have just outlined. Many believe that cooperation and a sense of community are more important than competition, that the immediate application of biomedical science to the problems of patients deserves a higher priority than research. Consequently, many of these students recently admitted are having enormous problems in medical school. Some of this is lack of adequate preparation, but too many of their difficulties stem from the fact that their values and aspirations are not those that we hold or have come to ex-*

pect of our medical students. They simply do not identify faculty who think their way, and they do not fit in our overly rigid system.

This is too bad. For I feel that while many of these men and women would be different kinds of doctors, they would not be second class. So I am increasingly turned off by faculty debates and rhetoric about which is the most difficult job—that of taking long term sensitive care of human beings, the management of episodic complex life threatening illness, or the lonely concerns of the research bench. Obviously they are all important, and we must offer now better preparation for the first.

FINANCIAL SUPPORT OF MEDICAL EDUCATION   The enormous amount of money that has been required to expand the system of medical education and the vast sums that are required each year to keep the system in operation have come from many different sources. The federal government has contributed large amounts, though many people believe not enough, in the form of construction grants, research grants and contracts, capitation allowances, and loans for medical students. There is a difference of opinion about the adequacy of the government's contribution to the operating expenses of the medical schools: Congressman Rogers estimates that it is greater than 50 per cent and quite generous, while Dr. Cooper, President of the Association of American Medical Colleges, estimates that it is only 20 per cent and far below what it should be (see Chapter 22). Most medical educators believe that the federal contribution must be increased in order to keep the schools in operation. In addition to the expenditures of the federal government, state and local governments have played a role in financing medical education. State governments in 1973 expended $364.6 million for this purpose. The largest state contributions in that year were California, $41.6 million; Texas, $37.0 million; Michigan, $28.3 million; and New York, $25.4 million. The smallest contributions were made by South Dakota ($900,000) and Nevada ($47,000). These funds were provided directly to medical schools located within the respective states (Bromberg, 1974). The funds for construction of new medical schools and for enlargement of the capacity of existing schools have come from federal and state governments, foundations, and individuals, and loans from banks, insurance companies, and other organizations.

The cost of medical education has increased greatly. It may be recalled that in the first century of American medicine the cost was no more than $100 to $200 per student. In 1974 a study by the National Institute of Medicine of the National Academy of Sciences placed the average cost at $12,650 per student per year. Since tuition fees are often nominal and rarely exceed one quarter of the cost, a very large proportion of the expense must be derived from other sources. A great part of the increase in the cost of medical education is attributable to postgraduate education—internships, residencies, and fellowships. In addition to the high educational costs, all of these graduate students are now paid salaries. Prior to World War II, interns got bed and board and a white uniform to wear, and some of them were fortunate to get as much as $25 per month. Residents rarely got more than $50 to $100 per month. Very few interns and residents were married, and

TABLE 6. AMA-APPROVED INTERNSHIPS AND RESIDENCIES*

Year	No. of Positions Offered	No. Filled by U.S. and Canadian Graduates	No. Filled by Foreign Graduates	Number Vacant
1950–51	28,734	19,453	2072	7209
1955–56	38,132	24,995	6033	7104
1960–61	45,333	27,627	9935	7771
1965–66	51,933	30,074	11,494	10,358
1970–71	61,938	34,708	16,307	10,923
1972–73	65,308	37,849	18,395	9064
1973–74	66,302	41,765	18,343	6189
1974–75	———	41,306	18,327	———

*Modified from Dublin (1974), with additional figures from Medical Education in the United States (JAMA) for years 1973–74 and 1974–75.

their living expenses were almost negligible. After the war, an increasing number of residents were married and were in greater need of funds. At first this need was met by small salaries and loans. During the 1960s, owing partly to the demands of the house staff and partly to the competition between hospitals to attract interns and residents, the salary levels increased rapidly. A recent study of the average house staff salaries paid by 107 hospitals (Painter and Carow, 1974) showed, among other things, that the salary of interns, which was $6161 in 1968, had risen to $9778 by 1972; during this same interval the salary of third-year residents had risen from $7785 to $11,730. In addition to the increase in salaries, there had been a marked increase in the size of the house staff. Table 6 shows that the number of approved internships and residencies offered increased from 28,734 in 1950–51 to 65,308 in 1972–73, while the number filled increased from 21,525 to 56,244. A 300-bed hospital which had a 15-member house staff in 1940 at a cost of $10,000 per year, in 1975 had a 50-member house staff at a cost of $550,000. Part of the heavy expense of a house staff is chargeable to the care of patients, but a large part of the expense is for education and on-the-job training. In a teaching hospital this cost is chargeable to the medical school budget, which has to provide funds for the teachers' salaries and other expenses.

FULL-TIME FACULTY

One of the great changes that has occurred in medical education in the past 50 years has been the increase in the number of full-time salaried faculty members. In the nation's first century it was rare for any faculty member to receive a salary; they had a small income from student fees but depended largely on their income from practice. By 1900 an increasing number of the teachers of the basic medical sciences were receiving full-time salaries. The first full-time salaries for clinical faculty were paid at Johns Hopkins in 1913. Subsequently, full-time positions at Johns Hopkins increased gradually, and by 1951 the number of senior faculty (assistant professors and above) who were on a full-time basis had reached 81. Although the increase at Johns Hopkins was probably greater than elsewhere, a similar trend was occurring at other medical schools. In a survey of medical faculties conducted by the Association of American Medical Colleges in 1974, it was found that in 106 medical schools there were 15,329 budgeted positions for "strict full-time salaries" for faculty members with a rank of assistant professor or higher. In 1973–74 the mean salary level for the clinical faculty was $32,600, while that of the preclinical faculty was $23,300. A sample of teachers at the instructor level indicated that members of the full-time clinical faculty had a mean salary of $18,600 and that those on the preclinical faculty received a salary of $13,300 (Fagan, 1974).

CURRICULAR INNOVATIONS After the medical schools had recovered from the dislocations resulting from World War II, the length of the medical curriculum was reestablished at four years. When it became evident that there was a need to speed up the production of physicians, various schemes were tried to shorten the eight-year period that most students devoted to college and medical school. This was accomplished for the most part by students' transferring to medical school at the end of their junior year in college, but more radical changes were introduced in some programs. For example, in 1958 Johns Hopkins revised its curriculum and offered a five-year medical program in which Year I was provided at the university campus and the other four years at the medical school. According to Dr. T. B. Turner, who was Dean of the medical faculty at the time this new program was inaugurated, "Its declared objectives were to accelerate the pace of medical education, to bring greater scientific content to the entire curriculum and to effect an overdue accommodation between the sciences and the humanities as they relate to medical education. These objectives were to be accomplished through three main provisions of the revised program; opportunity for early admission to the Medical School, opportunity for acceleration during the course of instruction, and a much larger segment of the curriculum allotted to elective type studies." The student with a bachelor's degree entered the course in Year II, but students with exceptional qualifications were admitted to Year I at the end of their sophomore year in college. After the revised curriculum became fully effective, about 20 per cent of the students graduated each year had entered the program in Year I. In addition to allowing entry into the medical program after only two years of college work, there was also an opportunity for completion of the course at the medical school in three rather than four years. Students could accomplish this by foregoing the usual elective periods and taking only the required work. Owing to the popularity of the electives, only about seven per cent of each class took the accelerated course which allowed them to obtain their medical degrees only six years after entering college.

When Joseph T. Wearn became Dean of the Western Reserve Medical School (now Case Western Reserve), he asked the faculty to take a hard look at the curriculum. After six years of intensive study and planning, and with generous financial support from the Commonwealth Fund, a new and radically altered curriculum was inaugurated in 1952. The student during his first two and a half years in medical school did not have to move from department to department. Instead, each student was assigned his own

411

desk and laboratory bench in a large teaching laboratory, and the teachers came to him. There was no formal division of the new curriculum into departmental courses such as anatomy, physiology, pharmacology, and pathology, the traditional pattern of medical curricula. Instead, the student began his first year with a study of the biology of cells and then moved on to the biology of organized tissues, then to metabolism, then to endocrine function, and then to study of an infant cadaver. Early in his course he was introduced to a woman who was about to have a baby; he was to be on hand for the delivery of the baby, and as part of his assignment for the next two years he was to visit the mother and her family from time to time and make a study of the growth and development of the infant.

The usual second year of the medical course was extended to a total of one and a half years in order to provide ample time for acquiring fundamental knowledge about disease. The first subject presented in the second year was infectious diseases, but after that diseases were studied in relation to organ systems, such as cardiovascular, urinary, gastrointestinal, respiratory; and as each system was taken up, the anatomical, physiological, pathological, pharmacological, and clinical aspects were presented by members of the appropriate departments, who came to the student laboratory to make their presentations and to discuss various aspects of the subject with the students.

At the end of the first two and a half years the student left his laboratory base and began his clinical clerkships and other studies in the wards and outpatient departments of the hospital. Thus, the preclinical portion of the curriculum was not organized departmentally but rather concentrated its attention on normal growth and development and dealt comprehensively with the effect of disease on various organ systems. The changes in the Western Reserve curriculum were undertaken deliberately as an experiment, and from time to time alterations were made when prompted by experience. However, the basic arrangement of the program has remained the same, and other medical schools have adopted some of its features.

In the 1960s most schools revised their programs to offer a "core curriculum," which all students were required to take; and simultaneously the elective time was increased so that a student could concentrate on courses that would prepare him to enter a chosen field in the basic sciences or a clinical specialty. With this type of curriculum, students could elect not to take a number of subjects that formerly had been part of the required course. In effect, the student started to specialize at an earlier stage in his professional development.

In 1967 the Harvard Medical School changed its program to offer a core curriculum, and it lengthened the elective time for students from four months to seventeen months. The time allotted to the basic sciences was reduced from two years to one and a half years, though students were encouraged to devote six months of their elective time to additional basic-science courses. The required time for clinical work was reduced from one and a half years to ten months, but students were expected to devote additional time to clinical electives. Only during the first half of the first year were subjects taught along traditional departmental lines. After that the core curriculum took over. It was designed to integrate the basic sciences with the clinical work that was to follow. The members of basic-science

412

departments joined with members of other departments, both basic and clinical, to participate in teaching courses centered around individual organ systems in the manner pioneered at Western Reserve. By 1973, the core curriculum seemed to have lost favor with many members of the Harvard faculty. It was particularly objectionable to the basic-science faculty, who felt that they were being disenfranchised by the removal from their departments of required courses for the students. They also believed that the students were going on to clinical studies without having been given a firm foundation in the basic sciences. To support this contention, they could point to the fact that since the introduction of the core curriculum Harvard students had done less well in the National Board examinations in the basic sciences.

In addition to the curricular changes that have just been described, every medical school changed its curriculum in one way or another. Indeed, changes were going on constantly because no one was really satisfied with the situation as it existed. No one knew how to fit the vast expansion of knowledge into the four-year span which once had accommodated it quite amply. There were always conflicting interests among the faculty and a running battle to obtain more student time for one's subject.

PROBLEMS IN GRADUATE MEDICAL EDUCATION

There were also problems in the field of graduate medical education. In 1962 the trustees of the AMA recommended that a commission, composed of both laymen and physicians, be formed to carry out a study and to submit a report on the graduate period of the education of physicians. As a result of this recommendation, the Citizens' Committee on Graduate Medical Education was formed, with John S. Millis, President of Western Reserve University, as chairman. In his Shattuck Lecture (1967), entitled "The Graduate Education of Physicians," President Millis stated that "medicine is the only learned profession that has turned to persons outside the profession for review of the process of education of its future practitioners." He pointed out that the study made by the Carnegie Foundation, which resulted in the publication of the Flexner Report, had been made by a layman with full cooperation of the AMA; and that the Citizens' Commission had been made up of a mixed group of citizens with a layman as chairman. In commenting on the studies of the commission, Millis said that to a layman the education of a physician appeared to be a discontinuum made up of several compartments with inadequate intercommunication. The compartments were the high school course, the college course, the two years of preclinical work in medical school, and then the two clinical years leading to work in a hospital. "The second aspect of medical education that strikes the layman educator is how little the teaching hospitals have adopted the form, the organization and the methods of higher education. . . . The process does not resemble that of the university but rather seems more like an institutionalization of an apprenticeship, much like undergraduate medical education in the pre-Flexner days before it became a university discipline. . . . In other parts of the university the completion of graduation is measured by actual accomplishment

413

of the student, not by the length of time for which he has been registered." Millis went on to say that those who were doing the teaching in some of the hospitals were not always abreast of new developments. "The necessity for adaptation to the forces of change should be more compelling in medical education than in medical practice. It is bad enough to become obsolete in practice, but it is worse to be the recipient of an obsolete education."

Millis said that the Citizens' Commission had pointed out the need for a "mechanism for continuous and evolutionary change and one based upon the voluntary principle. It, therefore, has recommended the creation of a standing commission charged with the responsibility of guiding the continuous improvement of graduate medical education."

The problems pointed out by Millis have not been solved: the educational discontinuum still exists; the postgraduate educational program in many hospitals is still of the apprenticeship type, involving little real responsibility; the completion of graduate education in hospitals is still measured by the length of time served rather than by accomplishment; and there is the ever-present problem of trying to keep the profession up-to-date. Great efforts have been made recently in the field of continuing education for physicians and all members of the health care team. This was given particular emphasis in the original legislation for the Regional Medical Programs (see Chap. 21). The AMA, the American College of Physicians, the American College of Surgeons, and many medical schools, specialty societies, and other organizations have taken part in this effort. In some areas there are regular educational radio broadcasts, and tapes are produced that can be circulated through the profession. Unfortunately, many physicians, because of lack of time or lack of interest, do not avail themselves of the opportunities that are offered. One of the devices recently developed to force continuing education has been the policy of recertification adopted by some of the specialist societies and by state legislatures.

EDUCATIONAL DILEMMAS

In 1975 the leaders of medical education were in deep doubt as to how to design curricula and select faculties for the future. The factors giving rise to the greatest concern were: the enormous size and complexity of the body of knowledge that had to be squeezed into a four-year course; the increasing emphasis on the training of specialists rather than of generalists; the enhanced need for continuing education of physicians; the crescendo of public protest against an educational system that seemed to have fixed its gaze on the starry skies of research rather than on the everyday health problems of the common person; and escalating educational costs. These problems had flowed ineluctably, one into the other: research was responsible for the enormity and complexity of the body of knowledge, which in turn made narrower and narrower specialization inevitable, and continuing education essential; and all of these factors contributed to the rising costs.

Most educators agreed that the emphasis placed upon research in the 1950s and 1960s, though beneficial to both medical science and medical practice, had been detrimental to medical education. Many faculty members were selected because of their ability as investigators rather than their in-

414

terest in education. The premium placed on research and the generous supply of research funds had a profound effect upon the motivation of both faculty and students. The model to which many of the best students aspired had become the great investigator rather than the great physician.

What was the educational system doing to cope with these problems and criticisms? To achieve a more balanced program, it was trying to gain a greater share of financial support for its educational, as opposed to its research objectives. It was playing a greater role in continuing education for those in practice. It was also paying more attention to the health problems of the general public. By 1974, some 80 medical schools had established departments of "family practice," and some schools had become deeply involved in dealing with the health problems of their communities. In addition, new categories of practitioners were being trained to fill some of the gaps in medical coverage. An educational and training program for "physicians' assistants," pioneered at the Duke University School of Medicine, had been taken up by many other schools; and there were also training programs for nurse-midwives and nurse-practitioners.

The problems and dilemmas of medical education were recently discussed by Dr. Paul B. Beeson in his Cartwright Lecture for 1974. This Lecture, with commentaries by several distinguished medical educators, was published in *Man and Medicine* (1975). Beeson dwells on the problems resulting from the extraordinary advances in medicine during the past 30 years; the great expansion of clinical departments, particularly departments of medicine; the more than tenfold increase in salaried clinical faculty; the fragmentation of departments as specialties and subspecialties came into being; the difficulty of maintaining in a free society a proper balance between specialists and general practitioners; and the problems involved in trying to arrange educational programs to meet national health needs. Beeson selects as an example of extraordinary medical progress the improvements in the diagnosis and treatment of cardiovascular diseases. Other examples might have been selected in which the progress has been just as spectacular. To emphasize one of the practical aspects of progress, Beeson notes that President F. D. Roosevelt suffered from severe hypertension and resulting heart failure, and he speculates that the course of history might have been different if today's drugs for the treatment of hypertension had been available then.

Beeson emphasizes that the multitude and magnitude of the advances during the past 30 years make it impossible to turn the clock back to those less hectic, more enjoyable days for the clinical faculty, especially the heads of departments of medicine. He suggests that a measure of improvement might be achieved by reducing the size of clinical departments and eliminating some of the teaching programs in affiliated hospitals over which a Department Chief has to exercise supervision. He is also inclined to agree with Eugene Braunwald, Physician-in-Chief of the Peter Bent Brigham Hospital, that research in a department of medicine should be carried on by "a highly skilled and sophisticated core group of biomedical investigators" and that it should be limited to a few carefully chosen fields.

Though an American citizen, Beeson's career has been similar to that of Osler. He graduated from McGill University Medical School, and after serving as Chairman of the Department of Medicine at both Emory and Yale universities he became Professor of Medicine at Oxford University. His ex-

415

perience in the smaller Department at Oxford impressed him with the disadvantages of the larger, more complex departments of medicine in the United States. He also noted that in the British health system, where the training and distribution of health manpower is controlled by the government, it is less difficult to maintain a proper balance between specialists and generalists: "General practitioners, who see patients only outside hospitals, outnumber hospital-based specialists by 2.5 to 1."

Beeson concludes his Cartwright Lecture:

Any suggestion that it is time to stop growing meets with a stock objection, namely, that when growth ceases the organism begins to deteriorate—I've used it myself. I realize that a no-growth policy is both difficult and risky, but it has to come. The problem is to find ways to keep infusing bright new talent in such a situation. One cannot deny that the greatest scientific achievements are likely to be made by young people, despite occasional exceptions like John Enders. If overall growth has to be limited, we must try to work out methods whereby some middle-aged members of the faculty can move gracefully on to other work, say, medical care or administration. This is difficult because it requires a tough institutional policy toward loyal friends. Decisions about appointment to posts which have a major research component ought to be based just as much on promise of future productivity as on past performance.

21

Federal Government in Medicine

Select scientific men of great power — men who are thus regarded by their colleagues — and see to it that they get every bit of support which they can utilize effectively, in their own undertaking, and in accordance with their own plans. Such an effort should cover every contributory field, and hence the entire science of man's physical and chemical constitution and growth.

(Statement on the strategy for supporting research. Vannevar Bush, 1946.)

In November, 1945, some seven months after taking office and three months after the end of World War II, President Truman delivered his first message to Congress. In it, among other matters discussed, he set forth what he considered to be the deficiencies in the field of medicine. He proposed that "Congress adopt a comprehensive and modern health program for the nation, consisting of five major parts each of which contributes to all the others." Briefly stated, the five parts were as follows: (1) construction of hospitals and related facilities through federal grants-in-aid to the states; (2) expansion of public health services, also through grants-in-aid to the states; (3) federal support of medical education and medical research; (4) a system of prepayment for medical care, financed through an expansion of "our compulsory social insurance system"; (5) protection against loss of wages from disability or sickness, again by expansion of the social insurance system.

The American Medical Association quickly expressed its strong opposition to the fourth and fifth of these proposals as steps toward compulsory health insurance and socialized medicine. It also objected to government support for medical education, because it saw in this proposal an attempt

417

by government to gain control of the medical schools. However, no objection was raised to grants-in-aid to the states for hospital construction and expansion of public health services.

The AMA had been expecting the liberal Democratic administration to launch a campaign for the adoption of compulsory health insurance, and in anticipation of waging war against this bugaboo, the Association had opened a Washington office in 1944. To gather data to defend its position, the AMA had also created, in 1946, a Bureau of Medical Economic Research and had hired Frank G. Dickinson, an economist on the faculty of the University of Illinois, to serve as Director of the Bureau. When the AMA gave its support to President Truman's recommendation for hospital construction, the Hill-Burton Act, providing substantial funding for this program, was adopted by Congress in 1946.

In October, 1947, the President's Scientific Research Board, headed by John R. Steelman, submitted its report, in which it stated that many medical schools, owing to inflation and a reduction in philanthropic contributions, were faced with the undesirable alternatives of restricting their programs or closing their doors, unless the nation met the financial crisis in medical education. The Board recommended a substantial increase in the allocation of federal funds for the support of medical education and medical research.

MEDICAL RESEARCH

Dr. Norman Topping had inserted into the Steelman Report specific mention of heart disease as a high priority item among research needs. The United States Public Health Service (USPHS) showed no real interest in sponsoring this type of research until Mary Lasker gave it her backing. Mrs. Lasker had done yeoman service in support of cancer research, and she had followed the work of the National Cancer Institute with great interest; she also had worked for the passage of the National Mental Health Act of 1946 and the creation of the Mental Health Institute for research in this field. Conversations between Mrs. Lasker and Surgeon-General Leonard A. Scheele of the USPHS led to the drafting of legislation to create a National Heart Institute similar to the National Cancer Institute. It provided for cardiac research to be conducted within the proposed Institute and for grants to outside institutions. It also provided training grants in both basic and clinical science as related to heart disease. Incorporated in this proposed legislation were two new provisions: (1) grant funds for construction of research facilities at cooperating institutions, and (2) admission of laymen to the Advisory Council. The AMA, which had shown little interest in the establishment of the Mental Health Institute in 1946, gave a rather cautious endorsement of the proposed Act to create a National Heart Institute. It urged that greater limitations be placed on the power that the measure granted to the Surgeon-General of the USPHS, and it voiced its opposition to the inclusion of laymen on the Advisory Council. The Congress moved rapidly, and on June 16, 1948, President Truman signed the measure into law. Mrs. Lasker had by then established her reputation as a remarkably successful lobbyist on behalf of medical research; she was the first layman to serve on a national medical research Advisory Council.

The concept of an organized national attack on major disease problems through the establishment of categorical institutes in a large research center gained momentum in the late 1940s. The Mental Health Institute was established in 1946, and both the National Heart Institute and the National Institute for Dental Disease were authorized in 1948. A so-called Omnibus Act was passed by Congress in 1950, giving to the Surgeon-General of the USPHS the power to establish institutes to deal with major disease problems. The National Institute of Neurological Diseases and Blindness, the National Institute of Arthritis and Metabolic Diseases, and the National Institute of Allergy and Infectious Diseases were founded in accordance with this legislation. This uniquely American approach to the advancement of medical science owes its solid foundation and its almost immediate success to the efforts of Mary Lasker and Dr. Scheele, who was Surgeon-General of the USPHS from 1948 to 1956.

Circumstances favored the very strong and constantly increasing financial support which the administration and Congress gave to the National Institutes of Health (NIH) during the next two decades. The AMA was conducting a vigorous and in many respects successful campaign against any form of compulsory health insurance and against the entry of government into the field of medical education or the delivery of health services. Congress could avoid these tough controversial issues, and at the same time show its concern for the advancement of medical science, by giving all-out support to medical research. When the authorities at the NIH realized that Congress was in a generous mood and that medical research had become politically popular on both sides of the aisle in the legislative houses, they began asking for more and more money. The executive and legislative branches of the federal government tried to outdo each other in providing the NIH not only with all that it asked for but also with additional sums which, they said, might be used to press ahead more rapidly. During the early years, the NIH had the strong support first of Congressman Frank Keiff of Wisconsin and then of Congressman John Fogarty of Rhode Island, both of whom utilized their positions as successive chairmen of the Labor-Federal Security Committee to assure generous appropriations.

The National Science Foundation (NSF), which had been recommended by Vannevar Bush in 1945, was finally created in May, 1950. The new Foundation had a Division of Biological and Medical Sciences, but the mission of this Division was to be limited to the support of basic research. It was not to compete with the NIH in clinically oriented research.

In addition to providing funds for the NIH and NSF, Congress allocated $5 million in 1950 to the Atomic Energy Commission for the specific purpose of relating atomic research to the treatment of cancer. Moreover, the Veterans' Administration, which previously had shown no interest in such matters, became very actively involved in clinical research after World War II, and Congress provided generous support for this work.

A brief pause in the steady rise in the medical research budget was occasioned by the Korean War, but in 1952 the upward trend was resumed. The NIH received unfaltering support from Congressman Fogarty's skillful legislative maneuvers in the House of Representatives and from the equally skillful handling of health appropriations in the Senate by Lister Hill. Hill had a background that drew him to the field of health. His father had been

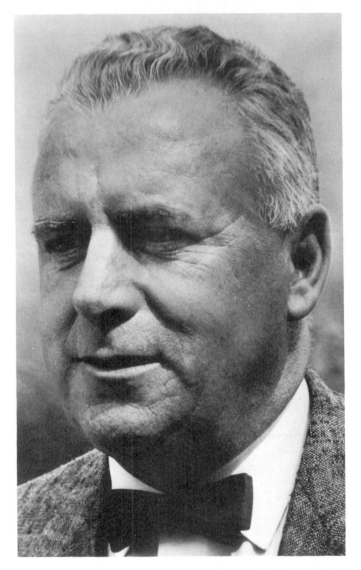

Figure 91. Congressman John Fogarty of Rhode Island.
(Courtesy of Providence College, Providence, R.I.)

a pioneer heart surgeon (see p. 502), and he had already made a name for himself in the health field by sponsoring the Hill-Burton Hospital Construction Act in 1946. In January, 1955, he assumed the chairmanship of the Senate's Subcommittee on Labor, Health, Education and Welfare. During his tenure in that post some 60 health measures became law under his sponsorship. Both Hill and Fogarty constantly stressed the need for a bipartisan approach to health legislation, and they succeeded in keeping their legislative proposals from having to run the gauntlet of party politics.

During the first Eisenhower administration, Congress regularly added some $8 to $15 million to the amount proposed by the administration for

420

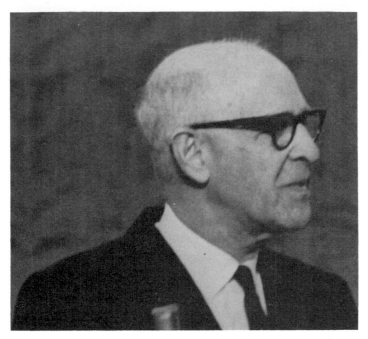

Figure 92.   Senator Lister Hill of Alabama. (National Library of Medicine, Bethesda, Maryland.)

the NIH budget. Fogarty was frank in stating that as long as it helped to save lives, he did not care how much it cost. By 1956 the annual NIH budget had risen to almost $100 million.

With the expansion of the NIH and the increasing size of its budget, Surgeon-General Scheele recognized the need to place the direction of the NIH in the hands of a capable administrator, a man of vision who could ensure a sound growth of the program and who would have the ability to keep Congress interested and favorably disposed toward its activities. He selected as Director of the NIH James A. Shannon, a physician and physiologist who had done outstanding work in renal physiology at the New York University College of Medicine before World War II and whose work on malaria during the war had earned him the presidential medal of merit. Before coming to the NIH in 1952 as Associate Director of the Heart Institute, Shannon had been Director of the Squibb Institute of Medical Research. Shannon was appointed Director of the NIH in August, 1955, and after Scheele retired in 1956, the Director of the NIH answered directly to Congress.

On the same day that Shannon became Director of the NIH, Marion B. Folsom became Secretary of the Department of Health, Education and Welfare (HEW). Soon after he was in office, Folsom met Mary Lasker and was impressed by her argument to give an even higher priority to the national medical research program. Shortly after this, Surgeon-General Scheele and Shannon informed Folsom that if they were required to keep the medical research budget at a level of $100 million for another year they would have to turn down grant applications from many excellent investigators. They

421

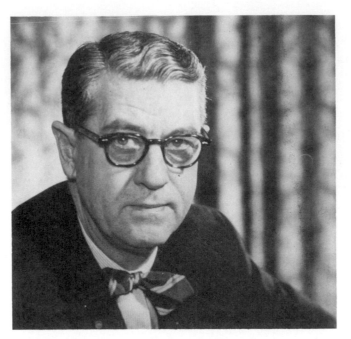

Figure 93. James A. Shannon. (National Library of Medicine, Bethesda, Maryland.)

recommended that the budget be increased by $30 million. A special committee, which Folsom appointed to look into this matter, assured him that the increase in budget was justified. At about the same time, a special congressional committee reported that there was a need for $50 million a year in matching grants for construction of research facilities, in order to rescue the medical schools from their difficult financial plight.

In September, 1955, President Eisenhower suffered a heart attack. Paul Dudley White, a Boston cardiologist who was called in for consultation, was a very articulate champion of increased federal appropriations for medical research, and while he was caring for the President he made his views known. The Secretary of the Treasury, George Humphrey, who had been a trustee of the medical school of the Case Western Reserve University, also became a strong advocate for increased spending for research. Several important members of Congress, including Senator Margaret Chase Smith, expressed similar views. With well-wishers on all sides, Secretary Folsom had little difficulty in persuading the various committees of Congress that the appropriations for medical research should be increased. In fact, these committees had become quite sophisticated in such matters, and some of their members voiced the opinion that the executive branch had consistently underestimated the medical research potential. Congress was evidently prepared to put medical research funding at a level that would ensure maximum progress.

However, it was Secretary Folsom's vision and intelligent leadership that made it seem logical to provide substantial budgetary increases for NIH at a time when the budgets of other departments were being cut. Folsom was also largely responsible for the enactment of the Health Research Facilities Construction Act of 1956, which contributed so much to the research capability of medical schools and related institutions. In addition, he encouraged expansion of the research fellowship and training-grant programs, which he considered essential to provide the scientists for the research programs of the future.

Although Secretary Folsom seemed to have a clear vision of what was necessary, his views did not have unanimous support in the executive branch, which by failing to propose a definite course of action, gave Congress an opportunity to seize the initiative. By skillful use of the hearings on appropriations, Senator Hill and Congressman Fogarty accumulated evidence to show that in the case of a number of major diseases, there were golden opportunities for research, provided funds were made available. In this manner they were able to persuade their colleagues that larger appropriations for medical research were fully justified.

With the rapid expansion of the NIH research program, Dr. Cassius J. vanSlyke introduced a new administrative system, which was designed to ensure high-quality research by grantees of the Institutes. *Study Sections* were organized under which grant proposals were reviewed by professional peers of the grant applicant to determine scientific merit and technical feasibility. These Study Sections passed judgment on proposed projects before they were presented to the Advisory Council of each Institute. The Advisory Council recommended final action. This "peer review" system was of great importance, for it kept politics out of the decisions and provided the best means of assuring quality control of the research expenditures. The scientific quality of the research assured by these controls encouraged Congress year after year to make increasing funds available. Many applications were rejected by the Study Sections because of lack of scientific merit or technical feasibility, but some of those found acceptable by the Study Sections had to be turned down at a later stage because of lack of funds.

One of the evidences of the sophisticated point of view that had grown up in Congress during the 1950s and 1960s was their willingness to provide funds without restrictions for both basic and applied research. The Senate Appropriations Committee Report on the Labor-HEW Appropriation Bill for 1967 contains the following extraordinarily liberal and understanding statement: "The committee continues to be convinced that progress of medical knowledge is basically dependent upon full support of undirected basic and applied research efforts of scientists working individually or in groups on the ideas, problems, and purposes of their selection and judged by their scientific peers to be scientifically meaningful, excellent, and relevant to extending knowledge of human health and disease" (Strickland, 1972).

One can see from the accomplishments in basic research (e.g., in genetics, immunology, and other fields) presented elsewhere in this volume that this policy resulted in unprecedented advancement in knowledge in the life sciences and that many of these advances led to new or improved methods for the treatment of disease.

The committees of Congress concerned with the NIH program did an excellent job in providing the members of Congress with reports on the important research developments. As a result, Congress was frequently better

423

informed than the executive branch in such matters, and it was willing to be more liberal in its provision of funds. For example, the Eisenhower budget for the NIH for fiscal 1957 was $126 million. Congress appropriated $183 million. The following year, the administration proposed $190 million and the Congress provided $211 million. Congress actually pushed the traditionally conservative research establishment far faster than it might have gone if left to its own devices. The liberality of Congress was a boon to many medical schools and university science departments, which had been hard pressed for funds. In later years the boon turned out to have some of the characteristics of a boomerang, but in the 1950s and 1960s the funds provided so generously by Congress enabled almost every medical school to enlarge its faculty and facilities, to pay better faculty salaries, and to upgrade its equipment in a manner that otherwise would have been impossible.

In addition to the efforts made by Congress to expand and hasten medical research, pressures in the same direction were being exerted by various lay groups. Mrs. Lasker and others like her believed that the members of the scientific community were overly cautious and that they had too narrow a view. The increased governmental support of cancer research served to stimulate private interest in this field. As the budget for the National Cancer Institute increased year after year, so did the public contributions to the American Cancer Society, and in 1970 the Society raised the unprecedented amount of $70 million. The success of the American Cancer Society served as an example to other private organizations interested in specific diseases and led to the creation of many new disease-oriented splinter groups. As new categorical Institutes came into being at the NIH, new associations and societies in these same specific health fields were organized in the private sector. These organizations were more worried about the slow progress of science than about how much money it would cost to get the job done. Surgeon-General Scheele said that it was hard to keep up with the enthusiasm of the lay members of the Advisory Councils of the Institutes. "We medical people are very conservative. These people constantly stimulate us and remind us of our responsibilities."

Mary Lasker and her friend Florence Mahoney were constantly pushing for a greater research effort. Mrs. Mahoney learned about Mike Gorman, who had run a journalistic crusade to improve the mental health institutions in Oklahoma, and she brought him to Florida to do the same thing there, using the facilities of the Miami *Daily News,* which was controlled by the Mahoneys. Gorman later became a full-time lobbyist in Washington, particularly in the mental health field, and he was appointed Executive Director of the President's Commission on the Health Needs of the Nation, under the chairmanship of Dr. Paul Magnuson. This Commission's report, written by Gorman, presented a well-documented case for enlargement of the federal efforts in medical research. Colonel Luke Quinn, when he retired from the Air Force, had many friends in Congress, and Mrs. Lasker increased her contribution to the American Cancer Society to enable them to employ Colonel Quinn, who also proved to be a very successful lobbyist in the cause of medical research.

During President Eisenhower's second term, questions began to be raised about the fiscal control of the NIH; some said that the supervision of

the funds was less rigorous than in other governmentally supported enterprises. Two committees were appointed to look into this matter, one by
President Eisenhower under the chairmanship of Stanhope Bayne-Jones,
the other by Senator Lister Hill under the chairmanship of Boisfuillet
Jones of Emory University. Both of these committees reported that the
money was being well spent by the NIH, and the Committee appointed by
Senator Hill went so far as to recommend that the NIH budget for the following year be increased by $264 million. Congress accepted this recom-
mendation and approved appropriations for the NIH in the amount
requested. In the first year of the Kennedy administration (1961), the
record-breaking sum of $738 million received Congressional approval, $155
million more than the executive branch had recommended. However, a year
later the Congress indicated that it was growing skeptical about whether
such large sums could be put to good use: the President's request for a
budget of $930 million for the NIH was reduced by Congress to $912
million (Strickland, 1972).

The American Medical Association, aside from its halfhearted support
of the National Heart Institute, made no effective contribution to the development of the nation's medical research program. It had supported the Hill-
Burton Act, but otherwise it had a record of opposing governmental sponsorship of medical care, health insurance, the training of physicians
through scholarships, and direct support of teaching in schools of medicine.
Gradually the AMA began to realize that this negative attitude kept them in
the background of the growing support for measures to advance the health
of American citizens. Finally, in June, 1964, the AMA Board of Trustees
created a Commission on Research, and the following year at a White
House Conference on health, Dr. James Appel, speaking on behalf of the
AMA, said that no one was more concerned than his organization "that
research be continued in the future on a wide and prudent course guaran-
teeing continued progress in the medical field." Shortly thereafter, the
Commission on Research recommended that the AMA support, in general,
the federal biomedical research program and that "the programs of the National Institutes of Health should be recognized for their contributions to
the national biomedical research efforts" (Strickland, 1972). This was rather
belated support for a program that already was spending over $1 billion an-
nually.

In contrast to the lavish provision of funds for medical research,
Congress did little to provide financial assistance for medical schools. To be
sure, the research grants to many of the schools enabled them to upgrade
their educational as well as their research programs, but much faculty time
and much floor space had to be given over to the research effort. Research
as a major academic function was relatively new in the universities. Prior to
World War II, there had been only very modest financial support, coming
largely from private donors and the institutions' own operating funds.
However, by 1965, research supported by government grants had moved
into a dominant position, and, as Shannon pointed out, there was "a persistent ambivalence concerning the extent to which research is an academic
function supported by public funds or a public function housed in universities." This ambivalence interfered with the universities' own planning

425

and development, their exercise of administrative responsibility, and their freedom to negotiate with other philanthropic agencies.

In 1959, a Subcommittee of the House Committee on Government Operations, chaired by Congressman L. H. Fountain of North Carolina, initiated a study of NIH activities, focusing on its research-grants management. In 1960, some 200 universities and medical schools were awarded $250 million by the NIH for the support of more than 10,000 research projects. The first report of the Fountain Committee (1961) stated that they had found that "NIH was not adequately organized to administer the grant programs with maximum effectiveness." Shannon took exception to this conclusion, stating his belief that the Committee had devoted too much attention to the financial aspects and not enough attention to the real purpose of the NIH program, which was to promote and support first-class research by the "selection of good men and good ideas—and the rejection of the inferior." "All subsequent administrative actions," he said, "having to do with the adjustments of budgets and so forth are essentially trivial in relation to the basic selection process" (Strickland, 1972). In June, 1962, the Fountain Committee restated their position that effective management of grants is a fundamental responsibility of a government agency charged with administering grant programs. They maintained that excellence is required both in the selection of the grantee and in the administration of the grant. They concluded that the NIH was guilty of loose administrative practices and that the pressure of spending increasingly large appropriations had kept the NIH from giving adequate attention to basic management problems.

As a result of the Fountain Committee's findings, Congress scaled down by $15 million the executive branch's request for NIH for fiscal year 1964. Early in 1964, President Johnson appointed a Committee headed by Dr. Dean E. Woolridge "to study how NIH spends its approximately billion dollar budget, to judge whether the American people are getting their money's worth from the expenditure, and to recommend any changes in organization or procedure that would increase the effectiveness of the program." This Committee spent a full year investigating NIH activities, visiting more than 600 NIH-funded scientists and 150 institutional administrators. The Committee's report in February, 1965, stated that the activities of the NIH were essentially sound and that its budget of a billion dollars a year was, on the whole, being spent wisely in the public interest. Nevertheless, there was a need, according to the Committee, to strengthen the organization and procedures of the NIH. Senator Hill and Congressman Fogarty interpreted the report of the Woolridge Committee as confirmation of the value and general competence of the NIH program. Under their leadership, Congress, which for two years had scaled down the requests of the executive branch, added $12 million to the $867 million proposed by the administration for the 1966 NIH budget.

In the meantime, Mrs. Lasker and the extragovernmental forces of which she was the leader were urging that the NIH give greater attention to research on specific major diseases. Shannon was opposed to emphasizing categorical at the expense of general research, but many members of Congress, faced with the need to "sell" medical research in terms understandable to their constituents, favored the categorical approach urged by the "medical research lobby." Pressures from congressmen and the lobbyists forced Shannon to make some concessions that he might otherwise not have made, but in general he succeeded in maintaining a balance between categorical and basic research (Strickland, 1972).

In February, 1964, President Johnson, who had manifested more than the usual executive interest in medical affairs and had given Mrs. Lasker easy access to the executive ear, delivered a Special Health Message to Congress. Among other things, he announced that he was "establishing a *Commission on Heart Disease, Cancer and Stroke* to recommend steps to reduce the incidence of these diseases through new knowledge and more complete utilization of the medical knowledge we already have." Thus, the President gave his backing to the categorical approach by ordering an attack on three specific categories of disease. When the Commission was appointed, Michael E. DeBakey, Professor of Surgery at Baylor University Medical College (Texas), was designated as Chairman. In the words of Dr. DeBakey, the Commission undertook "to develop a realistic battle plan leading to the ultimate conquest of three diseases—heart disease, cancer and stroke—which now account for more than 70 per cent of the deaths in this country."

In a preface to the 750-page report of the Commission, issued in February, 1965, Dr. DeBakey, in a buoyant mood, said,

Grateful beyond measure of expression for this Presidential mandate, we plunged into our assigned task—confident that the toll of these three diseases could in fact be sharply reduced now and in the immediate future. During the intervening months, as we sought and received testimony from scores of leaders in medicine and public affairs, our conviction mounted that we could chart a truly national effort—calling upon the full resources of Federal, State and local governments, the dedicated members of the health professions, and our great voluntary health organizations—leading to the increased control, and eventual elimination, of heart disease, cancer and stroke as leading causes of disability and death. . . .

In the early decades of this Republic, our people tended to view disease as an irrevocable and irreversible visitation from an implacable Fate. Our remarkable progress against many diseases over the past half century—the life span of the average American has been lengthened by 23 years since 1900—is vivid proof of the reversibility of any disease process.

[Among other things, the Commission found] that our government has a profound responsibility, which it is not yet fully discharging, for leadership, stimulation, and support in the protection of the health of the American people. . . . The nation can well afford and the people will enthusiastically support substantially increased expenditures intended to save lives today and produce more lifesaving knowledge for tomorrow.

The nation's resources are enormous and rapidly growing. Our Gross National Product passed $500 billion in 1960 and is spiraling upward toward $1 trillion. . . .

Against this gigantic backdrop, expenditures for health cast a small shadow.

Disease costs the American people $35 billion per year, but we are investing only about $1 billion of our national funds in medical research.

The report contained many recommendations, including legislation to permit forthright federal support of medical education; larger government

427

grants for construction of health research facilities; longer periods (up to five years) of support by government grants; reorganization of the Department of Health, Education and Welfare "to provide specific high-level policy direction and coordination of health programs."

Recommendations concerning heart disease, cancer, and stroke included not only greater emphasis on education and research but also, in order to narrow the time lag between the discovery and the application of new methods, "the establishment of a national network of Regional Heart Disease, Cancer and Stroke Centers for clinical investigation, teaching and patient care, in universities, hospitals and research institutes and other institutions across the country." Specifically, the Commission recommended that 25 centers for heart disease, 20 for cancer, and 15 for stroke be established over a five-year period.

The year 1965 was a dismal one for the AMA. In February, the DeBakey Commission, which was made up largely of doctors, recommended government support of medical education and the creation of many new centers not only for research but also for *treatment* of heart disease, cancer, and stroke. The Medicare Act, which had long been held up in committee, was finally approved by both houses of Congress and was signed into law by President Johnson in July. The Higher Education Act, adopted by Congress in October, provided some (very inadequate) support for medical education.

In fiscal 1967 the Congress finally got the NIH budget over the billion dollar mark by adding more than $64 million to the administration's request. However, for fiscal 1968 the President's budget prevailed. One reason was that in January, 1967, on the opening day of the Ninetieth Congress, John Fogarty died of a heart attack. For a full decade, Fogarty, Lister Hill, and James Shannon, supported by Mrs. Lasker's lay lobby, had made medical research a major enterprise of the federal government. With the death of Fogarty, the successful team had lost one of its key players.

In June, 1966, President Johnson invited the directors of the National Institutes of Health, the Surgeon-General of the USPHS, and John Gardner, Secretary of HEW, to the White House to discuss ways to convert research results into practical answers to disease problems. He suggested that they reshape their activities in order to get maximum practical results from the existing programs. Having no advance word of the President's intentions, the NIH directors were shaken. They quickly consulted their scientist friends, and it was concluded that the Lasker forces, which were close to Johnson, were trying to downgrade basic research. These suspicions were not entirely dispelled when Secretary Gardner held a meeting of the science-university community and told them that there was no change in the policy of supporting fundamental research.

Owing to the cost of the war in Vietnam, Congress decided to keep the lid on the NIH budget. They were made more comfortable in doing so by an additional Fountain Committee salvo at NIH management. The Fountain Committee, in 1968, charged NIH with weak central management, concentrating grants in a small group of institutions, inept handling of reimbursements to grantees for indirect costs, and general laxity in grant administration. They didn't like the NIH policy of obligating funds before they were appropriated, and they said that much of the work and many of the scientists were second-rate. The hardest blow to Shannon was what he considered to be the unjust charge against the quality of the scientists and research projects receiving support.

Fountain believed that Congress had been "overzealous in appropriating money for health research" and that this was the cause of the NIH's inability to keep up with the problems of management. He suggested that if the President wanted to reduce unnecessary federal expenditures he should turn his attention to the wasteful practices of the NIH. It was, therefore, no surprise when Congress reduced the NIH appropriation for fiscal 1969 to $1.1 billion, a cut of almost $20 million, the largest that the NIH had sustained in its relatively short history. The woes of the medical research advocates were increased when Senator Lister Hill, like Lyndon Johnson, decided not to run for re-election in 1968, and James Shannon, who had guided the NIH for 13 years, retired. With Nixon's election, the medical research lobby was hampered not only by the loss of allies in the Congress but also by lack of friends in the White House. When the terms of Mrs. Lasker and Mrs. Mahoney on the Advisory Councils of the Institutes expired in 1970, neither was reappointed. This was the first time in 18 years that Mrs. Lasker had not been sitting on the medical research councils.

Congressman Flood took Fogarty's place in the House, and Senator Magnusen, who had been the original sponsor of the cancer bill in 1937, assumed the chairmanship vacated by Lister Hill. In his first year, Magnusen added $112 million to the President's proposal for the NIH budget for fiscal 1970, $100 million more than the House had approved under the new team of Flood and Michel. The final figure appropriated was $56 million more than the executive branch had requested. For fiscal 1971, Congress increased the President's budget request by almost $100 million, giving the NIH a 9 per cent increase over the previous year; and for 1972 the House and Senate Appropriations Subcommittees added over $140 million to the President's request, a sizable portion of that being for research on aging. However, after the appropriations had been made for fiscal 1972, a reduction in funds, particularly for the training programs, created serious difficulties for all universities and other institutionally based government-supported research programs.

NIH was supporting in 1967–68 more than 67,000 senior research investigators. It supported research projects in more than 2000 universities and medical schools and helped provide advanced training in basic science and various clinical specialties for more than 35,000 individuals.

As a result of the NIH programs, the United States had become the acknowledged leader in the biomedical sciences. The research of the 41 Americans who won Nobel Prizes since World War II had been supported by the National Institutes of Health, and two recent Nobel laureates, Marshall Nirenberg, in 1968, and Julius Axelrod, in 1970, performed their research at the NIH research center in Bethesda. Today the NIH has eight intramural divisions which house the world's largest and most diversified concentration of biomedical investigators. The combination of internal and external research supported by the NIH is a healthy one. Both features of the system have contributed to the strong national biomedical research enterprise that exists today. The NIH has provided a training base for aspiring young scientists and has been most effective in creating a pool of excellent biomedical research workers. All would have to agree with the statement of Dr. John A. D. Cooper, President of the Association of American Medical Colleges, that "knowledge accumulated over the past 20 years has revolutionized the range of diagnostic, therapeutic and preventive capabilities of medicine, and has made it possible for physicians to offer more favorable prognoses to patients suffering from many diseases."

During the past three decades much fundamental knowledge has been gained about the structures and functions of cells, hormones, molecules, and enzymes, amounting to a virtual explosion of new knowledge. Apart from the many important discoveries made in the basic medical sciences, the research programs both at the National Institutes of Health and at other institutions supported by NIH grants have initiated or contributed significantly to major advances in the prevention and treatment of disease. If it had accomplished nothing else, its program would have been justified by a single great success: the development by the Division of Biological Standards (NIH) in the years 1965–69 of a vaccine for the prevention of rubella (German measles). Rubella, though a mild, almost insignificant malady, has devastating effects on the fetus when the mother contracts the infection in the early months of pregnancy. This important fact was not even suspected until 1941, when an Australian ophthalmologist, Norman M. Gregg, traced cataracts in newborn infants to a rubella epidemic that had occurred the previous year. Since then it has been learned that not only cataracts but also deafness, heart disease, mental retardation, and other defects can be traced to intrauterine rubella. Major epidemics of this disease account for many miscarriages and the birth of thousands of infants with serious congenital abnormalities. The rubella vaccine, which is highly effective in preventing the disease, has had and will continue to have tremendous social effects and will save millions of dollars annually in the care of defective children.

The NIH has also contributed to important new advances in the treatment of hypertension, rheumatic heart disease, and stroke. Antihypertensive drugs were first used in 1950; by 1968 the death rate from hypertensive heart disease had declined 59 per cent. Not only did NIH funds support the ultimately successful search for antihypertensive drugs but also they contributed materially to the development of new techniques for heart and vascular surgery. The artificial heart-lung machine is now used daily and was the keystone that allowed the development of open heart surgery. NIH funds also made cortisone available for clinical trials in 1948. The war against cancer is going slowly but is making steady progress. The National Cancer Institute has been effective in extending the life of children with acute leukemia to over three years after the diagnosis has been made, contrasted with only several months' survival in 1945. More than 50 per cent of patients with Hodgkin's disease (a malignant growth of lymph tissue) can now be cured by radiotherapy. Thirty-seven drugs that were developed in part with NIH funds can bring about temporary remission in 21 different types of cancer. The discovery of specific cancer viruses promises to open up new ways of treatment. The discovery of the genetic code was a giant step forward with profound implications for the health field. In 1970, scientists performed in rapid succession the critical steps of isolating one of the "fundamental units of inheritance"; then synthesizing a gene in the laboratory; and experimenting with "genetic surgery and genetic therapy." In

November, 1970, the secret of the hormone that makes bones strong or weak was deciphered.

Private research and research by other government agencies and pharmaceutical concerns have also contributed to the advance of medical science. The development of antituberculosis drugs and polio vaccines falls into this class. A new method for treating Parkinson's disease was developed under the auspices of the U.S. Atomic Energy Commission. The successful research and development of new therapeutic agents by the pharmaceutical companies has been described in Chapter 23. The National Institutes of Health has often assumed responsibility for the testing and further development of new techniques or new drugs after their original discovery by a private or pharmaceutical source.

The NIH programs have had a profound effect upon the medical schools. The funds made available for medical research have increased astronomically in the past two decades, and this phenomenon has had both favorable and unfavorable effects upon the educational function of the schools. Research has in many instances raised the quality of a faculty but at the same time has reduced the availability of that faculty for teaching. The NIH has also taken away many teachers from their jobs temporarily to work on Study Sections and Advisory Councils. In some instances a higher priority has been given to the research program than to the teaching program, and this has resulted in dissatisfaction among students. The detrimental effects have been greatest in the teaching of medical undergraduates. On the other hand, the standard of training for physicians in many important specialties has been improved greatly by the program of training grants. Within a 15-year period (1951–1966), the number of full-time medical faculty increased from 3500 to over 17,000, largely as a result of federal medical research and training expenditures. By 1970, one half of the total medical faculty of the country had received at least part of their salaries from federal sources. During this period, the total number of medical students increased, but the increase was of a lesser degree in the schools getting most of the research funds. Almost all medical schools had become increasingly dependent upon NIH grants for research and training, and for fellowships for their younger faculty members. Since the government, owing largely to the opposition of the AMA, provided very little for the direct support of medical education, the schools could pay their large faculties only by taking salary money from research and training grants. Robert H. Ebert, Professor of Medicine at Harvard, stated in 1973 that in his opinion "bootlegging the support of education from research dollars has been one of the most destructive by-products of NIH policy."

Soon after the Nixon administration took office, it was made known that there would be a drastic reduction in the NIH budget, that all training grants and research and training fellowships were to be discontinued, and that there was to be a shift in emphasis in the research programs. Greater emphasis was to be placed on categorical disease research, especially cancer research. The largest research budget cut experienced by any of the research institutes was that suffered by the Institute of General Medical Sciences and not by an Institute dedicated to the eradication of a particular disease. These changes in government policy resulted in the withdrawal of grant funds, which had become the lifeblood of the medical schools.

431

Before the Nixon administration began its program of retrenchment, but at a time when there were increasing pressures upon the NIH to devote more of its funds to categorical research, James Shannon summed up his views on medical research and its relation to medical practice in the following three paragraphs:

(1) Knowledge of life processes and of phenomena underlying health and disease is still grossly inadequate. In the absence of broad general theory, such as exists in the physical sciences, the development of diagnostic, therapeutic, and preventive capability will continue to be dependent upon empirical approaches, serendipity, and the intuitive brilliance of too few gifted individuals. Therefore, the hope of major advances lies in sustaining broad and free-ranging inquiry into all aspects of the phenomena of life, limited only by the criteria of excellence, the scientific importance, and the seriousness and competence of the investigator.

(2) Contrary to general impression, the whole scope of the medical and related sciences is pervaded by a purposeful concern for achieving mastery over the hazards to human life and health. Research in the biomedical sciences contains a high component of practical and problem-oriented activity, though there is no clear visibility as to the extent of this activity. Unfortunately, research with practical objectives is too often equated with organized national programs such as cancer chemotherapy, vaccine development, or drug trials. It must be emphasized that such ventures are the exception rather than the rule. In the present state of our knowledge, there are limited opportunities for highly organized research of a national nature with specific short-range goals. Both types of venture must be very carefully selected, for they will be expensive and, if undertaken in the absence of an adequate scientific base, may be unproductive and hence wasteful of limited resources.

(3) Despite the limitations of the base of biomedical knowledge, progress in our medical capability has been substantial. The benefits of this progress, however, are not universally available. This is evident in the differential between the quality of medicine offered in the nation's great centers of scientific and academic medicine and in too large a proportion of services at the community level. The solution lies not in medical science but in medical economics and sociology. In this area the private sector has heretofore been dominant. But the critical nature of these problems has generated growing public concern and action. If we are to preserve the private character of medicine in this country, the problems must be attacked with greater imagination, more concern for the public interest, and more willingness of diverse interests to cooperate than has characterized the private scene thus far.

MEDICAL EDUCATION

The Fogarty Committee warned the NIH in 1957 that funds for medical research were not to be spent for broad support of medical schools and medical education. In 1963, the passage of the Health Professions Educational Assistance Act provided for direct support of medical and paramedical education. Such support was limited to grants for construction of facilities and for student loans. The authority of the legislation was broadened in 1965 and 1966, and a more comprehensive means of federal support was provided by the Health Manpower Act of 1968. Under these authorities a total of more than $1.3 billion was appropriated between fiscal 1963 and fiscal 1971 for direct support of medical schools and allied health professional schools. In the same period, over $5.2 billion was appropriated for extramural research grants. In 1968, the Bureau of Health Professions Education and Manpower Training of the Department of Health, Education and Welfare was placed in the NIH. In 1970, it was designated the Bureau of

Health Manpower Education. However, the impact on medical education has remained slight, mainly because the monies appropriated for these new programs have been far below the level authorized. From 1969 through 1971 roughly $100 million less per year was appropriated than was authorized.

The termination of the training-grant program was a severe blow to the medical schools and to the training of future research workers and specialists. In fiscal 1960, about $125 million of the NIH budget—approximately one fourth of its total appropriation of $430 million and one half of its budget for extramural research grants—was being spent for training grants and fellowships. By 1970 the expenditure for these purposes was approximately $200 million, more than one third of NIH's extramural grant appropriation. In the academic year 1968--69, undergraduate medical students constituted less than half the total educational responsibilities of medical schools and their teaching faculties, owing to the number of biomedical research scientists whose training was being supported by the NIH programs. The policy makers, with their zeal for research and their persistent refusal to offer sufficient funds to support the undergraduate teaching functions of the institutions doing the research, have caused serious imbalances. Medical schools have often found it necessary to pay a significant part of the cost of doing research, and this has reduced the funds available for educational activities.

In February, 1971, President Nixon presented a broad health plan to Congress, in which he proposed several programs to increase the production of medical and allied health personnel. In November, 1971, the Comprehensive Health Manpower Act not only authorized direct federal support of medical education through institutional grants but also offered financial incentives to those medical schools willing to increase their enrollment of medical and other students. There were additional incentives to those that would do so by shortening their curricula. This was an effort to meet the increasing demand for better medical care in the country. The abolition of the research training programs and the incentives to increase medical student enrollment were deliberate efforts to keep young physicians out of the laboratory and to force them into medical practice. The major architect of this new federal approach was Congressman Paul G. Rogers of Florida; Senator Edward Kennedy led the effort on the Senate side.

The drive to create an effective program in the area of health care brought a new important lobbying force into the picture—the Association of American Medical Colleges. This organization had two major objectives: (1) protection of the interests of medical education, and (2) opposition to the creation of a new agency to deal with the cancer problem. As a result of the shifts in emphasis, the federal government's efforts in the health field are becoming more balanced in contrast to the earlier fixation on medical research, hospital construction, and public health programs. The high cost of health care and the "failure of the health system" to provide adequate medical care for all have now become dominant in the determination of federal policy. Medical research no longer occupies the center of the congressional stage. The major battle now deals with development of some type of national health insurance. It was apparent that the AMA had lost ground in its 60-year struggle against this ancient enemy. The old alliance of the 1940s (organized labor, liberal senators, and Mrs. Lasker) has reappeared with a

433

plan for health insurance that was introduced by Senator Edward Kennedy and 14 of his colleagues in the Senate. Their proposal provides comprehensive health insurance coverage for most citizens. The Nixon administration countered this proposal with a more limited form of insurance, covering the poor and near-poor, but relying on private health insurance for a large part of the coverage.

In a study of the cost of medical education in the academic year 1972–73, the Institute of Medicine of the National Academy of Sciences found that the educational cost per student per year was $9700. Dr. John A. D. Cooper, President of the Association of American Colleges, stated in August, 1975, that when this figure was adjusted for inflation it amounted to $11,630 in 1975. According to Dr. Cooper, the total educational costs for 56,000 medical students enrolled in 1973–74 was $651 million. The federal contribution toward meeting these costs was $85.8 million in the form of capitation grants to the medical schools based on the number of students enrolled. In addition, $44.4 million was provided through distress grants to permit schools in severe financial difficulties to remain open and for other special purposes. Dr. Cooper estimated that the federal government was contributing only about 20 per cent of the cost of educating a medical student. In 1974, the government also provided $27.7 million (7 per cent) of the $380 million which the medical schools spent that year for construction of facilities (Cooper, 1975). In commenting on Dr. Cooper's figures, Congressman Rogers pointed out that if one added the $2100 and $1300 per student in research and patient care revenues, respectively, provided by the federal government, the government's share of the cost per student rose from 20 per cent to close to 50 per cent. Rogers felt that it was reasonable to take this view of the magnitude of the federal share because "much of the research money provided to individual researchers and to medical shools is awarded directly to the school for the cost of faculty salaries, supplies, equipment and other items. Many researchers also engage in teaching of medical students. A significant portion of patient care revenues inures to the benefit of medical students, who learn from the patient care rendered by teaching hospitals" (Rogers, 1975).

Though Congressman Rogers's estimate of the federal share of the educational costs seems overly generous, if not exaggerated, it can certainly be said that the government contribution was far greater than it had been 10 years before and was a vital factor in keeping many medical schools in operation. Nevertheless, what the government provided was not enough to prevent mounting deficits, and for at least some of the schools the future seemed in doubt.

HOSPITAL CONSTRUCTION: THE HILL-BURTON ACT

During the depression of the 1930s, many hospitals found it difficult to make ends meet. There was little encouragement for new hospital construction, and many of the existing hospitals were allowed to deteriorate. More than 1000 counties in the nation had no hospital facilities of any type. During the war years, a number of small hospitals were built, often of flimsy construction, to deal with the emergency requirements of communities crowded with workers in the munitions and other wartime plants and in the shipyards.

In 1942, the Commission on Hospital Care was formed by joint action of the American Hospital Association and the U.S. Public Health Service, with financial support from several foundations. In 1946, Congress enacted the Hospital Survey and Construction Act (the Hill-Burton Act), which was based largely on the recommendations of the Commission on Hospital Care. The purpose of the Act was to provide funds to the states for the orderly planning and construction of hospitals. This piece of legislation was well conceived, and it made possible an almost ideal working relationship between federal and state governments. Each state requesting funds was required to have a State Advisory Council with consumer and professional representation, and large states were to be divided into regions, each with its own advisory body. Before requesting funds, the state was required to submit a survey indicating the need for hospitals in specific localities, and particular attention was to be paid to the need for hospitals to serve rural communities. The federal government provided only a portion of the funds required for each new hospital, determined by variable matching formulas. The Act expressly forbade governmental interference in the operation of the hospitals: "Except as otherwise specifically provided, nothing in this Title shall be construed as conferring on any Federal officer or employee the right to exercise any supervision or control over the administration, personnel, maintenance or operation of any hospital, diagnostic or treatment center, rehabilitation facility or nursing home, with respect to which any funds have been or may be expended under this Title."

In 1964, amendments to the original Hill-Burton Act were adopted that provided support for construction of nursing homes, diagnostic and treatment centers, chronic-disease hospitals, and rehabilitation facilities. Grants were also made available for research and demonstrations relating to the effecive utilization of hospitals.

By 1965, the federal government had provided almost $2 billion to match about $4 billion provided by sponsors for the construction of 6700 projects involving 285,000 hospital beds and 1880 health units of various types. Many of the hospitals were 50 to 100 bed units located in rural areas, more than half of the total being in areas which previously had possessed no hospital service. Through its architectural and technical services, the Hill-Burton administration also did much to improve the design of hospitals throughout the country.

Between 1965 and the end of fiscal 1974, Congress had appropriated another $2 billion in matching funds under the Hill-Burton program. The annual appropriations reached a maximum of $270 million in 1967. There was a sharp drop from $267 million in 1969 to $172 million in 1970. After 1970, the emphasis shifted from construction of new hospitals and nursing homes to modernization of existing hospitals and construction of facilities for the care of outpatients. The total Hill-Burton appropriation for 1974 was $185 million.

MEDICARE AND MEDICAID

The *Medicare* program was signed into law by President Johnson in July, 1965 (see Chap. 19), and became effective July 1, 1966. The processing of bills and payment of accounts was placed in

435

the hands of designated regional intermediaries such as Blue Cross and/or Blue Shield and/or commercial health insurance companies.

Before the program became effective, there were fears that Medicare might overtax hospital capacity and medical manpower. However, experience during the first three months allayed these fears, at least temporarily, when it was reported that hospital admissions had risen only 3 per cent. Nevertheless, there were problems: (1) hospital costs had risen more than expected; (2) patients, physicians, and hospitals complained bitterly about the number of forms that had to be filled out and the records that had to be kept; and (3) physicians were constantly under pressure from their elderly patients to admit them to a hospital unnecessarily and to keep them in the hospital longer than their condition required. This was owing to the fact that under the provisions of Medicare, hospital care was less costly to the patient than care in the home.

At the end of the first full year of Medicare, the Commissioner of Social Security reported that there had been 5 million hospital admissions at a cost of $2.4 billion. In addition, $60 million had been paid for extended (nursing home) care, $13 million for home care, $12 million for outpatient care, and $640 million under the supplementary plan, of which 90 per cent went for physicians' and surgeons' fees. At this time the chief problems were reported to be: (1) continued complaints about the time required for, and the additional cost of, the vast amount of paper work; (2) the insistence by many physicians that patients pay them directly and then collect subsequently from Medicare—a financial hardship to many patients; and (3) slow processing of claims, which made it necessary for some hospitals to borrow money to pay their bills while waiting for months for their Medicare accounts to be settled. To cope with the problem of the backlog in payments, the Social Security administration in January, 1968, agreed to pay each hospital a fixed monthly sum based on the estimated amount of care that the hospital would render to Medicare patients during the year, with the final settlement being made after all the claims for the period had been processed.

The *Medicaid* program, which had been enacted at the same time as Medicare, was in serious difficulty by the end of 1968. This program was to be financed jointly with the states, but when Medicare became effective only 19 states qualified for Medicaid matching funds. By 1968, 41 states and the District of Columbia were participating, and the cost that year was $2.5 billion, of which the federal share was $1.2 billion. Since it had been estimated originally that the federal share would be only about one fourth of this amount, Congress changed the formula for determining the amount of federal assistance that states would receive. Medicaid had been designed to assist the "medically needy" under the age of 65 in meeting the cost of their medical care. The federal government agreed to pay to the participating states 50 to 80 per cent of the cost of such care. The problem hinged on the definition of "medically needy"; each state adopted its own interpretation. Under the revised formula, families would have to have a lower income than was originally proposed in order to qualify as medically needy. When Congress changed the formula, most state legislatures, in order to reduce the financial burden on the states, went even further than Congress in reducing the family income level that would qualify for Medicaid.

The cost of both Medicare and Medicaid far exceeded the original estimates. The revised estimate for 1970, based on the prior three years' experience, put the cost of Medicare at $5.5 billion (original estimate, $2.9 billion) and the cost of Medicaid at $5.5 billion (original estimate, $3.5 billion). And the escalation continued. The major determinants of the rise in cost were inflation and the increase in hospital costs, which ever since World War II had risen at a rate exceeding that of the general price index. In addition, utilization of services was greater than expected, and there was an increase in physicians' and surgeons' fees. There were also growing suspicions of fraudulent abuse of the Medicaid program. To keep down the cost of Medicaid not only was the above-mentioned change in formula enacted but also the states were allowed to eliminate some of the benefits required by the original Medicaid law. To keep down the cost of Medicare, beneficiaries were required to pay a larger share of the hospital and nursing home costs, and the charges for the supplementary plan were increased almost yearly. In addition, greater efforts were made to obtain assurance that patients really needed the type of institutional care that was being provided. After several methods designed to achieve such assurance had failed, Congress in 1972 adopted Public Law 92–603 for the purpose of creating, on a regional basis throughout the nation, professional standards review organizations (PSROs). The opening paragraph of P.L. 92–603 reads as follows:

Declaration of Purpose

In order to promote the effective, efficient, and economical delivery of health care services of proper quality for which payment can be made, in whole or in part, under the Social Security Act and in recognition of the interests of patients, the public, practitioners, and providers in improved health care services, it is the purpose of this program to assure, through the application of suitable procedures of professional standards review, that the services for which payment would be made conform to appropriate professional standards for the provision of health care and that payment for these services will be made (1) only when, and to the extent, medically necessary, as determined in the exercise of reasonable limits of professional discretion; and (2) in the case of services provided by a hospital or other health care facility on an inpatient basis, only when and for the period these services cannot, consistent with professionally recognized health care standards, effectively be provided on an outpatient basis or more economically in an inpatient health care facility of a different type, as determined in the exercise of reasonable limits of professional discretion.

The AMA opposed the PSRO law, but in 1974 it agreed to assist in drawing up professional standards and formed committees for this purpose. However, the AMA did not withdraw its opposition to the legislation, which it considered to be unsound and probably unworkable, and it declared its intention to continue its efforts to have the law changed. The standards that were being prepared during 1975 were expected to define the type of care required for each illness and each surgical operation, the type of institution in which the care should be rendered, and the number of days of institutional care appropriate for each condition. The standards would have to be flexible enough to allow for individual variations in the course of an illness and for postoperative complications and other unpredictable happenings.

437

The primary purpose of the PSRO law is to lower the cost of institutional care provided for Medicare and Medicaid patients. The law is based on the assumption that a significant number of patients are hospitalized unnecessarily and that they are kept in a hospital longer than their illness or operation warrants. This assumption is probably correct, but the magnitude of the correctness is still to be determined. Furthermore, although a PSRO may help to reduce the overall cost of hospitalization, it introduces another costly factor: the cost of the very considerable amount of time that physicians and other professional personnel will have to devote to preparing, maintaining, and policing the standards.

The belief that PSRO or any other politically acceptable measure will prevent further increases in the cost of Medicare and Medicaid has very little to lend it support.

RMP AND CHP   The Regional Medical Program (RMP) was one of the major pieces of health legislation adopted by the Eighty-ninth Congress (see Chap. 19). It grew out of the recommendations made to President Johnson by the DeBakey Commission. However, the law (P.L. 89–239) as it finally emerged from Congress bore little resemblance to the DeBakey proposals, though it addressed itself to the same categorical diseases: heart disease, cancer, and stroke. The declaration of purposes was as follows:

> *(a) Through grants, to encourage and assist in the establishment of regional cooperative arrangements among medical schools, research institutions, and hospitals for research and training (including continuing education) and for related demonstrations of patient care in the fields of heart disease, cancer, stroke and related diseases:*
>
> *(b) To afford to the medical profession and the medical institutions of the Nation, through such cooperative arrangements, the opportunity of making available to their patients the latest advances in the diagnosis and treatment of these diseases; and*
>
> *(c) By these means, to improve generally the health manpower and facilities available to the Nation, and to accomplish these ends without interfering with the patterns, or the methods of financing, of patient care or professional practice, or with the administration of hospitals, and in cooperation with practicing physicians, medical center officials, hospital administrators, and representatives from appropriate voluntary health agencies.*

A medical school acting as fiscal agent was usually at the hub of each "Region" created under this program. The Department of Health, Education and Welfare administered the program, which was fully funded by the federal government. Money was provided for staffing and for projects approved by a Regional Advisory Group and by HEW. Initially, emphasis was placed on educational programs for physicians, nurses, technicians, and other health personnel, and on training in the use of specialized equipment, so that the most modern type of treatment could be provided for those suffering from heart disease, cancer, or stroke. With the passage of time, RMP lost its original character. In the early 1970s Congress became more interested in the delivery of general medical services than in upgrading education and facilities for the treatment of categorical diseases. Accordingly,

HEW mandated that a greater share of RMP funds be used for the development of pilot projects and other activities concerned with the delivery of health services to medically deprived urban ghettoes and rural communities.

The Comprehensive Health Planning Act, which also was adopted by the Eighty-ninth Congress, unlike the RMP law, did not provide full funding for its program. The funds were provided in the form of grants-in-aid, much like the funding of the Hill-Burton program. The law called for a state CHP agency to oversee the Health planning within its borders, but planning at the regional and local level was to be carried out by "areawide" CHP organizations. Unlike RMP, which was provider-oriented, it was intended that CHP should be consumer-oriented, and the law required that the governing board of an areawide CHP organization have a majority of "consumers" among its members. (Though all of us are consumers of health services, physicians, nurses, hospital administrators, and others earning their livelihood from such services were considered to be nonconsumers in relation to CHP.)

The CHP program was launched less quickly than the RMP owing to the interposition of a state agency between HEW and the areawide organization and owing also to the need to raise matching funds locally in order to obtain federal grants. By 1970, areawide CHP agencies were beginning to function in all parts of the country.

With the change in the goals and objectives of RMP which took place in 1971–72 it became clear that RMP and CHP had overlapping and sometimes conflicting functions. The planners often did not know what the implementers of RMP were doing, and the implementers frequently initiated projects which bore no relation to an overall CHP plan. An additional obstacle to coordinated operation was that the boundaries of the CHP and RMP areas often did not coincide.

To do away with overlapping and conflicting functions and to reduce the costly overhead of maintaining several independent health programs, Congress decided, in 1974, to combine RMP, CHP, Hill-Burton, and several other smaller programs into a single program of broader scope. Public Law 93–641, The *National Health Planning and Resources Development Act of 1974,* was signed by President Ford in January, 1975. When this Act becomes effective, presumably in 1976, RMP, CHP, and the Hill-Burton agencies will go out of existence, and their functions, together with additional functions, will be taken over by regional Health Systems Agencies (HSA), each responsible for a Health Service Area with a population of 500,000 to 3,000,000. The law provides that each state shall have a State Health Planning and Development Agency to coordinate the planning and operation of the HSAs within its jurisdiction. Each HSA will have a governing Board with a majority of its members in the consumer category. Federal support for the planning function of the HSA will be in the form of grants determined by the size of the population served. Grants for resources development are to be made on the basis of state allotments, and loans and loan guarantees are also provided for in the law.

In 1975 it seemed probable that Medicare, Medicaid, and the National Health Planning and Resources Development program would all soon become part of a national health insurance program.

439

THE CENTER FOR DISEASE CONTROL*

The Center for Disease Control (CDC), headquartered in Atlanta, Georgia, is one of six major agencies of the U.S. Public Health Service (USPHS). It was originally established as the Communicable Disease Center in July, 1946, as the first federal health organization ever set up to coordinate a national control program against a whole category of diseases. In this case, the diseases were those spread from person to person, or from animals (including insects), or from the environment to humans. Tuberculosis and venereal diseases were excluded initially because separate control programs already existed for them.

CDC grew out of the nucleus of its immediate progenitor, the Office of Malaria Control in War Areas (MCWA), an emergency World War II organization designed to reduce potential malaria transmission in the proximity of military establishments and essential war industries. Atlanta was selected for MCWA's home base because it was a conveniently central point of endemic malaria.

MCWA worked directly with state health departments through district (now regional) personnel to effect maximum control with the least cost in manpower and materials. The states carried out the actual operations through their own administrative channels. MCWA contributed trained personnel and specialized equipment and materials.

Although MCWA was set up originally to cope with just one disease, in 1943 it undertook measures against the mosquito *Aedes aegypti* in Hawaii to control dengue fever and in port cities in southeastern United States to prevent yellow fever. When DDT became available, malaria control was revolutionized, and an attack on other endemic insect-borne diseases became possible. In 1945 typhus control was added to MCWA's program, and rodent and rodent-ectoparasite control specialists joined the existing staff. As the war progressed, control activities were expanded, because many carriers of disease were found throughout the country among returning military personnel and prisoners of war.

Some research was carried out during these years, mostly on a cooperative basis with the National Institute of Health, the Tennessee Valley Authority, the Department of Agriculture, and university and state health departments. It was primarily related to malaria and typhus control methodolgy, anopheline ecology, and the infectivity of imported malaria parasites.

During its short life span, MCWA met new challenges in a way that demonstrated the inherent wisdom and efficiency of attacking related health problems with teams of specially trained and equipped scientists whose activities were coordinated within a single organization. This experience had a direct bearing on the decision of the USPHS to maintain the personnel and facilities for a peacetime operation of a much broader character.

On July 1, 1946, Dr. Thomas Parran, Surgeon-General of the USPHS, redesignated MCWA as the Communicable Disease Center, with headquarters in Atlanta. The working relationships with state health departments

---

*This account of the CDC is based on a historical sketch kindly prepared for us by Helen O. Neff, Writer-Editor, Office of Information, Center for Disease Control, Public Health Service, U.S. Department of Health, Education and Welfare.

that already had been established were maintained. Primary activities of the new Center included continued efforts toward malaria eradication, typhus control, technical development and training in insect and rodent control methodology, studies on the relationship of flies to diarrhea and poliomyelitis, and studies on arthropod-borne encephalitides. There was also concern for tropical, parasitic, and other diseases, such as amebiasis, schistosomiasis, ancylostomiasis, filariasis, hookworm, yellow fever, dengue fever, and sandfly fever. Plague control activities were transferred to CDC in 1947.

A substantial laboratory organization was developed, with personnel and facilities for methodology research, reference diagnosis, evaluation of public health laboratories, provision for diagnostic biological materials, laboratory consultation, and surveys. Laboratory services were also provided to the states.

The Epidemiology Division was established to determine the extent of various communicable disease problems through analysis of statistical and epidemiological data, to recommend and evaluate control methods, and to render epidemic aid (on request) to states. A broadly based training program was created, and technological activities were realigned to provide more comprehensive services. The famed Epidemic Intelligence Service, whose members are popularly known as "the disease detectives," was established in 1951. From the beginning, they were groomed to meet any epidemiological contingency in this country and abroad.

Advanced laboratory techniques that were developed during the 1950s and 1960s made it possible to identify many previously unknown strains and types of pathogenic micro-organisms. CDC played a major role in adapting the fluorescent antibody technique to the rapid diagnosis of a number of pathogens. Isolation and cultivation of the polio viruses led to the development of the Salk vaccine, with CDC assisting in the field trials that were conducted in 1954.

In April, 1955, two weeks after the Salk vaccine was released, six cases of polio in children who had received the vaccine were reported to the Public Health Service. In another two days, CDC's Poliomyelitis Surveillance Unit was established. It immediately began summarizing all available information about the occurrence of polio and its possible association with vaccine. More than 80 per cent of the vaccine-associated cases reported were related to the product prepared by a single manufacturer, although it composed less than 10 per cent of the total vaccine distributed. It was withdrawn at once. The other manufacturers of vaccine were encouraged to stay in production, and the immunization program proceeded. Surveillance and evaluation were maintained by CDC on the vaccine's safety and effectiveness.

The role of CDC in a national health emergency was clearly established during this incident, setting a precedent for the immediate development of similar surveillance programs. Urgency again called for prompt action two years later, when the new variant A2 Asian strain of influenza virus swept around the world.

The Asian flu pandemic of 1957–58 highlighted the value of global health activities. The United States had joined the World Health Organization (WHO) in 1948 to work with other countries toward achieving the highest possible level of health for all people. Even before the Asian influenza pandemic, WHO had established a network for the study of influenza strains in virus laboratories all over the world. Serving as the Center for the Americas, CDC distributed sets of typing reagents for the Asian and older influenza strains and shared current laboratory "know-how" with more than 160 laboratories representing 32 countries in the Western Hemisphere. WHO had also established an international intelligence network, of which CDC was a member. From this vantage point, and calling on its earlier experience with surveillance and reporting of polio and other diseases, CDC issued frequent reports on the status of Asian flu, which were of value to health workers here and abroad.

Practically all of CDC's operational services were put to work to some extent on the international health front through WHO, the Pan American Sanitary Organization, and our own Department of State's foreign aid program. CDC had been a pioneer in training foreign health workers, particularly those from developing countries, where infectious diseases were the major cause of death and disability and where advanced technology had not yet taken root. Now the philosophy behind CDC's assistance to state health departments was applied to all nations that sought its aid—to help them develop increasingly effective programs of their own for the prevention, detection, diagnosis, and control of infectious diseases.

By the end of the 1950s, CDC was the national resource through which new areas of knowledge in communicable disease control developed by research and other investigative activities—its own and those of other institutions—were converted rapidly and effectively into usable forms for public health practice. It had acquired a multidiscipline staff, whose professional and technical personnel were recognized internationally as experts in their specialties. It had established the Veterinary Public Health Division in 1947, and the Venereal Disease and Tuberculosis programs were transferred to CDC in 1957 and 1960, respectively. The first National Conference on Hospital-Acquired Staphylococcal Disease was held at CDC in 1957.

In 1960, CDC's new headquarters complex, adjoining Emory University in Atlanta's suburban northeast section, was dedicated. Until then, its activities had been carried out in scattered and often "make-do" facilities, not only around Atlanta but also in various remote field stations. It was now possible to bring together those functions that did not need to be separated geographically.

Responsibility for the *Morbidity and Mortality Weekly Report* was transferred to CDC in 1961, adding a new dimension to CDC's surveillance activities and further strengthening its partnership with the state health departments. The *Report* entails the weekly recording, analysis, publication, and distribution of data provided by state health departments and other sources concerning the occurrence of infectious diseases in this country. In addition, 121 major cities each week document the number of deaths from various causes.

Although the annual incidence of paralytic polio fell below 1000 for the first time in 1961, epidemics were still occurring all over the country. Unvaccinated preschool children in low socioeconomic areas were the major victims. Columbus, Georgia, was the first city to make a communitywide effort to wipe out the disease, with help from CDC and state and private health agencies. Atlanta was first to use the newly developed Sabin oral vaccine to avert a threatened epidemic. The incidence of paralytic polio fell from 13,850 cases in 1955 to 5 in 1975.

In 1962, Congress passed the Vaccination Assistance Act to help states and communities carry out intensive immunization programs against polio, diphtheria, whooping cough, tetanus, and other diseases as new vaccines became licensed. When funds were made available in 1963, CDC became responsible for administering the Act through project grants. By the end of the year, approximately 47 per cent of the population was covered. Measles vaccine was added to the program in 1965 and rubella vaccine in 1969. CDC has published studies showing the massive economic saving estimated to have come from widespread, federally funded use of these two vaccines. The saving in human suffering is immeasurable.

The Foreign Quarantine Division became a part of CDC in 1967. Today, captains of incoming ships and airplanes notify CDC by radio of any cause for suspicion on board; if there is none, they enter United States ports without delay. CDC has established "readiness" programs to cope with the possible importation of such diseases as smallpox and cholera.

WHO established a global program to eradicate smallpox within 10 years in 1966. With the Agency for International Development (AID) providing the funds, CDC gave direction to the program in 19 west and central African countries. The procedures it worked out were so successful that the goal was reached in those countries well ahead of time. By the fall of 1975, smallpox was endemic only in Ethiopia. By this deliberate, aggressive, and relentless effort, mankind for the first time in history was eradicating one of the world's greatest epidemic diseases.

During the 1960s, CDC began research in support of NASA's planetary quarantine activities. These resulted in the development of improved techniques for the microbial assay of spacecraft and the environment in which they were assembled and tested. Subsequently, CDC handled all quarantine measures in connection with the moon landings.

The national laboratory improvement program, begun by CDC in 1962, was oriented toward improving laboratory diagnostic procedures and standardizing tests. As the result of subsequent study, which showed that a high percentage of all clinical diagnostic tests were erroneous, Congress passed the Clinical Laboratories Improvement Act of 1967 (CLIA). It gave responsibility to the Department of Health, Education and Welfare to regulate and license clinical laboratories transacting business in interstate commerce. This task was delegated to CDC, which now examines and licenses laboratories that are not already accredited by bodies with standards at least as stringent as those required by the Act.

In order to reflect its broadened mission and open the door for action in other areas, CDC became the Center for Disease Control on June 24, 1970. It had already outgrown its headquarters facilities, requiring them to be expanded to more than twice their previous size, and had added an animal breeding and holding facility.

The 1970s became another era of transition for CDC—this time from control of infectious diseases only to an involvement with preventive medicine in its broadest sense. The Nutrition Program was transferred to CDC in 1970, and its report on the 10-State Nutrition Survey was delivered to Congress in 1972. The National Clearinghouse for Smoking and Health

443

was transferred in 1972, and the National Institute for Occupational Safety and Health in 1973. The Bureau of Health Education was established in 1974. By 1975, CDC's activities also included certain aspects of family planning, surveillance and investigations of congenital defects, leukemia epidemiology, lead-based paint poisoning, urban rat control, and prevention of dental disease.

CDC started as a field station of the Public Health Service in 1946; it became a bureau in 1968 and a full fledged agency in 1973. Its growth is both a continuum and a maturing of its earliest traditions, many inherited from MCWA. It provides leadership and direction to programs and activities designed to improve the health of the people of the United States by preventing or controlling diseases, improving laboratory performance, and assuring insofar as possible safe and healthful working conditions.

LOOKING AHEAD Charles C. Edwards, who for five years served within the federal health enterprise (during the last two years as Assistant Secretary of Health at HEW, the senior health professional position in the federal bureaucracy), wrote a thoughtful article for the *New England Journal of Medicine* in March, 1975, just after he had concluded his government service. He pointed out that close to one third of all expenditures for health came from federal funds: 70 per cent of all expenditures for medical research, 60 per cent of the cost of medical education, and 25 per cent of all payments for health services and supplies. He characterized the $2 billion research budget as a "political missile the aiming of which could simply not be left to the scientists," and he stated that the $650 million for cancer research in the proposed 1976 budget was based on "the politically attractive but scientifically dubious premise that a dread and enigmatic disease can, like the surface of the moon, be conquered if we simply spend enough money to get the job done." Edwards deplored the lack of leadership by health professionals and said:

> Biomedical research and health manpower are by no means the only, nor perhaps even the most important, areas in which a failure of leadership on the part of the health industry has led to politically motivated decisions of doubtful wisdom. In fact, I anticipate that we are about to see a failure of leadership whose consequences will be so vast and so pervasive as to dwarf everything that has come before it. I am referring, of course, to the enactment of a scheme of national health insurance.

> To say that the nation is not prepared for national health insurance is, in my judgment, just as certain as the fact that the United States must eventually adopt some form of universal, comprehensive health-care financing. Many millions of Americans have no protection whatever against the cost of health care, and those who do are likely to have inadequate coverage, especially for primary care and outpatient services. These factors, the consequences of which are made more ominous by the combined burden of inflation and recession, leave no doubt that we must move promptly and effectively toward a rational system of health-care financing that distributes the cost of care over the largest possible portion of the population and provides practical incentives for cost control and quality assurance. But to assume that the American health-care system is now capable of delivering the additional care that would certainly be demanded if national health insurance were enacted is, I believe, a dangerous and potentially disastrous mistake.

444

22

Modern Drugs

No one considers the prowling lion or the snake that poisons its victims before devouring them to be parasites. In such cases there is nothing equivocal; one creature destroys the life of another in order to preserve its own; the attacker is totally active and the attacked completely passive; the first is in absolute opposition to the life of the second. This concept is so simple that nobody has thought of giving it a name. This process, instead of being examined separately, may appear to be a factor in more complex phenomena. To simplify its terminology, we shall call it antibiosis.

(Villemin, 1889)

Some young officers were being instructed and examined by the commander of their regiment. He finally asked, "What, in a few words, is the object of the education given a soldier?" The answers were varied: to increase his intelligence, to make him hardy, to render him fearless, to train him in the art of war: but the commander still shook his head. At last someone suggested "to enable him to destroy his enemy." "That is correct," replied the instructor. "The aim of the soldier's training, from the marching routines taught the recruit to the instruction in higher mathematics given an artillery officer, is to enable him to destroy his enemy."

Suppose the question were put to a number of medical students about to graduate— "what is the object of medical education?" How should that question be answered? Some might reply "to enable the doctor to earn a living," some "to give him a knowledge of life and living things," some "to fit him to increase scientific knowledge of disease," but drowning out all other answers would surely come the vital one, "to enable him to destroy his enemy—disease." The practice of medicine, to prevent and cure disease, is the aim of medical education, from the first lesson in anatomy to the study of the most complicated disease problems in the hospital.

We have already seen the tremendous advances made during the first 40 years of the nation's second century in the prevention of disease, highlighted by the prevention that resulted from the birth of the new sciences of bacteriology and immunology. The story to be told now is that of the development of specific cures for disease. No chapter in this story is more impressive than that of how modern medicines were discovered. In the search for new cures, for every success there are many failures. Many thousands of new drugs must be prepared and tested each year in order to find the occasional one that reaches a stage of usefulness. The knowledge from many branches of scientific endeavor must be applied to the study of the abnormal function in the biochemical machinery of living systems caused by disease. The successful search requires elaborate teamwork, involving clinicians, chemists, and other basic scientists, and a multidisciplinary approach that has few equals in human endeavor (Clarke, 1973).

Many of the best drugs available today were developed from naturally occurring products that first came into use many, many years ago. One such example is the drug *morphine,* for which we still lack a rational theory to explain its action. Morphine is still widely used because the many efforts that have been made to modify it in order to obtain a product possessing its ability to moderate pain but lacking its addictive quality have been only partially successful. Important examples of the successful modification of natural products can be found among the antibiotics. The development of the tetracyclines and penicillins provides evidence of the great value of this approach.

The faculty of making a desirable discovery by accident is called *serendipity,* a word derived from Horace Walpole's fairy tale *The Three Princes of Serendip,* in which the characters make such discoveries. Many of the most useful drugs have been discovered in this fortuitous manner. Mass testing of many drugs, a process called screening, led to the discovery of the sulfonamides and their usefulness in the treatment of certain infections. When an effort was made to find out how these drugs work, it was learned that they compete with a constituent essential for the normal metabolism of certain bacteria. This "antimetabolite concept" led to the clinical testing of many other substances to find sulfonamide-like drugs with better characteristics. During such testing, serendipity revealed that these compounds are useful as diuretics. In a similar way, it was found that certain of the sulfonamides lower the blood glucose level and can be used as antidiabetic agents. Another example of serendipity was the discovery that certain of the antihistamines are potent depressants of the central nervous system. This was the birth of the tranquilizers and other drugs designed to have a specific effect upon the biochemistry of the brain.

New drugs may be discovered by modifying a natural product that has a desired therapeutic effect, or by starting with a rational concept of the nature of a disease and then seeking a therapeutic agent that will affect metabolically its natural course. Between these two extremes lies an area of research which has its basis in the pursuit of a new lead—often an accidental discovery—that results in the development of an agent which affects a potentially important biological activity.

Before a new drug is tested on humans, the investigator must have a reasonable basis for believing that it will perform the desired activity. The new drug should be able to accomplish something that cannot be accomplished by therapeutic agents already available; otherwise it will not be able to compete effectively in the marketplace. Clinical trials of a new drug should involve large numbers of patients so that its effectiveness and safety can be adequately assessed. Before a new drug is administered to pregnant women or women of childbearing age, tests should also be made of its effect upon the developing fetus of litter-bearing animals. If these studies all show that the drug is safe and effective, the data must be organized into a *new drug application,* and this application must be approved by the federal *Food and Drug Administration* (FDA) before the product can be prescribed by physicians. The process of review by the FDA may take months or even years, during which time additional studies may be required. Thus, in order to develop a new product for treatment of a disease in humans, a long, demanding, and costly procedure must be followed. Many times, drugs are taken a long way down this trail only to find that they are unsatisfactory for one reason or another, and there is no compensation for the costly and fruitless expenditure of time and effort. In spite of these complex procedures, which make drug development so expensive, the reward of success must be measured not only in dollars but also in the enhanced ability to control or cure human illness.

THE STORY OF THE "SULFA" DRUGS

The major killers of the nineteenth century were the infectious diseases. In the early years of the twentieth century, Paul Ehrlich in Germany sought with great imagination to find "magic bullets" that would kill the responsible micro-organisms. He coined the term "chemotherapy" to describe the destruction of bacteria by chemical agents that would not be too damaging to human tissues. In 1906, Ehrlich found an agent which would deal with the parasite that causes syphilis, but the chemotherapy of bacterial diseases remained an elusive goal for several more decades. The path that led to the conquest of the common infectious diseases began in the laboratories of the dye industry. Nineteenth-century bacteriologists initiated the staining of bacteria with dyes to make them more visible under the microscope. Such stains are still used today, and they provide the basis for an important classification (Gram stain) of bacteria.

The first breakthrough came in 1935 with the discovery that the red azo dye, *Prontosil,* protects mice against streptococcal infections. For this discovery, Gerhard Domagk was awarded a Nobel Prize in medicine in 1939. The azo dyes had been valued for their ability to bind tightly to the animal fibers, silk and wool, and were especially prized for their colorfastness in laundering. It was also widely known, even in Ehrlich's time, that bacteria are similar to wool in their binding of dyes. Two Americans narrowly missed making this discovery a number of years earlier; in 1917, W. A. Jacobs and Michael Heidelberger showed that sulfonamide-containing azo dyes have antibacterial activity, an observation that seems to have been smothered by the distractions of World War I.

The most puzzling thing about Prontosil was that it had greater antibacterial activity in the living animal than in the test tube. It seemed that the

447

drug underwent a change in the animal that made it more effective against bacteria, and this proved to be the case. Workers at the Pasteur Institute (Paris) discovered that the active component of the dye is *sulfanilamide,* a fragment of the Prontosil molecule. This finding was soon confirmed, and the modern era of antibacterial chemotherapy had truly been launched.

The major early American contributions to the use of the new agents were made by Perrin H. Long and Eleanor A. Bliss, who brought Prontosil to the United States and later employed sulfanilamide in wide-scale clinical applications at the Johns Hopkins Hospital, beginning in 1936. Participating in some of these studies, E. Kennerly Marshall, Jr., Professor of Pharmacology at Johns Hopkins, devised a method for determining the amount of sulfanilamide in the blood of patients receiving it. By studies of the blood level he was able to work out some of the basic principles involved in the use of chemotherapeutic agents, and he became one of the major architects of the modern age of chemotherapy.

Numerous derivatives of sulfanilamide were soon synthesized and tested for their clinical effectiveness against various infectious diseases. Sulfapyridine, sulfathiazole, and sulfadiazine came one after the other, each with more desirable qualities than the one which preceded it. After many other sulfonamides had been synthesized, some of them clinically useful, the major developments were (1) the introduction of congeners, including sulfaguanidine, which when taken by mouth are largely unabsorbed from the intestinal tract, and since they remain in the intestine they are particularly effective against intestinal bacteria; (2) the discovery of certain advantages of combinations of sulfonamides (triple sulfonamides); (3) the development of sulfonamides that are highly soluble in urine, thus

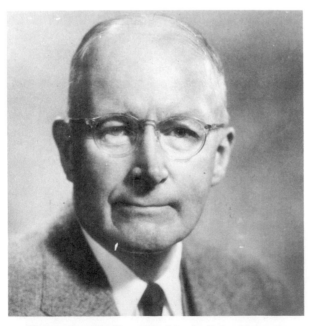

Figure 94. Eli Kennerly Marshall, Jr. (From the Archives Office, the Johns Hopkins Medical Institutions.)

reducing crystal formation in the urinary tract and renal toxicity; and (4) the establishment of the therapeutic value, in some instances, of combining sulfonamides with antibiotics.

There is an interesting story of the effect of sulfaguanidine (the congener developed for use in intestinal infections) on the outcome of the war in the southwest Pacific in 1941. The Japanese Army in New Guinea had crossed the Owen Stanley Range and was on the plains in front of the capital, Port Moresby. If Port Moresby had fallen, Australia would have been the next Japanese objective. While the Japanese were preparing to attack Port Moresby, an outbreak of bacillary dysentery occurred among the troops of both armies. Fortunately, a supply of sulfaguanidine (then one of the newest of the sulfa drugs) was available to the American and Australian troops, while the Japanese had only old and largely ineffective remedies. The sulfaguanidine enabled the Americans and Australians to remain in fighting trim and to drive the debilitated Japanese away from the approaches to Port Moresby and eventually back over the Owen Stanley Range.

Studies of the action of the sulfonamides disclosed that, unlike the older antiseptics, they do not kill bacteria outright; they merely arrest the growth and multiplication of the bacteria and allow the natural defenses of the body to do the job of mopping up. In 1940, D. D. Woods and T. Fildes of Great Britain independently found that the antibacterial action of sulfanilamide could be overcome by providing the bacteria with amounts of para-aminobenzoic acid, a natural substance required by many bacteria for normal growth. Para-aminobenzoic acid (PABA) has a close structural resemblance to a molecule of sulfanilamide. The sulfonamide enters the bacterium disguised, so to speak, as PABA and arrests the growth of the organism by preventing the incorporation of PABA. The PABA can compete successfully with the sulfonamide for its rightful place in the bacterium only if it is available in large amounts, as was shown by the experiments of Woods and Fildes.

The next serendipitous episode in the story of the sulfonamides came as the result of a chance clinical observation (Mahony, 1959). It was noted that individuals taking these drugs secreted a larger than usual volume of urine and that the urine was more alkaline than normal. It was soon discovered that sulfanilamide inhibits the enzyme carbonic anhydrase, which is found in many organs of the body, including the kidney, where its function is to acidify the urine. There had long been a need for a better and safer diuretic to promote the secretion of urine in patients who had become edematous as a result of heart failure or kidney disease. The chance discovery of the diuretic action of sulfanilamide prompted American pharmaceutical companies to go into action. They synthesized many new sulfonamides that inhibited carbonic anhydrase, some of which proved to be effective diuretic agents.

A group headed by R. H. Roblin at the Lederle Laboratories soon discovered that the best enzyme inhibitors and diuretics were found among the more acidic sulfonamides. This led them to manufacture and test a series of still more acidic heterocyclic sulfonamides. One of these, acetazolamide, was ultimately used in clinical practice as the first of a new class of diuretic drugs. We now have more effective diuretics, but the search that

449

led to the discovery of acetazolamide is one of the best examples of the correlation of a specific property (acidity) of the drug molecule with its biological activity. This has had a strong influence on the thinking of pharmaceutical chemists in their search for more rational approaches to the design of new drugs. Among the diuretics synthesized in this search was one called *carzenide,* which, although never marketed, proved to be the key to the future of diuretic research.

Another important American contribution to sulfonamide research came with the discovery of *probenecid,* which resulted from a rational and well-planned effort to attain a specific therapeutic objective. In spite of the efforts of the United States drug industry in 1942–45, penicillin remained in short supply throughout World War II and for a short period thereafter. This was due, in part, to the massive doses of penicillin that were employed to treat the more severe infections. A great part of this penicillin was wasted owing to its rapid elimination from the body by the kidneys. Penicillin is an organic acid, and a special transport system in the kidney speeds the elimination of such acids. Carl Beyer and his associates at the Sharp and Dohme Research Laboratories thought that it would be possible to find a simple organic acid that would compete with penicillin for use of the transport system, thus reducing the loss of penicillin in the urine. Starting with drugs belonging to the sulfonamide family, they found one — probenecid — with all the desired properties. As penicillin production increased, use of probenecid to prevent the loss of penicillin became less important. In the course of the experiments with penicillin, it had been found that the administration of probenecid brings about an increase in the urinary excretion of uric acid, and use was made of this discovery to lower the high level of uric acid in patients with chronic gout.

Probenecid is closely related structurally to the diuretic agent carzenide, mentioned above. All of the earlier sulfonamide diuretics had the disadvantage of causing the excretion of sodium bicarbonate, thus leading to an undesirable metabolic acidosis. The ideal diuretic should promote the excretion of equal amounts of sodium and chloride ions. The Sharp and Dohme group noted that carzenide, although primarily a carbonic anhydrase inhibitor, nevertheless produces a slight increase in chloride excretion. Systematic pursuit of this simple finding led to the discovery of the compound dichlorphenamide. The introduction of a second sulfonamide group in a specific position relative to the first greatly enhanced chloride excretion. It was then found that an analogue of dichlorphenamide, chlorothiazide, is an excellent diuretic in animals and humans. It produces a urine of almost normal ionic composition, thus avoiding the loss of bicarbonate that leads to acidosis. However, a large dose is required for a maximum effect in man. The organic chemists made variations of the molecule and soon had developed other diuretics that were more effective in smaller dosage. Recent studies have led to the synthesis of diuretics that are even more effective, including furosemide, another sulfonamide.

The principal use of the thiazides today is not as diuretics but for the treatment of high blood pressure. The effect of chlorothiazide on blood pressure was discovered in the preliminary clinical studies with this drug. Depletion of body salt and water by the use of low-salt diets had long been standard treatment for high blood pressure; so it was believed, initially, that the thiazides lower blood pressure by their diuretic action. However, evidence soon indicated that another factor is responsible for the effect on blood pressure.

Diazoxide, an experimental drug introduced by the Schering Laboratories, is a slightly modified analogue of chlorothiazide. It proved to be a more potent blood-pressure–lowering agent and not only is free of diuretic activity but also has some antidiuretic action. The antidiuresis can be prevented by the simultaneous administration of a thiazide, but this combination produces a rather serious side effect, namely, an elevation in blood glucose. Diazoxide is used for the emergency treatment of hypertension and also in those conditions characterized by low blood glucose. It lowers blood pressure by having a relaxant effect on the blood vessels.

Another observation illustrating serendipity was made in France by Ganbon and his co-workers in 1942. While studying patients with typhoid fever who were being given an experimental sulfa drug, they noted that the patients developed the symptoms of low blood glucose. Little attention was paid to this observation until 1955, when H. Franke and J. Fuch, while studying in humans the anti-infective properties of yet another experimental sulfonamide, also observed symptoms of low blood glucose. This time the practical therapeutic implications were not overlooked, and the compound *carbutamide* was soon available to physicians in Europe for the treatment of diabetes. Carbutamide is a sulfonylurea. The sulfonylureas have revolutionized treatment for the numerous diabetics who develop a mild form of the disease late in life. However, these drugs have not replaced insulin. Further studies indicated that the amino group of carbutamide, while essential for antibacterial properties, is not essential for its hypoglycemic action. The first drug that resulted from this finding, tolbutamide, also became the first sulfonylurea made available to diabetic patients in the United States.

THE ANTIBIOTIC STORY   No events of the twentieth century have had such a resounding impact upon both medical science and practical medical therapy as the introduction of penicillin and related agents. These marvelous substances are manufactured by lowly fungi and bacteria, which for eons have hidden their secrets in the dust and soil and stagnant pools that are their habitat. In past centuries, there was no more than a vague awareness of these secrets. Over 2500 years ago, long before microbes were known to exist, the Chinese learned to treat superficial infections, such as boils and carbuncles, by applying the moldy curd of soybean. But a vision of what miracles lay ahead did not occur until 1877, when Pasteur and Joubert reported that anthrax bacilli grew vigorously when placed in sterile urine but failed to multiply and soon died if the urine sample also contained one of the common bacteria of the air. This wholly unexpected turn of events led them to surmise that, among the lower species, life sometimes destroys life.

Farm soil abounding in decomposing organisms is the home of thousands of microbes, each struggling for survival. Each germ in this battle for survival uses chemical weapons, which the ingenuity of medical scientists

451

has turned to advantage in the struggle against the micro-organisms which produce the infectious diseases of man.

PENICILLIN In 1928, Alexander Fleming, in London, found that a mold had gained access to a culture plate on which he was growing colonies of a common staphylococcus. He noted that the colonies in the neighborhood of the mold, which previously had been developing normally, were now showing signs of dissolution. Since this was an unusual phenomenon, the mold was isolated and was identified as *Penicillium notatum*. Fleming later showed that this mold produces a substance that strongly inhibits the growth of the organisms which cause certain common infectious diseases. He named the substance *penicillin*. Ten years later, Howard W. Florey from Australia and Ernst B. Chain from Germany and some of their English associates at Oxford University began an intensive study of earlier scientific work, searching for ideas that might be carried further by the newer techniques and newer knowledge. During this search they ran across Fleming's almost forgotten paper (1929) about penicillin. They made some penicillin and tried to develop methods to improve the yield of this substance and to purify it without impairing its activity. They gradually accumulated a small store of pure penicillin for a trial on mice infected with a virulent strain of hemolytic streptococci (1940). All of the control (untreated) mice were dead within 16 hours, but the penicillin-protected mice survived.

The American part of the story came at this juncture. With the advent of World War II, there was great difficulty in obtaining supplies and apparatus in England. At the same time, there was need for improved medication to care for the war-wounded. Efforts were made to produce penicillin in larger quantities, but progress was slow. Making ingenious use of available apparatus, the Oxford group succeeded in producing enough penicillin for a clinical trial in 1941, when an Oxford policeman dying of septicemia was given the drug. There was marked improvement in his condition until the supply of penicillin was exhausted. English pharmaceutical firms were then unable to invest the time and equipment needed to perfect mass production of a new drug. Therefore, in 1941, Drs. Florey and Heatley came to the United States and were put in touch with Ross Harrison, then chairman of the National Research Council. Harrison, in turn, introduced them to Charles Thom of the Bureau of Plant Industry, who years before had identified Fleming's mold as *Penicillium notatum*. Ultimately they were sent to the Northern Regional Research Laboratory of the Department of Agriculture at Peoria, Illinois. There, on July 14, the problem of producing more penicillin was outlined to the Director of the laboratory, Orville E. May, and to the Director of the Fermentation Division, Robert E. Coghill. It was Dr. Coghill who suggested that the deep-tank fermentation methods then used to produce gluconic acid might be applied to penicillin production. Several measures to increase production were introduced at the laboratories in Peoria. For example, the addition of corn-steep liquor to the culture medium increased the output of penicillin 20 times. Substitution of lactose for glucose further improved output. A search for a more productive species of *Penicillium* was undertaken, and from a rotting cantaloupe found in a Peoria

452

market, a species of *Penicillium chrysogenum* was obtained that improved the yields of penicillin still further.

In addition to the work at Peoria, United States pharmaceutical manufacturers began to apply to the penicillin problem the experience gained in other industries using yeasts and molds, such as brewing and the manufacture of citric acid and other chemicals. By this time (1942), the United States had entered the war, which added a further stimulus to the effort. Finally, large quantities of penicillin began to be produced. The government took control of the entire penicillin output, assuring its availability for war needs and for the most urgent civilian needs. In 1942, there was barely enough penicillin to treat 100 patients; by late 1943, the United States was producing enough for its armed forces and those of our allies. In 1945, sufficient penicillin was being produced to meet civilian needs, and in 1958 more than 440 tons of crystalline penicillin were produced — enough to give penicillin in an amount of two million units to every individual in our population of 175 million people.

The inspiring story of the production of penicillin demonstrates what may be accomplished when a glint of hope, a strong stimulus, and a cooperative spirit are combined. In 1940, a biological curiosity of doubtful value was being produced in old whiskey and milk bottles. Little more than five years later, owing to the magnificent cooperation of biological scientists, agricultural specialists, government laboratories, and the pharmaceutical industry, an antibacterial agent of assured potency was being manufactured by the ton in assemblages of huge vats. Since this vast enterprise was part of the wartime effort, its coordination was entrusted to the Committee on Medical Research (CMR) of the Office of Scientific Research and Development. As mentioned in an earlier chapter, the chairman of the CMR, A. N. Richards, is credited with having kept the various cooperating agencies and individuals moving smoothly and rapidly toward their common goal.

DUBOS, WAKSMAN, AND CREATURES OF THE SOIL

The Lord hath created medicines out of the earth; and he that is wise will not abhor them.

(Ecclesiasticus, XXXVIII, 4)

René Dubos was born in Saint Brice, France, in 1901 and immigrated to the United States in 1924. He had spent six years as a student at the National Institute of Agronomy in Paris, from which he had received the equivalent of a master's degree in soil science. On the boat from France to America he met by chance Selman A. Waksman, a soil bacteriologist on the faculty of the College of Agriculture of Rutgers University. Waksman suggested that Dubos come to Rutgers to take a doctorate. Dubos did so, and two and a half years later he received his doctor of philosophy degree. He then applied for a National Research Council fellowship. When this was refused because Dubos was not an American citizen, he decided to seek a job at the Rockefeller Institute. His French compatriot, Alexis Carrel, took him to lunch at the Institute, and there he met Oswald T. Avery. When Dubos said that he was writing his thesis on the decomposition of cellulose by soil bacteria, this interested Avery, who had been trying without success

453

to decompose the capsule of the pneumococcus. Dubos said that he thought he could find a microbe in the soil that would decompose the capsular substance. He further surmised that if he should succeed in finding such a micro-organism, he could probably extract from it an enzyme that would do the job.

Dubos returned to Rutgers and soon thereafter accepted a job at an agricultural experiment station at Fargo, North Dakota. On the day of his arrival in Fargo, he received a telegram from the Rockefeller Institute, offering him a fellowship under Avery at $1800 a year. He quickly accepted, though it meant a reduction in salary of $1200. He was attracted by the great reputation of the Institute and by the opportunity to participate in the very important work that was then in progress in Avery's laboratory. Dubos was confident that something could be found in nature to solve Avery's problem. He reasoned that if the pneumococcus capsule had failed to decompose during its millions of years of existence, the earth would have been smothered by it.

In 1930, less than three years after his appearance in Avery's laboratory, Dubos isolated the microbe whose existence he had postulated. In seeking it, he had realized that he was dealing with a capsular substance that was composed of a gummy polysaccharide. He knew that such gummy stuff accumulates in bogs and that there was a cranberry bog near New Brunswick, New Jersey, the home of Rutgers. He felt confident that some kind of microbe would be found there that attacked substances like this capsular polysaccharide, and his hunch was correct. He extracted the enzyme from the microbe and showed in many ways that it does decompose the polysaccharide, that it actually removes the capsule from the pneumococcus. He infected mice with

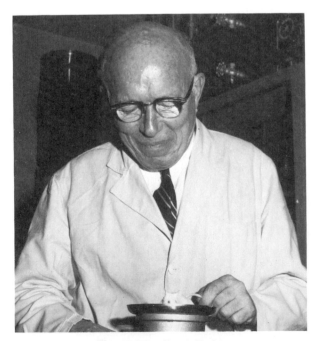

Figure 95. René Dubos.

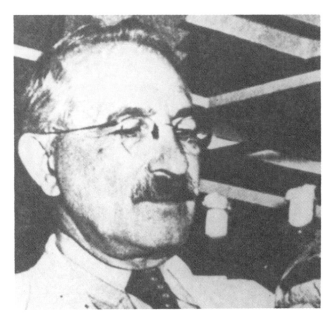

Figure 96. Selman A. Waksman. (National Library of Medicine, Bethesda, Maryland.)

type 3 pneumococcus and then gave them the enzyme. It cured them without fail. He wrote to Avery, who was on vacation. Avery rushed back, and they repeated the experiment, and again the infected mice were cured. The results, published in 1931, created a sensation.

It should not be forgotten that Dubos discovered that the organism which produces the enzyme that decomposes the capsular polysaccharide does so only when the polysaccharide is the only available food. He therefore called it an *adaptive enzyme,* a term which he invented. The discovery of this phenomenon was of great biological importance. It was the first demonstration that organisms produce certain enzymes only when they are compelled to do so. Dubos could not carry the work very far at that time because there were then serious gaps in the understanding of genetics and biochemistry. By the time Dubos had completed his work on the adaptive enzyme in 1935, the sulfa drugs were available, and they were much easier to use in the treatment of pneumococcal pneumonia.

TYROTHRICIN AND GRAMICIDIN

Since he had found a microbe that would attack polysaccharides, Dubos decided to search for one that would attack a whole bacterium. He chose the staphylococcus as his target, since there was no effective therapy against this organism. He isolated a soil bacterium, *Bacillus brevis,* from which he extracted a soluble principle called *tyrothricin.* Later, working with Rollin Hotchkiss, an organic chemist, a crystalline substance called *gramicidin* was isolated and proved to be the active fraction. Tyrothricin and gramicidin were the first drugs of the antibiotic class to be produced (1939 and 1940) on a commercial scale. These substances killed not only the staphylococcus but

455

also all the gram-positive bacteria, namely, pneumococcus, streptococcus, staphylococcus, and others. Gramicidin was used widely for the treatment of infected wounds during the early part of World War II. It also found a place in veterinary work for the treatment of mastitis in cows, a disease caused by a streptococcus.

It was the success of gramicidin that encouraged the British to revive the study of penicillin, and Florey gave Dubos full credit for this. Once penicillin was produced in quantity, it proved to be much more practical and less toxic than gramidicin, which could not be used internally because it produces kidney damage. The importance of the gramicidin work was twofold: (1) it encouraged the English workers to pursue the study of penicillin; (2) it made everyone aware that by going to the soil there was a fair chance that one could find other micro-organisms capable of producing antibiotics. Dubos believed that the possibility of finding specific enzymes to decompose certain tissues was also a reasonable possibility.

An interesting sidelight on the manner in which science progresses is cast by Dubos's comments on his life at the Rockefeller Institute during his early years there. This provides some insight into how original and productive ideas take shape. He said that the dining room at the Institute was the "greatest educational institution" that he had ever known. He came to the Institute knowing nothing about medicine, but every day in the dining room at lunch he learned something about viruses from Thomas Rivers and his group. He knew little organic chemistry, but as he sat with Hotchkiss and other people, he soon learned. The biochemist Alfred Mirsky had very broad philosophical knowledge of science, and Dubos sat with him for hours. Of course, he read and studied, but the dining room talks gave him perspective, and his success in science would not have developed so rapidly without this important influence.

STREPTOMYCIN   The significance of what happened next is dramatized by the following statement, which appeared on the front page of the New York *World Telegram:* "Saranac Lake, New York, October 12, 1954 (AP)—The Trudeau Sanatorium credited with pioneering in tuberculosis will close on December 1 as a treatment center because of deficits and a decline in patients."

This simple news item spells out dramatically the development of effective antibiotic treatment for the "great white plague." It was no longer necessary to enter a special sanatorium for a prolonged period of rest in order to deal with this widespread infection. The chain of events that led to the closing of the Trudeau and many other sanatoria began in 1943, when a strain of *Streptomyces griseus* capable of producing a new antibiotic, streptomycin, was isolated in the laboratories of Rutgers University under the direction of Selman A. Waksman. The story of this development is a thrilling one.

Less than a year after emigrating from Russia, Waksman entered Rutgers College in 1911. He had left the town of his birth in the Ukraine in search of a better education and a better opportunity than was available in his native land. After receiving his B.A. degree in agriculture in 1915, he joined the New Jersey Agricultural Experiment Station as a research assistant, while continuing with his graduate work. A year later, he received a research fellowship at the University of California, where in 1918 he obtained a doctorate in biochemistry, after which he returned to Rutgers as a microbiologist at the Experiment Station. In 1930, he was made a full professor of the university. Soil bacteriology was Waksman's major field of study, and his monograph on this subject (1927) is a classic, but in his own words: "Little did I dream at that time that there was gold in those ditches in the form of microbes many of which had never been seen before by the human eye."

By 1939, Waksman had examined thousands of soil samples. He was concerned with how the microbes lived, how they brought about radical changes in the soil, their varied chemical activities, and their influences on each other. The announcement by Dubos, his former pupil, that he had trained a microbe to feed on the capsule of the pneumococcus changed the whole course of Waksman's research.

In contrast to the chance discovery of penicillin, the isolation of streptomycin was the result of a long, systematic, plodding effort by a large group of workers under the leadership of Waksman. In 1939, one year before the rediscovery of penicillin by the Oxford group, Waksman began his highly organized study aimed at determining the nature of the substances by which the various soil microbes destroy each other. He had been interested in the *actinomycetes* (a genus of fungi) for 25 years, and it was natural that he should turn his attention first to these organisms.

Certain facts, known to Waksman, had indicated that soil is able to kill tubercle bacilli. In 1932, William Charles White, chairman of a Committee on the Microbiology of the Soil of the National Research Council and also chairman of the first research committee of the National Tuberculosis Association, asked Waksman to undertake a study of the fate of the tubercle bacillus in natural environments, especially in soils and in water systems. Waksman assigned the problem to one of his graduate students, Chester Rhimes. This study lasted for three years, and from it the following conclusions were drawn: (1) the *avian strain 531* of the tubercle bacillus has a very slow death rate in sewage and in stream water; (2) certain protozoa have the capacity to ingest large numbers of acid-fast bacteria (the tubercle bacillus is acid-fast); (3) the avian bacillus is able to multiply in sterile soil, even in association with some common soil bacteria, but it is slowly destroyed in nonsterilized soil; (4) certain fungi are able to suppress the development of the tubercle bacillus in soil, especially in manured soil. At that time, Waksman was not advanced enough in his thinking to take advantage of these findings nor of one that followed soon afterward, when the poultry pathologist of the New Jersey Agricultural Experiment Station brought him an agar slant of a culture of the tubercle bacillus which had been killed by a fungus growing in the culture medium. At that time Waksman's major interest was in other matters.

The first antibiotic to be isolated by the Rutgers team (1940) came from a culture of a soil actinomyces and was named *actinomycin*. It had a beautiful red color and either killed or prevented the growth of a large number of bacteria, including *M. tuberculosis* (the tubercle bacillus), but it was extremely toxic. (Incidentally, it was noted that actinomycin caused the spleen and other lymphatic tissues to shrink in size in experimental animals, and years later it was found that it had a marked inhibiting effect on the growth of human tumors of lymphatic tissues, such as Hodgkin's disease.)

In 1942, a second active compound, *streptothricin,* was isolated from a strain of soil actinomyces. This substance had great antibiotic activity and was less toxic than actinomycin, but before it could be clinically evaluated, *streptomycin* had been isolated (1943), and all attention was directed toward it. The streptomycin-producing culture of actinomyces originally was obtained by swabbing a chicken's throat in August, 1943. The organism belongs to a group of actinomycetes described in 1916 as *Actinomyces griseus.* In January, 1943, Waksman and Henrici had decided to create a new genus, to which they gave the name *Streptomyces.* As a result of this change, *Actinomyces griseus* became *Streptomyces griseus,* and when the discovery of the new antibiotic was reported in January, 1944, it was called *streptomycin.*

A fortunate circumstance made the experimental and clinical testing of streptomycin easier than it might otherwise have been. In 1939, after it had been reported by Arnold R. Rich and Richard H. Follis of the Johns Hopkins Medical School that sulfanilamide had a limited suppressive effect on experimental tuberculosis in the guinea pig, H. Corwin Hinshaw drew the attention of his collaborator at the Mayo Clinic, William H. Feldman, to the greater effect of sulfapyridine in the treatment of pneumonia and suggested that they explore its effectiveness against experimental tuberculosis. This was their first attempt to suppress a tuberculous infection with a drug, and the results indicated that additional work with the sulfonamides would not be rewarding.

In 1940, Hinshaw learned of a new compound, *Promin,* which had been synthesized in the research laboratories of Parke, Davis and Company. This drug was being tested against a variety of bacterial infections, but not tuberculosis. Hinshaw received some Promin, presumably for a trial against pneumonia, but he and Feldman diverted a portion of the supply to study its effect upon experimental tuberculosis. The results revealed a notable inhibition of a human-type tuberculous infection in guinea pigs. These results, published in October, 1940, convinced Hinshaw and Feldman that tuberculosis was vulnerable to chemotherapy. Promin has great historical significance in that it was the first antimicrobial substance which was proved unequivocally effective in suppressing an experimental tuberculosis infection induced by the human-type tubercle bacillus. In addition, this demonstration was soon followed by the use of Promin at the Leprosy Hospital in Carville, Louisiana, in the treatment of another disease, leprosy, that is caused by an acid-fast mycobacterium. Its later use against leprosy in various parts of the world has had a tremendous impact on the social and medical aspects of this disease, which for centuries had made social outcasts of its victims.

Hinshaw and Feldman's studies of sulfapyridine and Promin resulted in the development of scientifically sound experimental procedures for the laboratory testing of antituberculous agents. In 1943, they were aware of Waksman's work, and they wrote to ask him whether *clavacin,* a highly potent antibiotic that Waksman's group had recently discovered, might be available for experimental testing. Waksman replied that clavacin was too toxic for use in animals. In November, 1943, while visiting the Rutgers laboratories, Feldman told Waksman about the work which he and Hinshaw were doing in an effort to find a drug for the treatment of tuberculosis.

In his studies of streptomycin, Waksman had found that *M. tuberculosis* is susceptible *in vitro* to the antagonistic action of this drug. Following this lead, he wrote to Hinshaw and Feldman in March, 1944, inquiring whether they were prepared to undertake a test of streptomycin in the experimental tuberculosis of guinea pigs. The answer was affirmative, and 10 grams of streptomycin was received at the Mayo Clinic in April. The first experiment, on only four guinea pigs, was started April 27 and terminated June 20, 1944. The results were highly promising. The drug had not destroyed all of the bacilli, indicating that its action is largely bacteriostatic rather than bactericidal.

Clearly, additional studies were indicated, but in wartime it was difficult to get supplies of any drugs, let alone unproven ones. After a visit to Rutgers in early July to seek the help of Waksman, Hinshaw and Feldman decided to inoculate a large group of guinea pigs with tubercle bacilli, hoping that if the supplies were forthcoming, a more rapid answer could be obtained. Waksman arranged a meeting with Merck and Company on July 10, and Merck agreed to make the streptomycin available. Experiment No. 2 was highly successful and in every way confirmed the effect of streptomycin against tuberculous infection in the guinea pig. This was a short-term experiment. A third and crucial experiment extending over a period of seven months was terminated in January, 1945. The results fully justified the planning of a clinical trial in human patients, in view of the reversal of the lethal course of the guinea pig infection and the relatively low toxicity of the purified streptomycin.

Beginning in December, 1944, the production of streptomycin by Merck and Company had progressed sufficiently to enable Hinshaw, in collaboration with Karl H. Pfuetze, then Medical Superintendent of the Mineral Springs Sanitorium, Cannon Falls, Minnesota, and several associates at the Mayo Clinic, to begin a series of preliminary observations on the effect of the drug in cases of clinical tuberculosis. In September, 1945, a preliminary report on 34 cases was published. By June, 1945, the number of patients under treatment had increased to 75. The results were very encouraging, but during these early trials it became evident that the drug has a selective toxic effect on the eighth cranial nerve (the nerve of hearing and balance). It was also found that the usefulness of the drug in clinical tuberculosis depends on continuation of the suppressive action for an indefinitely long period. It was apparent that extensive and prolonged clinical investigation would be required to determine the place of streptomycin in the treatment of human tuberculosis.

Since the clinical potentialities of streptomycin had been demonstrated and production of the drug had reached sufficient volume for limited distribution for investigative purposes, the Committee on Medical Research (CMR), which controlled the distribution and use of drugs in wartime, arranged a conference in June, 1945, under the chairmanship of Chester S. Keefer, at which the experimental and clinical results of Hinshaw, Feldman, and their associates were presented. Later in the same month, a similar conference was arranged by Merck and Company. Impressed by the favorable

459

results and future possibilities, Merck authorized the construction of a new plant at Elkton, Virginia, for the production of streptomycin.

Hinshaw and Feldman presented their findings at the forty-second annual meeting of the National Tuberculosis Association in June, 1946. During the discussion that followed this paper, Walsh McDermott and Carl Muschenheim announced that they and their associates at Cornell University Medical College had fully confirmed Hinshaw and Feldman's observations. This was in marked contrast to the skepticism with which Hinshaw and Feldman's reports on Promin had been received at the annual meeting of the same organization four years previously. After the 1946 meeting, a conference with military and Veterans' Administration authorities was held in Washington, D.C. Soon thereafter, the initiative for large-scale, controlled clinical studies was taken over by the Veterans' Administration, under the leadership of John Barnwell and Arthur M. Walker. These studies, involving hundreds of investigators and many thousands of patients, grew and prospered, to become an unparalleled exhibition of cooperative medical research. The results indicated that streptomycin had a highly favorable effect upon pulmonary tuberculosis, amounting in many cases to a cure. The effect upon tuberculous meningitis and miliary tuberculosis, which previously had been almost invariably fatal, was even more dramatic and gratifying, because so many of these patients could be restored to health.

In spite of its great therapeutic value, streptomycin had its drawbacks. The toxic effect on the eighth nerve, mentioned above, became a serious problem. It was found that the toxicity is related to the dose of the drug; the larger the daily dose, the greater the toxic effect. Finally, after trials in many patients, a dose was found that was effective against tuberculosis and largely free of toxicity. Another problem has been the development of strains of bacteria which are resistant to the effect of streptomycin.

Streptomycin proved to have a more extensive antibacterial action than that against the tubercle bacillus, being effective against a large number of pathogenic bacteria, many of which are not influenced by penicillin.

For his ingenious, systematic, and successful study of micro-organisms of the soil, which resulted in the discovery of streptomycin, Waksman was awarded a Nobel Prize in 1952. Folkers and Wintersteiner worked out the chemical formula that led to the isolation of streptomycin in pure form.

The production of streptomycin grew into a great industry. In 1953 in the United States alone, nine companies were manufacturing it. There were by that time two companies producing streptomycin in Great Britain, one in Sweden, one in Denmark, three in France, one in Germany, three in Italy, two in Spain, and four in Japan as well as companies in several of the Iron Curtain countries. During this period, the bulk price of streptomycin had dropped from $24 per gram in 1946 to 25 cents.

ISONIAZID   Of the many stories told about the risks run by pharmaceutical concerns in the development of new drugs, there is none more dramatic than that related to the discovery of isoniazid. The pharmaceutical firm E. R. Squibb and Sons, in their research laboratories at the Squibb Institute, set out in 1946 to find a new antituberculous drug. In the next five years, almost five thousand compounds were synthesized and tested by a new technique for rapid screening that they had developed, using infected mice rather than guinea pigs as test animals. In 1951, after 50,000 mice had died in the course of the search, a compound, *isonicotinic acid hydrazide,* was tested and found to protect mice from a dose of tubercle bacilli that usually caused a fatal infection. Tests indicated that this new product had a very low toxicity, and its effect against tuberculosis was so striking that the production of the drug was speeded up. It was given to Walsh McDermott and Carl Muschenheim of the New York Hospital–Cornell Medical Center, who found it promising in the treatment of tuberculous patients. The Squibb Company named the drug *nydrazid,* and they were making plans to market it when the front pages of New York's newspapers, in February, 1952, heralded the "discovery of a new antituberculous drug," which was also isonicotinic acid hydrazide. This drug had been produced by the Hoffmann-La Roche research laboratories and had been given the short name *isoniazid.*

By an extraordinary coincidence, both the Squibb organization and Hoffmann-La Roche, working independently, had discovered the antituberculous effect of the same drug at almost the same time. To avoid litigation and undue delay in marketing their new product, the officers of the two companies got together and placed the dated notes of their chemists in a hat. It was agreed that the company with the earlier date would receive the patent rights, and the other company would be granted a royalty-free license to manufacture and market the product. The Hoffmann-La Roche notes were earlier by a few days. When the application was submitted for a patent on isoniazid, it was discovered that the compound had been synthesized, but not used, by two German chemists in 1912, so that only a "use" patent was granted. Hoffmann-La Roche realized little from the patent, and the Squibb Company, which had spent $1,250,000 in the course of its five-year search, gained even less. However, both companies received in 1955 an Albert Lasker Medical Research Award, the first to be granted to the scientists of a pharmaceutical company.

Isoniazid is the most effective drug yet found against the tubercle bacillus, both in the test tube and in patients. Its toxicity is very low—considerably less than that of streptomycin—so that it is an ideal therapeutic agent. In the treatment of tuberculosis, particularly the more serious types of infection, a multiple drug program is frequently employed. In such a program, isoniazid is commonly combined with streptomycin, each drug seeming to enhance the effectiveness of the other. When combined with isoniazid, the dose of streptomycin can be kept at a lower level, thereby avoiding toxic effects. A third drug, frequently employed in multiple drug programs, is para-aminosalicylic acid (PAS). Though this drug is a less potent antituberculous agent, it possesses certain advantages when given in combination with either isoniazid or streptomycin. For example, when given in combination with streptomycin, it delays the emergence of streptomycin-resistant tubercle bacilli.

BROAD-SPECTRUM ANTIBIOTICS

Typhus fever, as was described in Chapter 12, is caused by organisms called rickettsias, named after the American scientist Howard Taylor Ricketts. In 1947, when a typhus epidemic flared up along the border between Peru and Bolivia, Dr. Eugene H. Payne arrived from the United States with a supply of a new drug sufficient to treat 22 patients. The patients selected for its use were those with the most severe form of the disease, including some who had been in coma for as long as three days. In the case of one patient, Gregorio Zalles, the burial arrangements had already been made, since he had been in coma for three days, and it was thought that he had no chance of recovering. Forty minutes after being given an injection of the new drug, Señor Zalles aroused from his coma and asked for a drink of water. This was the first use in humans of *chloromycetin* (later renamed *chloramphenicol*), the first antibiotic to merit the term "broad-spectrum" because of its ability to cure a wide range of infectious diseases. Dr. Payne was a clinical investigator for the manufacturer of the drug, Parke, Davis and Company of Detroit. As was evidenced by the case of Señor Zalles, chloromycetin proved to be highly effective in the treatment of typhus fever. A short time later, Dr. Payne returned to South America to test the effect of chloromycetin against Carrión's disease (also known as Oroya fever or verruga peruana), which is caused by an organism of the genus *Bartonella*. The mortality from this disease varies, but in some epidemics it runs above 50 per cent. The effect of chloromycetin on Carrión's disease was found to be just as dramatic as its effect against typhus. And this was soon found to be the case in many other types of infection.

The chloromycetin story began with a moonlight walk of two scientists at a Chemical Society meeting on Gibson Island in the Chesapeake Bay in 1943. One of the strollers was Paul R. Burkholder, a microbiologist on the faculty of Yale University, and the other was Oliver Kamm, research director of Parke, Davis and Company. Dr. Kamm was widely known for his research on the hormones of the pituitary gland, and he had participated in the development of gramicidin, the antibiotic discovered by Dubos in 1939. Stimulated by his experience with gramicidin, Dr. Kamm hoped to find in soil micro-organisms antibiotics of greater effectiveness. He succeeded in interesting Dr. Burkholder in this endeavor. Burkholder began to collect soil samples and screen their organisms for antibiotic activity against virulent bacteria. People in many parts of the world were sent plastic mailing tubes in which to return soil samples to Burkholder in New Haven. Of 7000 samples received, 4 produced organisms that appeared to be unusually active. One of these organisms, which was grown from a sample received from Venezuela, was named *Streptomyces venezuelae*. From this organism the Parke, Davis researchers ultimately produced chloromycetin.

The effectiveness of chloromycetin against human diseases was proved not only by Dr. Payne's trips to South America but also by Dr. Joseph E. Smadel of the Army Medical Service Graduate School, in an epidemic of scrub typhus on the Malay Peninsula. A short time later, Smadel and Theodore Woodward of the University of Maryland found that chloromycetin is also effective against typhoid fever.

Meanwhile, back in Detroit, a research team including Harry M. Crooks, Jr., Loren M. Long, John Controulis, and Mildred Revstock worked out the chemical formula of chloramphenicol and succeeded in synthesizing it. This was the first commercial synthesis of an antibiotic. In 1949, chloromycetin was made available for general use (Mahony, 1965).

While Parke, Davis and Company was developing chloromycetin, an antibiotic search was also being conducted by the Lederle Laboratories. This search began with an effort to obtain a compound that was more effective than streptomycin for the treatment of tuberculosis. The research effort was placed under the direction of Benjamin M. Duggar, a retired botany professor from the University of Wisconsin. Duggar screened soil samples that came in from all parts of the world. From a sample received from Columbia, Missouri, he isolated a hitherto unknown species of actinomycete. At first, this did not appear to be a very promising organism, and Duggar's associates urged him not to pursue it any further. However, he continued his work on this organism and ultimately succeeded in obtaining an antibiotic, which was named *Aureomycin,* or *chlortetracycline.* Tests carried out in 1947 indicated that Aureomycin has a very wide range of activity against many different bacteria and also against rickettsiae and some of the large viruses. The discovery of this antibiotic was announced in July, 1948; by that time, it was possible to show that it was useful against the organisms causing more than 100 diseases. The Lederle Laboratories rushed the production of Aureomycin, and it soon became the most frequently prescribed antibiotic (Mahony, 1965).

During the decade following World War II, many thousands of organisms were tested for antibiotic production, and there were reports of hundreds of antimicrobial agents. Experience indicated that only about one out of several hundred agents tested in the research laboratories proved to be worthy of advancing to the stage of clinical trial. The search still goes on, and from time to time, a new antibiotic is discovered that has a different type of activity or can be used as a better substitute for one of the older ones. The fight against the bacteria is not altogether one-sided: bacteria have a way of developing resistance to antibiotics, either by mutations or by internal metabolic rearrangements. The bacteria are sometimes helped in their fight for survival by the fact that patients develop hypersensitivity to certain antibiotics so that they cannot be used in a dose adequate to overcome the micro-organisms. Bacterial resistance and individual hypersensitivity make it desirable to have a large supply of antibiotics to choose from in the treatment of any given patient. Fortunately, the world has an almost inexhaustible biotic reservoir from which antibiotic substances may be sought. At least 50,000 kinds of molds are known, and the antibiotic-producing potentiality of these and other natural organisms is far from exhausted. In addition, as research workers learn the mechanism of action of antibiotics and determine their precise chemical structure, the synthesis of new compounds becomes possible. An example of this type of development was announced in November, 1959, when the production of new synthetic penicillins was made known. The credit for this unique and important advance belongs to John C. Sheehan, in the United States, and E. B. Chain, in England, who developed the fermentation techniques, and to the English investigators Doyle and Rolinson, who uncovered the economically feasible method of making these compounds in fermentation broths. More than 500 synthetic penicillins have been made, and some of these are superior to any produced by the natural activity of the molds. This chapter in medical research is still evolving.

The antibiotics are of too recent origin and their development has been

463

too spectacular to allow any historical evaluation of them until sometime in the future. However, one thing seems clear today: the beneficial effects of the antibiotics in the treatment of formerly fatal diseases has contributed to widespread social changes. Hudson (1967) has pointed out that medical discoveries sometimes have negative effects; with apologies to Newton, he puts the matter this way: "For each action in medical discovery there is an equal and opposite social reaction." In 1900, pneumonia was a major killer of the population. Nevertheless, it was often referred to as "the old man's friend," because it spared so many old people months of hopeless illness. Today, pneumonia is frequently a curable disease; it has fallen to sixth place among the causes of death. The success of penicillin in treating this disease has created new problems for society. The economic burden of an increase in the proportion of elderly individuals in the population has radically affected the role of government in our lives. In 1948, President Truman backed away from health insurance legislation because of widespread sentiment against further socialization of medicine. Two decades later, the Medicare Bill breezed through Congress. Indeed, the passage of Medicare indicates that more has changed than the public attitude toward big government. The American people have come to consider health a natural right. Thus, the antibiotics have certainly been responsible, at least in significant part, for many of the changes in the age distribution of the population and the social phenomena associated with it (Hudson, 1967).

ANTITHYROID DRUGS
In 1927, Alan M. Chesney, Director of the Syphilis Division of the Johns Hopkins Hospital, was carrying out some studies of experimental syphilis in rabbits, when serendipity intervened. The rabbits developed syphilis as expected; but they also developed large goiters, which were not expected. Because of this development, Chesney, for the next several years, with the assistance of Bruce Webster and T. A. Clawson, shifted much of his time and interest from experimental syphilis to experimental goiter. It turned out that the goiters had nothing to do with the syphilis but were due to the cabbage diet that the rabbits were fed in the laboratory. Those who tried to repeat Chesney's experiments found it difficult to obtain consistent results, but in 1936 C. E. Hercus and H. D. Purves obtained a clear-cut and reproducible goitrogenic effect by feeding rabbits the seeds of plants belonging to the cabbage family.

The first two pure chemical compounds shown to produce goiter were also discovered, serendipitously, at Johns Hopkins. Julia and Cosmo Mackenzie, working in E. V. McCollum's laboratory in the School of Hygiene and Public Health, were engaged in the study of a nutritional problem in weanling rats. They fed sulfaguanidine to some of the animals in order to inhibit the growth of micro-organisms in the intestinal tract. While receiving the sulfaguanidine over an extended period, the rats developed enlarged thyroids. These goiters differed from the Chesney variety, and from the naturally occurring goiters of dogs which David Marine had observed in Ohio, in that the thyroid glands did not shrink in size when iodine was administered. The Mackenzies fed rats guanidine and sulfanilic acid in order to determine which moiety of the sulfaguanidine molecule was responsible for the effect on the thyroid. The administration of these two chemicals, either separately or together, had no effect on the thyroid. It then occurred to the Mackenzies that the latter effect might be governed by the spatial relation between the sulfur and the guanidine in the molecule. To test this hypothesis they fed rats *thiourea* and found that it not only produced goiters but also had a more powerful goitrogenic effect than sulfaguanidine. By determining the basal metabolic rate in these animals, it was shown that they were hypothyroid.

While the Mackenzies were working in McCollum's laboratory, Curt Richter and Katherine Clisby were working independently in the research laboratory of the Department of Psychiatry. They were trying to test taste-discrimination in rats, and they were using *phenylthiourea* as a test substance. To their surprise, the animals receiving this substance developed goiters and severe edema.

Edwin B. Astwood was the first physician to test the effectiveness of thiourea in the treatment of patients. Astwood had spent two years (1935–37) as a research fellow at Johns Hopkins and another year there (1939–40) as assistant obstetrician. While in Baltimore he had become acquainted with Richter and had done some work in his laboratory. In 1940, Astwood joined the staff of the Peter Bent Brigham Hospital in Boston. He established there an endocrine laboratory that was well equipped to study various hormones, including the thyroid hormone. After a few months' work with thiourea, Astwood concluded that it acted by inhibiting the synthesis of thyroid hormone and that it should, therefore, be useful for the treatment of hyperthyroidism. His first experiments with the use of thiourea in hyperthyroid patients were disappointing, but after further experimentation, a satisfactory treatment program was developed. In a short time thiourea, or rather its cousin propylthiouracil, had become the drug of first choice for the treatment of hyperthyroidism, either for continuous long-term therapy or to prepare patients for thyroidectomy.

As a result of the work of Astwood and others, we now know that the thiourea family of antithyroid chemicals act by preventing the iodination of the thyroid hormone. The hormone is, therefore, biologically inactive. Enlargement of the thyroid (goiter) apparently is due to thyrotropic stimulation of the gland which, though designed to make the gland secrete more hormones, succeeds only in making it grow larger.

The basic studies of this new family of antithyroid drugs were completed just before the United States entered World War II. Not until after the war did they become available for general clinical use.

DRUGS THAT INHIBIT ENZYMES

The term "intermediary metabolism" embraces those reactions concerned with the formation and breakdown of the biochemical components of the body. During the past 50 years, the metabolic pathways involving the sugars, fatty acids, amino acids, cholesterol, hormones, nucleic acids, and certain proteins have been revealed. Many diseases of humans are the result of a "metabolic disorder" in which a normal component or metabolic product is produced at an abnormal rate. Often, this results when one or more enzymes — those unique substances that regulate metabolic activity — get out of control. The study of enzymes (Chap. 24) has resulted in many advances in the understanding and treatment of diseases. If one seeks to control a

465

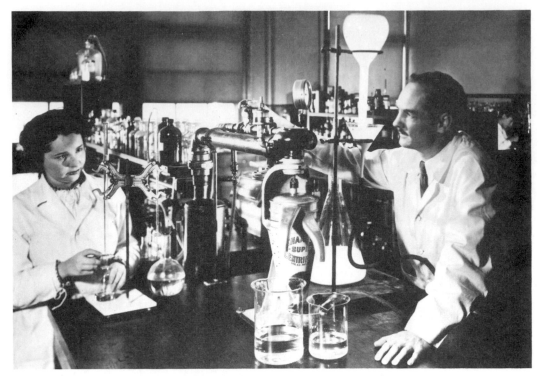

Figure 97. Gertrude Elion and George H. Hitchings. (Courtesy of Iris Evans.)

disease that involves the abnormal production of a metabolic substance in one of these pathways by means of an enzyme, it is first necessary to understand the process involved. There are many examples of diseases that arise when the body produces too much or too little of a normal constituent. For example, too little insulin results in diabetes; too much stomach acid may give rise to a gastric or duodenal ulcer. By controlling the rate of formation of the body constituent, one may be able to control the disease. This may be accomplished by suppressing or enhancing the effect of an enzyme involved in the formation of the constituent.

Outstanding work in the development of agents to inhibit specific enzymes has been performed by George H. Hitchings. Hitchings received his Ph.D. in biochemistry from Harvard in 1933. After serving on the faculty, first at Harvard, and then at Western Reserve University, he became Research Director in 1942 at the laboratories of Burroughs Wellcome and Company, Tuckahoe, New York, where the work that concerns us here was carried out. Hitching's work on gout serves as an example of his approach to the treatment of metabolic disorders. In gout, urates are deposited in the tissues, especially in the joints. The body gets rid of its nitrogen partly by excreting uric acid in the urine. When too much uric acid accumulates, or when its elimination is reduced by disease of the kidneys, urates are deposited in the joints, giving rise to the painful symptoms of gout. Hitchings approached this problem not by making a blind search for compounds that might promote the excretion of uric acid but by focusing on the intermediary metabolism of uric acid. The immediate precursor of uric acid is a purine called xanthine. Xanthine is converted to uric acid by the en-

466

zyme *xanthine oxidase;* so Hitchings searched for a drug that would inhibit this enzyme, thereby reducing the formation of uric acid in the body. The search was successful, and the drug that was developed, *allopurinol,* is very useful in the treatment of gout.

Hitchings has made a remarkable series of contributions to therapy by his masterful studies of the metabolic inhibitors of enzymes involved in the metabolism of purines and pyrimidines—substances that are a vital part of the basic materials making up cell nuclei. The discovery of sulfanilamide gave a great stimulus to the search for specific remedies. At the time this drug came on the scene, workers in the field of chemotherapy were sharply divided; some hoped that by testing enough compounds, they would run across one that did more damage to the infecting organism than to its host. Others felt that it would be more profitable to concentrate on the basic physiology and biochemistry of host and parasites, hoping that this information would enable them to design drugs on a rational basis.

Hitchings and his group adopted a middle course; they exploited the "antimetabolite" theory, which had developed as a by-product of the discovery of sulfanilamide. It was found that sulfanilamide's effect on bacteria could be nullified by a naturally occurring substance, para-aminobenzoic acid (PABA), which is closely related chemically to sulfanilamide. Primitive organisms make the essential vitamin folic acid from small building blocks, one of which is PABA. A sulfonamide displaces PABA and inhibits the synthesis of folic acid. Higher organisms, including man, are unable to make their own folic acid; they must, therefore, get it preformed in their food. At some time during evolution, the biosynthetic mechanism, the sulfonamide-sensitive metabolic step, was eliminated, leaving a clear-cut exploitable difference in biochemical make-up between parasite and host. Sulfanilamide acts as a counterfeit PABA. Hitchings proposed to make and use other metabolites in a similar way; that is to say, his work would be centered on a study of enzymes and metabolic pathways. He hoped to detect differences between hosts and parasites that would lead to chemotherapeutic agents with known mechanisms of actions. He chose to work in the field of nucleic acids. This seemed an appropriate target for chemotherapy for several reasons. Parasites live in a hostile environment and often depend for survival on a rapid rate of multiplication, which in turn requires a rapid turnover of nucleic acids. Some information tied nucleic acids to sulfanilamide and to a vitamin called folic acid, which had been detected but not at that time isolated. Thus, nucleic acids, folic acid, PABA, and sulfanilamide all seemed to have interrelationships.

Folic acid blocks a reaction that is critical to the parasite (e.g., bacteria) but is nonexistent in the host (e.g., humans). All cells and organisms use a form of folic acid, tetrahydrofolate, as a tool in the nucleic-acid assembly line; but in performing one of its functions, tetrahydrofolate itself is converted to dihydrofolate and has to be regenerated. This requires a separate system, using an enzyme called dihydrofolate reductase. Hitchings had already found that some of his analogues interfered with the utilization of folic acid. It became clear in time that they were inhibitors of the enzyme dihydrofolate reductase. What was important and exciting was that they were highly selective. These compounds could be shaped to inhibit an enzyme in one species but not in another. Thus Hitchings introduced with his work the broad principle of selective toxicity. Sulfonamides depend on

467

qualitative differences between host and parasite, and qualitative differences between species are rare. The pyrimidines depend on a selective inhibition of a function that is common to all organisms and take advantage of the kind of evolutionary changes that probably have occurred in all enzymes and functions. In recent years, Hitchings has found it possible to quantify this selectivity by working with a group of inhibitors and dihydrofolate reductases from a large range of species. The evolutionary changes in this enzyme have been very great indeed. In enzymatic terms, the antimalarial drug *pyrimethamine* is 2000 times as toxic to the malarial parasite as to the human host, and the antibacterial *trimethoprim* is 100,000 times more active on a bacterial than on a human enzyme. Substances such as pyrimethamine and trimethoprim are chemotherapeutic agents in their own rights, but both are much more effective when used with sulfonamides. Not only is trimethoprim with a sulfonamide a better antibacterial agent than either drug alone, but also this combination played a major role in the control of the drug-resistant malarias of Southeast Asia. The sulfonamide inhibits the synthesis of folate, and the pyrimidine blocks its utilization. Hence, in the malarial parasite there is a double blockade of a vital biochemical pathway.

Pursuing similar principles of investigation in chemotherapy, two other vitally important drugs were developed. One was the first important antileukemic agents 6-*mercaptopurine,* and the other was the immunosuppressive drug *azathioprine.*

A research program in which knowledge and skill rather than luck were the vital ingredients led to the development of these new and very important agents for the management of disease. As more and more biochemical knowledge accumulates, the possibilities for other programs of rational drug design are coming into being.

To the biochemically oriented chemotherapist, it is not only a matter of faith but also a fact that every cell type must have a characteristic biochemical pattern and therefore must be susceptible to attack at some locus critical for its survival and replication. The existence of cancer chemotherapeutic agents, however unsatisfactory at the present time, is evidence that exploitable patterns of metabolism exist in various types of cancer cells. Empirical methods continue to prevail in the search for new drugs, but the purposeful exploration of enzymes, metabolic pathways, and cell receptors would seem to hold the promise of the future.

ORAL ANTICOAGULANTS

The coagulation of blood is the body's protection against hemorrhage. It is an intricate process involving a number of chemical reactions, which must be carried out in the proper sequence. When all of the required substances are present and in perfect working order, the entire chain of reactions can be completed in a time span of no more than a few minutes. One may describe this complicated process in an oversimplified manner by beginning with the final step and working backward, as follows: the matrix of a blood clot is fibrin. Fibrin, which is both visible and palpable, is formed from the invisible chemical substance fibrinogen, which is present in the circulating blood. The conversion of soluble fibrinogen to insoluble fibrin is brought about by the action of thrombin, which is not constantly present in the blood but must be formed, as needed, from prothrombin (the role of vitamin K in the formation of prothrombin was described in Chapter 12). The conversion of prothrombin to thrombin is activated by thromboplastin, which is not a discrete chemical substance but an expression to represent the appropriate interaction of a number of different plasma proteins, which are known as "coagulation factors." These factors are required for normal blood coagulation. For example, a deficiency of one of them, *Factor VIII,* is responsible for the inherited bleeding disorder, hemophilia. In addition to the other substances calcium must also be present for normal coagulation to occur.

Highly sophisticated laboratory methods have been developed for detecting and measuring the individual factors, but in general the clinician relies on three not very precise tests for determining the general nature of a coagulation defect: *the bleeding time; the clotting time* and the character of the clot; and the *prothrombin time,* which provides an index of the availability of prothrombin and its level in the blood plasma. Usually, we are concerned with trying to keep all of these measurements within a normal range, but there are occasions when it is desirable to do the reverse and deliberately retard the normal process of coagulation; this is what is meant by the term *anticoagulation.*

The formation of undesirable blood clots within the blood vessels is known as thrombosis, and for a long time scientists have been searching for a substance that would prevent thrombosis. Reference was made in earlier chapters to Abel's use of hirudin in his first experiments with an artificial kidney, and Howell's discovery of the anticoagulant heparin. One of the objections to these anticoagulants is that they have to be given by injection, because they are not absorbed when given by mouth. The first lead toward the development of an oral anticoagulant came from the barnyard.

Early settlers in the Great Plains area of the upper midwestern United States and Canada impoverished the soil by overfarming. To this tragedy was added the corn borer scourge of the early 1900s. When it was discovered that sweet clover could grow on relatively barren land, this plant became a popular crop between 1910 and 1920. At about this time, a new cattle disease began to appear. In one reported instance, 65 of 80 cattle bled to death after dehorning. In another instance, 12 of 25 bulls died as the result of hemorrhage after they had been castrated. Pregnant cows tended to abort, and newborn calves bled to death during their first few days of life.

Frank W. Schofield, a veterinary pathologist in Ontario, first recognized that this hemorrhagic disease of cattle occurred in animals that had eaten spoiled sweet clover; notably when the clover was in the form of moldy silage. Schofield fed some of the spoiled sweet clover to rabbits and found that they developed hemorrhages and that their bleeding time and clotting time were prolonged. In 1929, Lee M. Roderick, another veterinary pathologist, demonstrated that the plasma prothrombin level was depressed in the hemorrhagic disorder of cattle.

The interest of Karl Paul Link, a biochemist at the University of Wisconsin, was aroused one day when a farmer strode down the corridors of the Wisconsin Agricultural Experiment Station, sloshing unclotted blood from a pail onto the floor. The farmer demanded prompt action because his castrated and dehorned cattle had been bleeding to death. Two years later,

469

in 1940, Link and his associates had isolated the toxic agent from sweet clover, had crystallized it, and soon identified it as two coumarin molecules, linked by formaldehyde. This substance was called *"dicumarol,"* and when they reported its discovery in April, 1941, Stahmann, Huebner, and Link stated, "In view of the prothrombin-reducing or inactivating properties of this dicoumarin, and the spread between detectable and lethal doses, together with the relative ease with which it may be synthesized and administered, it would appear that its anticoagulant properties merit consideration from the physiologist and hematologist." A few days later, Dr. Link received a request from the Mayo Clinic for a supply of dicumarol, and within several months Hugh R. Butt, Edgar C. Allen, and J. L. Bollman of the Mayo Clinic published the first report on the successful clinical use of this new oral anticoagulant. Finally, Dr. Link and his associates produced a water-soluble oral anticoagulant, which was effective in very small doses and was given the name *warfarin.*

The hemorrhagic disorder produced by the ingestion of spoiled sweet clover or dicumarol, like that of vitamin K deficiency, is characterized by a depression in the plasma prothrombin. It is not surprising, therefore, that the administration of vitamin K was found to overcome the effect of dicumarol. This has added a safety factor to the use of dicumarol as an anticoagulant agent, since if its administration is carried to the point of producing hemorrhages, its effect can be reversed quickly by the administration of vitamin K.

Not only did the discovery of dicumarol and related agents provide clinicians with a useful and easily administered drug to prevent or retard thrombus formation but also it helped to clarify some of the obscure aspects of the coagulation process. For example, it was found by Charles A. Owen, who was then working as a Resident in J. L. Bollman's laboratory (1946–47) at the Mayo Clinic, that dicumarol acts primarily by depressing a factor that is responsible for the conversion of prothrombin to thrombin and only secondarily by depressing the prothrombin level. It was found subsequently that the conversion factor affected by dicumarol is not *Factor V,* which already had been recognized as a conversion factor, but another factor still to be discovered. The discovery was finally made in 1951 by Benjamin Alexander and his associates, who were treating a patient who lacked this specific factor; they were able to identify the factor by the effect of its absence and gave it the name *Factor SPCA* (Serum Prothrombin Conversion Accelerator). Hougie and associates soon discovered that Factor SPCA is, in fact, two distinct factors, now usually identified as Factors VII and X. Both of these factors are depressed by vitamin K deficiency and by oral anticoagulation therapy.

NEW DRUGS FOR THE CONQUEST OF DISEASE— SOME ASPECTS OF THE AMERICAN PHARMACEUTICAL INDUSTRY

At the close of the nation's first century, American drug manufacturers were still engaged in making and selling innumerable pills, powders, salves, lotions, tinctures, extracts, etc., etc. Most of these substances were inactive and useless. Even the drugs that possessed some type of activity were of unknown and variable strength. There was no requirement that drugs be assayed for their potency, or for their toxicity. Some companies had a better reputation than others for ethical dealings, but very few adhered to proven facts in their advertising. An effort was made to avoid mixing incompatible substances, but this was about the extent of the research conducted at any drug manufacturing plant.

The situation is, of course, altogether different at the close of the second century of American medicine. Some of the pharmaceutical concerns are at the very forefront of the advances in medical science. They have large research budgets, large and able research staffs, fine laboratories, and quantities of sophisticated equipment. Reference has already been made to the research and development work carried on by such organizations as Merck, Parke-Davis, Lederle, Eli Lilly, E. R. Squibb, Burroughs Wellcome, Hoffmann-La Roche, Smith Kline and others. There are still many companies of a different type, which devote all their energies to making, advertising, and selling their products, frequently capitalizing on the research and development of other companies without themselves contributing in any way to the advance. Sometimes these companies devote their entire effort to the manufacture of one or two products, for which they conduct high-powered advertising campaigns in the press and on radio and television. Their advertisements are often slyly misleading. For example, one can think of advertisements which are designed to make people think that certain vitamins, iron, and other ingredients should be taken daily in medicinal form, when in fact these substances are adequately supplied by the ordinary diet.

Many of the more obvious avenues for unethical practices have now

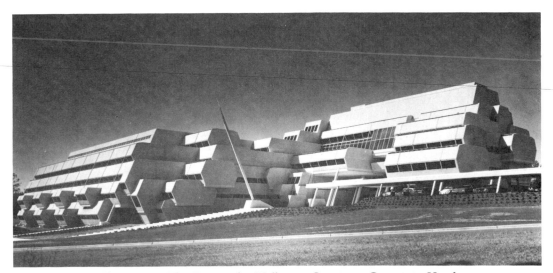

Figure 98. The Burroughs Wellcome Company Corporate Headquarters and Research Laboratories, Research Triangle Park, North Carolina. Burroughs Wellcome has no stockholders. All profits are used to support medical research and education. (Courtesy of Iris Evans.)

471

been blocked by the food and drug laws. Drugs must contain what they are said to contain, and the grosser forms of deception by dilution and adulteration can no longer be practiced as they were in the past. Mahony (1965) tells a story about the adulteration of senna in the last century. Senna, a popular nineteenth century laxative, is derived from a plant that grows both in India and Egypt, but the Egyptian product was superior in quality and higher in price. When a customer complained that the Egyptian senna which he had received contained camel dung, the dealer laughed. "Of course it's camel dung," he replied; "this proves it is genuine Alexandrian senna. There are no camels in India."

It was not an easy matter to put an end to the deceptive practices of the nineteenth century. It took several catastrophes to persuade the public that better regulation of the manufacture of pharmaceutical products was required. One of these catastrophes occurred in 1901, when 10 children died because they had been injected with contaminated tetanus antitoxin. This episode, followed by agitation by the AMA and other interested parties, brought about the passage of the first Food and Drug Act, in 1906, at the height of the reform administration of Theodore Roosevelt. The Act prohibited the sale in interstate commerce of adulterated or misbranded products. No serious effort was made to enforce the Act, partly because misbranding had not been clearly defined. The Shirley Amendment of 1912 classified a product as misbranded if claims of therapeutic or curative effects on the labels of drugs were false or fraudulent. But here again, enforcement was difficult, because the government was required to prove a deliberate intention to defraud before regulatory action could be taken.

In 1927, the Food and Drug Administration (FDA) became an independent regulatory agency. Between 1906 and 1927, the main emphasis of control legislation had been on foods, in part because little was known about the dangers of drugs and very few effective drugs were available. Dangerous drugs continued to be sold legally prior to 1927, because testing for safety before marketing was not required. Flagrant violations by manufacturers were identified, but the government was not empowered to take action against them. Moreover, the control of drug advertisements was the responsibility of the Federal Trade Commission rather than the FDA. The establishment of the FDA as an independent agency was designed to eliminate the previously existing deficiencies in the testing and marketing of drugs.

Little need was felt, and no serious effort made to enlarge the FDA's responsibilities again until about 1960, when concern about the high prices of drugs prompted an investigation by the Antitrust and Monopoly Subcommittee of the Senate Judiciary Committee under the chairmanship of Senator Estes Kefauver. This committee reached the following conclusions: (1) that certain drug manufacturers were making exorbitant profits; (2) that the drug companies were exploiting certain proprietary products not only by advertising but also by personal representations to physicians; (3) that there was widespread lack of knowledge about the actions and the adverse effects of drugs. The committee's hearings were given wide publicity in the press, and some of them were broadcast "live" on television. As a result of all this, the public was made aware, as never before, of the inadequacies of the drug laws. In the midst of this controversy, the thalidomide disaster occurred,

472

and with this added stimulus, the greatly strengthened Drug Amendments of 1962 were adopted by Congress. This new legislation required the registration of drug manufacturers and the periodic inspection of their factories, records, and testing procedures. Drugs had to be approved by the FDA in terms of both safety and effectiveness before they could be marketed. Drugs that were already on the market could be withdrawn if they were found to be unsafe or ineffective. Testing of new drugs in human subjects required "informed consent," and those who were doing the testing had to be registered by both the manufacturer and the FDA. Official names of drugs had to be approved, and when drugs were sent to physicians for use they had to be accompanied by valid and proven statements of efficiency and safety, and the conditions for which the drug should not be administered had to be clearly spelled out.

Since the end of the nineteenth century the AMA has played a major role in improving the safety and efficacy of drugs. It has tried to eliminate from its own publications advertising in which false claims are made. The AMA's Council on Pharmacy and Chemistry, established in 1905, whose efforts to eliminate nostrums and quackery have already been described, became the Council on Drugs in 1956. Its several publications on drug information have been very useful to the profession. Concern about the incidence of aplastic anemia attributed to the administration of chloramphenicol led the Council in 1953 to establish a Committee on Blood Dyscrasias, which solicited from physicians reports of unfavorable reactions to this drug. In 1960, the Registry was broadened to include adverse reactions to other drugs. The AMA was trying to develop a nationwide system for the reporting of adverse drug effects, in the hope that this would facilitate earlier recognition of serious drug-induced disease. Much valuable and timely information was obtained, but when the FDA assumed responsibility for monitoring adverse drug reactions in 1960, the AMA program ceased to function. In recent years, extensive epidemiological studies have shown the immensity of the problem of adverse drug reactions, and increasing attention has been given to influencing sound drug utilization practices in order to diminish the problem of drug-induced disease (Cluff, Caranasos, and Stewart, 1975).

Space cannot be given to a full discussion of the history of the pharmaceutical companies that have contributed so handsomely to the development of useful therapeutic agents. The history of a few of them will be sketched briefly in order to indicate how they have entered the research and development field.

Not only was Philadelphia the cradle of American liberty but also it became the first home of an American pharmacy when Christopher Marshall, an Irishman turned Quaker, established his apothecary shop at the "Sign of the Golden Ball"; his son Charles was the first President of the Philadelphia College of Pharmacy, and his daughter, Elizabeth, was the first American woman pharmacist. The Smith Kline and French firm (there is no comma between Smith and Kline because a typist left it out in preparing the articles of incorporation) began its operations in the old tradition of nineteenth-century Philadelphia. In the 1920s, it was still marketing an enormous number of products, ranging from aspirin to liniment, having had great success with *EsKay Neurophosphates* as a "stimulant." In the late 1920s,

473

the firm decided to venture into making specialty items for sale by pharmacists only when prescribed by physicians. In 1929, the wholesaling and jobbing of proprietary products was relegated to a subsidiary division, and the parent company, Smith Kline and French Laboratories, was organized to devote itself to research and manufacturing.

In the depression year 1936, S. K. and F. began to concentrate on developing, manufacturing, and selling specialties. During this period, leadership was provided by C. Mahlon Kline, son of the founder, and Francis Boyer, who joined the company in 1919 and was its president from 1951 to 1958. To find new specialties, the company established close working relations with research scientists in the Philadelphia area. To sell them, they pioneered new ways to reach the prescribing physician. They were the first company regularly to send doctors samples of new drugs through the mail. They developed an entirely new philosophy of management in their research and development enterprise. They employed well-qualified research scientists, and these men in turn came up with products that were both new and useful. They were the first to develop the use of amphetamines to shrink the swollen mucous membranes of the millions of victims of hay fever and the common cold. However, the benzedrine inhaler, which they introduced, had troublesome side effects. It stimulated the patients so greatly that it interfered with the action of narcotics and spoiled the appetite. Many people found that by taking apart the inhaler and using its contents, they could get a "cheap jag." These difficulties were overcome when an inhaler product was developed that shrank the membranes without producing stimulation. The related products, *Dexedrine* and *Dexamyl*, proved to be capable of relieving varying degrees of depression, and they also curbed the appetite, which made them useful for the treatment of obesity.

When the French chemical firm Rhone-Poulenc reported the development of a new allergy drug that "slowed down" bodily processes, S. K. and F. scientists, particularly Francis Boyer, were impressed by this drug's capacity to block what might be called psychoneurotic behavior in laboratory animals. Boyer acquired patent rights to the drug in 1952 and introduced it to the medical profession as the tranquilizer *Thorazine*. This drug had a remarkably beneficial effect on the finances of S. K. and F., but it had an even greater impact on mental hospitals. In 1956, following the Thorazine success story, *Compazine* was introduced, and both of these drugs were found to be effective in the treatment of patients with nausea and vomiting, including the "morning sickness" of pregnancy.

S. K. and F. also introduced some novel technical developments in the manufacture of drugs. They found that when drugs are put up in a mixture of tiny pellets variously coated to dissolve at different time intervals, the period of the drug's action is lengthened considerably. This type of preparation, a capsule containing many pellets, was called a "spansule." Under the research-minded leadership of Boyer and his successor, Walter A. Munns, S. K. and F. devoted between a fifth and a quarter of its profits, its personnel, and its floor space to the search for new and better drugs. In addition to spending over $10 million a year on their own research staff, the company made grants totaling $1 million to academic research scientists. In 1952, the Smith Kline and French Foundation was created to administer some $600,000 in grants ranging from $100 for the National Safety Council to a three-year $100,000 award to the American Psychiatric Association (Mahony, 1965).

After World War II, a Czech scientist, Frank A. Berger, was looking for a better preservative for penicillin. As a by-product he found *mephenesin,* a muscle relaxer. One variation of this, which he called *meprobamate* for short, quieted mice in an interesting way. "They were relaxed alright," he reported, "but they looked straight at you and obviously knew what was going on around them." This information was seized upon by Wallace Laboratories, a division of Carter Products (of "Little Liver Pill" fame), which hired Berger and trademarked his compound as *Miltown.* The drug became almost embarrassingly popular, and as a result the Wyeth Company bought a license from Wallace to make *Miltown* by a name that had a less provincial sound — *Equanil.* Wyeth paid Carter $1.9 million in royalties in 1957.

An important man to Parke, Davis, and Company was Jokichi Takamine, who has been mentioned several times in earlier chapters of this history. He was trained at Anderson College in Scotland, where he studied the chemistry of brewing and became interested in ferments. In 1884, he came to the United States for the first time, married an American woman, and returned to Japan, where he established the first artificial-fertilizer industry in that country. He also developed a potent starch-splitting enzyme which he called Taka-diastase. He returned to the United States in 1890, and after trying unsuccessfully to interest the distilling industry in this new enzyme, he finally succeeded in 1895 in inducing Parke, Davis and Company to market it as a digestive product, and at the same time he became a consultant to the company. Because of this association, he later turned over to Parke, Davis a more marketable product. This was epinephrine, which he had learned how to isolate and purify after his visit to Professor Abel's laboratory in Baltimore. He obtained patents on this product and on the process for extracting it from the adrenal glands of animals. Beginning in 1900, Parke, Davis marketed it under the trade name *Adrenalin.* This was the first hormone to be marketed in pure form. Much of the money that Takamine received from his royalties on Adrenalin was used to develop better Japanese-American relations. When the wife of President Taft gave the city of Washington 80 Japanese cherry trees as symbols of "loyalty and purity," Takamine persuaded the city of Tokyo to present to Washington 2000 additional trees. Parke, Davis developed many other drugs. They backed E. A. Doisy of St. Louis in his work on hormones. *Dilantin,* one of the most important drugs for the control of epilepsy, was introduced by Parke, Davis in 1938. *Promin,* a Parke, Davis product that was described earlier, was the first modern drug to be used in the treatment of leprosy (1944). The same decade brought *Benadryl,* one of the first and most versatile of the antihistamine drugs (Mahony, 1965).

An important phase in the development of the Eli Lilly Company came after World War I, when George Henry Alexander Clowes, an English chemist, became its research director. When Dr. Clowes learned that Banting and Best had succeeded in extracting insulin from the pancreas, he at once offered to make it. These efforts began in May, 1922, when a group of 100 workers at the Eli Lilly plant in Indianapolis were set to work on the problem. A clinic was established nearby to test each new batch of insulin as it was produced. By August, they had obtained a pure and stable prod-

475

uct. By the spring of 1923, George B. Walden had perfected a method of isoelectric precipitation, which greatly increased the yield of insulin, though it was still necessary to use the pancreases of 6000 cattle or 24,000 hogs to produce a single ounce of the hormone. Shortly after Minot's discovery of the value of liver in the treatment of pernicious anemia, the Eli Lilly Company took over the job of purifying and marketing liver extract. Their liver extract number 343 was the first recognized and standardized specific for the treatment of pernicious anemia. The Lilly Company also developed and introduced the drug *Darvon,* a non-narcotic analgesic, which could be used in place of codeine. The development of Darvon required 10 years of research.

A striking example of the role that serendipity plays in finding new uses for drugs occurred in 1948. Leslie N. Gay, chief of the Allergy Clinic at Johns Hopkins, was in charge of the clinical research on a new drug, an antihistaminic, which was expected to be useful for the treatment of hives. Gay gave some of this drug to a woman and told her how to use it. On her next visit to the clinic, the woman reported that the medicine had not helped her hives very much but that her motion sickness seemed to be cured; for the first time, her ride to the hospital on the streetcar gave her no discomfort. This aroused the curiosity of Dr. Gay and his assistant, P. E. Carliner. They thought they would fool the patient by giving her a placebo instead of the medicine. When she came back to the clinic the next time, she reported that her motion sickness had returned. Another trial of the new drug again brought relief of symptoms. Excited by this experience, Gay solicited the cooperation of the Army in carrying out an experiment. On one of the Army's transatlantic troop ships, the drug was given to some of the soldiers, for whom it made bearable the rough and stormy passage across the North Atlantic. This drug was *Dramamine;* it was one of the first important research discoveries in the laboratories of G. D. Searle and Company. After introducing Dramamine as a motion-sickness remedy in 1949, the sales of this drug increased rapidly. It was soon put aboard ocean liners and commercial airplanes and was made available at rail and bus terminals. During the first five years, it was sold by prescription only, but in 1954, the Food and Drug Administration asked Searle to make Dramamine directly available to the public.

Shortly after Dramamine was launched, research workers at Searle in 1950 introduced *Banthine,* which brought about a whole new approach to the treatment of gastric and duodenal ulcers. Then, in 1957, Searle's research workers were responsible for the development of the controversial synthetic steroid, *Enovid,* which was offered first for the treatment of menstrual disorders but soon proved to be successful as an oral contraceptive.

Yella Pragada Subbarow, a Hindu educated at Harvard, who had once planned to become a Buddhist priest, became research director of the Lederle Laboratories in the 1940s, when they were interested in the development of better liver preparations. In one of the steps in the process of purification, charcoal was added to the liver extract, but the chemists found that they had to keep this mixture hot; otherwise the potency of the liver was lost. Subbarow perceived that if the potency was lost under these circumstances, the potent factor must have been taken out of the mixture by the charcoal. He therefore withdrew some of the charcoal from the mixture,

476

treated it with a solvent, and obtained a solution that had the potency in concentrated form. From this, a liver extract was produced, which was more pure than previous products and was effective against pernicious anemia when it was administered in a very small dose.

It was recognized that animal livers contain a growth-promoting ingredient, the lack of which results in the development of anemia in experimental animals. The same substance is also present in brewers' yeast and in certain leafy plants. Because of its origin from leafy plants, it was named folic acid. Starting with a ton and a half of liver in the fall of 1941, Lederle scientists, after a laborious effort, had isolated one third of a gram of pure folic acid by 1943. The synthesis of this substance was finally achieved in August, 1945, a few days ahead of a similar achievement by another firm. By this time, Lederle had invested $500,000 in the folic acid project and another $200,000 on clinical trials.

Some of the early lots of folic acid tablets were sent to Tom D. Spies at the Hillman Hospital in Birmingham, Alabama, and to William J. Darby at Vanderbilt University. These workers soon demonstrated that folic acid would cure patients with what was considered to be hopelessly severe sprue and other macrocytic anemias. Further research disclosed that a daily supply of folic acid is essential for the formation of the nucleic acids necessary for the growth and survival of all cells. Since cancer is essentially a wild growth of cells, research workers in this field conceived the notion that some chemical closely related to folic acid might be substituted for it in cellular metabolism and thereby starve, or otherwise halt the growth of cancer cells. By substituting other chemicals for various parts of the folic acid molecule, Lederle research workers produced a series of folic acid antagonists. One of these, *aminopterin,* first made in 1947, was found by Sidney Farber at the Children's Hospital in Boston to produce temporary remissions in children with acute leukemia. *Methotrexate,* a less toxic folic acid antagonist, was developed the following year. In 1958, workers at the National Cancer Institute found that this drug would suppress the growth of a solid malignant tumor: 10 women with choriocarcinoma, a rare but usually fatal cancer of the uterus, were treated successfully with methotrexate, and after more than two years the growth had not recurred.

Merck and Company has also made many outstanding contributions. In 1933, the Merck Institute for Therapeutic Research was built in Rahway, New Jersey, for chemical and biological research in an environment where "genuinely creative minds" could be "so protected that their mental powers of thought, study and imagination can concentrate on problems of great difficulty." After World War II, two outstanding research workers, Randolph T. Major of Princeton University and Hans Molitor of the University of Vienna, were induced to join the staff of the Institute at Rahway. One night in 1934, R. R. Williams of the Bell Laboratories called Dr. Major to ask whether Merck was interested in crystalline vitamin B_1, which he had isolated recently, and whether they could supply him with concentrates of vitamin B_1 so that he could try to work out the formula of the molecule and synthesize it. Merck agreed to cooperate, and for more than a year they obtained a vitamin B_1 concentrate from hundreds of tons of rice bran, and as the concentrate was prepared it was sent in small batches to Williams. Finally the formula of the vitamin B_1 molecule was established, and it was

477

synthesized. Merck was granted a license by Williams to manufacture the product and by 1937 was manufacturing B_1 from simple organic compounds.

As a result of the experience with Williams, Merck become interested in vitamins and among other things produced nicotinic acid (niacin) for the treatment of pellagra. In the spring of 1948, a team of five Merck research workers, headed by Karl Folkers, announced the discovery of vitamin B_{12}, which is the substance in liver that combats pernicious anemia. This vitamin in its pure state is the most powerful medicine known; 1/30 of a millionth of an ounce per day is enough to keep a normal person healthy; and 1/3 of a millionth of an ounce checks pernicious anemia. In the fall of 1948, the Merck chemists announced that vitamin B_{12} could be obtained from a strain of *Streptomyces griseus,* which strangely enough is the same species of mold that produces the antibiotic streptomycin. In February, 1949, less than 11 months after the first announcement, Merck placed pure crystalline vitamin B_{12} on the market.

PROBLEMS OF DRUG DEVELOPMENT

The sulfonamide story clearly illustrates that in the final analysis, the evaluation of drugs *in humans* is essential to drug discovery. Any obstacles in the way of well-conceived, well-controlled human experimentation will almost certainly hinder drug discovery and the development of new drugs for clinical use. There has been a recent tendency to impose social and legal barriers to human experimentation beyond those necessary for the safety of the patient. There is little doubt that this trend has already slowed progress in the discovery of new and needed drugs. Drugs must be evaluated in humans in order to determine their true effectiveness in the treatment of human disease. The preliminary screening in animals is important, but frequently a new use for a drug is found as the result of a serendipitous incident during the testing of the drug in human subjects. The sulfonamide story provides a classic example of how such things happen. The diuretic and hypoglycemic actions of these drugs were discovered quite by accident when their antibacterial effect was being tested in human subjects. It is very difficult to find an animal model which faithfully reproduces human disease. Fortunately, there are animal models for many infectious diseases. If an antibiotic drug destroys or prevents the growth of bacteria *in vitro* and in the experimental animal infected with the organisms, it is reasonably predictable that it will perform similarly in humans. However, in many other types of disease, there is no satisfactory animal counterpart for the human malady, and the results of treatment are not so easily measured as they are in microbial diseases.

The thalidomide episode in Germany, in which this drug was administered to pregnant women without having been adequately tested for its effect on the fetus, has served to place many barriers in the way of therapeutic studies on human subjects. Now much more care is taken in getting the informed consent of the patient. New rules with respect to human experimentation were needed for the protection of the individual involved. As the result of the Kefauver-Harris Amendment, essentially every step of clinical investigation must be either directly or indirectly sanctioned by a federal employee. This has placed many difficulties in the path of the well-trained and conscientious investigator. It has made studies much more difficult and much more expensive, and barriers have been erected that are higher than those necessary for sound and safe use of human subjects in the study of new drugs.

In addition to the professionals in medical schools and research institutions, who furnish much of the innovative input for the discovery of new drugs, the ethical pharmaceutical industry plays a most important role in this enterprise. The industry is now spending several hundred million dollars a year for research and development, the highest percentage of income devoted to these activities by any industry in the United States. The new rules make it far more difficult for the industry to develop new and original drugs. Moreover, it is discouraging to the discoverer and producer of a new drug when Congress and the medical profession agitate for the use of generic rather than proprietary names in prescribing drugs. Generic drugs are cheaper because the companies that make them do little, if any, productive research and certainly are not in the business of developing new products. However, one cannot expect the FDA to be sympathetic toward this point of view. Its job is not to increase the freedom and productivity of clinical investigation but to ensure that the laws governing the manufacture, testing, and sale of drugs are observed. It has no responsibility to serve as a motivator of drug discovery. The law, and the FDA regulations, consistently refer to safety and efficacy but not to the promotion of new drug discoveries.

There is great concern about the possibility of injury to volunteers, even when the drugs being tested are designed for the treatment of serious human disease and have been fully tested for safety in experimental animals. In this connection, the voice of the responsible scientist often seems to carry less weight than that of ill-informed interests. Most of the members of Congress have found it difficult to acquire the knowledge essential for assessing the technological issues that come before them. A few congressmen who understood the problems of modern medicine were able to persuade their colleagues to establish and support the NIH. This was a magnificent contribution to the advancement of medical science, but few in Congress today understand the intricate principles of drug discovery. It is easier to understand safety than to comprehend science. Safety is important, but it should not be permitted to strangle the testing of new drugs when this is conducted under properly controlled conditions. There is an obvious contradiction between the agitation to prevent human experimentation and the almost frantic public pressure to find cures for cancer, heart disease, muscular dystrophy, multiple sclerosis, etc., etc.

23

Cardiovascular Diseases

It were disgraceful, with this most spacious and admirable realm of nature before us, and where the reward ever exceeds the promise, did we take the reports of others upon trust, and go on coining crude problems out of these, and on them hanging knotty and captious and petty disputations. Nature is herself to be addressed; the paths she shows us are to be boldly trodden; for thus, and whilst we consult our proper senses, from inferior advancing to superior levels, shall we penetrate at length into the heart of her mystery.

(William Harvey)

CORONARY ARTERY DISEASE

In the late nineteenth and early twentieth centuries, leading clinicians, many of them also trained in pathology, were interested chiefly in clinical-pathological correlations and the description of new clinical entities. In the latter part of this period a few physicians, no longer content with mere descriptions of disease, shifted their interest to clinical investigation and experimentation. The transition from one approach to the other is well illustrated by the evolution of our knowledge of coronary artery disease.

The first case of occlusion of a coronary artery to be diagnosed correctly during life was reported by *Adam Hammer* of St. Louis, who had received his medical training at the University of Heidelberg. In 1848 he took part in a revolution in Germany, and when it failed he was forced to seek asylum abroad. He reached St. Louis in October, 1848, began practice there, and was soon impressed by the need for reform in American medical education. In 1850 the legislature of Missouri chartered an institution organized to carry out Hammer's ideas. It was the first medical school in the United States to have high entrance requirements, a graded curriculum, and four courses of lectures. Hammer's school was too advanced for the students of

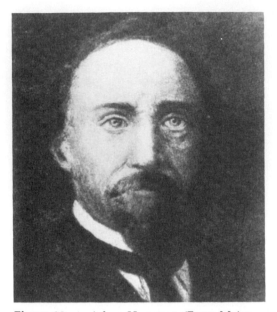

Figure 99. Adam Hammer. (From Major,
R. H.: Classic Descriptions of Disease, 1932.
Courtesy of Charles C Thomas, Springfield,
Illinois.)

his day; it survived for only one year. In 1877 Hammer returned to Europe
and died there the following year (Ball, 1909).

In 1878 a paper appeared in the *Wiener Medizinische Wochenschrift,* entitled "A Case of Thrombotic Occlusion of One of the Coronary Arteries of
the Heart: Diagnosed at the Bedside and Communicated by Dr. A. Hammer,
Professor of Surgery from St. Louis, at present in Vienna." On May 4, 1876,
Hammer had been taken by a colleague to see a patient, 34 years old, who
had suffered from attacks of articular rheumatism, and while recovering
from one of these attacks, he insisted on getting out of bed and suddenly
collapsed. One-half hour later his physician found the patient to be cyanotic
and short of breath; his pulse was weak, 40 beats to the minute. Over the
next few hours the pulse rate dropped to 16 per minute.

Hammer made a thorough examination of the patient and was particularly impressed by the sudden collapse and steady deterioration in his condition. "I thought that only a sudden progressively increasing disturbance
in the nutrition of the heart itself, such as a cutting off of the supply of
nourishment, could produce such changes as this case showed, and that
such an obstruction could be produced only by a thrombotic occlusion of at
least one of the coronary arteries. I mentioned my conviction to my colleague at the bedside; he, however, had a non-plussed expression and burst
out, 'I have never heard of such a diagnosis in my whole life.' And I answered, 'Nor I also.' " The patient died a few hours later. At autopsy, a large
thrombus was found in the right sinus of Valsalva, which, when it extended, occluded the lumen of the coronary artery. Hammer believed that
the progressive diminution in the pulse rate was caused by the constant
growth of the thrombus until complete closure of the coronary artery oc-

curred. He noted that Cohnheim, in his lectures on general pathology in 1877, had stated the following: "In fact Bezold, by closing the coronary arteries with a clamp and Panum by producing an embolus in the same with a thin, waxy emulsion, were able to stop the heart; but whether a similar event in human pathology will ever be observed, is to me improbable enough." Cohnheim did not know that this occurrence had, indeed, been observed 18 months before (Major, 1932).

Other physicians became aware of a relationship between angina pectoris and disease of the coronary arteries and that thrombosis of a coronary artery was sometimes associated with sudden development of acute pain in the chest. Notable among these was *George Dock*. Dock was an outstanding internist, teacher, and investigator, who served as Assistant in Medicine at the University of Pennsylvania, his alma mater, under William Osler. In 1891 he was called to the Chair of Medicine at the University of Michigan, where he remained until 1908. While there (in 1896) he published an account, the first to appear in America, of a case of coronary thrombosis diagnosed during life and confirmed by autopsy (Dock, 1896). From 1908 until 1910, Dock was Professor of Medicine at Tulane University, and in 1910 he became Professor of Medicine at Washington University, St. Louis.

Osler also was aware of the relationship between angina pectoris and disease of the coronary arteries, as described in his Lumleian Lectures on angina pectoris, delivered before the Royal College of Physicians of London in 1910. Among the cases that he had studied at autopsy, some had occlusion of a coronary artery.

The first physician clearly to characterize the clinical manifestations of coronary occlusion was *James B. Herrick*. One of the most distinguished clinicians of his day, Herrick was born in 1861 and graduated from the Uni-

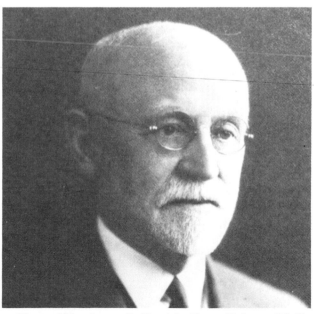

Figure 100. James B. Herrick. (From Holmes, W. H.: James Bryan Herrick. Privately printed, 1935.)

483

versity of Michigan in 1882. He received his M.D. in 1888 from Rush Medical College, Chicago, where he became Professor of Medicine in 1900. His outstanding contributions were his original description of sickle cell anemia and his classic work on coronary occlusion. He believed, at first, that coronary artery occlusion was almost always fatal, and he referred often to Parry's writings on angina pectoris and its relation to coronary artery disease. The tragic death of the great Danish sculptor, Bertel Thorvaldsen, in a theater in Copenhagen with the finding of a plugged coronary artery, had also attracted Herrick's attention to the relationship between blockage of the coronary arteries and sudden death. Cohnheim, he knew, felt that the coronary arteries were end-arteries and that sudden occlusions of one of these vessels would lead to death within a few minutes.

Herrick's famous paper giving the first full description of the clinical manifestations of coronary occlusion was entitled "Clinical Features of Sudden Obstruction of the Coronary Arteries." It appeared in 1912 in the *Journal of the American Medical Association*. In this article and others which followed it, Herrick clearly differentiated coronary occlusion from "prolonged angina pectoris" with which it generally had been confused by Osler and others. The key paragraphs in Herrick's paper were the following:

> *Obstruction of a coronary artery or any of its large branches has long been regarded as a serious accident. Several events contributed toward the prevalence of the view that this condition was almost always suddenly fatal. . . .*
>
> *But there are reasons for believing that even large branches of the coronary arteries may be occluded—at times acutely occluded—without resulting in death in the immediate future. Even the main trunk may at times be obstructed and the patient live. It is the object of this paper to present a few facts along this line and particularly to describe some of the clinical manifestations of sudden yet not immediately fatal cases of coronary obstruction. . . .*
>
> *A study of cases of this type shows that nearly all are men past the middle period of life. Previous attacks of angina have generally been experienced, though as shown by my first case, the fatal thrombosis may bring on the first seizure. The seizure is described by patients who have had previous experience with angina as of unusual severity, and the pain persists much longer.*

Coronary heart disease is so common today that it is difficult to understand how coronary occlusion went for so many years without being recognized. One explanation is that physicians did not know how to make the diagnosis until Herrick showed them the way. But it is hard to believe that alert diagnosticians of the last two decades of the nineteenth century such as Austin Flint and William Osler and others like them could have overlooked such a spectacular association of clinical symptoms and pathological findings if it had occurred as frequently then as it does today. Flint and Osler and their peers certainly recognized angina pectoris when they encountered it, but they all considered it to be an infrequent occurrence. When they did encounter it, it was usually in their more prosperous patients. Flint, in his medical textbook in 1866, described it as a rare disease; and so did Osler in his *Practice* in 1892. Paul Dudley White, who graduated from the Harvard Medical School in 1911 and began the practice of cardiology in Boston shortly thereafter, said that angina pectoris was still uncommon at that time. White states that when the automobile gained popularity in the 1920s and more people became fat and prosperous, coronary heart disease began to appear in younger and younger men (White, 1974).

METHODS FOR THE DIAGNOSIS OF HEART DISEASE, WITH PARTICULAR REFERENCE TO MYOCARDIAL INFARCTION

When a coronary artery is occluded, the heart muscle that had received its blood supply from the obstructed artery dies and ceases to function, a condition known as *myocardial infarction*. It is the infarction of the heart muscle rather than the obstruction of the artery that causes the symptoms. The infarction may be large or small, depending on how much of the blood supply has been blocked off; the larger it is, the more threatening it is to life and health. Though Herrick made his diagnoses of coronary occlusion largely on the basis of signs and symptoms observed at the patient's bedside, we now know that if we had to rely solely on such simple observation, many cases of myocardial infarction would escape detection, and appropriate methods of treatment would not be applied.

ELECTROCARDIOGRAPHY   Since the 1920s physicians have been relying principally on the *electrocardiogram* to verify the diagnosis of myocardial infarction.* The contraction of the muscles of the heart occurs in response to a minute electrical current, which is generated in neuromuscular tissue near the base of the heart and passes from there to the atria and through special conducting bundles to the ventricles. When the current reaches the muscle cells, it causes them to contract. The electrocardiogram records the sequence of electrical events that accompanies each cycle of cardiac contraction (i.e., each heartbeat). Luigi Galvani (1737–1798) of Bologna, Italy, who began his professional career as an anatomist, was one of the early experimenters with electricity, and he was the first to observe that when an electric current is applied to the nerve of a frog's leg, it causes a contraction of the muscles supplied by that nerve. He was also the first to discover that animal tissue is capable of generating an electric discharge (actually, ancient peoples, though they were unaware of its significance, had observed this fact when they first made contact with a torpedo fish or electric ray).

Kölliker and Müller in Germany demonstrated in 1855 that the heart generates an electric current: they placed the nerve of a frog's leg on the surface of a beating heart and found that the muscles of the leg gave a twitch with each beat of the heart. This was followed by other experiments on the

---

*The fascinating history of the development of electrocardiography is beautifully related in an article written by Louis N. Katz and H. K. Kellerstein in Fishman and Richards (1964). Reference may be made to that article for the many interesting details which must be omitted from this necessarily brief account.

electrical phenomena exhibited by the exposed heart in experimental animals. However, the detection of the very small currents generated by the unexposed heart in intact animals and man had to await the development of a more sensitive instrument. In 1875 Gabriel Lippmann, a German physicist interested in the study of electricity, invented the *capillary electrometer,* which allowed him to magnify and record minute fluctuations in electrical potential. Using this instrument, Augustus V. Waller at St. Mary's Hospital in London made the first records of cardiac electrical current in an intact human being by placing the two electrodes of the electrometer on the front and back of the chest. He demonstrated his method in 1887 to a group of distinguished physiologists, including Willem Einthoven of Leiden.

Intrigued by Waller's demonstration, Einthoven returned to his laboratory in Holland and began a series of experiments in which he improved and refined the records produced by the electrometer. He found that during each heartbeat there is a series of electrical waves, which he designated by the letters P, Q, R, S, and T. Einthoven realized that the electrometer lacked the sensitivity (frequency response) required for accurate recording of the small currents coming from the heart, and he was on the alert to find a more sensitive recording instrument.

In the latter part of the nineteenth century many submarine cables were being laid to transmit long-distance telegraph messages. Since the signals lost strength in transmission, efforts were made to find new instruments that would respond to very weak signals of high frequency. In the course of this search Clement Ader, a French inventor, developed an instrument in 1897, the *string galvanometer,* based on an entirely new principle. This device had a frequency response considerably higher than that of the electrometer, and Einthoven quickly realized that it might be a superior instrument for recording the electrical signals emanating from the heart.

The string galvanometer is based on the principle that a magnet and a conductor of electric current will interact. A fine, threadlike, metallic-coated quartz filament (the string) is stretched between the two poles of a powerful electromagnet. When the two ends of the string are connected with electrodes appropriately placed on the body of a resting subject, the fluctuations in electrical potentials coming from the heart cause the string to move in the magnetic field. With a source of illumination and a system of lenses, the shadow of the string can be photographed on moving film. The tracing of the moving string which Einthoven was able to obtain on his photographic film was sharper, more precise, and more reliable than that which he had obtained with the electrometer, but the same P, Q, R, S, and T waves were there. The strip of film with its wavelike tracing of the moving string constitutes the electrocardiogram.

Einthoven and his co-workers in Leiden carried out many of the basic studies in electrocardiography. They found that when the electrodes were placed on various parts of the body, the tracing of the shadow took on certain forms, and they endeavored to understand what these differences meant in terms of the origin and propagation of the electrical currents in the heart. They found it useful to place one electrode on the right forearm, another on the left forearm, and a third on the left lower leg. Much of the early work with clinical electrocardiography was carried out with the electrodes placed in these locations. Three tracings were made, using three different "standard leads"; lead I (right arm—left arm), lead II (right arm—left leg), lead III (left arm—left leg).

The first electrocardiographic apparatus was heavy and clumsy and took up a lot of laboratory space, but with the advent of vacuum-tube amplification and, more recently, of the transistor, the modern apparatus is easily portable and fits into a carrying case no larger than an overnight bag. The tracings are now made with a stylus on specially prepared paper so that the records can be examined immediately without having to wait for the development of photographic film.

In the early clinical work with the electrocardiogram (EKG), attention was focused principally upon the more obvious abnormalities in cardiac rhythm. Then attention shifted to the conduction system within the heart, and it was at about this time that the first American contributions to electrocardiography were reported. In 1909, three institutions in the United States, two in New York and one in Baltimore, acquired at about the same time a rather flimsy electrocardiographic apparatus made in Germany by Edelmann. One of these pieces of equipment was set up at Mount Sinai Hospital, New York, under the direction of Alfred E. Cohn. Cohn had graduated from the College of Physicians and Surgeons, New York, in 1904, and after that had taken six years of graduate training, two of which were spent abroad in Germany and in England, where he worked under Thomas Lewis, the English pioneer in electrocardiography. The other electrocardiograph in New York was set up at the old Presbyterian Hospital under the direction of Dr. Walter B. James, Professor of Medicine at The College of Physicians and Surgeons. In establishing the apparatus at the Presbyterian Hospital, Dr. James had the assistance of Horatio B. Williams of the Department of Physiology.

When Alfred Cohn joined the staff of the Hospital of the Rockefeller Institute in 1911, he had become discouraged by some of the inadequacies of the Edelmann apparatus, and he solicited the help of Dr. Williams. Together they planned and put together the first American-designed electrocardiograph. This apparatus was installed at the Rockefeller Hospital in March, 1911, and it was so well made that it continued in operation for the next 32 years.

The third Edelmann electrocardiograph was set up at the Johns Hopkins Hospital. This appears to have been the first of the three to be placed in operation (October, 1909), and like the one at Mount Sinai, it proved to be unreliable. These early Edelmann models were compact and did not require much space, but they had a number of faults, and after Drs. Arthur D. Hirschfelder and George S. Bond had spent a frustrating six months working with the apparatus in Baltimore, they ordered from Edelmann a new and considerably larger model, which was delivered in October, 1910. Figure 101 shows the Heart Station (cardiac laboratory) at the Johns Hopkins Hospital shortly after the new apparatus was installed. The original Edelmann model is on the small table to the left, and the larger model is on the table to the right. By that time, the small model had been redesigned to record the heart sounds which were projected on the moving film simultaneously with the electrocardiographic tracing. The first American papers on electrocardiography were published in 1910 by James and Williams of New York and Barker, Hirschfelder, and Bond of Baltimore.

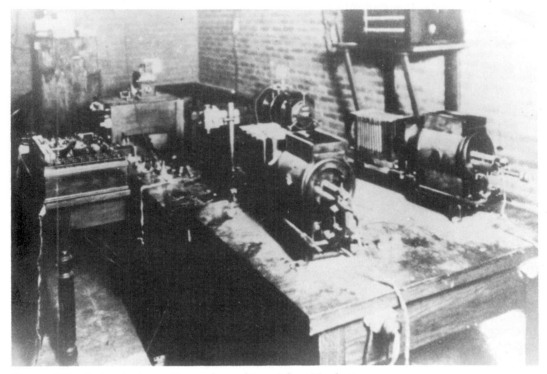

Figure 101. Early electrocardiograph machine. Johns Hopkins Hospital, 1909. (From the Archives Office, the Johns Hopkins Medical Institutions.)

In the early years of electrocardiography in the United States a great deal of interest was centered on conduction defects within the heart. In 1912, Cohn and Lewis described the EKG and post-mortem findings in a patient with complete heart block. In the same year the same authors presented the EKG of a patient in whom there were both atrial fibrillation and complete heart block. The following year Cohn published the first EKGs of a patient with complete dissociation of the contractions of the atrium and ventricle resulting from digitalis intoxication. J. A. E. Eyster and W. J. Meek, in 1914, showed that the atrioventricular node is the site of impulse formation in what is known as nodal rhythm. Simon and Robinson in 1917 published the EKGs of a patient with intermittent complete heart block.

Frank N. Wilson was the foremost American contributor to the theory of electrocardiography and the practical interpretation of EKGs. Wilson received both his undergraduate and his medical degrees from the University of Michigan, the latter in 1914. For several years after graduation he worked at Washington University, St. Louis, under George Dock, whose early observations on coronary occlusion were previously cited. Wilson was largely a self-taught electrocardiographer; his first papers on this subject were published the year after he graduated from medical school. During World War I, Wilson was in England, where he carried out electrocardiographic studies under Sir Thomas Lewis. The great contributions of Wilson and his colleagues came during the 1930s and 1940s, when he was

488

Professor of Medicine at the University of Michigan. During that period the Michigan group carried out a series of brilliant studies on normal human subjects, on patients with various types of heart disease, and on experimental animals. Their work extended that of Einthoven and was based in part on the observations of W. H. Craib on the electrical field surrounding strips of cardiac and skeletal muscle. As a result they were able to describe with greater precision than had been possible before the laws that govern the distribution of the electromotive forces in the heart.

Though Wilson and his group were concerned for the most part with gaining a better understanding of the basic principles of electrocardiography, their work cast new light on many of the abnormalities observed in the EKGs of patients. Their theoretical concept led to the introduction of unipolar leads derived from an *indifferent* electrode (formed by combining the three standard limb electrodes) and an *exploring* electrode, which could be placed on the body in various strategic locations. As a direct result of Wilson's work the electrocardiogram today consists of tracings made by using successively 12 different leads: the 3 standard limb leads of Einthoven, and 9 unipolar leads made with the exploring electrode applied in sequence to the right arm, left arm, left leg, and 6 points on the chest overlying the heart. The use of the 12-lead technique allows one to record the cardiac electrical events in a series of two-dimensional planes. By combining these records one can derive an approximate three-dimensional representation of the events. The 12-lead electrocardiogram provides a vast amount of information about the electrical activity of the heart and is particularly useful in diagnosing, localizing, and following the progress of myocardial infarcts.

While Wilson's work was still in its early phases, observations by several different groups were bringing to light the possible usefulness of the electrocardiogram for the diagnosis of myocardial infarction. In 1919 J. B. Herrick, following up his original observations on coronary occlusion, published the first paper describing abnormal T waves in leads II and III in a patient who clinically had a myocardial infarction. Herrick suggested at that time that the EKG might be useful in the diagnosis of myocardial infarcts. Even before this paper appeared, Herrick had suggested to Fred M. Smith that he ligate the coronary arteries in a dog, making electrocardiograms before and after the operation, in hopes of detecting some change in the EKG record. Smith reported these experiments in 1918. In the same year Brousfield, in England, directed attention to the alterations in the EKG tracings that occurred during an attack of angina pectoris, and in 1920, H. E. B. Pardee of New York described "an electrocardiographic sign of coronary obstruction." Pardee's sign consists of a "cove-like" inversion of the terminal portion of the ventricular complex of the electrocardiogram.

J. Parkinson and D. E. Bedford, in 1928, and A. R. Barnes and M. B. Whitten, in 1929, obtained EKG records which led them to believe that they could distinguish between an anterior and a posterior infarction by the reciprocal changes in the S-T segments and T waves in standard leads I and III; when the changes occurred in lead I, the infarction was likely to be anterior, and when they occurred in lead III, the infarction was likely to be posterior. The studies of Wilson and his co-workers, reported in 1933, directed attention to the abnormalities in the Q wave, which were also diagnostic of myocardial infarction; a prominent Q wave in lead I being associated with a T-I type curve and a prominent Q wave in lead III being associated with a T-III type curve.

In clinical practice, the value of electrocardiography was only dimly realized even in the 1920s. It was used principally to distinguish abnormalities in rhythm and conduction, and many of these distinctions could be made just as satisfactorily with mechanical recording devices. In the 1925 edition of Osler and McCrae's *Principles and Practice of Medicine,* electrocardiography is not described, though three short EKG tracings are reproduced (without labeling them as such) to demonstrate one abnormal rhythm and two types of heart block. The fourth edition of Sir James Mackenzie's *Diseases of the Heart* appeared at about the same time as the Osler and McCrae text, and this widely used treatise on cardiology gave a brief description of Einthoven's apparatus and technique, illustrated by a single short EKG tracing, and then went on to cast doubt on the significance and clinical utility of the electrical record. Mackenzie devotes only 4 of 483 pages to this subject.

Though the studies of Sir Thomas Lewis and Frank Wilson had demonstrated that much could be learned about cardiac electrical phenomena by placing electrodes directly over the heart (precordial leads), clinical electrocardiographers continued to employ only the three standard limb leads until the 1930s. Francis C. Wood and Charles C. Wolferth of the University of Pennsylvania were the first to point out that information valuable to the clinician could be obtained by employing a precordial lead. Their paper on this subject, which appeared in 1932, was entitled "An electrocardiographic study of coronary occlusion: The inadequacy of the three conventional leads in recording certain characteristic changes in action currents." When this paper was written, Wood was a young assistant in Wolferth's laboratory. They had been making a study of angina pectoris and were taking EKGs before, during, and after attacks of anginal pain. They suspected that the pain and the accompanying changes in the electrocardiogram might be due to ischemia (reduced blood flow) of the heart muscle. To obtain further information on this question, Wood had embarked on some experimental studies in dogs, taking EKGs before, during, and after brief periods of obstruction of the coronary arteries. Wood's interesting account of how the work in the experimental laboratory eventually led to the publication of the paper in 1932 follows (Burch and DePasquale, 1964):

> In the animal laboratory I first clamped the anterior descending and right coronary arteries and got nothing very much. Then one day I wanted to get through so I decided to terminate the experiments by clamping all three coronary arteries: the left anterior descending, the right, and the circumflex as well. I was astonished to find that whereas the anterior descending and the right coronary arteries had produced relatively little change in the EKG, when I clamped all three I got a sudden, dramatic, rapidly appearing change in Leads II and III which disappeared promptly when I took the bulldog clamp from the coronary arteries. Further fiddling around demonstrated that you could always get a change when you clamped the posterior descending artery without clamping any other vessels. This puzzled me a great deal because when I clamped the anterior descending artery, I got a dramatic change in the appearance of the heart which was as dramatic as the change which occurred when clamping the posterior descending artery, but got no EKG change. . . . [then] I

490

tried putting an electrode directly on the anterior wall of the heart and clamping the anterior vessel. This made a dramatic change in the EKG as recorded from the heart surface even though nothing much had appeared in the limb leads. I went back to the hospital after seeing this and told Dr. Wolferth about it. The next morning he said to me, "You know, I've been thinking about this overnight. There are a lot of patients who have coronary occlusions which don't show up in the EKG, somewhat similar to the situation in the dog, and although we can't put an electrode right on the heart the way you did in this dog, we might put an electrode near the heart, right on the chest surface over the heart, when we see the next patient of this sort, and see what happens."

That very afternoon, on September 14, 1931, the patient appeared. . . . The patient, M.K., had a perfect history of acute cardiac infarction, so I put an electrode right on the precordium and connected it to the right arm wire, and put one opposite on the left side of the chest at the back and connected it with the left arm lead wire and took a tracing. Much to our delight and astonishment, it showed a dramatic change in the S-T interval of this lead, which we called Lead IV, whereas nothing diagnostic had appeared in the limb leads.

During the next several years, most electrocardiograms were taken with lead IV in addition to the standard limb lead. In 1934 Wilson introduced other precordial leads, which he designated with Roman numerals. From this point on, there was a great improvement in the electrocardiographic diagnosis and localization of myocardial infarcts, and it became possible to recognize the current of injury arising from fresh infarcts and the scars left behind by old infarcts. Further improvement in electrocardiographic interpretation resulted from the introduction of unipolar leads, and finally, a little more than a decade after World War II, the 12-lead technique described earlier came into general clinical use.

CARDIAC RESUSCITATION AND THE DEVELOPMENT OF THE CORONARY CARE UNIT

Each year more than 1.5 million Americans suffer heart attacks, and of these, about 600,000 die. In most instances these attacks are due to coronary occlusion leading to myocardial infarction. The sudden-death characteristic of a heart attack has been compared to the halting of a pendulum of a clock. When the pendulum is halted, the clock stops ticking even though its internal machinery is still in good working order. It has long been known that the heart may stop beating either because of power failure or because of electrical failure. The electrical failure responsible for many of the deaths from coronary attacks is due either to asystole (sudden cessation of the heartbeat) or to ventricular fibrillation. Asystole is caused by a breakdown in the pacemaking mechanism that generates the electric current, which initiates the contraction of the heart muscle. On the other hand, ventricular fibrillation is due to excessive electrical activity conducted through the heart in a random, uneven, and uncoordinated manner; the heart is unable to contract effectively, and death quickly ensues. Ventricular fibrillation is not peculiar to coronary occlusion. It has long been recognized as a terminal event in experimental animals in which the heart is exposed and the uncoordinated twitching of

491

the heart muscle can be observed. The occurrence of this condition in living patients could not be recorded until the advent of electrocardiography. The first American electrocardiogram showing ventricular fibrillation was obtained at the Rockefeller Institute in 1912 by G. Canby Robinson in a patient dying of poliomyelitis.

Cardiac resuscitation has a long history. In 1883 Sidney Ringer, while a student at Cambridge University, described the antagonistic effects of calcium and potassium ions on myocardial contractility. Calcium increases and potassium decreases the force of contraction of heart muscle. Maurice d'Halluin used this information to treat ventricular fibrillation. To produce fibrillation he injected a 5 per cent solution of potassium chloride into the jugular vein and massaged the heart. To stop the fibrillation and reestablish normal cardiac contraction, he then injected Locke's solution (a balanced salt solution containing calcium in physiological concentration) into an artery. If normal cardiac contraction did not return promptly, he gave an intravenous injection of 5 per cent calcium chloride. Following a different line of research, two French workers, Prevost and Battelli, observed that a strong electrical current would cause ventricular fibrillation and that if another shock were administered, the fibrillation would cease. Even earlier (1775) Peter Christian Abildgaard, a Danish veterinarian and physician, conducted experiments on the effect of electrical countershock on animals. He succeeded in first rendering fowl lifeless by an electric shock and then reviving them by a countershock applied to the thorax (Driscol et al., 1975).

CARDIOPULMONARY RESUSCITATION   In the 1920s the electric utility companies became concerned about the increasing number of linemen killed by electric shock, and they decided to support research on this problem. The Consolidated Edison Company of New York City, in 1925, appealed to the Rockefeller Institute for help. As a result of this appeal five investigations were started, one of which was conducted by Professor W. H. Howell in Baltimore. The work there began under the supervision of William B. Kouwenhoven, Professor of Electrical Engineering at Johns Hopkins, and O. R. Langworthy, a member of the faculty of the Medical School. Using rats as experimental animals, they studied the effects of direct current (DC) and alternating current (AC) shock of high and low voltages as well as lightning discharges. Analysis of the problem in human subjects revealed that ventricular fibrillation occurred mainly from low-voltage shocks and that paralysis of respiration resulted from higher voltage shocks. In 1930 Howell called attention to the experiments of Prevost and Batelli, in which ventricular fibrillation had been arrested by a strong electric shock, and he suggested that Kouwenhoven and Langworthy try to repeat this work and verify the results. In 1933 Kouwenhoven and Langworthy reported that they had confirmed the earlier work and that they were able to make a dog's fibrillating heart resume normal contraction by administering a strong electric shock (Kouwenhoven et al., 1973).

Patients who are undergoing surgery occasionally develop ventricular fibrillation on the operating table, and Carl J. Wiggers, Professor of Physiology at Case Western Reserve University, conceived the idea of applying Kouwenhoven's findings to such patients to restore normal cardiac activity.

Working on experimental animals with R. Wégria, Wiggers found that an AC shock would produce fibrillation and that a stronger "countershock" would stop the fibrillation. Wiggers and Wégria went further and found that fibrillation could be most readily induced if the shock were applied at a particular point in the cardiac cycle, which they termed the vulnerable period. Claude Beck, a surgeon working with Wiggers, was the first to report the successful use of AC countershock to halt ventricular fibrillation which had occurred in a patient undergoing surgery. In this case the countershock was delivered by electrodes applied directly to the surface of the exposed heart.

For some years after this, on the basis of Beck's experience, it became standard procedure, whenever the heart stopped beating or began to fibrillate during a surgical operation, to open the chest immediately, and to begin squeezing the heart rhythmically. The rhythmic squeezing of the heart would maintain the circulation temporarily, and sometimes after a brief period of this type of massage the heart muscle would resume normal contraction. If the heart failed to respond spontaneously, the circulation could be maintained long enough to get apparatus into position to apply countershock. The success of this type of procedure at the operating table led to its being applied more widely. It was recommended that whenever a patient's heart stopped beating while a physician was near at hand, the physician should cut open the chest and begin squeezing the heart to maintain the circulation until spontaneous contractions were resumed or countershock could be applied (Johnson, 1970).

For a long time it had been known that a sharp blow to the chest over the heart occasionally would restore activity to a heart that had stopped beating, without having to open the chest. In 1946 two Russians, Gurvich and Yuniev, reported that a strong electric shock applied externally across the closed chest would halt ventricular fibrillation. Following this lead, Paul M. Zoll of the Harvard Medical Faculty at Beth Israel Hospital first confirmed the Russian results in a series of experiments on dogs and pigs, and then in 1952 he applied external shock to restore cardiac activity in a patient whose heart had stopped beating. In his work with patients Zoll found that ventricular fibrillation could be halted most successfully by an AC shock of 0.15 second's duration. He began with a shock of 180 volts, and if this did not work, stronger shocks (not exceeding 720 volts) were applied until the fibrillation ceased. For restoration of normal rhythm in cases of simple cardiac standstill, a weaker ("pacemaking") current of only 0.003 second's duration and 25 to 100 volts was found to produce the best results. If the heart did not resume rhythmic contraction after defibrillation, the external pacemaker delivered small shocks rhythmically to maintain regular activity. Zoll also found that a number of other types of abnormal cardiac rhythms could be brought to a halt by externally applied AC shocks, sometimes followed by a brief period of external pacemaking in order to reinstitute normal rhythm.

While Zoll's work was going forward at Harvard, Kouwenhoven's group at Johns Hopkins was also experimenting with various types of external defibrillation and other methods of cardiac resuscitation. In 1954 G. Guy Knickerbocker, a member of Kouwenhoven's staff, suggested that it might be possible to squeeze the heart by applying pressure rhythmically to the

493

chest over the heart. This was tried with dogs, and it was found that by applying rhythmic pressure to the lower third of the sternum with a force of 80 to 100 pounds at a rate of 1 per second, a dog whose heart had been rendered inactive could be kept alive for a period of at least ten minutes. In February, 1958, Henry T. Bahnson, a surgeon who had been associated with Kouwenhoven, had the first opportunity to try this technique on a patient. He successfully resuscitated a two-year-old child whose heart was in ventricular fibrillation. This method of resuscitation became known as external cardiac massage, and it came into wide use to maintain the circulation for brief periods until the heart spontaneously resumed contraction or electrical methods could be applied. It is combined with mouth-to-mouth breathing, which provides aeration of the lungs and oxygenation of the blood. The mouth-to-mouth method of lung ventilation was perfected shortly after World War II by James Elam and Peter Safer. The great advantage of external cardiac massage and mouth-to-mouth breathing is that they can be applied immediately by any person trained in the technique. Life can be maintained for an hour or more without having to open the chest. One of the unfavorable aspects of external cardiac massage is that the firm pressure on the chest frequently results in fracture of the ribs (Kouwenhoven et al., 1960).

During the 1950s and 1960s the methods and equipment for cardiac resuscitation were improved. Capacitors were developed that would deliver a DC rather than an AC shock. In 1962 Bernard Lown of the Harvard School of Public Health introduced a method for delivering the direct current shock to the heart in a safe period of the cardiac cycle. The capacitor was synchronized with the electrocardiogram so that it was tripped by the QRS complex to deliver a countershock of 0.004 second's duration. This assured the delivery of the shock before the vulnerable period that had been demonstrated some years before by Wiggers (Zoll, 1975).

Along with the advances in methods of cardiac resuscitation, there were advances in the development of cardiac pacemakers. These devices are particularly useful in patients who have Stokes-Adams attacks. The latter are characterized by sudden episodes of fainting, which are due either to a very slow heart rate (less than 20 beats per minute) or to prolonged failure of the heart to contract. The patient faints because not enough blood is being pumped to the brain to preserve consciousness. In 1952 Zoll used his external electric pacemaker in a patient who had severe coronary artery disease and periods of prolonged ventricular standstill with loss of consciousness. By keeping a close watch on the patient and using the pacemaker to prevent or control the fainting episodes, the patient was carried through this difficult period and recovered sufficiently to go home and live without the pacemaker. It was Zoll's interest in preventing Stokes-Adams attacks that led him to develop the monitoring equipment which is now used all over the world. He found that in patients who had frequent Stokes-Adams attacks, it was impossible to prevent attacks even with the most devoted attendants watching the patient. "We quickly realized the need for a reliable electronic machine that would not get bored or distracted or walk out of the room seconds before an unpredictable episode of cardiac arrest" (Zoll, 1975).

The "reliable electronic machine" that was devised by Zoll and his colleagues was the first automatic cardiac monitor. The external pacemaker was kept in position with its electrodes on the patient's chest, and it was connected to an electronic mechanism that used the patient's electrocardiograph as a signal-processing device. Whenever the heart stopped beating, an audible alarm was sounded, and within ten seconds the pacemaker was automatically activated.

The external pacemaker required cumbersome equipment and could be used only in patients who were virtually immobilized. But its success in the management of Stokes-Adams attacks led to the development of pacemakers that could be used over long periods of time in ambulatory patients. It had long been known that cardiac pacing could be accomplished in experimental animals with electrodes implanted in the heart muscle. Joseph Erlanger, in 1912, started an animal's heart which had stopped beating by passing a platinum electrode through the chest wall into the heart and causing it to resume beating by the stimulating effect of an electric current. The first internal pacemakers to be used in human patients were of two types: electrodes were either implanted directly into the heart by a cardiac surgeon, or an electrode was introduced into the cavity of the right ventricle via a vein. The pacemaking current was generated by a battery device which the patient could carry around with him. In the early 1960s, by using transistors and small mercury batteries, it became possible to reduce the size of the pacemaker to that of a package of cigarettes. Much of the work in improving and miniaturizing the pacemaker was accomplished by William M. Chardack, a physician in the Veterans' Administration, and his engineer associate, Watson Greatbatch.

In 1960 Chardack, Gage, and Greatbatch introduced a transistorized, self-contained pacemaker that could be implanted under the skin. Since then a number of improvements have been made in implantable pacemakers, and by 1975 many different models were being produced commercially in this country. The pulse-generating unit in most of these models is light in weight, about 6 centimeters long, 4 centimeters wide, and 2 to 3 centimeters in depth. They are designed to be implanted under the skin overlying the chest. The power is generated by batteries that have a long life so that the unit can be left in place for two to three years, after which it has to be replaced. The electrodes through which the electric pulse is transmitted to the heart are either placed directly in the heart muscle through a small surgical incision or are introduced by way of a vein into the cavity of the right ventricle. The wires connecting the pacemaker with the electrodes are placed beneath the skin. The pacemaker can be set to deliver its electric pulse at a fixed regular rate of about 70 per minute, or it can be set to go into action only when the heart stops beating or the heart rate falls below a certain level. Pacemakers have also been designed that can be recharged through the intact skin by electromagnetic induction. These units have the advantage of being smaller and lighter in weight, and it is estimated that they can be left in place for up to 50 years.

Nuclear-powered pacemakers also have been developed. The first of these to be used on patients was devised in the early 1970s by Chardack and his associates at the Veterans' Administration Hospital in Buffalo, New York. The pulse-generating mechanism in these units is actually quite small, but since the units generate heat and emit injurious rays, they have

495

to be insulated and shielded. Hence the size of the unit is about the same as that of the commonly used battery-powered pacemakers.

THE CORONARY
CARE UNIT

The various devices which have just been described — the defibrillators, the electronic monitoring equipment, the various types of pacemakers, and external cardiac massage — all were developed to deal with cardiac emergencies such as ventricular fibrillation or cardiac standstill, or for the treatment of patients with Stokes-Adams attacks, heart block, or a pulse rate too slow to maintain a normal circulation. It was gradually realized that all of these devices and methods could be put to good use in the care of patients who had had a myocardial infarction. During the first week after a coronary heart attack, the heart is prone to develop various abnormalities in rhythm, or it may suddenly cease beating or develop ventricular fibrillation. In most instances, if these problems can be dealt with adequately, the patient will recover. The desirability of keeping these patients in an area of the hospital where the equipment and trained personnel for their care can be concentrated gave rise to the coronary care unit (CCU). The patients in these units are all connected with monitoring devices, which record their electrocardiographic tracings continuously and which give an audible and visible alarm if the pulse rate exceeds a certain level, if irregularity develops, or if the heart stops beating. Defibrillating equipment and external pacemaking equipment are available for immediate use. The most important ingredient of a coronary care unit is the nursing staff. These nurses have had special training in electrocardiography and in the use of the important cardiac drugs, defibrillators, pacemakers, and other specialized equipment. By keeping close watch on the patient and his electrocardiogram, a well-trained nurse can often anticipate trouble and take appropriate action before the alarm sounds. The monitoring equipment and the alert and well-trained nurse have saved the lives of thousands of patients suffering from myocardial infarctions.

The development of CCUs was a major advance in the prevention of deaths from coronary heart disease, but unfortunately many patients who have had a coronary occlusion die before they ever reach the hospital. Some die quite suddenly, immediately after the attack begins; others die at home before the doctor arrives; and others die in the automobile or ambulance that is transporting them to the hospital. In some communities, special mobile coronary care units have been developed consisting of an ambulance equipped with an electrocardiograph and other specialized apparatus, manned by a specially trained team of attendants. These units also have two-way radio equipment so that they can communicate with the hospital and get advice as needed, or forewarn the hospital to make appropriate preparations to receive the patient.

**CARDIAC CATH-
ETERIZATION**

As the heart performs its work, blood is forced by the right ventricle through the vessels of the lungs, where it picks up oxygen and releases carbon dioxide; the blood then flows back to the left side of the heart, where the

496

left ventricle forces it through the arteries to all parts of the body to oxygenate and nourish the tissues and to pick up waste carbon dioxide; it then flows back through the veins to the right side of the heart to begin the circuit over again. Two factors are decisive for determining the efficiency with which the heart is performing its work: one is the pressure conditions in the various chambers of the heart; the other is the amount of blood which the heart forces out in a given period of time. The latter is usually expressed in milliliters (ml) of blood flow per minute, or "minute volume." If the amount of oxygen taken up by the lungs in a specified period of time is known, and if the oxygen content of the blood entering and leaving the lungs during that period is also known, it is possible to calculate the amount of blood passing through the lungs in that period. This calculation is made by using a formula first proposed in 1882 by the German physiologist Adolf Fick. Fick's formula says that the blood flow is equal to the oxygen uptake by the lungs divided by the difference between the oxygen content of the blood entering and that of the blood leaving the lungs. If the oxygen content of the blood entering the lungs is 140 ml per liter and that of the blood leaving the lungs is 180 ml per liter, each liter of blood has absorbed 40 ml of oxygen. If 200 ml of oxygen is absorbed by the subject's lungs in one minute, then (200 divided by 40) 5 liters of blood must have flowed through the lungs in a minute in order to absorb this quantity of oxygen. Under normal circumstances the blood flow through the lungs in one minute closely approximates the minute volume output of the heart. Thus the cardiac output can be calculated by means of the Fick formula.

For many years it has been possible to measure in experimental animals both the pressure in the cardiac chambers and the factors required for the calculation of cardiac output. However, in human subjects it was not possible to measure pressures within the heart, and since the oxygen content of the blood entering the lungs could not be measured, the Fick formula could be calculated only approximately. Hence, as late as 1928, physiologists and physicians had to be content with indirect and untrustworthy estimates of intracardiac pressure and cardiac output.

A way to solve some of the problems in human cardiac physiology was indicated in 1929 by *Werner Forssmann,* a 25-year-old surgical resident in a hospital in Berlin, Germany. After performing some preliminary experiments on cadavers, Forssmann had the courage to insert a small catheter into a vein in his own arm and pass it up the vein into the right side of his heart. He watched the progress of the catheter in a mirror held in front of a fluoroscopic screen. In reporting this experiment, Forssmann said that he had experienced no discomfort and had had no untoward reaction. The importance of Forssmann's feat was not immediately realized; in fact, it was generally scoffed at as a foolhardy and impractical venture. Neither Forssmann nor his German colleagues made any effort to pursue the matter further, and it was forgotten for more than a decade.

André Cournand and *Dickinson W. Richards, Jr.,* were the first to make practical use of Forssmann's pathfinding experiment. These two clinical investigators, working at Bellevue Hospital, New York, had studied the circulation under many different conditions. They were, therefore, quite familiar with the limitations of current methods, and they appreciated what might be learned by gaining direct access to the right side of the heart.

497

They made some minor improvements in Forssmann's technique and in 1941 reported their early experiences with cardiac catheterization in humans (Cournand and Ranges, 1941; Richards et al., 1941). These reports indicated the safety and the potentialities of the method, and it soon came into widespread use. The advent of cardiac catheterization, as will be seen later, coincided with great advances in the technology of cardiac surgery, and the two working hand in hand opened wholly new vistas in the treatment of heart disease. In 1956 the Nobel Prize in physiology and medicine was awarded to Cournand, Richards, and Forssmann for their development of cardiac catheterization. By that time Forssmann, having forsaken any interest in cardiac physiology, had become a urological surgeon; but Cournand and Richards were still hard at work on studies of the physiology and diseases of the heart and lungs.

Richards was a graduate of Yale College, and he received his M.D. degree from Columbia University in 1923. After completing his residency training at the Presbyterian Hospital, New York, he went to England and became a research fellow at the National Institute for Medical Research under Sir Henry Dale. On his return to the United States he began research in pulmonary and circulatory physiology, working first under Lawrence J. Henderson, Professor of Biochemistry at Harvard. Shortly after Richards's return to New York, he became engaged in research on the Chest Service of the Columbia University Division at Bellevue Hospital. In 1931 one of the residents on that service was a young Frenchman, *André Cournand,* who had received his medical degree in Paris in 1930 and had come to the United States for additional training. During his residency, Cournand seized the opportunity to work with Richards on pulmonary physiology, and they began a collaboration which was to continue for many years.

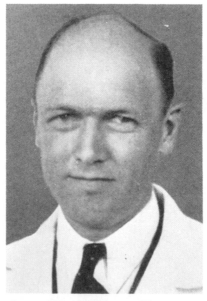

Figure 102. Dickinson W. Richards, Jr. (From Riesman, D.: A History of the Interurban Clinical Club, 1905–37. Philadelphia, The John C. Winston Co., 1937.)

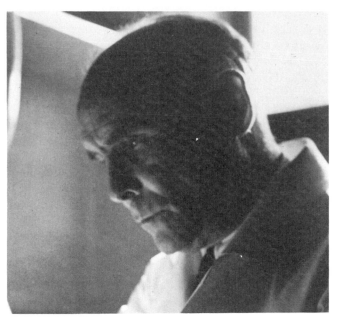

Figure 103. André Cournand. (Courtesy of Dr. Richard Riley.)

Cournand and Richards's early work with the cardiac catheter was limited to studies of the pressure in the right atrium, the chamber of the heart most easily reached by the catheter. They were the first to prove what had been long suspected; that in congestive heart failure the right atrial pressure may be four or five times higher than normal.

During the war, the development of cardiac catheterization went forward slowly, but after the war there was a great burst of activity in many medical centers. It was found that the catheter could easily be introduced into the right ventricle and, under favorable circumstances, into the pulmonary artery. Several techniques were also developed for introducing a catheter into the chambers of the left side of the heart, either by puncture or by introduction of the catheter in retrograde fashion up the aorta and into the left ventricle. With the catheter in the heart chambers or in the aorta or pulmonary artery, it became possible to record pressure curves, to withdraw blood for measurement of oxygen content, to detect an abnormal passage such as a septal defect, to inject indicator substances for the detection of cardiovascular shunts or regurgitation through valves, or to introduce contrast material for visualization of selected portions of the heart or vessels. Electrocardiographic leads could be introduced into the heart for taking intracardiac electrocardiograms, and as was mentioned earlier, electrodes could be introduced into the right ventricle for intracardiac pacemaking. One of the more recent important developments has been the use of catheters to introduce radiopaque material directly into the coronary arteries for the purpose of cineangiography. So many people in so many different institutions have been involved in the development and elaboration of cardiac catheterization, both in the United States and in foreign countries, that it is not feasible even to list them here.

Cardiac catheterization has resulted in more precise cardiac diagnosis and greatly improved methods of treatment. Perhaps the greatest advance has been in the diagnosis of congenital malformations of the heart. Prior to World War II, most of these conditions were considered to present a hopeless problem from the point of view of both diagnosis and treatment. The studies of Helen B. Taussig (see also The Blalock-Taussig Operation, p. 505) in the 1930s and early 1940s threw much new light on this difficult subject. Taussig's treatise, *Congenital Malformations of the Heart,* appeared in 1947 just as cardiac catheterization was coming into wide use. In this first edition of Taussig's work, there is bare mention of cardiac catheterization and angiocardiography (X-ray pictures of the heart taken after the injection of a radiopaque substance). In the second edition, which appeared in 1960, much space was devoted to both of these techniques, and one can readily see what a vast improvement they had brought about in the diagnosis of congenital defects.

Among those who made noteworthy contributions to the early catheterization studies of congenital heart disease were Richard J. Bing and his associates at Johns Hopkins (1947), Lewis Dexter and his associates at the Peter Bent Brigham Hospital (1947), Earl H. Wood and his associates at the Mayo Clinic (1948), and André Cournand and his associates at Bellevue Hospital. Bing's work is of particular interest. He showed how the Fick formula could be utilized to calculate the blood flow through both the pulmonary and the systemic circulations and that one could thus determine the quantity of blood that is short-circuited from one side of the heart to the other. He also introduced the concept of "effective pulmonary blood flow," which is calculated by a modified Fick formula and which provides an estimate of the proportion of blood that is fully oxygenated in its passage through the lungs. In another series of studies, Bing and his associates found that the tip of a catheter could be guided into one of the large veins of the coronary circulation, the coronary sinus. This made it possible to examine a sample of blood just after it had passed through the heart muscle and so to find how much oxygen the muscle had consumed and what foodstuffs it had utilized. Prior to that time, the metabolism of heart muscle had been studied only in slices of heart tissue and in a heart completely removed from the body of an experimental animal. However, the biochemical changes that take place under these circumstances are not necessarily the same as those in the living, actively beating heart. Bing's technique made it possible for the first time to calculate the heart's efficiency in converting the energy of its fuel into useful work.

This technique of intravascular catheterization of individual organs has now been greatly extended. It can be used to study the circulation and metabolism of the brain, the liver, the kidneys, various endocrine glands, and other organs. These studies can be carried out during both health and disease and thus provide information that is helpful for correcting organic abnormalities.

Angiocardiography, which was mentioned earlier in connection with the second edition of Taussig's book, was developed during the late 1930s. In October, 1937, at a medical meeting in Havana, Cuba, Castellanos and his associates described a new technique for visualizing the heart and great vessels by injecting a radiopaque substance into a vein in the arm and then taking X-ray pictures to visualize the chambers of the heart. At about the same time, a similar technique was developed by George Robb and Israel Steinberg in New York. By careful timing of the X-ray exposures, they were able to obtain the first clear pictures of the left atrium, left ventricle, and thoracic aorta in man.

An important addition to cardiovascular instrumentation was the optical manometer developed by W. F. Hamilton and his associates in 1934. This is a sensitive high-frequency manometer with a metal diaphragm, which gives accurate recordings of intravascular pressure. By using an optical system and moving film, one could make long continuous records of pressure. In the early years of cardiac catheterization, the Hamilton manometer was frequently used to record the blood pressure in the chambers of the heart.

CARDIOVASCULAR SURGERY

Fifty years ago, surgeons had a "hands-off" attitude toward the heart. Occasionally, when the heart was injured, a surgeon might be bold enough to try to repair some minor damage. But the results were usually discouraging, and the surgeon was not anxious to repeat the experience. The earliest elective cardiac operations involved the functioning portion of the heart only minimally, if at all. They were directed usually at a disease of the membranes surrounding the heart, the pericardium. In the late 1930s, with improved surgical techniques and better methods of anesthesia, operations were undertaken to correct congenital abnormalities in the great vessels close to the heart. Blalock's operation (see p. 505) was the first (1944) that had been devised to deal specifically with an abnormality within the heart, but it did so by carefully avoiding the heart itself and rearranging the vessels in the chest so as partially to compensate for the abnormality. Though it failed to correct the underlying cardiac defects, Blalock's operation converted "blue babies" into pink ones and enabled them to lead relatively normal lives. Some 12 to 15 years later, surgeons began to open the heart and correct the defects that made the babies blue.

Though the first great triumph of cardiac surgery was in the treatment of congenital abnormalities, progress was being made almost simultaneously in operations for other forms of heart disease. By 1976 it had become possible to treat surgically many patients with coronary artery disease and acquired disease of the valves of the heart. Methods had also been devised for the surgical treatment of serious and often fatal diseases of the larger arteries: aneurysms (ballooning of the arteries), which often rupture with resulting fatal hemorrhage, could be removed and replaced by plastic tubes; partially obstructed carotid arteries, which lead to strokes, could be reamed out or bypassed; partially obstructed renal arteries, which lead to high blood pressure, could be similarly treated. In a little more than 30 years cardiac and vascular surgery had grown from techniques of little practical importance into two major surgical specialties.

EARLY CARDIAC SURGERY

In 1891, H. C. Dalton, Professor of Surgery at Washington University, St. Louis, sutured the pericardium, the membrane enveloping the heart, in a young man who had been stabbed in the chest. Two years later, a simi-

501

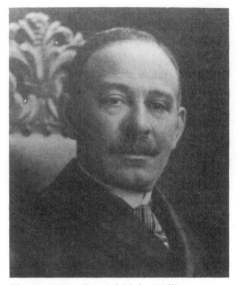

Figure 104. Daniel Hale Williams.
(From Buckler, H.: Doctor Dan, Pioneer
in American Surgery. Boston, Little,
Brown and Co., 1954.)

lar operation was performed in Chicago by *Daniel Hale Williams*. Williams
was a black physician, one of the first of his race to graduate from the medical college of Northwestern University (1883). He had been instrumental in
founding the Provident Hospital on Chicago's South Side. While he was at
the hospital on July 10, 1893, a young man was brought in near death from a
stab wound in the chest. Dr. Williams had the courage to open the man's
chest and sew up a rent in the pericardium. The young man made a
complete recovery. In 1902, Dr. Luther Hill of Montgomery, Alabama (father
of Senator Lister Hill, see Chap. 21) was called to see a 13-year-old boy who
had been stabbed five times in the chest. Dr. Hill operated, and when he
had exposed the heart, he found that one of the stab wounds had penetrated one of the heart chambers. The wound was successfully sutured, and
the boy recovered. This operation was performed by the light from two kerosene lamps on an old kitchen table in a slum district shack.

About 1930, surgeons began to recognize a new type of problem resulting from cardiac wounds. When a weapon penetrates the heart, the contractions of the heart may force blood out into the pericardial sac. With each
beat of the heart, more blood is forced out, and since the pericardium is
inelastic and cannot expand, the accumulation of blood in the sac gradually
squeezes the heart until it loses its ability to pump blood into the circulation. Unless something is done to relieve the pressure in the pericardial sac,
the patient dies, not from loss of blood but from loss of circulation. This
condition is known as cardiac tamponade. When the cause and symptoms
of cardiac tamponade became generally recognized, surgeons found that the
symptoms could be relieved promptly and dramatically by inserting a
needle into the pericardium and applying suction to withdraw the accumulated blood. There were many reports of successful operations of this

type. For example, Rettig A. Griswold and his surgical associates at the University of Louisville reported only three deaths in 36 cases (Johnson, 1970).

At about this same time, surgeons also began to drain the pericardial sac when fluid accumulated in it as the result of an inflammatory infection such as tuberculosis. Sometimes the drainage could be accomplished through a needle, but at other times it was necessary to cut through the chest wall and open a small window in the pericardial sac for drainage and irrigation.

There is another type of inflammation which is chronic and during which the pericardium gradually shrinks and thickens, thus constricting the heart and preventing enough blood from entering the heart to maintain an adequate circulation. E. Delorme, a French surgeon, suggested in 1898 that this condition might be amenable to surgical treatment. He said that he had not performed the operation because his medical colleagues would not allow him to do so on their patients. The first successful operation on constrictive pericarditis was carried out in Germany in 1920 by L. Rehn. Edward D. Churchill was the first to perform this type of operation in the United States, on a patient in whom Dr. Paul D. White had made a diagnosis of chronic constrictive pericarditis. This operation was performed at the Massachusetts General Hospital on an 18-year-old schoolgirl who was very ill and barely able to walk. Churchill removed a portion of the thickened pericardium to give the heart room to work, and the patient made an excellent recovery. Churchill's classic article describing this case and the technique of pericardial resection appeared in 1929. Since that time surgeons have saved many lives with this type of operative procedure. In 1946 George Heuer, Professor of Surgery at Cornell, reported a series of 18 such operations with no deaths and with cure or substantial improvement in 83 per cent of the cases.

Another advance in the treatment of traumatic cardiac injuries occurred during World War II. When American troops were involved in the cross-channel invasion of France in June, 1944, some of the casualties were treated at the 160th General Hospital, which was based in Cirencester, England. A group of surgeons at that hospital, led by Dwight E. Harken of Boston, performed a series of 134 cardiac operations without a single fatality. Harken was convinced that foreign objects such as shell fragments in or about the heart were a source of peril to the patient, since they might result in fatal embolism or lead to infection or other serious complications. To remove an intracardiac missile, the heart was often split wide open, with tremendous loss of blood. Rapid massive blood transfusions were needed to keep the patient alive. In the 10 months following D-day, this surgical team removed 13 missiles from the heart muscle, 17 from the pericardium, 13 from within the chambers of the heart, and 78 in or about the large blood vessels entering or leaving the heart.

OPERATIONS FOR CONGENITAL CARDIO-VASCULAR DEFECTS   The contributions of two individuals—Maude E. Abbott of McGill University and Helen B. Taussig of Johns Hopkins—helped to prepare the way for the surgical treatment of congenital abnormalities. Abbott made a comprehensive study of congenital defects of the heart

503

and great vessels, using the material from 142 hearts which she collected at autopsy. In 1936 these studies were brought together in an *Atlas of Congenital Cardiac Disease*. Taussig's work, on the other hand, was in the clinical field; in a series of articles published during the 1930s and 1940s, she demonstrated how it was possible to make more accurate diagnoses of congenital defects, and her great treatise, *Congenital Malformations of the Heart,* appeared in 1947. In addition to the work of these two individuals, the development of angiocardiography and cardiac catheterization after World War II greatly improved the diagnosis of congenital malformations. The better understanding of congenital defects and the improvements in methods of diagnosis enabled surgeons to undertake operations knowing in advance the precise nature of the problem with which they would have to deal.

Before birth, the fetus does not need to circulate its blood through its lungs. Its lungs are uninflated and its blood is oxygenated in its mother's circulation. The blood of the fetus bypasses its lungs and flows through a special shortcut, the ductus arteriosus, a short vessel that carries the blood directly from the main artery of the lungs (pulmonary artery) into the aorta. When the baby is born and begins to breathe, the ductus arteriosus normally closes, and the blood begins to circulate through the lungs. Occasionally, however, the ductus fails to close, and since the pressure is higher in the aorta than in the pulmonary arteries, part of the blood that is pumped out by the left ventricle flows back into the pulmonary circulation. The abnormal pressure relations that result cause dilatation of the heart. Although an individual may live for many years with a small patent ductus, the usual result is gradual cardiac failure and premature death. In addition, patients with this anomaly are subject to the development of a serious infection known as subacute bacterial endocarditis. In 1937, John W. Strieder of Boston made an unsuccessful attempt to ligate a patent ductus in a patient who had bacterial endocarditis. Two years later the first successful ligation of a ductus was performed at the Children's Hospital in Boston by Robert E. Gross. Within the next two years Gross performed nine successful ligations of the ductus. By then, the operation was being performed successfully in many other medical centers.

Another congenital anomaly that attracted the attention of surgeons at a relatively early date was coarctation of the aorta. This consists of a narrowing of the aorta at about the point where the ductus arteriosus normally enters it. The narrowing may vary from slight to complete occlusion of the aorta. Since the narrowing occurs at a point below that at which the arteries to the head and arms emerge, the blood pressure in the upper part of the body is high while that in the legs is low. The effect of coarctation of the aorta on the heart is much like that of hypertension: the heart has to work against increased pressure, and in time it fails. This abnormality is particularly conducive to surgical treatment because it is easily diagnosed, it does not involve the heart itself, and it is always at approximately the same location, one which affords a good surgical approach and exposure. Successful operations for resection of the constricted portion of the aorta were performed at almost the same time in 1945 by C. Crafoord in Sweden and Robert E. Gross in Boston. In these operations, after the narrow portion of the aorta had been removed, the two ends of the vessel were brought together and sewn in place. At about this same time, Alfred Blalock performed a dif-

504

ferent type of operation, in which he fashioned a bypass around the constricted part of the aorta. The type of operation devised by Gross is the one generally used at the present time. If the area of constriction is so long that the cut ends of the aorta cannot be brought together, a plastic tube is used to bridge the gap.

THE BLALOCK-TAUSSIG OPERATION   *Helen Taussig* graduated from the Johns Hopkins Medical School in 1927. She then spent a year working as a fellow in the old "Heart Station" of the Johns Hopkins Hospital. From 1928 to 1930 she was a pediatric intern at the Harriet Lane Home. At the end of her internship, E. A. Park, Professor of Pediatrics, had the good judgment and courage to appoint this young woman as Director of the Pediatric Cardiac Clinic. Shortly thereafter, Taussig's studies and papers began to illuminate the whole field of congenital heart disease. She became particularly interested in those defects which are associated with cyanosis—a blue color of the skin—which is due to the fact that part of the blood in the circulation has not been oxygenated by passage through the lungs. Oxygenated blood is bright red, and it gives the skin a pinkish hue; unoxygenated blood is bluish-purple, and this produces the skin color which is characteristic of "blue babies."

Alfred Blalock graduated from the Johns Hopkins Medical School in 1922. From 1927 to 1942, he was a member of the Surgical Department at Vanderbilt University, the last three years of this period as Professor of Surgery. During his years at Vanderbilt, he had become particularly inter-

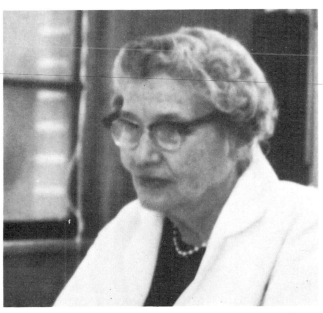

Figure 105. Helen B. Taussig. (From the Archives Office, the Johns Hopkins Medical Institutions.)

ested in thoracic surgery, had performed operations for removal of tumors from the chest, and had operated successfully on three patients with a patent ductus arteriosus. In addition, he had carried out a number of operations on experimental animals, in order to improve his technique in vascular surgery. In 1942 Blalock came to Baltimore as Surgeon-in-Chief of the Johns Hopkins Hospital. Shortly thereafter he developed his bypass operation for coarctation of the aorta.

About 1940 Dr. Taussig began to wonder about the possibility of an operation to increase the blood flow to the lungs in blue babies. She made a trip to Boston to try to interest Dr. Gross in her idea, but at that time he was too deeply involved in other problems. After Blalock came to Baltimore, he and Taussig had a number of conversations about possible surgical operations for the treatment of cyanotic heart disease. When Taussig suggested that one might increase the blood flow to the lungs by hooking up the subclavian artery with the pulmonary artery, Blalock said that he thought this might be possible. During the two years after this suggestion had been made, Blalock carried out some 200 experiments on dogs, and at the end of this period he told Dr. Taussig that he was ready to undertake the operation on a suitable baby.

Blalock's first operation was performed in November, 1944, on a baby slightly more than a year old who weighed only 10 pounds. The subclavian artery was joined to the side of the pulmonary artery. The infant not only survived the operation but also improved and began to gain weight. After allowing time to evaluate the results of this operation, a similar operation was performed on an 11-year-old girl in February, 1945. This was also highly successful. Thereafter, the operations were performed with increasing frequency. Patients came from all over the world, and after they had

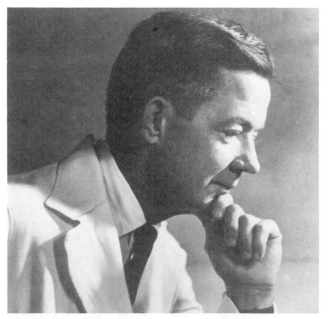

Figure 106. Alfred Blalock. (From the Archives Office, the Johns Hopkins Medical Institutions.)

been subjected to thorough study by Taussig, the suitable children were turned over to Blalock for operation.

During the six years 1945 to 1950, more than 1000 cyanotic patients were subjected to operation by Blalock and his associates. Most of these patients had multiple congenital defects, the commonest being a combination of four defects known as the tetralogy of Fallot. The one factor that all patients had in common was cyanosis. With improvements in surgical technique and better selection of cases, the operative mortality fell steadily; it was 20.3 per cent in 1945 and only 4.7 per cent in 1950. In follow-up studies on 685 patients (1945–50) who survived the Blalock-Taussig operation for the tetralogy of Fallot, 432 were known to be alive 15 years after operation, and 376 were known to be alive 20 years after operation. Of 319 on whom occupational information was available 20 to 28 years after operation, 75.6 per cent were gainfully employed, and others were working as housewives, students, etc. (Taussig et al., 1975).

One of the earliest improvements in the Blalock operation came when the Chicago heart surgeon Willis J. Potts devised an ingenious clamp that closes off a small section of an artery, permitting the surgeon to operate on this section while blood continues to flow through the main channel. Using this technique, Potts was able to join the pulmonary artery directly to the aorta, thus obviating the need to sever the subclavian artery.

Blalock's operation was a great pioneering achievement, and it restored many very ill children to a relatively normal existence. However, it relieved the cyanosis only partially, and it left behind the basic defects in the heart. The hesitation about intracardiac operations was due to the fear of hemorrhage when the heart was opened and the realization that the flow of blood through the heart would obscure the surgeon's vision so that he could not see what he was doing. Nevertheless, a few operations were performed successfully in the late 1940s and early 1950s to cover over septal defects (holes in the septum) between the two cardiac atria.

OPEN-HEART SURGERY   Experiments in animals had shown that by placing clamps on the vessels that lead blood into the heart, it was possible to obtain a clear dry field for work within the heart. However, if the circulation was shut off for more than about two minutes, the animal's life was endangered. The brain cannot withstand having its circulation and oxygen supply shut off for more than a brief period. Additional experiments in animals demonstrated that when the body temperature was reduced to about 83° to 86° F (28° to 30° C), the oxygen requirement of the brain and other tissues was reduced substantially so that the circulation could be shut off without harm for 15 to 20 minutes. The surgeon would, therefore, have this amount of time to work in a dry field with good visibility. A few operations were performed using this technique in the early 1950s, but by the mid-1950s the whole field of cardiac surgery had undergone a tremendous change as the result of a new technical development—the *heart-lung machine*.

The development of the heart-lung machine was the achievement of John H. Gibbon, Jr. Gibbon graduated from Jefferson Medical College in 1927. In 1930, while he was working as a research fellow in surgery under

507

Dr. Edward C. Churchill at the Massachusetts General Hospital, he watched a patient die of a pulmonary embolus which obstructed the blood flow through the lungs. It occurred to him that he might have been able to save the patient's life if he had had a machine to draw off the patient's blood, oxygenate it, and return it to the circulation. After working with many different types of equipment, Gibbon and his wife finally devised an apparatus with which they successfully bypassed an obstructed pulmonary artery in an experimental animal. In 1935 they demonstrated for the first time that life could be maintained by an extracorporeal (outside the body) blood circuit with a pump acting as an artificial heart and a device for oxygenating the blood. They also demonstrated that after the blood had been excluded from the animal's own heart and lungs for a period of 39 minutes, these organs resumed normal activity when the artificial circuit was shut off and normal circulation was restored.

At this point, Gibbon returned to Philadelphia, where he worked in the surgical research laboratories at the medical school of the University of Pennsylvania for six years, until the United States entered World War II. During the war his research was interrupted for four years, but after the war it was resumed at Jefferson Medical College. The problem at this point was to build an artificial lung with an oxygenating capacity great enough to be used in human subjects. Through an association for six years with the IBM Corporation, engineering help was provided in the design of a machine appropriate for use in patients. The entire cost of this engineering

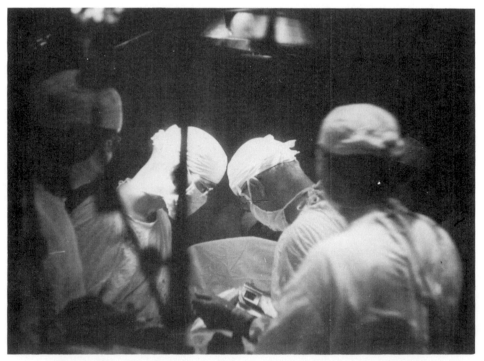

Figure 107. The first successful open heart operation in the world, using a heart-lung machine. Dr. J. H. Gibbon, Jr. (center right) and Dr. F. F. Albritten, Jr. (center left) performed the operation at Jefferson Medical College in 1953. (Courtesy of Mrs. J. H. Gibbon, Jr.)

work was contributed by IBM. They did not succeed in achieving their objective until two assistants, Stokes and Flick, working in Gibbon's laboratory, discovered that the creation of turbulence in the blood passing through the oxygenator increased the oxygenation approximately eight times. After testing the new oxygenator thoroughly on experimental animals, Gibbon used it in May, 1953, on an 18-year-old girl with a large opening in the atrial septum. All the patient's cardiopulmonary functions were maintained by the heart-lung machine for 26 minutes while Gibbon closed the opening in the septum. This successful operation on a congenital cardiac defect was the first to be accomplished with an extracorporeal heart-lung machine.

During the next 10 years, the heart-lung machine was greatly improved, particularly by the work of C. Walton Lillehei and his group at the University of Minnesota. They ultimately developed a fully mechanical extracorporeal pump-oxygenator, the so-called helix-reservoir system, which was introduced in 1955. This heart-lung machine, which bypasses the patient's heart and lungs, affords the surgeon ample time for work in the heart in a dry field with good visibility. After this, it became possible to develop effective operations not only for many forms of congenital heart disease but also for defects of heart valves that had been affected by acquired disease.

OPERATIONS ON HEART VALVES Even before the heart-lung machine had been perfected, a great deal of work had been done on valvular defects. Most of the early work was centered around mitral stenosis, i.e., scarring and narrowing of the mitral valve, which lies between the left atrium and left ventricle. In the 1920s several daring surgeons inserted a knife into the left ventricle and tried to cut through the scarred mitral valve. When Elliott C. Cutler and Claude Beck, who had worked together on this subject at the Peter Bent Brigham Hospital in Boston, reviewed the reported operative experience with valve surgery up to 1929, there were seven cases with only one survivor.

During the 1940s Charles Bailey, a young surgeon at Jefferson Medical College, developed an operation which became known as mitral commissurotomy. This operation involved slipping the finger through the left atrium, pushing a knife along the finger and cutting the lateral commissure of the mitral valve. Bailey performed his first successful operation in June, 1948, and a few days later Dwight Harken at the Peter Bent Brigham Hospital performed a somewhat similar operation for relief of mitral stenosis.

The next important contribution to this type of cardiac surgery was the development of artificial heart valves. After much experimentation with various animal tissues and plastic materials, Charles Hufnagel and his colleagues at the Georgetown University Medical Center developed a ball-and-socket type of valve, which in a long series of experiments on dogs they found to be a satisfactory substitute for the aortic valve. The first operation in which this valve was inserted in a patient was performed by Hufnagel in September, 1952. Hufnagel's work helped to trigger a large-scale assault on valvular heart disease, and in the years since then much progress has been made in the design of prosthetic heart valves. Valvular surgery as well as the surgery of congenital heart defects has been greatly advanced by the use of the heart-lung machine.

In the early years of cardiac surgery, the operator had to contend not

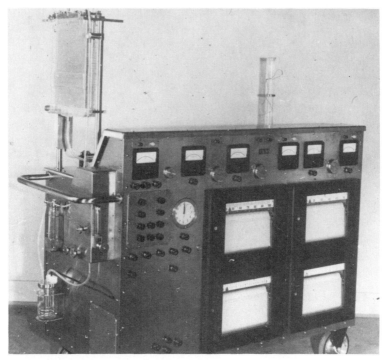

Figure 108. Apparatus for extracorporeal circulation. (Courtesy of Mrs. J. H. Gibbon, Jr.)

only with the problem of blood flowing through the area where he wished to work but also with the unremitting to-and-fro movement of the heart. It is essential particularly in open-heart surgery to arrest the cardiac contractions. This was accomplished at first by the use of chemicals such as potassium citrate or acetylcholine, which halt muscular activity, or by shutting off the coronary blood flow so that the muscle would not have the oxygen required for contraction. These methods were gradually abandoned because it became apparent that they often caused irreversible myocardial damage so that normal contractions could not be reestablished. Henry Swan and his associates at the University of Colorado found that they could obtain a relatively quiet operative field by employing electric shock to induce ventricular fibrillation. Though this resulted in multiple small twitches of the muscle, it eliminated the gross rhythmic contractions, and normal cardiac activity could be restored by defibrillation. Cardiac arrest may also be induced by hypothermia, and this is the method that has been most frequently employed in recent years. It has the advantage of reducing the metabolic requirements of the heart muscle and therefore serves to protect it against the damage resulting from a reduced supply of oxygen.

SURGICAL TREATMENT OF CORONARY ARTERY DISEASE The history of the surgical treatment of coronary artery disease goes back many years, but it has gained such momentum during the 1970s that in 1975 far more operations were being performed for coronary disease than for all other types of heart disease together.

There have been three main surgical approaches to coronary artery disease: (1) providing the heart muscle with an alternative supply of blood, (2) repairing or replacing a diseased artery, and (3) repairing the damaged heart muscle. The early work in this country was carried out by Claude S. Beck of Cleveland, who made an effort to create a new blood supply for the heart. He removed the pericardium from the heart and grafted adjacent tissues directly to the heart muscle. He hoped that the blood vessels of the grafted tissues would grow into the heart and thus increase its blood supply. Though some of the patients on whom this type of operation was performed seemed to get better, the improvement was rarely striking, and there were many failures.

No significant advance in the surgical treatment of coronary artery disease occurred until better diagnostic methods had been developed. A unique advance in radiological technique, known as image intensification, set the stage for what was to follow. The use of an image intensifier not only made it possible to obtain sharper X-ray images but also greatly reduced the time of exposure required to produce a good result. Prior to the introduction of this new technique it had not been possible to take satisfactory pictures of the moving image on a fluoroscopic screen. However, when one could intensify the image and reduce the time of exposure, motion pictures became possible. This new technique gave birth to cineangiography and cinearteriography and laid the groundwork for further advances in coronary artery surgery. Important contributions in this new field were made in the late 1950s by *F. Mason Sones, Jr.*, of the Cleveland Clinic, and Charles T. Dotter of the University of Oregon Medical School.

To obtain X-ray pictures of the coronary arteries, Sones inserted a flexi-

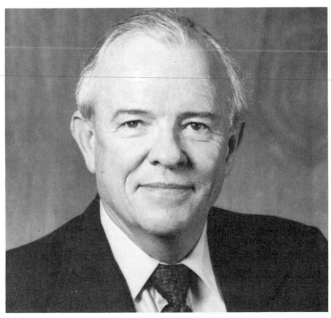

Figure 109.   F. Mason Sones, Jr.   511

ble catheter into a major artery and passed it retrograde into the aorta and thence into the mouth of a coronary artery. He could then inject an opaque substance into the coronary circulation and, using an image intensifier and a motion-picture camera, could take moving pictures of the coronary arteries, showing their condition in precise detail. Employing the same technique with the tip of the catheter in the left ventricle, he could obtain moving pictures of the ventricular cavity as the heart contracted and expanded. This gave an indication of whether the muscle of the ventricular wall was performing normally. The techniques of cineangiography and cinearteriography developed by Sones, Dotter, and others soon came into use in many medical centers. These methods enabled cardiologists not only to see whether there was narrowing or obstruction of a coronary artery but also to locate precisely the narrowing or obstruction. With such exact information available, surgeons could turn their attention toward developing new methods to deal with the problem.

The first surgical efforts to deal directly with obstructed or partially obstructed coronary arteries were not satisfactory and were attended with a high surgical mortality. The first truly successful surgical attack on coronary artery disease was the coronary bypass operation that was introduced at the Cleveland Clinic by René G. Favaloro.

Favaloro's history is an interesting one. He was born in 1923 in LaPlata, Argentina, where he received his baccalaureate before he was 18 years old. After serving for several years as an officer in the Argentine Army, he entered medical school and received his M.D. degree in 1949. He served an internship and surgical residency at the Policlinic Hospital in LaPlata and took graduate courses in general surgery at Rawson Hospital in Buenos Aires before he entered private practice.

In 1951 Favaloro and his brother, who was also a physician, opened a clinic in a small rural community, where they provided medical and surgical care and attended to accidents and other emergencies for the farmers of the area. Though isolated from an urban medical center, Favaloro managed to keep abreast of medical and surgical advances as they were reported in the literature.

Early in 1962, after having served for 11 years as a rural practitioner, Favaloro decided to visit the United States. He was particularly interested in learning something about the modern developments in surgery of the heart, and he decided to go to the Cleveland Clinic because he knew that work of this type was being conducted there. His "visit" to Cleveland lasted for a decade. At the Cleveland Clinic he was first an observer, then a junior fellow, then senior fellow, and finally chief resident. He learned thoracic and cardiovascular surgery from Dr. Donald B. Effler and spent long hours studying cinearteriograms in Dr. Sones's vast film library.

In May, 1967, Favaloro operated on a woman who had suffered typical angina pectoris for three years. The coronary arteriograms had shown a complete occlusion of the right coronary artery. In his operation Favaloro took a segment of saphenous vein from the woman's leg, and after exposing the heart and finding that there was a good arterial channel beyond the point of obstruction in the coronary artery, he sewed one end of the saphenous vein into the aorta and the other end into the coronary artery beyond the point of obstruction. Thus, the vein bypassed the point of obstruction and reestablished the blood flow in the obstructed artery. The patient made an uneventful recovery from the operation and had no further attacks of angina pectoris.

Having demonstrated the success of his method, Favaloro operated on a succession of patients with angina pectoris in whom cineangiograms had shown narrowing or obstruction of coronary arteries. He developed a routine technique for bypassing all the areas in the coronary circulation by single or multiple bypasses. In 1968 he began to perform emergency bypass operations on patients with impending or acute myocardial infarction. Before Favaloro left Cleveland, he and his associates at the Clinic had performed 2200 coronary bypass grafts with an operative mortality of only 3 per cent.

Favaloro returned to Argentina in 1971 and became Associate Professor of Surgery at the University of Cordoba and Chief of Thoracic and Cardiovascular Surgery at the prestigious Guëmes Clinic in Buenos Aires. There he has continued to perform his coronary bypass operation and has been teaching his techniques to young surgeons who come to Buenos Aires from many South and Central American countries and from Spain.

There have been some modifications in Favaloro's operation since it has been taken up by surgeon after surgeon throughout the country. For example, some surgeons prefer to use arteries rather than veins for the bypass vessel. In 1972, the year after Favaloro left Cleveland, a survey by the Joint Commission on the Accreditation of Hospitals disclosed that approximately 50,000 open-heart operations had been performed in that year and that of these, 25,000 were for coronary bypass surgery. This is a modest figure when one considers that coronary artery disease kills more than 500,000 Americans each year, and it has been estimated that another 3.5 million people are more or less incapacitated by this disease. It has also been estimated that upwards of 20 million people have some inadequacy of the coronary blood supply.

Coronary artery bypass grafts (CABG) appear to offer a better chance of immediate and complete relief of severe symptoms than can be hoped for from medical treatment. Modern medical treatment for angina pectoris is quite successful in most patients if they are willing to restrict their activities. But a number of patients do not like to be dependent on medicines and resent having to lead a quiet life. They are the ones who prefer surgery, and for them CABG appears to be the best type of treatment.

There is still doubt about the effect of CABG on the length of survival of those who have coronary disease. We do not yet know enough about the natural history of coronary disease. We do know that the outcome depends upon a great many variables over which we have little control. Some of these variables, such as the number of coronary arteries involved, the location and extent of the involvement, the amount of damage to the heart muscle, and the amount of collateral circulation, are all-important, but until the advent of CABG we had no way to evaluate them.

In brief it may be said that although coronary artery bypass grafts are capable of improving the quality of life for 70 to 90 per cent of patients with uncomplicated angina pectoris, surgeons in 1975 still did not agree on the indications for the operation, and some feared that it might hasten the progression of coronary disease. Collaborative studies are now under way

513

in many medical centers to assess the long-term benefits of the procedure and the criteria that should be used in selecting patients for the operation.

HYPERTENSION   Mortality statistics gathered by life insurance companies over the course of the past six decades show quite clearly that the average individual with an elevated blood pressure has a shorter life expectancy than a comparable individual with a normal blood pressure; and that the higher the blood pressure, the greater is the shortening of life. The statistics also show that an elevated diastolic pressure is more ominous than an elevated systolic pressure.

Serious disability or death associated with hypertension is usually due to either cerebral hemorrhage or heart failure, but the latter is far more common than the former. Heart failure in hypertensive individuals may be caused by coronary artery disease, but more commonly it is due to a gradual loss of the heart's ability to work effectively against the increased head of pressure in the aorta. Hypertension is the leading cause of congestive heart failure. According to P. D. White (1951): "The most common and important of all types of heart disease by and large the world over is that due to systemic hypertension with elevation of the diastolic blood pressure."

In 1733 Stephen Hales, an English clergyman who performed many ingenious experiments on plants and animals, introduced a glass tube into an artery in a horse. The blood in the tube rose vertically to a height of nine feet. This was the first record of an animal's blood pressure. A French physiologist, J. L. M. Poiseuille, in 1828, introduced the mercury manometer, which made it possible to measure the blood pressure in experimental animals with a tube of more practical length (6 to 12 inches). Following this, many experiments were performed on animals in which the blood pressure was recorded by means of a mercury manometer with a tube inserted in an artery. This type of blood pressure measurement could not be applied safely to human subjects, and the clinical determination of blood pressure had to await the development of new apparatus.

The study of human blood pressure began in 1876 when Ritter von Basch, a German physiologist, developed the sphygmomanometer. Though von Basch's first apparatus was crude and not very accurate, it introduced the important principle of measuring human blood pressure by indirect means, without having to introduce a tube into an artery. Physicians were slow to appreciate the potential value of this new method for determining blood pressure. In the 1886 edition of Austin Flint's widely used *Practice of Medicine,* the sphygmomanometer is not mentioned. Blood pressure determinations rarely were made in clinical work until 1896 when the Italian, Scipione Riva-Rocci, introduced an improved sphygmomanometer which was more accurate, easier to apply, and more portable. Riva-Rocci's method was more accurate because he used an inflatable rubber bag encircling the arm in place of von Basch's small pressure diaphragm; and the apparatus was made portable by substituting a metal dial-type manometer for the mercury manometer. As mentioned in Chapter 14, when Harvey Cushing returned from a trip to Europe in 1901 he brought with him a Riva-Rocci apparatus and was the first to employ it in the United States. This apparatus

514

made blood pressure determinations easy, and doctors soon started to carry the sphygmomanometer around with them when they called on their patients.

In the first few years following the introduction of the Riva-Rocci apparatus, the blood pressure was determined in patients by feeling the pulse at the wrist and pumping up the pressure in the arm cuff until the pulse disappeared. The pressure was then slowly lowered until the pulse could be felt again. The cuff pressure at this point was considered to be the "blood pressure." Actually it was the maximal pressure or "systolic pressure." In 1905 a Russian physician, N. S. Korotkoff, introduced the method by which clinical blood pressure determinations are made today. He placed a stethoscope over the artery below the cuff and found that as the pressure in the previously inflated cuff was gradually lowered he could suddenly hear pulse sounds and that as the pressure was lowered further, the sounds suddenly disappeared. Korotkoff surmised, and we now know, that the pressure at which the sound appears is systolic pressure and that the pressure at which the sound disappears is diastolic pressure. The systolic and diastolic pressure as determined clinically are not precisely accurate; they are affected by a number of variables, an important consideration being the size of the arm in which the blood pressure is being determined. However, the Korotkoff method provides figures which, in the vast majority of subjects, are reasonably accurate and reliable.

Even before the sphygmomanometer was introduced, physicians had suspected that the blood pressure was elevated in certain conditions. Richard Bright, in his studies of diseases of the kidneys, spoke of the increased thickness of the left ventricle in patients who had contracted kidneys. Austin Flint, in the textbook mentioned above, observed that in patients having apoplexy the pulse was "full and hard, the artery striking against the finger like a metal rod." In spite of these suspicions no one had any concept of the wide prevalence of hypertension until blood pressure determinations had been made in thousands of individuals.

The first treatise on human blood pressure written in the United States was that of Theodore C. Janeway. This volume of some 300 pages, entitled *The Clinical Study of Blood-Pressure — A Guide to the Use of the Sphygmomanometer,* appeared in 1904. Janeway at that time was practicing medicine in New York City and was on the faculty of New York University–Bellevue Hospital Medical College. His book presents an excellent review of the work up to that time and contains many original observations which he made on animals, in healthy individuals, and in patients. He introduced the term "essential hypertension," but he used it to mean merely a permanent elevation in blood pressure. Subsequently, essential hypertension was the expression used to denote that form of hypertension which is not associated with renal disease or other known causes.

THE RELATION OF THE KIDNEY TO HYPERTENSION

The early studies of blood pressure in patients divided those with hypertension into two broad groups: those with disease of the kidneys and those with essential hypertension. It gradually came to light that patients who started with what was thought to be essential hypertension not infrequently ended up with disease of the kidneys. For many years there was controversy about whether the hypertension in such cases led to secondary development of renal disease or whether the renal disease was there all along but was not identifiable by the methods of examination then available. Pathologists often remarked that in autopsies of patients with a history of hypertension it was rare not to find some disease of the kidneys though this might not have been recognized clinically.

Harry Goldblatt, a pathologist on the faculty of Western Reserve University, Cleveland, had been impressed by the fact that high blood pressure was frequently associated with obstructive disease of the renal arteries. It occcurred to him that the hypertension might be secondary to a reduction in blood flow through the kidneys. With this hypothesis in mind, Goldblatt began a series of experiments on dogs, in which he tried to devise a method of reducing the blood flow to the kidneys in a way that might simulate the situation in patients. Finally, after four years of experimentation, he succeeded in inventing an ingenious silver clamp, so constructed that all degrees of narrowing of the main renal artery could be accomplished. The design of this clamp was such that it could be left on the artery permanently, or removed later, according to the desire of the experimenter.

In 1932 Goldblatt and his associates reported that they had succeeded in producing hypertension in dogs by narrowing the renal arteries and reducing the blood flow to the kidneys. They found that in some animals this could be accomplished by reducing the blood flow to one kidney only. Since Goldblatt's dogs showed no evidence of kidney disease, they had the counterpart of essential hypertension. In cases where narrowing of one renal artery had caused hypertension, release of the clamp or removal of the

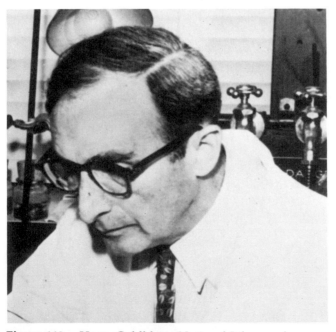

Figure 110. Harry Goldblatt. (National Library of Medicine, Bethesda, Maryland.)

kidney was followed by a drop in blood pressure to normal. It was not long before Goldblatt's discovery began to bear fruit in the treatment of patients. In 1937 Alan Butler of the Massachusetts General Hospital reported the cure of severe hypertension in a child with unilateral pyelonephritis by removal of the single diseased kidney. Butler's paper awakened great interest in the subject of hypertension in patients with disease of one kidney. In the next few years many nephrectomies were performed for the relief of hypertension. However, most of these operations were unsuccessful. When Homer Smith reviewed the subject in 1948, he found that among the many patients subjected to nephrectomy, the hypertension had been definitely relieved for a period of at least one year in only 47 cases.

Several years after the publication of Goldblatt's first paper, the significance of his results was given strong support by the pathological studies of Alan R. Moritz and Ruth Oldt. These authors carried out an objective study of the occurrence of obliterative arterial disease in various organs in 100 patients who had had essential hypertension and 100 in whom the blood pressure had been normal. Only in the kidneys was there a striking difference in the occurrence and severity of arterial disease. In the hypertensives there was pronounced renal arterial disease, but significant disease of the renal arteries was found in only 1 of the 100 subjects with normal blood pressure. They reached the conclusion that in individuals with arterial disease, hypertension develops only if and when the arteries of the kidneys become involved to a sufficient degree.

HUMORAL REGULATION: THE RENIN-ANGIO-TENSIN-ALDOSTERONE SYSTEM   In 1898 two German investigators, R. Tigerstedt and P. G. Bergman, extracted from kidneys a substance, *renin*, that raised the blood pressure in experimental animals. Others tried to confirm their findings, largely with negative results, but in 1938 G. W. Pickering and M. Prinzmetal reaffirmed the existence of a pressor substance in renal extracts and aroused new interest in renin. The first significant progress toward identifying the existence of a humoral mechanism was made by Irvine H. Page. Working first with Franz Volhard in Germany, then with Donald Van Slyke at the Rockefeller Institute, and later with Oscar Helmer, Kenneth Kohlstaedt, and A. C. Corcoran at the Indianapolis City Hospital, Page succeeded in isolating a pressor substance from extracts of kidney tissue. Further work with this substance, still called *renin*, disclosed that it is an enzyme that causes the release of a hypertensive substance in the plasma. The discovery of the latter substance, named *angiotensin*, was reported in 1939 by Page and Helmer. By a remarkable coincidence, the same substance was discovered in the same year by E. Braun-Menéndez and his co-workers in Argentina and was given the name *hypertensin*.

Leonard T. Skeggs and J. R. Kahn of Western Reserve University succeeded in separating two forms of angiotensin: *angiotensin I*, which is the direct product of the action of renin on the plasma substrate; and *angiotensin II*, which is formed from angiotensin I by the action of a blood protease which they called *converting-enzyme*. Angiotensin was first isolated in pure

517

form in 1955 by W. S. Peart. Later (1956) Peart and Elliot identified the 10 amino acids that make up angiotensin I, and Skeggs and his co-workers showed that angiotensin II is formed from this polypeptide by the deletion of two amino acids at one end of the chain. The synthesis of angiotensin II was accomplished in 1957 by F. M. Bumpus, H. Schwarz, and Page. The vast amount of work which went on in the 30 years following the discovery of angiotensin is well described in the book *Renal Hypertension* by Irvine H. Page and James W. McCubbin, which appeared in 1968.

A third element involved in the regulation of blood pressure is aldosterone, the salt-retaining hormone produced by the adrenal cortex. In recent years frequent reference has been made to the renin-angiotensin-aldosterone system. Hypertension is one of the manifestations of aldosteronism. This condition was first described by Jerome W. Conn of the University of Michigan Medical School, who demonstrated that discrete tumors made up of aldosterone-secreting cells cause hypertension, which is relieved by the removal of the tumors. The exact role that the renin-angiotensin system plays in the day-to-day regulation of blood pressure is still not fully understood. However, it is clear that this system has a reciprocal relationship with aldosterone. In aldosteronism, renin is low in the plasma. On the other hand, in Addison's disease, in which aldosterone is low or absent in the plasma, renin is high.

It is now known that renin is synthesized in the kidney by a group of cells located in the juxtaglomerular apparatus of the renal cortex. This apparatus apparently is sensitive to changes in pressure and to variations in the concentration of blood electrolytes. Tumors of the renin-secreting cells of the kidney (reninomas) are associated with hypertension.

A classification of hypertension which served a very useful purpose in relation to prognosis was the one proposed in 1939 by N. M. Keith, H. P. Wagener, and N. W. Barker of the Mayo Clinic. This classification is based on the ophthalmoscopic appearance of the retinal arteries and other changes in the retina, and it divides patients into four groups, ranging from mild hypertension with a good prognosis to severe hypertension with a very limited life expectancy. The distinction between these types of hypertension is neither precise nor enduring; frequently with the passage of time one type is transformed into another. Though the milder types of hypertension are frequently (and usually erroneously) considered to be benign, there is one type, "malignant hypertension," in which the prognosis, until recently, was uniformly gloomy. The diagnosis of malignant hypertension is a clinical one; it refers to a condition in which very high diastolic blood pressure is accompanied by advanced changes in the retina and rapid deterioration in renal function. The striking finding in autopsies on most patients with this form of hypertension is necrotizing disease of the small arteries (arteriolar necrosis), particularly in the kidneys. Malignant hypertension is not a disease but a phase, usually the terminal phase, of an illness which at the outset might have presented quite a different picture. "Benign" essential hypertension, renal hypertension, Cushing's disease, and pheochromocytomas (see Chap. 14) may, as they advance, present the picture of malignant hypertension. Prior to the advent of modern forms of therapy, malignant hypertension was almost invariably fatal within a period of a year or two.

EVOLUTION OF THE
TREATMENT OF
ESSENTIAL
HYPERTENSION

F. A. Mahomed of Guy's Hospital in London was one of the first physicians to use a sphygmograph to estimate the blood pressure in patients. He recognized that there are two forms of high blood pressure. He associated one of these forms with Bright's disease; the other he referred to as the prealbuminuric stage of Bright's disease. The latter we would now call essential hypertension. Mahomed knew that veratum and nitrites are capable of reducing the blood pressure, but he believed that their action was too transient to be of much use in the treatment of hypertension. The treatment that he recommended in the 1870s and 1880s was dietary restriction, particularly restriction of protein. A low-protein diet was still being recommended by many physicians throughout the first half of the twentieth century. Two Frenchmen, Ambard and Beaujard, in 1904, were the first to suggest a low-salt diet for hypertension. It was known that the administration of salt results in the retention of water and that a low-salt diet results in the elimination of water. In 1909, Blum pointed out that it was the sodium rather than the chloride in salt that is the chief factor in water retention; but actual proof of this did not come until 1920 through the work of Blum and Magnus-Levy. During the 1920s, F. M. Allen of New York was the great champion in the United States of salt restriction for the treatment of hypertension. After the 1920s, salt restriction seemed to fall more and more into disregard until the 1940s, when Walter Kempner of Duke University introduced his rice diet for the treatment of high blood pressure.

Kempner was born in Germany and received his M.D. degree from the University of Heidelberg. Before coming to the United States he had worked at the Kaiser Wilhelm Institute in Berlin and had written extensively on metabolism. In 1948 Kempner published his data on dietary therapy in 500 patients with high blood pressure. He demonstrated that a diet consisting or rice and fruit (both of which are very low in sodium) would considerably reduce arterial pressure in many hypertensive patients. In 1955 Newborg and Kempner published their data on the use of the rice-fruit diet as the only treatment for a large group of patients with severe hypertensive disease and advanced changes in the retina. In 83 of the 120 patients there was evidence of impairment of renal function. Forty-seven of these patients survived for one year; 26 were living an average of 4.25 years after treatment was started. These results gave strong support to the use of low-sodium diets in the management of hypertension. Such diets are used as an adjunct to most forms of antihypertensive therapy today, but the reduction in the sodium content of the diet is usually not as drastic as that employed by Kempner.

Surgical Treatment of Hypertension. Surgery has been employed for the treatment of those rare forms of hypertension that are due to tumors which secrete pressor substances: pheochromocytomas, reninomas, and aldosteronomas; and bilateral adrenalectomy is now the standard treatment for Cushing's disease. Surgery employed for the treatment of essential hypertension has been of two types, both originally designed to reduce the constrictor tone of the small arteries and arterioles. One of these surgical procedures is sympathectomy; the other, adrenalectomy.

The original rationale for adrenalectomy was that the adrenal glands

519

secrete the pressor substance epinephrine and that patients with Addison's disease have a low blood pressure. George Crile of Cleveland, in 1914, attempted to relieve hypertension by unilateral adrenalectomy, cervical sympathectomy, and ligation of the thyroid arteries. This drastic type of surgery did not achieve the hoped-for results and was abandoned. Interest in adrenalectomy was aroused again by Goldblatt, who found that the blood pressure in hypertensive dogs could be lowered by removing the adrenal glands. After the discovery of cortisone and other adrenal hormones, it became possible to sustain life in human subjects after both adrenals had been excised, and for a time bilateral adrenalectomy was performed for the relief of the more severe forms of hypertension. Very satisfactory results were reported in a few patients with malignant hypertension. However, when increasingly effective methods of chemotherapy became available, adrenalectomy, which involves such difficult problems in postoperative care, was quickly abandoned.

Leonard G. Rowntree and A. W. Adson of the Mayo Clinic were the first (1925) to report the use of sympathectomy for the treatment of hypertension. This type of surgery came into use throughout the country after Adson, Craig, and Brown reported their results with a more extensive operation. Sympathectomy as a method of treating hypertension gained strong support from the work at the Mayo Clinic and from the reports of the neurosurgeons M. M. Peet of the University of Michigan and R. H. Smithwick of Boston, each of whom developed his own type of operation. Smithwick's two-stage bilateral thoracolumbar sympathectomy (1940) became extremely popular in many medical centers. Though some very good results were reported following sympathectomy, the beneficial effects were for the most part temporary—a few weeks to a year or two—and many patients underwent these extensive operations without deriving any appreciable benefit. The results were so unpredictable and usually so short-lived that when effective drugs became available, sympathectomy gradually went out of use.

Chemotherapy for Hypertension. The level of the blood pressure in many individuals is quite labile. It tends to rise when a person is tense or excited and to fall during periods of relaxation. The first visit to a doctor's office is often attended by enough anxiety and excitement to cause an appreciable elevation in blood pressure. Owing to the lability of the pressure and its tendency to fall to a lower level as patients feel more at ease in the doctor's office, physicians often were misled into believing that certain medicines had antihypertensive effects. Many drugs which seemed at first to have a beneficial effect were finally abandoned after their ineffectiveness had been demonstrated by more carefully controlled observations. In addition to the drugs that had an honest though temporary popularity, a host of quack hypertension remedies came and went throughout the first half of the twentieth century.

In a discussion of the treatment of hypertension at a meeting of the Royal Society of Medicine in 1947, only two types of drugs were mentioned: sedatives and cyanates. Sedatives had established their usefulness through their ability to moderate the upward fluctuations in a labile blood pressure. Cyanates were first recommended for the treatment of hypertension in 1903. The early use of thiocyanate was terminated by a high incidence of serious toxic reactions. In the United States it enjoyed its greatest popularity in the 1930s and 1940s after M. Herbert Barker had demonstrated that the incidence of toxic reactions could be reduced if blood cyanate determinations were made and if the dosage was adjusted to keep the cyanate in the blood below a certain critical level. Thiocyanate does unquestionably lower the blood pressure, but when it is given in non-toxic doses this effect is not very great. The popularity of the cyanates faded as safer and more effective chemicals became available.

At the end of World War II, surgical sympathectomy was the popular method for the treatment of hypertension. Dr. Robert W. Wilkins of Boston was working with Smithwick to assess the cardiovascular and circulatory results of this operative procedure. James Shannon, then Director of the Squibb Institute for Medical Research, asked Wilkins and Chester S. Keefer to work with the Institute in an effort to develop a chemotherapeutic agent for the treatment of hypertension. The clinical evaluation of any drug that might emerge in this project was assigned to a fellow in Dr. Wilkin's group, Edward D. Freis.

The first drug tested, *pentaquine,* was an outgrowth of the World War II antimalarial program. When given to normal volunteers, it had been shown to produce orthostatic hypotension. Dr. Shannon suggested that it be tried in hypertensive patients. This drug turned out to be too toxic in the doses required to lower the blood pressure, but in the course of this trial it was given to a patient with malignant hypertension, whose diastolic pressure dropped from 150 to 100 accompanied by relief of headache, cessation of hematuria, regression of papilledema, and clearing of the signs of congestive heart failure. This encouraged the investigators to proceed with the testing of other antihypertensive agents. The next drug to be tried, *veratrum viride,* had been used by nineteenth-century physicians to "soften" the pulse. Again, this was not a satisfactory drug for long-term treatment, as the emetic dose was too close to the therapeutic dose.

At this time the "rice diet" of Kempner came into popularity, so Freis combined a low-sodium diet with veratrum and observed an enhanced antihypertensive effect. Veratrum was also used in patients who had failed to respond to sympathectomy. As a result of these experiences Wilkins, Freis, and their associates began to search for agents that would reproduce the effects of sympathectomy and low-sodium diets.

Early studies of the sympathetic nervous system were puzzling in that it was found that epinephrine, when injected in low concentration, caused a drop in blood pressure while higher concentrations caused the blood pressure to rise. This seeming paradox was explained by Raymond P. Ahlquist of the Medical College of Georgia, who showed that there are two types of sympathetic receptors—the alpha and beta types. Ahlquist's concept was based on the different effects of three closely related catecholamines: epinephrine, norepinephrine, and isopropylnorepinephrine (isoproterenol). The receptors have a certain molecular configuration for which the various catecholamines have an affinity, depending on their size and shape. The resulting interaction causes affected cells to react in a specific manner. There are also blocking agents of alpha and beta types, which have an affinity for the receptor, but their interaction with it does not activate the cell. The blocker impedes access of the particular activator to the receptor, thus blocking the response of the cell.

521

The first compounds to receive consideration as antihypertensive drugs were alpha-adrenergic blocking agents. It was hoped that these agents, by blocking the binding sites of the alpha receptors, would block the constricting action of norepinephrine on the small arteries. Two alpha-adrenergic blockers, *phentolamine* and *piperoxan,* were studied in the late 1940s. They were not successful in the treatment of essential hypertension, but they caused a marked fall in the high blood pressure of patients with pheochromocytomas. Thus they have served as useful agents to differentiate essential hypertension from the hypertension of pheochromocytomas.

Dale and Burn, in 1915, had shown that *tetraethylammonium (TEA)* has a powerful effect in blocking the ganglia of the autonomic nervous system. In the late 1940s Eugene B. Ferris of the Cincinnati General Hospital and Sibley W. Hoobler at the University of Michigan tested the effect of TEA in patients with hypertension. They found that although it lowered the blood pressure, its effect was too fleeting to be of practical therapeutic value.

Shortly after this, W. D. M. Paton and E. J. Zaimis (1948), in England, reported the blocking effect of methonium salts on autonomic (sympathetic and parasympathetic) ganglia. Paton and Walker and several other workers in England quickly demonstrated that salts of *hexamethonium* are capable of lowering the blood pressure in hypertensive patients. In 1948 Harvey and his associates reported dramatically favorable effects of hexamethonium on patients with malignant hypertension, and Freis and Finnerty and others demonstrated that it was a reliable antihypertensive drug. Hexamethonium has certain unfavorable side effects owing to the fact that it blocks parasympathetic as well as sympathetic ganglia and therefore affects vision, gastrointestinal motility, contraction of the urinary bladder, and sexual function (impotence in the male). Patients also develop tolerance to hexamethonium so that the dose has to be gradually increased. For the treatment of hypertension, hexamethonium has been most useful when given with hydralazine (see below). The use of these two drugs in combination is described at length in the book by Henry A. Schroeder of Washington University, *Hypertensive Diseases, Causes and Control* (1953).

In 1946 Drake and Peck at the University of Maryland, in a search for better antimalarial drugs, studied certain phthalazines. Chemists at Ciba Laboratories (Basel, Switzerland), in carrying out screening tests for antihypertensive drugs, found that some of the phthalazines lowered the blood pressure in animals. One of these compounds, hydrazino-phthalazine *(hydralazine),* when tested in normal man and hypertensive patients was found not only to lower the blood pressure but also to increase the blood flow through the kidneys. Francois C. Reubi, a Swiss physician who had been working with Schroeder in St. Louis, wrote to his former chief about the Ciba experiments. Schroeder obtained a supply of hydralazine and began at once to test it in animals and in hypertensive patients. The drug was also promptly investigated by Freis and Finnerty. Hydralazine and hexamethonium were the first truly effective drugs for the treatment of the more serious forms of hypertension. They are still used in special cases, but they are not usually employed until some of the safer and less toxic drugs have been found to be ineffective.

The powdered root of the plant *Rauwolfia serpentina* had been used in India for centuries for the treatment of mentally disturbed patients. An Indian cardiologist, Ruston Jal Vaskil, in 1949, found it to be effective for the treatment of hypertension. His observations were confirmed in this country by Wilkins. *Reserpine,* the active alkaloid of the rauwolfia root, was extracted by Müller and Schlittler of Ciba in 1952. Subsequent studies have shown that reserpine acts on the cardiovascular system by reducing the activity of the entire sympathetic nervous system, including the beta receptors. Reserpine is one of the drugs that is now widely used in the treatment of hypertension. Its action in safe doses is rather mild but there are few toxic symptoms, and it has the advantage of being effective when given by mouth.

Guanethidine, another of the drugs which is still in use for the treatment of hypertension, was prepared in 1959 by Robert Mull of Ciba and was evaluated biologically by Robert Maxwell and Albert Plummer. Its cardiovascular effect results from a depleting action on the supply of norepinephrine at the sympathetic nerve endings. Guanethidine has a more powerful antihypertensive effect than does reserpine, but it is also more toxic, and its dosage has to be carefully controlled.

Theodore L. Sourkes of McGill University, in 1954, discovered *alpha-methyldopa,* the first effective inhibitor of the synthesis of norepinephrine. It was introduced into clinical practice for the treatment of hypertension by Oates and Sjoerdsma in 1960.

In 1957, in the course of a search for inhibitors of the enzyme *carbonic anhydrase,* F. C. Novello and J. M. Sprague at the Merck Laboratories synthesized a new chemical, *chlorothiazide.* They found that this substance had what they called a "novel" diuretic action. At about the same time the closely related chemical, *hydrochlorothiazide,* was synthesized at the Ciba Laboratories. These thiazide diuretics act by promoting the renal excretion of sodium. Since it was believed that this action would enhance the effect of a low-sodium diet, Freis and his associates in Washington and Wilkins and his associates in Boston immediately began to test the effect of the thiazides in the treatment of patients with hypertension. Their studies, among others, have demonstrated that these agents not only lower the blood pressure in hypertensives but also are remarkably free of unfavorable side effects, though one has to guard against too great a loss of body potassium as a consequence of their diuretic action. It is now known that the antihypertensive effect of the thiazides is due to a relaxing effect upon the small blood vessels as well as to their promotion of sodium excretion. In addition, these drugs serve to increase the responsiveness to other antihypertensive agents.

Thus, within a span of 10 years, the chemotherapy of hypertension advanced from cumbersome methods applicable only to patients with the most severe forms of the disease to a choice of drugs which, as single entities or combined, are suitable for the treatment of all forms of hypertension. Guanethidine has replaced the ganglion-blocking agents for the treatment of more severe forms of hypertension. Alpha-methyldopa has proved valuable in the treatment of all forms of hypertension from mild to severe. Thus, at the present time the five antihypertensive agents available in the United States which have withstood the test of time or have replaced less effective drugs are the thiazide diuretics, reserpine, hydralazine, guanethidine, and alpha-methyldopa. Each acts through a somewhat different mechanism to lower blood pressure.

523

Although the decade from 1950 to 1960 was characterized by the use of these agents for reducing an elevated blood pressure, it remained to be demonstrated that they favorably affect morbidity and mortality. For this there was needed a well-controlled, prospective therapeutic trial. This came about by a cooperative study that is a model of what can be done with good planning. In 1956 a group of physicians at the Veterans' Administration hospitals organized a study group to evaluate antihypertensive agents under well-controlled conditions. This project was under the direction of Edward D. Freis, who received the Albert Lasker Award for Clinical Research in 1971. These studies have contributed greatly to documenting the effectiveness of long-term chemotherapy for hypertension and in formulating the guidelines as to when treatment should be instituted. This trial was important in demonstrating that antihypertensive treatment is effective in patients exhibiting evidence of cardiovascular damage and in those with diastolic pressures averaging 105 mm Hg or higher. Treatment reduced dramatically the incidence of strokes, congestive heart failure, and progressive renal damage but did not prevent myocardial infarction and sudden death. This indicates that coronary artery disease is a separate problem, caused by atherosclerosis and aggravated by hypertension.

Hypertension is a major public health problem. The prevention of the complications such as stroke is less expensive than the care of the invalids that result. In making the public aware of high blood pressure and the availability of effective treatment, much can be done to prevent some of the more serious consequences of this major health hazard.

Renal Surgery to Relieve Hypertension. In the early 1950s two developments served to renew interest in the association of hypertension and renal disease. One was improvement in the technique of translumbar arteriography and demonstration of its value in visualizing renal arterial lesions, and the other was a report by J. E. Howard and his collaborators in 1954 of six patients with hypertension associated with impaired blood flow to the kidney, dramatically improved by nephrectomy. This report showed that renal arteriography could be diagnostic; that the intravenous urogram could suggest the presence of the lesion; and that the affected kidney has a pattern of water and sodium excretion that is quantitatively and qualitatively different from that of the unaffected kidney. In the ensuing years the importance of renal arterial disease as a cause of hypertension has become more widely appreciated. Operations to remove obstructions in the larger renal arteries have been highly effective in some cases. These operations represent an attempt to eradicate a cause of high blood pressure and not merely to treat the elevated pressure itself by surgical means.

524

24

Enzymes
and Hormones

One must always be prepared to recognize that but a hair above the underbrush may mean a large mammal is at hand.

(George R. Minot, 1926)

In Chapter 12 we gave an account of the early studies of the endocrine glands and the part played by research workers in the United States and Canada in the discovery of such important hormones as those of the pancreas and the adrenal, pituitary, and parathyroid glands. Since World War II there have been many significant developments in our knowledge of enzymes and hormones. Important discoveries have resulted from the exploitation of new techniques for the study of proteins and polypeptides; from the measurement of hormones in minute amounts by radioimmunoassay; and from new knowledge of receptor substances and the mechanisms by which hormones produce their effect. New hormones have been identified; new forms of previously recognized hormones have been brought to light; and much has been learned about the structure and function of both known and newly discovered hormones. Of basic importance has been the acquisition of detailed knowledge about enzymes and how they engineer the complex biochemical reactions involved in the metabolic activity of the human organism.

ENZYMES   Enzymes act as catalysts to "fire up" the mechanisms that regulate the biochemical reactions within cells. A rapid molecular turnover is constantly taking place within the cells of solid tissues as well as in the circulating blood. Even deposits of fat, which were once believed to be no more than storehouses for food

525

reserves, are involved in ceaseless activity similar to that of highway traffic at rush hour. Fatty tissues are teeming with biochemical reactions, in which breakdown and synthesis of the various substances neatly balance each other so that within a few months, entirely new fat deposits are created. These incessant and rapid changes take place in all of the tissues as the component chains of molecules are split apart and welded together again in a beehive of metabolic activity.

Much of our knowledge of these complex biochemical events was accumulated by the modern techniques of labeling molecules with isotopic (radioactive) tracers. These studies have disclosed that the governing influence that makes life possible is *catalysis*. The proteins that serve as catalysts or regulators are the *enzymes*. The understanding of how all this chemical machinery functions has come from the discovery of what enzymes are, how they work, and how they are involved in human health and disease. Enzymes are unaffected by the reactions for which they are responsible, and they operate in amazingly small concentrations. A single cell, too small to be seen by unaided vision, has been estimated to contain some 100,000 enzyme molecules, which accelerate 1000 to 2000 intracellular chemical reactions, or an average of about 50 to 100 molecules for each reaction.

THE DISCOVERY
OF ENZYMES

Until the eighteenth century the process of digestion was thought to be of a purely mechanical nature—like that of a meat grinder. The situation changed abruptly when the French scientist René-A.-F. de Réaumur fed to his pet falcon pieces of meat enclosed in a perforated metal tube to protect them from the mechanical effects of stomach friction. When he removed the tube a few hours later, it was intact, but the meat had been digested. Obviously the digestion had taken place as the result of chemical rather than mechanical action. John R. Young, who graduated from the University of Pennsylvania in 1803, added further information to the digestion story. Young was one of the very few Americans of that period who took an experimental approach to the problems of physiology. His graduation essay (1803) was entitled "An experimental inquiry into the principles of nutrition and the digestive process." In it he described experiments on frogs and snakes and on himself which disclosed for the first time that the gastric juice contains a strong acid. Young believed, and he gave evidence to support his hypothesis, that the digestive action of the juice is due to its strong acidity. However, in 1835 the German physiologist Theodor Schwann discovered a non-acid digestive substance in gastric juice, which he called *pepsin*. Pepsin was later shown to be an enzyme.

A quarter of a century after Schwann's discovery, Pasteur, in his studies of the souring of wine, found that wine did not become sour if it were kept under sterile conditions; that the souring was due to the action of micro-organisms that produce lactic acid. This led to a thorough investigation of the process of alcoholic fermentation, which proved to be the work of yeast cells digesting sugars for their own nourishment. A great controversy ensued on the nature of this process, in the course of which the German physiologist Willy Kühne, in 1878, invented a new term, *enzyme*, which means "in yeast." For the next two decades biologists used two words, *enzyme* to designate substances such as pepsin, and *ferment* for the chemical activity produced by living organisms. Then in 1897 a lucky laboratory accident led Eduard Buchner, another German scientist, to discover that fermentation actually does not require the presence of *living* yeast cells but will occur in their absence as a result of the action of a substance (which he called *zymase*) that he was able to extract from the cells. This accidental discovery ultimately won Buchner the 1907 Nobel Prize in chemistry.

Much work was done to gain an understanding of the nature of enzymes, but it was not until 1926 that James B. Sumner of Cornell University, after nine years of research, isolated an enzyme from the jackbean. This enzyme, *urease,* decomposes the metabolic waste product, urea. (Urease, like many other enzymes, bears the name of the substance on which it acts, plus the suffix -*ase*.) Sumner's work emphasizes how "absurdly simple" the key steps in a great discovery sometimes may be. One day in April, 1926, he mixed jackbean meal with acetone, a solvent that was suggested by his former biochemistry professor at Harvard, and he allowed the solution to filter overnight. The next morning he examined the filtrate under a microscope and saw tiny crystals. He demonstrated that these crystals had a strong action in decomposing urea. That afternoon he called his wife to give her the news: "I have crystallized the first enzyme" (Pfeiffer, 1948).

Unfortunately, the crystallization of enzymes is not always so simple. Schwann had discovered and named *pepsin* almost a century before anyone was able to isolate it in pure crystalline form. This feat was accomplished by John H. Northrop of the Princeton branch of the Rockefeller Institute in 1930, but he found it necessary to employ a process far more complex than that used by Sumner. In his early efforts he was plagued by the fact that the chemical manipulations denatured the enzyme (that is, destroyed its proteolytic activity). This obstacle was finally overcome by a series of exceedingly sensitive precipitations, and pepsin at last crystallized out in pure form.

As will be described in Chapter 27, Wendell M. Stanley, who also worked at the Rockefeller Institute in Princeton, adapted Northrop's method to obtain in crystalline form the virus of the mosaic disease of tobacco. In 1946 Sumner, Northrop, and Stanley were joint recipients of the Nobel Prize in chemistry.

ENZYMES AND DISEASE   Enzymes not only are important in normal metabolic processes but also play a role in disease. Some bacterial toxins have been identified as enzymes: for example, *Clostridium perfringens (C. welchii)* releases an enzyme called lecithinase, which destroys red blood cells by disintegrating the lecithin in their capsules. Moreover, certain diseases can be treated by employing agents that inhibit enzymes; for example, neostigmine, which is used in treating myasthenia gravis, a disease associated wtih severe muscle weakness, acts by strongly inhibiting the enzyme cholinesterase.

In 1932 it was found that an essential part of the coenzyme I molecule is nicotinic acid. (A coenzyme is the nonspecific portion of an enzyme that is responsible for its fermentative or digestive action, called zymolysis.) Three years later, C. A. Elvehjem and his associates at the University of Wisconsin

527

identified this substance as the antipellagra vitamin. Other vitamins definitely known to be part of coenzyme molecules include B_1, B_2, and B_6. There is a strong possibility that factors concerned in nutrition that are needed in only trace quantities are all parts of coenzymes: 1/10,000,000 of an ounce of vitamin B_{12} is sufficient to produce measurable rises in the red blood count of patients with pernicious anemia. Vitamins are as necessary to pathogenic bacteria as they are to human life. This fact opened the way for putting to medical use the competitive inhibition of enzymes.

ENZYMES AND
CARBOHYDRATE
METABOLISM

Carl F. Cori and *Gerty T. Radnitz* were born in Czechoslovakia in 1896. They both enrolled as medical students at the University of Prague at the age of 18 years. In 1920, shortly after receiving their degrees, they were married, and in 1922 they came to the United States, where they began their work together at the New York State Institute for the Study of Malignant Diseases, in Buffalo. In 1931 they moved to St. Louis to become members of the faculty of the Washington University School of Medicine. There they worked first in the Department of Phar-

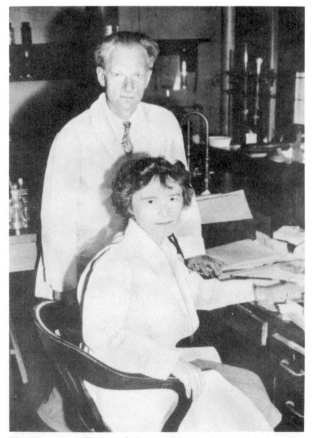

Figure 110. Carl and Gerty Cori. (National Library of Medicine, Bethesda, Maryland.)

macology, but in 1942 Carl Cori became Professor of Biochemistry, and his wife became an Associate Professor in the same department.

In the year of the Coris' arrival in the United States, Banting reported the discovery of insulin (Chap. 12), and though he had shown that this hormone, extracted from the pancreas, would rectify the carbohydrate metabolism in diabetic patients, there was no knowledge of how insulin acts. The metabolism of glucose (sugar) supplies energy for all bodily activities. With the slightest muscular movement, one burns an appropriate amount of sugar. In the mid-nineteenth century the great French physiologist Claude Bernard discovered that the liver and muscles contain a starchlike material which he called *glycogen*. Each molecule of glycogen is composed of a large number of smaller sugar molecules, which are united together and stored until they are needed. When the moment of need arrives, the glycogen is broken down into glucose. In this manner the glucose content of the blood — the "blood sugar" — can be kept fairly constant in spite of variations in the intake of carbohydrates.

In the 1920s the British biochemist Robert Robison and the German biochemist Gustav Embden had discovered that sugar in living cells and tissues, under certain circumstances, appears to be bound to phosphoric acid. Further work revealed that this combination with phosphoric acid occurs at the sixth atom in the chain of six carbon atoms of the sugar molecule. Between 1932 and 1936 the Coris showed that when a piece of muscle tissue was washed with water, the washed tissue could still bind with free phosphoric acid but that under these circumstances the phosphoric acid was linked with the first carbon atom rather than the sixth carbon atom of the sugar. This compound became known as the *Cori-ester*. The Cori-ester is found only in washed muscle, because the washing removes an enzyme whose catalytic action is required to move the phosphoric acid from the first to the sixth carbon atom of the sugar. This enzyme, which was soon crystallized, is known as *phosphorylase*. It is found in different tissues, and if allowed to act on glycogen in the presence of phosphoric acid, the whole glycogen molecule is split up into glucose molecules, each bound to phosphoric acid. The same process may also proceed in the opposite direction so that glycogen can be formed from the Cori-ester, the direction of the reaction being determined by the relative amounts of the components.

If under extreme conditions all glycogen were broken down, the individual would permanently lose his capacity to form glycogen. A special protective mechanism, discovered by the Coris, prevents this from happening. When the glycogen supply is threatened, another enzyme intervenes which, for the time being, inactivates the glycogen-splitting phosphorylase and thus preserves the last traces of the glycogen.

The Coris also accomplished the remarkable feat of synthesizing glycogen in a test tube, with the help of a number of enzymes which they had prepared in pure form and whose action they described. The Cori enzymes made the synthesis possible, since the phosphorylases first isolated formed unbranched compounds resembling starch, and only with the help of additional enzymes were the branched chains characteristic of glycogen obtained.

Blood and tissues contain free glucose. The chemical changes in metabolism are always initiated by coupling of the free glucose to phosphoric

529

acid, which is transferred from a nitrogenous phosphoric acid compound, adenosine triphosphate (ATP). This reaction is catalyzed by the enzyme *hexokinase*. In 1945 the Coris, together with Price, Colowick, and Stein, discovered that the hexokinase reaction is promoted by insulin but is checked by another hormone found in extracts from the anterior lobe of the pituitary gland.

L. M. Davidoff and Harvey Cushing at Harvard had observed in 1927 that when diabetes was produced in dogs by the removal of a part of the pancreas, the symptoms were moderated if part of the hypophysis (pituitary gland) were also removed. Additional evidence indicating a relationship between the pancreas and the hypophysis was gathered in 1931 when Herbert M. Evans and his co-workers in California, in their work on the growth hormone of the hypophysis, found that when they injected an extract of the anterior pituitary, it provoked diabetes in the experimental animals. It was later shown by Frank G. Young of London that the injection of growth hormone from the pituitary gland into dogs resulted in the development of permanent diabetes mellitus.

Much of our knowledge concerning the relationship between the pituitary and carbohydrate metabolism has come from the work of B. A. Houssay and his associates in Argentina. In view of the fact that the earlier experiments of Davidoff and Cushing were not entirely conclusive, Houssay and his assistant A. Biasotti decided to perform a crucial experiment. They first removed the whole hypophysis from an experimental animal and subsequently removed the entire pancreas. When the pancreas is removed from an animal whose hypophysis is intact, sugar quickly appears in the urine, and the animal continues to excrete sugar. However, in the experiment of Houssay and Biasotti, the animal's urine remained free of sugar. Houssay also found that animals whose pituitary gland had been removed were abnormally sensitive to insulin and that they died with symptoms of hypoglycemia (low blood glucose) from doses of insulin that were quite harmless for normal animals (Houssay, 1942). A corresponding situation exists in patients who have a condition known as Simmond's disease. This disease occurs when the anterior lobe of the hypophysis has been destroyed. These patients are also abnormally sensitive to insulin. Thus the work of Houssay and others showed clearly that a hormone of the anterior lobe of the hypophysis is antagonistic to the hormone of the pancreas, insulin.

For their elucidation of the factors involved in carbohydrate metabolism, Carl Cori, Gerty Cori, and B. A. Houssay were awarded the Nobel Prize in physiology and medicine in 1947.

ENZYMES AND INTERMEDIARY METABOLISM

During the first half of the twentieth century, biochemists had learned much about the individual processes that are concerned in the functions of living cells, but this knowledge was fragmentary, and there was need for new information and new concepts that would tie the fragments together and construct a complete picture of how food is used by cells to carry on the work of the body. Two research scientists, Hans Adolf Krebs and Fritz Lipmann, went far toward uniting the fragments. Both of these scientists received their education and did their early work in

Germany, but both became refugees from their native land in the 1930s. Krebs fled to England in 1933, and his most important work was done there. Lipmann, after receiving his M.D. degree in Berlin in 1924, worked in a series of laboratories, developing his biochemical skills, and in 1926 he became an assistant to the famous biochemist Otto Meyerhof, at the Kaiser Wilhelm Institute in Berlin. In 1931 and 1932 he was a Fellow in the laboratory of P. A. Levene at the Rockefeller Institute in New York. After spending seven years in Denmark doing biological research, he returned to the United States in 1939 and became a research associate in the Department of Biochemistry at the Cornell Medical College. Two years later he moved to Boston to join the research staff of the Massachusetts General Hospital. In 1949 he became Professor of Biological Chemistry at the Harvard Medical School and in 1957 moved back to New York as a professor at the Rockefeller University (Riedman and Gustafsen, 1963).

Krebs concentrated his attention on the breakdown products from both the food and the cell components to determine how these are utilized as building material for the working machinery of the cell. He discovered how the individual reactions are linked to each other in a cyclic process. His work provided a much clearer picture of how the energy released within a cell is used for the building processes that take place. The energy that powers the intracellular machinery is liberated by the oxidation of a two-carbon compound to carbonic acid and water. This two-carbon compound is derived from the foodstuffs and is introduced into the cycle of chemical events that became known as the *Krebs cycle*. The cycle incorporates two simultaneous processes: the degradation reactions, which yield energy, and the building-up processes, which use up energy.

Thus, out of the chaos of isolated reactions, Krebs pieced together the basic system that constitutes the essential pathway of oxidative processes within the cell. It is necessary to introduce compounds from the outside into the Krebs cycle in order to keep it in operation, although theoretically the integral components are not used up in the process. The incorporation takes place mainly through the introduction into the cycle of the two-carbon compound mentioned above.

Lipmann's great contribution was his discovery of the nature of the two-carbon compound that is essential for the operation of the Krebs cycle. Most scientists had assumed that this compound was closely related to acetic acid. For several years Lipmann himself had maintained that acetyl phosphate, a compound formed from acetic acid and phosphoric acid, was the active principle. Then quite suddenly Lipmann discovered coenzyme A, a small molecule which, when united with the specific enzyme-protein, acquires the ability to bind acetic acid. Though acetic acid is normally quite unreactive, when bound in this manner it takes on increased reactivity and combines with a four-carbon compound to form the citric acid of the Krebs cycle. This great discovery explained how the mysterious two-carbon compound promotes the transmission of energy in the cell. It soon became clear that Lipmann's discovery had even wider applications; he and others found that acids other than acetic acid are activated by coenzyme A when bound to different specific enzyme-proteins. Some of these enzymes belong to the class of vitamins. Lipmann's coenzyme, for example, is related to the B vitamins.

531

In 1953 the Nobel Prize for physiology and medicine was awarded jointly to Krebs for his discovery of the citric acid cycle and to Lipmann for his discovery of coenzyme A and its importance for intermediary metabolism.

ENZYMES AND
CHOLESTEROL
METABOLISM

In 1964 the Nobel Prize for physiology and medicine was awarded jointly to Konrad E. Bloch of Harvard University and Feodor Lynen of the University of Munich. These two investigators independently studied how animal cells produce *cholesterol,* the substance from which the body manufactures the steroid hormones (those of the sex glands and the adrenal cortex). Bloch and Lynen discovered that animal cells manufacture cholesterol from the simple acetate ion in a complex sequence of some 36 steps.

Cholesterol is a universal constituent of animal tissues and is characterized chemically by four rings of carbon atoms, fused together, with various other attached groups that specify the particular steroid compound and its physiological activity: cholesterol itself, the sex hormones, the bile acids, and the adrenal cortical hormones. Vitamin D is derived from certain steroids by ultraviolet irradiation. Because of these relationships, it was believed that when the mechanism of cholesterol formation was discovered, the biological synthesis of the related hormones and vitamins would also be unraveled.

It was demonstrated by David Rittenberg and Rudolf Schoenheimer at Columbia University, in 1937, that these steroids are constructed by the interaction of numerous small molecules and that acetic acid furnishes the building blocks. This process was described for cholesterol in animal tissues by Bloch and Rittenberg in 1942, using isotopic atoms to label the acetic acid molecule, thus permitting the identification of the atoms derived from acetic acid in the finished sterol product. In 1953, Langdon and Bloch identified squalene as an intermediate in cholesterol biosynthesis. In 1958 Bloch and Lynen simultaneously identified a phosphorylated compound made up of five carbon atoms, called isopentenyl pyrophosphate, as a precursor of the sterols. After determining the 30-carbon structure of squalene, Bloch studied the transformation of this substance, which is an open-chain compound, into the cyclic steroid structures leading to cholesterol.

Acetic acid enters the metabolism by being phosphorylated and converted to the active form. Lynen discovered in 1951 that this active form is a product of acetate and coenzyme A, which Lipmann and his co-workers had discovered. In 1958 it was found that the conversion of acetyl-coenzyme A to long-chain fatty acids requires the B vitamin biotin as a participant in the reaction. Through the work of many investigators, it was learned that biotin enables the acetyl-coenzyme A to take up a molecule of carbon dioxide to form malonyl-coenzyme A and that this substance is actually the source of the carbon atoms in the fatty acids.

A basic discovery in this chain of events was the isolation of a soluble enzyme system from yeast that was found to catalyze the conversion of mevalonic acid to squalene, in the presence of ATP, divalent manganese ions, and reduced pyridine nucleotide. It was these investigations of the mechanisms of squalene synthesis from mevalonic acid that led to the awarding of the Nobel Prize to Bloch.

Konrad Emil Bloch was born in Germany and studied chemical engineering in Munich. Like so many of his fellow scientists, he left Germany for the United States during the Nazi period (1936). He received his Ph.D. in biochemistry at Columbia University where he worked with Rudolf Schoenheimer on a metabolic problem, using compounds that had been labeled with deuterium, at that time a highly novel technique. After serving successively on the faculties of Columbia University and the University of Chicago, he went to Harvard University in 1954 to become Higgins Professor of Biochemistry.

The discoveries that have just been described are of great importance to medicine, because many diseases are known to be due to disorders of lipid metabolism. Cholesterol is an important constituent of the arterial plaques of atherosclerosis, which occlude circulation through the coronary arteries, the arteries of the brain, and elsewhere. The metabolism of cholesterol and fat is upset in diabetes mellitus and accounts for some of the serious complications of this disease. Some gallstones are made up almost entirely of cholesterol. An intimate knowledge of the manner in which specific lipids are formed and broken down in the body should ultimately provide a better understanding of these important diseases. Compounds have been developed that can inhibit the biological formation of cholesterol in the body at one stage or another. Unfortunately, the compounds that have been developed thus far are too toxic to be used clinically. Nevertheless, their action gives hope that similar, less toxic compounds will become available for use in patients. It should be noted also that an aberration of fat metabolism, namely, obesity, has been labeled as the major nutritional problem in the United States today.

THE DISSECTION AND SYNTHESIS OF ENZYMES AND HORMONES

Proteins are key components of all living organisms; they play a vital role in almost every aspect of biology. Large complex molecules, they are major constituents of blood, muscle, skin, bone, nerve, and, in fact, of every tissue and organ of the body. All of the enzymes, and many of the hormones that regulate them, are proteins. If we are to understand and eventually to control the events that occur in the body, we must first understand the composition, structure, and function of the proteins.

In 1959 Linus Pauling made a prediction which at the time seemed rather extravagant:

Twenty-five years from now we shall probably know the complete structures of 100 protein molecules and a few nucleic acid molecules. We shall then have a detailed understanding of the ways in which a few enzymes carry out their specific activities, the way in which genes duplicate themselves and accomplish their individual tasks of precisely controlling the synthesis of protein molecules with well-defined structures, the way in which abnormal molecules give rise to the manifestations of

533

the diseases that they cause, the ways in which drugs and other physiologically ac-
tive substances achieve their effect. When this time comes, medicine will have made
a significant start in its transformation from macroscopic and cellular medicine to
molecular medicine.

Though only 17 of the 25 years have passed since that statement was made, the prediction has moved rapidly toward fulfillment.

In Chapter 25 an account will be given of the important role played by ribonucleic acid (RNA) in instructing ribosomes in the preparation of specific genes. In the metabolism of the cell, the decomposition of RNA is accomplished by hydrolysis, and the enzyme that catalyzes this reaction is ribonuclease. Ribonuclease is of particular interest because it was the first enzyme whose amino acid structure was precisely determined, and it was the first enzyme to be synthesized. The chemical dissection of ribonuclease moved forward over a period of 30 years, advancing step by step as new physical and chemical methods of analysis became available.

The story began in 1941 with the isolation of ribonuclease by M. Kunitz. During World War II, the enzyme was obtained in large quantities by Armour, Inc., of Chicago, as a by-product of their work on the fractionation of the proteins of blood plasma. This was part of the protein fractionation project that was organized and supervised by Professor E. J. Cohn of Harvard University. Armour made the enzyme available to research chemists at low cost.

In the mid-1940s Frederick Sanger reported his determination of the amino acid sequence of the two polypeptide chains of insulin. His studies confirmed the peptide hypothesis of protein structure and stimulated chemists to undertake studies of other biologically active proteins. His investigations also provided an exciting example of the application of *paper chromatography,* a technique originated in England a few years earlier by A. J. P. Martin and R. L. M. Synge (Nobel Prize, 1952). *Column chromatography,* another new technique of analysis which was soon to come into wide use, also was being perfected at this time.

At about the time of Sanger's report, Stanford Moore and William H. Stein of the Rockefeller Institute began their studies of amino acids, peptides, and proteins. With new techniques, such as chromatography and the use of ion-exchange resins, they undertook the complete separation and quantitative analysis of various amino acid mixtures. Along the way, they invented the fraction collector, and in collaboration with D. H. Spackman, they developed the completely *automatic amino acid analyzer*. Utilizing this new analytical technique, Stein and Moore, together with C. H. W. Hirs, determined the sequence of amino acids in ribonuclease. This work, which was completed in 1959, provided the first determination of the full sequence of amino acids in an enzyme. It disclosed that ribonuclease is made up of 124 amino acids, and the precise location of the 1876 atoms contained in these acids was determined.

While Moore and Stein were working on amino acid sequences, Christian B. Anfinsen was working on another aspect of the ribonuclease problem. His work was carried out largely at the National Institutes of Health, with interludes at the Carlsberg Laboratory in Copenhagen and at Harvard University. Anfinsen concentrated his attention on the disulfide bonds of the enzyme. He found that enzymatic activity was lost when the four disulfide bonds were fully reduced. His key observation was that the totally reduced protein began to recover enzymatic activity merely on standing. Anfinsen immediately recognized that the enzyme is capable of refolding itself into its native structure and reestablishing its disulfide bridges by simple atmospheric oxidation, thus regaining fully its catalytic activity. In other words, all of the "information" needed for the self-assembly of the three-dimensional structure of this native protein is present in the sequence of the linear polypeptide chain. The concept that the information contained in the linear sequence will, by itself, result in the rapid formation of a unique, biologically active structure is of basic importance in modern biochemistry and molecular biology (Richards, 1972). The 1972 Nobel Prize for chemistry was awarded jointly to Stanford Moore, William H. Stein, and Christian B. Anfinsen.

Without attempting to mention all of the many recent technical advances in protein chemistry, one advance may be cited that has been of great importance to endocrinology and the study of metabolism. This development came in 1969 when Robert Bruce Merrifield at Rockefeller University devised a method for the total synthesis of polypeptides and proteins. The unique feature of Merrifield's method, which accounted for its success, was that he kept the peptide chain attached to a solid substance, whereas in previous methods the reactants were in solution.

Merrifield and his colleagues designed and constructed an apparatus for carrying out what became known as "solid phase peptide synthesis." The extraordinary effectiveness of this apparatus in synthesizing biologically active proteins was clearly proved when the group at Rockefeller University succeeded in synthesizing hormones such as insulin, angiotensin, and bradykinin. They also brought the ribonuclease story to a glorious end by synthesizing this enzyme. Merrifield's technique has wide application to medical science and, potentially, to the therapeutic aspects of medical practice (Merrifield, 1969).

HORMONES

THE ANTERIOR PITUITARY

In Chapter 12 there was a description of the early work of Harvey Cushing on the pituitary gland and of the subsequent research by H. M. Evans, P. E. Smith, and others that resulted in the identification of the following anterior pituitary hormones: growth hormone (GH), adrenal cortical stimulating hormone (ACTH), thyroid-stimulating hormone (TSH), mammary-gland–stimulating hormone (prolactin or LTH); and the hormones acting on the sex glands — follicle-stimulating hormone (FSH) and luteinizing hormone (LH). An additional anterior pituitary hormone, not mentioned in the earlier chapter, is melanocyte-stimulating hormone (MSH). Though the action of MSH on the pigment cells of some of the lower animals has been well documented, its function in human physiology remains obscure. It has been detected in high titer in the blood and urine of patients with Addison's disease, in whom there is hyperpigmentation of the skin.

Though the anterior lobe of the pituitary is so small that it can be con-

535

tained in the cavity of a thimble, it stands first in importance among the glands of internal secretion. Its hormones control growth, sexual development, reproduction, and thyroid activity and, to an important degree, govern the body's general response to stress and disease. The pituitary exercises its control by a two-stage process: its hormones regulate the output of the effector hormones produced by other endocrine glands such as the thyroid, testes, ovaries, and adrenals. For example, ACTH induces the adrenal cortex to produce and release half a dozen different steroid hormones. In humans, the hormones produced by the adrenal cortex include cortisol, corticosterone, aldosterone, and lesser amounts of the sex hormones. Apart from the sex hormones, the chief functions of the adrenocortical substances are (1) regulation of carbohydrate metabolism and (2) control of the balance of electrolytes, such as sodium, in the blood and other body fluids. Cortisol is the principal steroid serving the first of these functions, whereas aldosterone is the steroid chiefly involved in controlling electrolyte balance.

Adrenocorticotropic Hormone (ACTH). The investigations of Choh Hao Li at the University of California, which began in the early 1940s, have led to knowledge of the complete molecular structure of ACTH and to the chemical synthesis of various active portions of the molecule. As this work has progressed it has been aided by many important contributions from workers in other biochemical laboratories.

The productive work of Li and his colleagues began in 1942 when they obtained from sheep pituitaries an apparently homogeneous protein that possessed ACTH activity. Its molecular weight was 20,000, indicating that it had about 200 amino acid subunits. In the following year, George Sayers, Abraham White, and Cyril N. H. Long of Yale University reported the isolation from pig pituitaries of a highly purified protein with the same molecular weight.

In the late 1940s and early 1950s, major advances were made in methods for isolating polypeptides and other large molecules. These methods included electrophoresis, chromatography, and countercurrent partitioning. The workers chiefly responsible for these advances were Arne W. K. Tiselius of Sweden, A. J. P. Martin and R. L. M. Synge of England, and Lyman C. Craig of the Rockefeller Institute. In 1954, utilizing these new procedures, Li and his associates obtained from sheep pituitary extracts an entity smaller than the one isolated in 1942 but having greater ACTH activity. This was a straight-chain peptide with 39 amino acid subunits and a molecular weight of about 4500. Within a few months Paul H. Bell, Robert G. Shepherd, and their co-workers at the American Cyanamid Company announced the purification and the partial determination of the structure of ACTH obtained from the pituitaries of pigs. By 1955 the complete sequence of amino acid subunits in both sheep and pig ACTH had been reported by the American Cyanamid workers.

In 1960 Li's group synthesized a peptide composed of the first 19 amino acids of natural ACTH and demonstrated that it possessed all the biological properties of the natural hormone. In subsequent months Klaus H. Hofmann and his co-workers at the University of Pittsburgh School of Medicine and R. Schwyzer and his associates at the CIBA Company, in Switzerland, also announced the synthesis of a polypeptide 19 to 24 subunits in length and having ACTH activity.

The 19-unit synthetic product caused a greater darkening of the skin (MSH effect) than did the natural product when injected into live frogs whose pituitaries had been removed. This led to the first important correlation between chemical structure and hormonal activity. The complete chemical structures of two skin-darkening anterior pituitary hormones, alpha-MSH and beta-MSH, were established soon after the structure of ACTH was determined.

THE POSTERIOR
PITUITARY

In 1895, George Oliver and E. A. Schafer of London demonstrated that the intravenous injection of an emulsion of the whole pituitary gland produced a striking rise in blood pressure. Three years later, W. H. Howell of Baltimore reported that this pressor effect could be obtained with extracts of the posterior lobe of the gland but not with extracts of the anterior lobe.

The posterior pituitary contains two polypeptide hormones known as oxytocin and vasopressin. The former stimulates the contraction of the uterus, and the latter raises the blood pressure and regulates the excretion of water by the kidneys. They both have immense practical importance in clinical medicine: oxytocin helps to prevent hemorrhage after childbirth, and vasopressin is useful in the treatment of shock and in the control of the excessive urinary excretion in patients with diabetes insipidus.

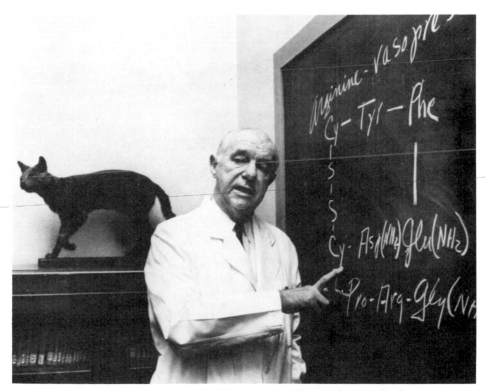

Figure 111. Vincent du Vigneaud. (Medical Archives, New York Hospital–Cornell Medical Center.)

As was mentioned in Chapter 12, one of the most important American contributions in the field of endocrinology came when *Vincent du Vigneaud* of Cornell Medical College succeeded in synthesizing the two polypeptide hormones of the posterior pituitary. Du Vigneaud's work on this subject went back to the 1930s, when he found that some rather impure extracts of the posterior lobe contained a high percentage of sulfur, which seemed to be related to the physiological activity of the extracts. After much additional work he succeeded in isolating both hormones in a pure state and found that they had a similar structure: both contained eight amino acids, connected in a chain that was curled up at one end to form a ring. The molecule had some resemblance to the figure 6, with the circular loop containing five amino acids and the tail containing three. Two sulfur atoms, linked to each other, formed a part of the ring. With this information in hand du Vigneaud concentrated first on the synthesis of oxytocin. Step by step the amino acid chain was built up, with the two sulfur atoms in the proper positions, one at the end of the chain and the other near the middle. Finally, the ring was closed by the formation of a bond between the sulfur atoms. Then came the thrilling moment of testing the synthesized product to be sure that it possessed the physiological activity of natural oxytocin. The test proved that it was in every way identical to the natural product. This was the first synthesis of a polypeptide hormone, and it demonstrated that substances with important physiological properties could be built up from well-known amino acids according to well-known chemical principles.

THE HORMONES OF THE HYPOTHALAMUS

The activity of the anterior pituitary, which controls the peripheral endocrine glands, is itself regulated by "releasing factors" originating in the brain. Several of these releasing hormones have now been isolated and synthesized.

The pituitary gland is attached by a stalk to a region at the base of the brain known as the hypothalamus. In the late 1960s, after nearly 20 years of effort in many laboratories, two substances were isolated from animal brain tissue that proved to be long-sought hypothalamic hormones. Because the molecular structures of these new hormones are relatively simple, they can be synthesized readily. Their availability has opened a new chapter in endocrinology.

As early as 1924 it was realized that the hormones secreted by the posterior lobe of the pituitary are also found in the hypothalamus. Later it was found that the two hormones of the posterior pituitary are actually manufactured in specialized nerve cells in the hypothalamus. Once formed, the hormones slowly flow down the pituitary stalk to the posterior lobe through the axons, or long fibers, of the hypothalamic nerve cells. They are then stored in the posterior pituitary and are secreted into the bloodstream under appropriate physiological stimulation.

These observations led Ernst and Berta Scharrer to the concept of "neurosecretion" (the secretion of hormones by nerve cells). They suggested that specialized nerve cells might secrete true hormones, which would be carried by the blood and exert their effect on remote target organs. The ability to manufacture hormones had traditionally been assigned to endocrine glands such as the thyroid, the gonads, and the adrenals. The suggestion that nerve cells could synthesize and secrete hormones that affect the function of distant organs would endow them with a capacity far beyond their known ability to liberate neurotransmitters, such as epinephrine and acetylcholine, at the microscopic regions (synapses) where they make contact with other nerve cells.

In 1945 G. W. Harris of Oxford University proposed that hypothalamic control of the secretory activity of the anterior pituitary is neurochemical. He suggested that substances manufactured by nerve cells in the hypothalamus are released into the capillary vessels that run from the hypothalamus to the anterior pituitary, where they are stored in the endocrine cells until needed.

By 1960 it had been clearly established that crude extracts of hypothalamic tissue were able to stimulate the secretion of at least four anterior pituitary hormones: ACTH, thyrotropin (TSH), and the two gonadotropins (LH and FSH). Results obtained between 1960 and 1962 were best explained by assuming the existence of three separate hypothalamic releasing factors: TRF (the TSH-releasing factor), LRF (the LH-releasing factor), and FRF (the FSH-releasing factor). Two groups of workers in the United States responded to the challenge of trying to isolate and characterize these releasing factors: a group headed by A. V. Schally at the Tulane University School of Medicine and one headed by Roger Guillemin, first at the Baylor University College of Medicine in Houston and then at the Salk Institute in La Jolla, California.

Over a period of four years the Tulane group worked with extracts from approximately two million pig brains. Guillemin's laboratory collected, dissected, and processed close to five million hypothalamic fragments from the brains of sheep. Since one sheep brain has a wet weight of about 100 grams, this meant handling 500 tons of brain tissue. From this enormous mass they removed 7 tons of hypothalamic tissue. Semi-industrial methods had to be developed in order to handle, extract, and purify such large quantities. Finally, in 1968, one milligram of a preparation of TRF was obtained. Chemical analysis showed that this entire milligram of physiologically active material was made up of just three amino acids: histidine (His), glutamic acid (Glu), and proline (Pro), present in equal amounts. The biological activity of the sequence Glu-His-Pro, and of that sequence alone, was qualitatively indistinguishable from the activity of natural TRF. When the synthetic Glu-His-Pro-OH was modified to pGlu-His-Pro-NH$_2$ by replacing the hydroxyl (OH) with an amino (NH$_2$) group to produce the primary amide, the latter proved to have the same biological activity as the natural TRF. Finally the complete structure of the natural TRF was obtained by high-resolution mass spectrometry. It turned out to have the structure pGlu-His-Pro-NH$_2$. This result was achieved late in 1969. From the side-fractions of the programs to isolate TRF, a polypeptide composed of ten amino acids was isolated which proved, in 1971, to be LRF.

The hypothalamic hormones TRF and LRF have both been synthesized and are now available in unlimited quantities. TRF has already become a powerful tool for exploring pituitary function in several diseases characterized by an abnormality of one or several of the pituitary secretions. There is increasing evidence that most patients with such abnormalities (primarily

539

children) actually have normally functioning pituitary glands, since they respond promptly to the administration of synthetic hypothalamic hormones. Evidently their abnormalities are due to hypothalamic rather than pituitary deficiencies. For example, some deficiencies in thyroid function can now be treated successfully by the administration of the hypothalamic polypeptide, TRF.

Similarly, an increasing number of women who have an anovulatory menstrual cycle and who show no pituitary or ovarian defect begin to secrete normal amounts of the gonadotropins LH and FSH after the administration of LRF. The administration of synthetic LRF should, therefore, be the method of choice for the treatment of those cases of infertility in which the functional defect resides in the hypothalamus-pituitary system. Indeed, ovulation can be induced in women by the administration of synthetic LRF. Moreover, knowledge of the structure of the LRF molecule may open up an entirely novel approach to fertility control. Synthetic compounds closely related to LRF in structure may act as inhibitors of the native LRF. Two such analogues of LRF, made by modifying the histidine in the hormone, have been reported to be antagonists of LRF. This suggests that LRF antagonists could serve as contraceptives.

SOMATOMEDIN   In 1921, H. M. Evans and J. A. Long of the University of California (Berkeley) showed that repeated injections of an anterior pituitary extract into rats produced gigantism. The factor that had this effect, growth hormone (GH), regulates the growth of the skeleton by acting on the epiphyseal cartilages. Some years later Li and his co-workers succeeded in establishing the sequence of amino acids in human growth hormones.

W. D. Salmon, Jr., and W. H. Daughaday of Washington University, St. Louis, reported in 1957 that the incorporation of radioactive sulfate into cartilage was stimulated when normal serum was incubated with rat cartilage and radioactive sulfate. From this fundamental observation came the concept that growth hormone does not induce skeletal growth directly but acts by stimulating the formation of a secondary growth-promoting substance, which became known first as "sulfation factor" but later was renamed *somatomedin*.

DIABETES MELLITUS— NEW CONCEPTS   Diabetes mellitus is a health problem of steadily increasing magnitude. The number of diabetics in the United States has increased from 1.2 million in 1950 to an estimated 5 million in 1975, an increase of more than 300 per cent, while the population was increasing only about 50 per cent. In spite of treatment with insulin, special diets, and oral antidiabetic agents, diabetes is the fifth leading cause of death in the United States and the second leading cause of blindness. There was little progress in research in relation to this disease in the 1950s and early 1960s; but the advent of new approaches and new techniques has stimulated a marked increase in the study of diabetes in recent years.

SOMATOSTATIN
AND GLUCAGON

The traditional view of diabetes is that the disease is a simple metabolic disturbance resulting from impaired insulin production. But recently new factors have come to light, and much of the investigation of the molecular biology of diabetes during the past decade has been focused on glucagon. This substance was discovered in 1923 by John R. Murlin and C. P. Kimball of the University of Rochester. Whereas insulin is normally deficient in diabetes, glucagon may be present in excess.

In 1955 another aspect of this problem came to light when Rolf Luft of Stockholm, Sweden, introduced hypophysectomy (removal of the pituitary gland) for the treatment of the vascular disease of the optic retina, which leads to blindness in diabetics. This operation seemed worthy of trial because it had been observed that severe diabetic retinitis improved when anterior pituitary deficiency developed.

The hypothesis had been advanced that hypersecretion of growth hormone by the pituitary is responsible for the disease of small arteries that causes blindness and other serious complications of diabetes. It became possible to test this hypothesis in 1973 when Roger Guillemin and his colleagues isolated an inhibitor of hypothalamic growth hormone, which they named *somatostatin*. In the course of studies of somatostatin (which was synthesized in 1973 by D. H. Coy and co-workers at Tulane University School of Medicine) it was found to suppress the release of both insulin and glucagon, again emphasizing a possible role for growth hormone in the pathophysiology of diabetes.

In 1974 M. Vranic of Toronto and S. Pek of the University of Michigan found glucagon-like activity in the blood of dogs from which the pancreas had been removed. R. H. Unger and his associates at Southwestern Medical School in Texas discovered that a substance apparently identical to glucagon is also released by tissues in the stomach and upper intestine of dogs. Unger and others have stated that three lines of evidence support the conclusion that glucagon plays a role in human diabetes: (1) an increase in the concentration of glucagon has been observed in association with an increase in the concentration of glucose in the blood; (2) when the secretion of both glucagon and insulin is suppressed, an elevation in blood glucose is not observed unless the concentration of glucagon is restored to normal; (3) the somatostatin-induced suppression of glucagon release in diabetic animals and humans lowers the blood glucose concentration and alleviates certain other symptoms of diabetes.

Matlack and his co-workers at the University of Washington School of Medicine observed that the concentration of glucose in baboons fell during the administration of somatostatin. They then discovered that the secretion of both insulin and glucagon could be inhibited completely and quickly by somatostatin, and they concluded that the site of action of this agent is the pancreas. The important aspect of these observations is that when the release of insulin is suppressed, the blood glucose does not rise to high levels if there is a simultaneous suppression of the release of glucagon. These studies of the action of somatostatin suggest that glucagon may play a vital role in controlling the level of glucose in the blood.

The action of somatostatin in diabetes is at present too ill-defined to allow for any important therapeutic role. However, new synthetic analogues

541

may be found that have a more prolonged and more specific action. The discovery of a long-acting preparation with selective suppressive effects on glucagon might offer an advance in the management of diabetes (Editorial, Lancet, 1975; Maugh, 1975b).

There are other possible therapeutic uses for somatostatin. S. S. Yen, at the University of California (San Diego), found that the administration of somatostatin sharply reduces the amount of somatomedin in the blood of individuals afflicted with the form of gigantism known as acromegaly. It therefore seems likely that somatostatin may be useful in the treatment of this disorder. Somatostatin also inhibits the increased secretion of thyrotropin caused by thyrotropin-releasing hormone (TRF), and under certain circumstances it inhibits the secretion of prolactin (LTH).

VIRUSES AND DIABETES   In 1864 a Norwegian physician, J. Stang, reported that diabetes developed in a patient shortly after an attack of mumps, and he suggested that there might be a link between these two events. Since that time there have been scattered reports of a temporal association between a wide variety of viral infections and the onset of diabetes. Recently, more persuasive evidence has come forth as a result of the identification of high concentrations of viral antibodies in newly diagnosed cases of diabetes. The accumulated information points toward a viral role in the initiation of diabetes, particularly in children.

Strong evidence for a relationship between mumps virus and diabetes was presented in 1974 by Sultz and his associates at the State University of New York at Buffalo. They found that the epidemiological pattern of mumps varied through three cycles of high and low incidence, with the peaks occurring approximately every seven years. The incidence of juvenile diabetes paralleled the incidence of mumps, but with a lag period averaging 3.8 years after the peaks. This lag period may reflect the time required for the virus to produce permanent damage to the pancreas. These workers located 118 children who were diagnosed during that period as having juvenile diabetes. Of the 118, 59 either had had mumps or had been exposed to mumps, and an additional 29 had been vaccinated against mumps, prior to the onset of diabetes.

GENETIC FACTORS   If, in fact, viruses are involved in the etiology of
IN DIABETES   diabetes, the current interpretation of their role is that they cause pancreatic damage only in individuals who are genetically predisposed to such damage. This predisposition appears to be more evident in children than in adults. Recent studies indicate that the genetic elements associated with juvenile diabetes differ from those associated with the adult type. The juvenile form appears to be linked to histocompatibility antigens that may be associated with certain genes controlling immune responses. The adult form appears to be linked to a different and as yet unknown set of genes that are primarily responsible for familial inheritance of diabetes, although the onset of this form is probably precipitated by environmental factors.

Additional evidence on the genetics of diabetes has come from the studies of twins conducted by Priscilla White and her associates at the Eliot P. Joslin Research Laboratory in Boston and by other groups. Among 176 pairs of identical adult twins of which one member had diabetes, this disease occurred in the other member in 45 per cent of the pairs. Among 416 pairs of non-identical adult twins, diabetes occurred in both members of a pair in only 8 per cent of the pairs. The studies of Tattersall and Fajans in Michigan have indicated that there are stronger genetic links among patients with the adult type of diabetes than among those with the juvenile type (Maugh, 1975a).

RADIOIMMUNOASSAY   In 1960, *Rosalyn S. Yalow* and *Saul A. Berson* of the Veterans' Administration Hospital, New York City, introduced the technique of radioimmunoassay, which has been utilized for the measurement of minute quantities of hormones. This technical development has made possible the study of insulin secretion under various physiological and pathological conditions. Prior to 1960, information about insulin secretion had been obtained by means of *in vitro* and *in vivo* bioassays. However, this technique lacked the sensitivity, precision, specificity, and ease of performance required for the determination of the plasma and tissue insulin levels in large numbers of patients and laboratory animals.

The radioimmunoassay technique has been widely used in endocrinology, and the outstanding progress that has been made in the last decade in

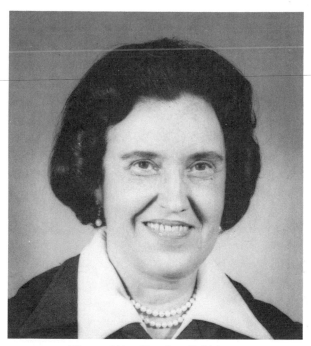

Figure 112.   Rosalyn S. Yalow.   543

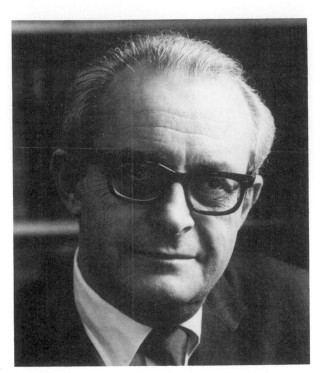

Figure 113.   Saul Berson. (Courtesy of Public
Relations Department, The Mt. Sinai Medical Center,
N.Y., N.Y.)

the study of diabetes and other endocrine disturbances would not have
been possible without this procedure. Immunoassays are available for many
hormones and other specific polypeptides; their use has greatly expanded
our understanding of the molecular mechanisms involved in many disease
processes.

NEW FORMS OF INSULIN   It is now known that the chemical form in which
AND OTHER HORMONES   certain hormones exert their effect on their target
tissues differs from the form in which they are
synthesized in, or secreted from, their glands of origin. Certain peptide hormones are synthesized as large-molecule "pro" hormones which, either
before or after their secretion into the blood, are modified to yield smaller
moieties of great biological potency. *Proinsulin* serves as a good example of
this new development in endocrinology (Rubenstein and Steiner, 1971).

Until 1967 it was accepted that insulin synthesis occurs within the beta
cells of the pancreas through the union of two separately synthesized
polypeptide chains. *In vitro* experiments with separated natural or synthetic
chains had shown relatively efficient resynthesis of insulin in the presence
of the enzyme glutathione-insulin-transhydrogenase. It was further believed that insulin is assembled from small oligopeptides, some of which
contain cystine to provide the disulfide bridges.

544   In 1965, D. Givol and R. R. Porter at St. Mary's Hospital, London,

suggested that the amino acid sequences of the single-chain proteins, ribonuclease and chymotrypsinogen, direct the folding of the molecule so as to permit the disulfide bonds to form spontaneously. After cleavage of their polypeptide chains at one or more sites, the stability of the proteins under conditions of disulfide-sulfhydryl exchange was markedly diminished, as had already been observed with insulin. By analogy, these authors suggested that the insulin chains might be formed as part of a larger single polypeptide from which insulin could be released by proteolysis after the native conformation had been established. Various workers searched without success for such an insulin precursor in pancreatic extracts (Rubenstein and Steiner, 1971).

In 1967 proinsulin was discovered by D. F. Steiner and P. E. Oyer of the University of Chicago during an investigation of insulin biosynthesis in an islet-cell tumor removed from a patient with an extremely depressed level of blood glucose. When slices from this tumor were incubated with tritiated leucine or phenylalanine, the amino acids were incorporated not only into insulin but also into a protein of higher molecular weight and having a higher specific activity than insulin and a strong reaction with insulin antisera. Incubation of the latter protein with low concentrations of trypsin resulted in its conversion to insulin or a closely related form, whereas cleavage of its disulfide bonds by sulfatolysis did not yield separate A or B chains but indicated the presence of a polypeptide chain larger than insulin. These and other data led to the conclusion that this protein, later named proinsulin, is a precursor of insulin and consists of a single polypeptide chain similar to insulin but having an additional polypeptide interposed between the A and B chains. These observations were confirmed in later experiments using isolated islets of Langerhans obtained from rat pancreas by collagenase digestion (Rubenstein and Steiner, 1971). The existence of proinsulin and an enzymatic system necessary for its conversion to insulin raised new possibilities in the search for genetically determined abnormalities that might account for inherited diabetes.

Studies have now been made of the other hormones in the blood, using similar fractionation techniques, and the results with gastrin, glucagon, growth hormone, parathyroid hormone, and others have proved to be equally exciting.

TRANSPLANTATION OF INSULIN-PRODUCING TISSUE   The advances that have been made in the past decade have led to a better understanding of diabetes mellitus and have raised hopes of better methods of management, but thus far there have been no dramatic therapeutic developments.

One new approach to treatment, not previously mentioned, may or may not have a bright future. This approach, which has taken several forms, is designed to provide for the diabetic individual a more natural source of insulin. To this end, efforts have been made in animals with experimental diabetes, to transplant the pancreas, or the islets of Langerhans, or pancreatic beta cells which have been grown in tissue culture. None of these methods has yet reached the stage of clinical application, but this is another promising area of research (Maugh, 1975b).

MECHANISMS OF HORMONAL ACTION

A challenging problem in endocrinology has been that of determining the manner in which hormones serve as regulators of biochemical processes in the tissues. Two general patterns of hormone-cell interaction have been recognized. The first, illustrated by epinephrine and by many types of peptide hormones, involves hormone-reaction with membrane-bound nucleotide cyclase systems to stimulate the conversion of a nucleoside triphosphate such as adenosine triphosphate (ATP) to the corresponding monophosphate; for example, cyclic adenosine monophosphate (cAMP). In the second pattern of interaction, which appears to be operative with the various steroid hormones, the hormone enters the cell and binds to a specific intracellular receptor-protein characteristic of the responsive or target cell. The resulting steroid-protein complex then migrates to the nucleus, where specific RNA synthesis is initiated or accelerated.

CYCLIC AMP

This relatively small molecule is the "second messenger" between certain hormones and their effects within the cell. It plays a key role in regulating the speed of chemical processes in organisms as distantly related as bacteria and humans. Its proper chemical name is cyclic-3',5'-adenosine monophosphate, but it is more widely known as cyclic AMP. (The term "cyclic" refers to the fact that the atoms in the single phosphate group of the molecule are arranged in a ring.) Among the many functions served by cAMP in humans and other animals is that of acting as a chemical messenger and regulating the enzymatic reactions within cells that store sugars and fats. Cyclic AMP has

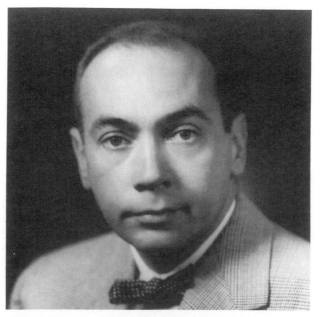

Figure 114. Earl Sutherland. (National Library of Medicine, Bethesda, Maryland.)

also been shown to control the activity of genes. Moreover, a precondition for the uncontrolled growth of cells characteristic of cancer appears to be an inadequate supply of cAMP.

The Nobel Prize for physiology and medicine for the year 1971 was awarded to *Earl W. Sutherland, Jr.,* for his "discoveries concerning the mechanisms of action of hormones." Sutherland's crowning achievement was the discovery of cyclic AMP.

At the time of his death, Sutherland was Professor of Physiology at the Vanderbilt University School of Medicine, but he began his investigations of hormone action at Washington University, St. Louis, in the laboratory of Carl and Gerty Cori. The work of the Coris and others had already resulted in the identification of the enzymes involved in glycogen breakdown, and Sutherland began to investigate how the hormone epinephrine (Adrenalin) stimulates the degradation of glycogen in liver and muscle. By measuring the levels of various intermediates in the pathway of glycogen degradation, he established that the initial step in glycogen breakdown is catalyzed by the enzyme phosphorylase, and he then found that the activity of phosphorylase is increased in liver cells that have been exposed to epinephrine. In liver extracts, Sutherland discovered a second enzyme that converts active phosphorylase into an inactive form, with the release of inorganic phosphate. In association with Rall, he then found that the inactive form of phosphorylase could be converted back to the active form by still another enzyme present in liver extracts. With this step, phosphate is reincorporated into the phosphorylase molecule. A similar enzyme was discovered simultaneously in muscle and was named phosphorylase kinase.

Thus, the degradation of glycogen is controlled by the relative amounts of active and inactive enzymes. Sutherland and his co-workers also found that, in cell-free extracts, both epinephrine and glucagon promote the accumulation of the active form of phosphorylase. This was the first demonstration of a physiologically significant effect of a hormone in a cell-free extract, and it opened the way to an understanding of how hormones act.

Accumulating in the cell-free extracts of liver, following epinephrine treatment, was a small heat-stable molecule (later identified as cAMP). It was this molecule that promoted the conversion of inactive phosphorylase to the active form. Cyclic AMP did not accumulate, however, if the cell-membrane fraction was removed from the extract. Later studies showed that epinephrine and many other hormones act on the outside of the cell membrane to promote the synthesis of cAMP, which is then released on the inner surface of the cell membrane.

The fact that cAMP could activate phosphorylase and stimulate glycogen breakdown provided the basis for Sutherland and his co-workers to assay cAMP and to make a number of revolutionary observations that were fundamental not only to endocrinology but also to all aspects of biology, for it was learned that cAMP plays an important role in almost all cells.

Since glycogen is found mainly in liver and muscle, it seemed likely that the cAMP in the other tissues controls other processes. When Sutherland examined cAMP accumulation in other hormonally dependent tissues, he found that many hormones increase cAMP synthesis in their target tissues. The various hormones act by increasing the activity of the enzyme adenyl cyclase, thereby increasing cAMP synthesis.

547

Sutherland's contributions made possible a unifying concept of the mechanism of hormone action. Hormones may be considered as "first messengers," leaving their site of synthesis and circulating to their target tissues, where they are recognized by specific receptors. Sutherland suggested that after the hormone combines with the receptor, the activity of adenyl cyclase present in the cell membrane increases, and the common "second messenger," cAMP, is generated inside the cell, where it can stimulate cAMP-sensitive enzymes already present in the tissue to carry out their specialized functions.

Sutherland was also interested in the role of cAMP in human disease. Because cAMP serves primarily a regulatory function, it seemed likely that a great variety of disorders might be related to defects in the formation or action of this nucleotide. One of the first disorders to be studied was pseudohypoparathyroidism, a hereditary disease in which parathyroid hormone appears incapable of stimulating cAMP formation in target tissues. Other hereditary disorders in which cAMP has been implicated include bronchial asthma, diabetes mellitus, and certain affective disorders. Cyclic AMP is also involved in some bacterial infections, of which an interesting example is cholera. The toxin responsible for the symptoms of this disease produces an apparently irreversible increase in adenyl cyclase activity, leading to prolonged high levels of cAMP in intestinal epithelial cells, which in turn leads to the outpouring of fluid and electrolytes into the intestinal canal—the characteristic feature of this disease. Finally, there is now evidence that defective cAMP formation may be involved in the growth of tumors. To date, our knowledge of cAMP has not led to improved methods of therapy. However, many drugs already in use appear to act through the cyclic AMP mechanism (Pastan, 1971; Sutherland, 1972).

THE STEROID-HORMONE MESSENGER   As mentioned earlier, the pattern of interaction of the steroid hormones does not involve the cyclic AMP mechanism. Instead, these hormones enter the target cell and bind to a specific extranuclear receptor-protein, and the resulting steroid-protein migrates to the nucleus and initiates the synthesis of specific RNA. In the case of the estrogens, the hormone-induced translocation to the nucleus involves an alteration of the receptor-protein ("receptor transformation"). For this reason, it has been proposed that estrogen acts to induce conversion of the receptor-protein to a biochemically functional form (Jensen and DeSombre, 1973).

All steroid hormones appear to have a similar subcellular mechanism of action. Although differences may exist in the details, a generally accepted sequence of events applicable to all steroid hormones has been postulated: "(A) binding of the hormone to cytoplasmic receptors in target cells and subsequent translocation of this steroid-receptor complex to a nuclear acceptor site; (B) activation of the genome by an as yet unknown mechanism leading to increased RNA synthesis and resulting in the induction of new protein; and (C) mediation of the biological effects of the hormone by the induced protein" (Jensen and DeSombre, 1973).

Thus, hormones provide a means of external control, enabling the cells composing the tissue to act in concert. A recurring question has been:

Exactly how does a hormone activate the genes? Pioneering work elucidating the mechanism of action of the hormones that affect the uterus was done by E. V. Jensen of the University of Chicago, J. Gorski of the University of Illinois, and T. H. Hamilton of the University of Texas. A group at Vanderbilt University (B. W. O'Malley and others) added to this work by finding evidence that in the cells of the chick oviduct, the hormone (progesterone) which activates genes that give rise to the production of the protein *avidin* is bound to a receptor-molecule of protein in the cytoplasm of the target cells. The hormone-receptor complex then moves into the nucleus of the cell, where it becomes associated with *chromatin,* the material that incorporates the genes. Thereafter there are changes in the synthesis of nuclear ribonucleic acid, leading ultimately to the synthesis of avidin. The Vanderbilt group concluded (1972) that in "the oviduct, receptor-protein is essential for nuclear binding of progesterone" and that "oviduct nuclei but not spleen, lung, intestine or liver nuclei can bind the progesterone-receptor complex" (O'Malley et al., 1972). Since the hormone-receptor complex binds much better to target cell chromatin than to other chromatins, the Vanderbilt workers suggested that "perhaps the target cell genome contains specific 'acceptor sites' which receive the inducer complex as it enters the nucleus."

A clear example of the activation of genes by an adrenocortical hormone was demonstrated in the studies of I. S. Edelman, R. Bogoroch, and G. A. Porter, of the University of California School of Medicine. They demonstrated that the hormone aldosterone regulates the passage through the cell membrane of sodium and potassium ions. Tracer studies with radioactively labeled aldosterone showed that when the bladder cells of a toad were exposed to the hormone, the molecules of hormone penetrated all the way into the nuclei of the cells. About an hour and a half after aldosterone had reached its peak concentration within the cell, the movement of sodium ions across the cell membrane increased. The evidence indicates that this facilitation of sodium transport is brought about by proteins that the cell is induced to make. These experiments suggest that aldosterone activates genes in the nucleus to synthesize proteins (enzymes) that speed up the passage of sodium ions across the membrane.

VITAMIN D: INVESTIGATIONS OF A NEW STEROID HORMONE

We have seen earlier how rickets was eliminated as a significant disease by the discovery of vitamin D. Recent research has focused attention on a new steroid "hormone" derived from vitamin D that regulates the level of calcium in the blood.

Calcium enters the bloodstream from the intestine, or from the bones by the mobilization of the calcium stored in the skeleton. Absorption from the intestine and mobilization from bones are controlled by the steroid hormone 1,25-dihydroxy vitamin D_3, which is metabolized from vitamin D. This hormone is secreted into the bloodstream by the kidney and then is transported to the intestine or bone, where it acts to promote absorption or mobilization. Most investigators agree that parathyroid hormone is in-

549

volved in signaling the kidney to release the steroid hormone. Research in this area gained momentum when Hector F. DeLuca and his colleagues at the University of Wisconsin, in the early 1960s, began a long series of experiments to elucidate the role of the kidney in calcium metabolism. One of their discoveries was that rats deficient in parathyroid hormone also lack 1,25-dihydroxy-D_3 in their blood. Since then much additional research has been carried out in this area by DeLuca, by Anthony Norman and his associates at the University of California, by Haussler at the University of Arizona, and by Wasserman at Cornell University. Since 1,25-dihydroxy-D_3 is a steroid hormone, efforts have been made to learn whether its mode of action is similar to that of estrogen, which serves as a model for other steroid hormones (Kolata, 1975).

There is now evidence to support the hypothesis that 1,25-dihydroxy-D_3 binds to a protein when it enters the cytoplasm of a receptive intestinal cell and, in a manner similar to the action of estrogen, stimulates the synthesis of a calcium-binding protein. However, it is questionable whether the synthesis of this specific protein is adequate to explain the major effect of 1,25-dihydroxy-D_3 on calcium transport by the intestinal cells. Although much remains to be learned about vitamin D metabolism, the discovery of the sequence of chemical modifications that this vitamin undergoes when 1,25-dihydroxy-D_3 is produced is already proving its value in the study and treatment of human disease (Kolata, 1975).

Since vitamin D is modified in the liver, diseases of the liver may distort the chemical conversion of vitamin D and thus lead to defective production of the hormone 1,25-dihydroxy-D_3. For example, it has been noted that anticonvulsant drugs, such as phenobarbital and diphenylhydantoin, apparently affect the metabolism of vitamin D in the liver and, when administered for long periods of time, result in the development of rickets, osteomalacia, or hypocalcemia. Chronic alcoholics may also suffer diseases of calcium deficiency because of impaired liver function. Avioli and his associates at Washington University, St. Louis, have successfully treated calcium deficiencies of this type with large doses of vitamin D. Moreover, patients with chronic kidney disease cannot synthesize 1,25-dihydroxy-D_3 and often develop bone disease and hypocalcemia. Coburn and his associates at the University of California (Los Angeles) have successfully dealt with this problem in more than 50 patients with renal failure by giving them 1,25-dihydroxy-D_3 (Kolata, 1975).

HORMONES AS ORAL CONTRACEPTIVES

The first demonstration of an ovarian hormone occurred in 1896 when Emil Knauer of Vienna transplanted ovaries into immature and castrated male animals and found that they developed female sexual characteristics. In 1917 Charles R. Stockard and George N. Papanicolaou demonstrated that the vaginal epithelium of certain mammals undergoes characteristic changes during each phase of the estrous cycle.

In 1923 Edgar Allen and Edward Doisy of St. Louis used the bioassay method of Stockard and Papanicolaou, in rats whose ovaries had been removed, to show that there is present in the fluid of the ovarian follicles an estrus-producing substance. That appreciable amounts of this substance are present in the urine of pregnant females was shown by S. Ascheim and B. Zondek in Germany in 1927. This discovery stimulated intense activity by the chemists, and two years later the estrogenic hormone, *estrione,* was isolated from the urine in crystalline form, independently by Doisy in St. Louis and Adolph Butenandt in Germany.

It had long been suspected that the ovary secretes a second hormone in addition to the estrogenic hormone. As far back as 1897 John Beard, an anatomist at the University of Edinburgh, had postulated that the corpus luteum, the yellowish nodule which is left behind in the ovary after the follicle has discharged its egg, must serve some function during pregnancy. Evidence supporting this view was offered in 1903 by L. Fraenkel in Germany when he found that destruction of the corpora lutea in pregnant rabbits caused abortion. But it was not until 1929 that the work of G. W. Corner and W. M. Allen firmly established the hormonal role of the corpus luteum. The luteal hormone has since been named progestin or progesterol.

The foregoing discoveries and observations provided the background for the development of hormonal contraceptives, a major medical and social achievement of the twentieth century. An additional important observation was made in 1898 by Professor Zschokke, a veterinarian in Zurich, Switzerland, who stated that for many decades it had been the practice of veterinarians manually to crush persistent corpora lutea in sterile cows, since as long as a corpus luteum remained, further development of follicles was inhibited. Restating this observation in modern terms, a persistent corpus luteum produces a hormone that inhibits ovulation.

By 1909, Leo Loeb in Philadelphia had observed that ovulation in guinea pigs occurred earlier than usual when corpora lutea were removed, and he also came to the conclusion that the growing corpus luteum suppresses ovulation. The next important development occurred in 1916 when Herrmann and Stein of the Institute of Anatomy in Vienna reported that lipid extracts of corpus luteum suppressed ovulation in rats.

Credit for formulating these observations into a concept that led to intentional contraception belongs to Ludwig Haberlandt, Professor of Physiology at Innsbruck, Austria. In March, 1919, he transplanted ovaries from pregnant rabbits under the skin of fertile adult female rabbits and found that they became infertile. In the following 13 years, he proved that extracts of corpora lutea from pregnant cows rendered rabbits infertile, and in 1927 he reported that ovarian extracts given *orally* to mice produced temporary sterility (National Science Foundation, 1973). Haberlandt was always aware of the clinical implications of his work; by 1930, he was talking about "Geburtenregelung"—birth control. In 1931 he said, "Of all the methods available, hormonal sterilization, based on a biological principle, if it can be applied unobjectionably in the human, is the ideal method for practical medicine and its future task of birth control" (National Science Foundation, 1973).

Seven years later, Otfried Fellner presented additional experiments that confirmed Haberlandt's findings; but Fellner's results were with the estrogenic hormone rather than with progesterone. Similar results were obtained in guinea pigs by Loeb and Kountz in St. Louis, who knew nothing about Fellner's work.

551

After convenient bioassay methods had been developed by Allen and Doisy in 1923 for study of estrogenic activity and by Corner and Allen in 1929 for study of progestational activity, and after Doisy had isolated estrogen in 1929, the pharmaceutical companies expanded their efforts to find synthetic compounds with improved properties, such as longer duration of action and greater oral potency. No less than four groups of chemists isolated the active component of the corpus luteum, and in 1934, Karl Slotta and his associates at Breslau identified its structure. Three years later, A. W. Makepeace and his co-workers at the University of Pennsylvania reported that corpus luteum preparations or pure progesterone completely inhibited postcoital ovulation in the rabbit, and Dempsey at Brown University obtained similar results in guinea pigs. The highly potent estrogenic hormone ethinyl estradiol was synthesized in 1938.

In 1935, Russell Marker developed an efficient method for converting certain plant sterols (sapogenins) into progesterone, and then he began an active botanical search for a good source of this material. The search brought to light a compound, diosgenin, available from the root of several species of *Dioscorea,* called cabeza de negra in southern Mexico, which appeared to Marker to be the key material. In 1943, working in complete isolation for two months, he produced 2000 grams of progesterone. Since progesterone was then selling at $80 a gram, he had no difficulty in forming an association with a small Mexican pharmaceutical firm, which adopted the name Syntex, S.A. Later Marker broke off his connection with Syntex, taking the secrets of his process with him. As a result of a case of accidental hemolysis caused by barbasco root, Marker's associate Norman Applezweig found that this root was a rich source of the desired sterol, and the barbasco root ultimately proved to be the best raw material for the production of progesterone.

After Marker's departure, Syntex, S.A., hired George Rosenkranz, a well-qualified chemist, who within two months had deciphered Marker's methods, and Syntex was back in production. At first, the Syntex management refused to enter the field of biological application of steroid hormones. When Alejandro Zaffaroni joined Syntex in 1951, he tried to direct research toward the synthesis of new steroid hormones of biological potency.

As a result of this newly directed effort at Syntex, Carl Djerassi began a series of fruitful experiments. Progesterone has minimal activity when taken by mouth, and efforts were made to enhance this action. The synthesis of *ethisterone* was reported by L. Ruzicka and his co-workers in 1937. This substance is potent when administered, but when it was placed on the market in 1941 it proved to have undesirable androgenic properties. In 1944, M. R. Ehrenstein of the University of Pennsylvania synthesized a mixture that contained 19-norprogesterone, and bioassay in rabbits indicated that it was a powerful progestational agent. Djerassi synthesized 19-norprogesterone early in 1951 and then modified it by adding a 17-ethynyl group and produced *norethindrone,* for which a patent application was entered in November, 1952. At about the same time, Colton synthesized *norethynodrel.* Both of these substances proved to have potent progestational effects when administered by mouth.

At a conference on Contraceptive Research and Clinical Practice held in New York in December, 1936, Raphael Kurzrok of The College of Physicians and Surgeons, Columbia University, presented a paper on "The prospects for hormonal sterilization." Kurzrok apparently was unaware of Haberlandt's work and of much of the information on the antiovulatory activity of the corpus luteum and its hormone. He specifically mentioned that estrone, by inhibiting ovulation, was a possible modality for hormonal sterilization, and concluded with the opinion that "the potentialities of hormonal sterilization are tremendous." His opinion attracted little attention at that time.

In 1938, Wilson and Kurzrok concluded that functional dysmenorrhea signifies ovulation, for it occurs only in patients with a functioning corpus luteum. This led others to explore the inhibition of ovulation as a means of treating dysmenorrhea, and in 1940, S. H. Sturgis and Fuller Albright, at the Massachusetts General Hospital, reported that frequent injections of estradiol benzoate prevented cramps when ovulation was successfully inhibited. In the same year K. J. Karnaky in Texas "produced a physiologic sterility" with continuous daily doses of the synthetic estrogen, *stilbestrol.*

In 1945, *Fuller Albright* clearly specified the potential of ovulation-inhibiting doses of estrogen as a contraceptive method. His comment appeared in a section within a chapter in a large textbook of internal medicine, where it commanded no special attention.

A brief digression must be made at this point to say more about Fuller Albright, who has sometimes been called the father of American endocrinology. He would have received more attention in this history if we had chosen to devote greater space to bone disease and disorders of the

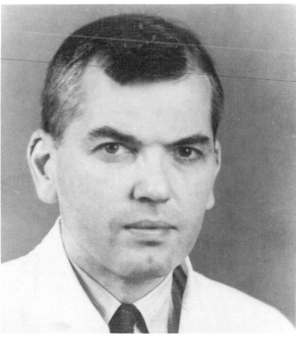

Figure 115. Fuller Albright. (Courtesy of Dr. Harry Klinefelter.)

parathyroids, areas in which he was an undisputed master. Albright was a graduate of the Harvard School of Medicine (1924), and he spent most of his professional life in the wards and laboratories of the Massachusetts General Hospital, except for a year at Johns Hopkins and another year as a traveling Fellow in Europe.

In his presidential address to the Association for the Study of Internal Secretions, in 1947, he gave a charming historical account of the development of knowledge about the parathyroid glands prior to his entry into the field in the mid-1920s. The first operations for parathyroid tumors were carried out in Europe in 1925 and in the United States in 1926. From that point on, the study of parathyroid pathology and physiology was dominated by Albright. There was no better example of a clinical investigator; he never strayed far from the practical problems presented by sick individuals. His interest in the parathyroids and their effect upon calcium and phosphorus metabolism made him an expert in the diagnosis and treatment of metabolic bone disease and urinary calculi. He recognized idiopathic hypoparathyroidism and showed how it could be treated with AT-10 (dihydrotachysterol). He also was the first to recognize the osteomalacia resulting from steatorrhea; the changes in bone that result from kidney disease; and the type of rickets that is resistant to treatment with vitamin D.

Cushing's disease had attracted little attention until Albright delivered his Harvey Lecture (1942) on "Cushing's syndrome: Its pathological physiology, its relationship to the adrenogenital syndrome and its connection with the reaction of the body to injurious agents (alarm reaction of Selye)." The concepts expressed in that lecture have become such standard features of steroid therapy that most people have forgotten who was responsible for introducing them. A method for the quantitative assay of follicle-stimulating hormone was developed in Albright's laboratory, which allowed him to distinguish gonadal dysgenesis from other forms of primary amenorrhea and which made possible the differential diagnosis of Klinefelter's syndrome from other forms of eunuchoidism. When these two genetic diseases were characterized in 1943, they helped to fuel the snowballing knowledge of human chromosomal defects. In this same year Albright described pseudohypoparathyroidism, which introduced the concept of target-organ resistance to the effect of hormones.

Albright's laboratory was the first in this country to measure the urinary excretion of steroids. In his Ovarian Dysfunction Clinic he introduced the "medical D and C" and demonstrated the safety and wisdom of replacement therapy for the menopause. By showing how to suppress ovulation with estrogen, while preventing metropathia with progesterone, he laid the foundation for development of the contraceptive pill, and as mentioned above he was one of the first to be aware of its potential usefulness.

Albright had the misfortune to develop signs of Parkinson's disease when he was in his thirties. The disease progressed slowly and relentlessly, and by the time he reached the age of 50, he was having great difficulty in getting about, though his intellectual brilliance and inquisitiveness seemed unimpaired. Troubled by his increasing physical dependence upon others, he decided to risk a brain operation which offered an outside chance of ameliorating some of his symptoms. The operation not only failed to achieve its objective but also put an end to his intellect and left him wholly out of touch with his surroundings for the remaining 15 years of his life.

With all his physical troubles, Albright, prior to his unfortunate operation, retained his delightful whimsical sense of humor. He was even able to make fun of his own tremors and difficulty in walking. In his 1947 presidential address, mentioned earlier, he outlines how information about hyperparathyroidism was developed by pathologists in Europe and by clinical physiologists in the United States:

> *The pathologist uncovers new truths by a tearing-down process, the physiologist gets at his new truths by a building-up process. The pathologist asks "What"; the physiologist asks "How" and "Why." The pathologist resorts to observation and correlation; the physiologist resorts to observation and correlation but, in addition, to the formulation of working hypotheses. The pathologist moves along step by step on solid ground; the physiologist loops along, albeit part of the time in thin air.*

Though they approached the subject from different directions, and with very little intercommunication, both groups arrived independently at the same point at about the same time when the first operations were performed for parathyroid tumors. "All of which proves," said Albright, "that there are two ways of killing a cat." Beneath this statement was the drawing shown in Figure 116; and beneath the drawing Albright added, "At the Massachusetts General Hospital we prefer 'A'" (Albright, 1948).

In 1950 Margaret Sanger, the noted feminist, decided that birth control technology needed advancement. She enlisted the aid of *Gregory Pincus,* a reproductive biologist at the Worcester Foundation in Massachusetts. Pincus and his associates decided to explore the potentialities of progesterone and began by repeating Makepeace's observations in rabbits. By 1952, Pincus was ready to give progesterone a clinical trial, and he secured the collaboration of John Rock, a gynecologist with a special interest in the endocrine therapy of infertility (National Science Foundation, 1973). Pincus and his associates carried out extensive tests on the synthetic hormone

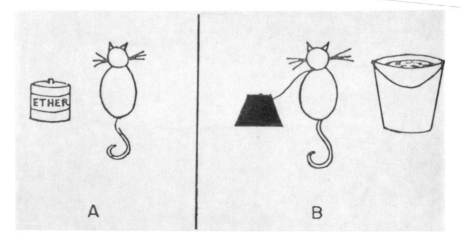

Figure 116. See text page 555 for explanation. (From Albright, F.: A page in the history of hyperparathyroidism. J. Clin. Endocrinol. *8:* 656, 1948.)

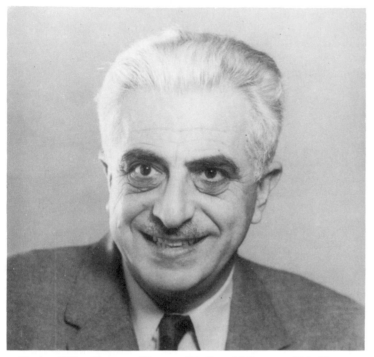

Figure 117. Gregory Pincus. (National Library of Medicine, Bethesda, Maryland.)

norethynodrel in rabbits late in 1953. Samples for clinical use were made available to Rock at the end of 1954. The first report of the studies with this compound in infertile women appeared in 1956. Except for a paper on the inhibition of ovulation by progesterone, which Pincus presented in Tokyo in 1955, the interest in contraception was well concealed.

Norethynodrel was marketed for gynecological indications in 1957, but the management of the G. D. Searle Company, which had actively collaborated with Pincus in the development of this product, refused to promote it as a birth-control pill. At this critical point, the reassurance that was needed was provided by Dr. Rock, who in addition to being a noted Boston gynecologist and member of the Harvard faculty, was a prominent Roman Catholic layman.

In order to increase the sale of its norethindrone, the Syntex Company arranged with several gynecologists in the United States to carry out clinical tests. They also established working relationships first with the Charles Pfizer Company and then with Parke, Davis, hoping to increase the use of their product. However, the management of both of these American companies refused to promote norethindrone as a contraceptive. In 1956, the Syntex Company was sold to the Ogden Corporation and subsequently became an independent company under the direction of Rosenkranz and Zaffaroni, who were committed to contraceptive research. Zaffaroni arranged for Rice-Wray, who had been working along these lines in Puerto Rico, to come to Mexico City as Director of a private family-planning center, which became a focal point for the evaluation of contraceptive agents over the next decade and a half (National Science Foundation, 1973).

During the period 1957 to 1960, Syntex supplied J. W. Goldzieher, Rice-

Wray, and Edward Tyler with norethindrone-mestranol formulations for contraceptive evaluation. A number of marketed preparations resulted from this activity and from programs supported by other pharmaceutical concerns.

In the meantime, an entirely different class of orally active progestational compounds, the 17-acetoxyprogestins, had been developed. One of these, chlormadinone acetate, had been synthesized by Syntex and licensed to the Eli Lilly Company. Since the policy of the Lilly Company excluded contraceptive research, Ray Rice, the Medical Director, and Goldzieher began preliminary unpublicized clinical trials jointly with Rice-Wray in Mexico City in 1960.

The possibility that ethinyl estrogens might have unique advantages was quickly affirmed, and a suitable daily dose of mestranol (an ethinyl estradiol) for consistent inhibition of ovulation was established. The concept of "sequential therapy," based on the extraordinary potency of mestranol with respect to pituitary inhibition, provided the culmination of the studies of Otfried Fellner.

The early preparations of norethynodrel were contaminated with a minute amount of mestranol. Clinical studies with purified norethynodrel showed poor menstrual-cycle control, and it was found that the best results were obtained by adding to the pure product a fixed amount of the "contaminant." In the early phases of this work, no effort was made to assess the contribution of estrogen to the overall contraceptive effectiveness of these combined formulations. However, clinical studies of side effects and considerations of cost led to a gradual reduction in the dosage of both estrogen and the progestational component.

This trend was given impetus by a joint British-Scandinavian epidemiological study in the early 1970s that indicated that the higher dosages were associated with thromboembolic disease. As a result, combination oral contraceptives were formulated that contain a small amount of ethinyl estradiol combined with submilligram amounts of the progestational agent. The two steroids act synergistically as hypothalamopituitary inhibitors of gonadotropin release.

A National Science Foundation study (1973) throws light on the scientific aspects of the development of contraceptives. The earliest relevant knowledge was derived from pragmatic veterinary medicine. Later, the basic research and far-sighted observations of such individuals as Haberlandt and Fellner, who perceived a contraceptive role for the ovarian hormones, were virtually ignored. The use of steroids as oral contraceptives probably would have emerged, in any event, when clinicians explored progestational compounds newly synthesized by the pharmaceutical concerns, if a positive motivational force for contraceptive development had existed. The lack of incentive accounts in part for the failure of nearly two decades of gynecoendocrine research to address itself to contraceptive development. The "climate of disrepute" in which contraception was held by society certainly retarded progress. The initiative of Sanger and Stone was crucial, but "the pill" became a reality only because of the timely developments in steroid chemistry and the activity of vigorous advocates who overcame the hesitancy of the pharmaceutical industry to venture into such an emotionally charged arena (National Science Foundation, 1973).

557

PROSTAGLANDINS   The prostaglandins are hormone-like substances that affect a wide range of physiological processes, from contraction of the uterus to secretion of gastric juice. In the early 1930s several investigators discovered that human semen and animal seminal tissues contain physiologically active substances. Two gynecologists in New York, Raphael Kurzrok and Charles C. Lieb, examined the effects of fresh semen on strips of uterus from hysterectomized women and found that the seminal fluid caused the uterine muscle to relax or contract, depending on whether the woman was fertile or sterile. At about the same time Maurice W. Goldblatt in England and Ulf S. von Euler in Sweden were experimenting with human semen and with extracts from the seminal vesicular gland of sheep. They reported that they had obtained an active substance which would stimulate muscle tissue to contract, or, when injected into an animal, would lower the blood pressure. To this previously unknown substance, von Euler gave the name *prostaglandin*. Prostaglandins are found in other body fluids and tissues and are now known to be a family of substances having a wide diversity of biological effects. In contrast to other known hormones, they are fatty acids (Pike, 1971).

By the late 1950s it was known that the prostaglandins are 20-carboxylic acids and are synthesized in the body from certain polyunsaturated fatty acids. The enzymes involved in their synthesis are widely distributed. One of the common fatty-acid precursors of prostaglandins is arachidonic acid, present as a component of the cell membrane. Consequently it appears that the conversion of arachidonic acid to prostaglandin may play an important role in regulating the function of cell membranes. It was soon found that a fatty acid extracted from seeds of the borage plant (a European herb) could be converted into a polyunsaturated fatty acid that would serve as a precursor for prostaglandin biosynthesis. Enzymes for the biosynthesis were obtained from the seminal vesicular glands of sheep. In 1968 chemists of the Upjohn Company and Elias J. Corey and his co-workers at Harvard University developed methods of total synthesis of prostaglandins from more common materials. Remarkably high concentrations of a prostaglandin isomer were found by Alfred J. Weinheimer and Oredell Spraggins of the University of Oklahoma in a type of coral, the sea whip or sea fan, which is found in reefs off the Florida coast. This isomer has been successfully converted into biologically important prostaglandins by Gordon Bundy, William P. Schneider, and their co-workers in the Upjohn laboratories (Pike, 1971).

The prostaglandins are remarkably versatile and have a wide range of effects. For example, one prostaglandin, PGE_2, lowers blood pressure, whereas a closely related member of the family, PGF_2-alpha, raises blood pressure. Intravenous injection of a small amount of either PGE_2 or PGF_2-alpha was shown by Mark Bygdeman to stimulate contraction of the uterus. This finding, together with the discovery by S. M. M. Karim that prostaglandins are present in the amniotic fluid and in the venous blood of women during the uterine contractions of labor, suggests that the prostaglandins play an important role in parturition. Prostaglandins have therefore been used to facilitate labor in thousands of women. Infusion of PGE_2 at a rate of 0.05 microgram per kilogram per minute has been found to induce delivery within a few hours. The possible use of prostaglandins as agents for abortion and for inducing menstruation is also being investigated. Kenneth T. Kirton found that PGF_2-alpha, when infused into female monkeys after mating, produced a dramatic reduction in the secretion of progesterone by the corpus luteum of the ovary. This effect prevents pregnancy, since progesterone is needed to insure implantation of a fertilized ovum in the wall of the uterus. Hence, prostaglandins or their synthetic analogues may also be useful for population control.

André Robert of the Upjohn Company has shown that prostaglandin E_1 or E_2 can inhibit gastric secretion in dogs. It is believed to produce this effect by changing the chemical activity within the cells of the stomach that are responsible for the production of gastric juice. Further experiments have shown that these two prostaglandins can prevent gastric and duodenal ulcers in rats. This suggests that they may have a similar effect in humans.

Other potential uses for prostaglandins include the following: opening the air passages of the lungs in asthmatic subjects; regulating blood pressure; clearing the nasal passages; and regulating metabolism. Recent experiments by a group in Sweden have demonstrated a clear interrelation between the prostaglandins and the substances involved in the transmission of nerve impulses. They found that infusion of prostaglandin E_2 markedly inhibited the release of norepinephrine in response to nerve stimulation. These results suggest that prostaglandins are part of the mechanism that normally controls transmission in the sympathetic nervous system. Vane and his co-workers in London have obtained results suggesting that the anti-inflammatory action of aspirin and certain other agents may be due to the fact that they block the synthesis of prostaglandins.

Thus, the diverse biological effects of the prostaglandins have opened a new chapter of hormone research, and it appears that they may be leading us to the meeting ground of two main systems of communication in the body: the hormones and the nerves. It would seem that the two systems meet most directly in the cellular membrane, which controls the selective transport of all kinds of materials into and out of the cell. The membrane also governs many aspects of the formation of products within the cell and is responsible for a cell-to-cell communication, particularly the chemical transmission of signals across the synapses in the nervous system. The discovery of the prostaglandins lends new significance to the fact that the cell membrane is made up largely of phospholipids and proteins. Phospholipids supply the fatty acids out of which prostaglandins are built; further study of this relationship may explain how the prostaglandins influence the function of cell membranes. In their effect upon the membrane, the prostaglandins may play an important role in the formation of cyclic AMP, the "second messenger," which is a key factor in translating the messages of specific hormones and in regulating the growth and differentiation of cells.

25

Medical Genetics

Genetics is to biology what the atomic theory is to the physical sciences. Human genetics has implications not only for all aspects of the science of man, but also for the cultural, political and social aspects of human activity.

(Victor A. McKusick)

Genetics is that branch of biomedical science which is concerned with the study of heredity and variation. Its development in relation to medical science has occurred almost entirely during the period of the nation's second century, and Americans have made impressive contributions to that development. Prior to 1876, a few fundamental but poorly understood aspects of the inheritance of disease had been reported. The most significant of these early reports was that of John Conrad Otto of Philadelphia, whose investigation (1803) of a family of "bleeders" first brought to light the sex-linked inheritance of hemophilia. Two other American families in which the bleeding tendency exhibited the same hereditary pattern were reported by Hay in 1813 and Buels in 1815. In 1876, Horner in Germany found that colorblindness also passes from one generation to the next in a sex-linked pattern.

The modern concept of genetics got its start not with a study of disease but with the painstaking experiments of the Moravian monk Gregor Johann Mendel. His experimental subject was a plant, the common garden pea. He began his work with 34 different kinds of peas that had been grown in the monastery garden under close observation for two years to make sure that each plant was a pure strain. Of these proven strains he chose 22 for his experiments. Seven pairs of contrasting characteristics were selected for study (e.g., red blossoms vs. white blossoms, tall plants vs. short plants), and in each of his seven experiments 287 crosses were made on 70 plants. He worked with these large numbers in order to prevent pure chance from affecting his results.

Mendel reported his experiments and his conclusions in 1865 at a meeting of a small society of naturalists in the Czech village of Brúnn (now Brno), where his monastery garden was located. His audience, confused by Mendel's mixture of botany and mathematics, is said to have shown little interest in his paper (Woglom, 1949). The paper, published in the Transactions of this insignificant society, was quickly forgotten in Brúnn and received no attention elsewhere. Yet what Mendel had reported formed the very foundation of the science of genetics. He had shown that when two pea plants with contrasting characters were mated, the hybrid offspring resembled one or the other parent, depending upon which character was dominant. For example, if a plant with red blossoms was mated with one that had white blossoms, all of the first generation of hybrids had red blossoms. This is because in garden peas the red color is dominant over white. However, the factor for white had not been lost, for some of the second generation of hybrids were white. In later experiments performed by Mendel with snapdragons the results were quite different: when a plant having red blossoms was crossed with one having white blossoms the hybrids had pink blossoms. This was interpreted as being due to the fact that in snapdragons neither red nor white is dominant, and thus the resulting color is intermediate between the two. But here again neither the white nor the red factor was lost, since in the second generation of hybrids, some of the blossoms were red, some white, and some pink.

The behavior of these two unit characters, red and white, led Mendel to the discovery of an important law of inheritance; namely, the independent character of the units that are responsible for traits such as color. The unit for color remains intact. Though it may appear at times to blend with other units, this is not truly the case, for each unit is passed from generation to generation without losing its character. Mendel concluded that the material responsible for inheritance is transmitted as a series of discrete units, which he called elements (now called genes).

Mendel also found that if a pea plant with the factor *tallness* (TT) is crossed with one with a factor for *shortness* (SS), on the average, one quarter of the first generation will be tall (TT), one quarter will be short (SS), and one half of them will be intermediate in height (TS). The exact height depends upon the relative dominance of these two factors. In both TT and SS, the elements for height are homozygous (identical units yoked together), whereas in TS they are heterozygous (contrasting units yoked together). TT's mated with TT's produce only their own kind, and this is also true of SS to SS matings. However, matings between two TS's result in the production of offspring made up of one quarter TT's, one quarter SS's, and one half TS's. Like the color of snapdragons, this is the pattern of inheritance of *recessive* traits. In the *dominant* pattern of inheritance, the trait may come down from one parent only (e.g., red blossoms in peas), while in the *recessive* pattern the trait must be present in both parents, although neither parent may exhibit the trait in overt form.

Mendel's important observations did not reach the attention of the scientific community until 35 years later, when the report in the obscure Transactions was "discovered." After its discovery in 1900, three European botanists, Hugo deVries, Carl Correns, and Erich Tschermak, simultaneously repeated his experiments and confirmed his results.

In the meantime, other work had been going on in the field of heredity, much of it stimulated by Charles Darwin's *On the Origin of Species by Natural Selection* (1859) and *The Descent of Man* (1871). Francis Galton, Darwin's cousin, began to investigate inheritance experimentally. His book *Natural Inheritance* (1889) contained many interesting observations, including his experiments on the inheritance of certain traits in basset hounds. Galton was an ingenious and original thinker: he coined the expression "eugenics" (Greek *eugenes* = well-born), and in 1892 he introduced the use of fingerprints for identification purposes.

William Bateson did much to focus and elucidate the main points at issue in his book, *Variations* (1894). It was Bateson who introduced the term "genetics." As the result of some experiments that he had conducted on inheritance in primroses, deVries advanced the hypothesis of mutation (1901), or the abrupt or spontaneous origin of species.

Mendel had found that the inheritance of traits is governed by rather simple mathematical rules. His observations could best be explained by a simple biological mechanism. This mechanism was found to be associated with the chromosomes of the sex cells (egg and sperm) when they unite to initiate the development of a new organism. Early in the twentieth century, two scientists, Sutton at Columbia University (1903) and Theodor Boveri of Frankfort, Germany (1904), provided evidence to indicate that the hereditary material (Mendel's elements) resides in the chromosomes.

After Mendel, the next major contributor to our understanding of ge-

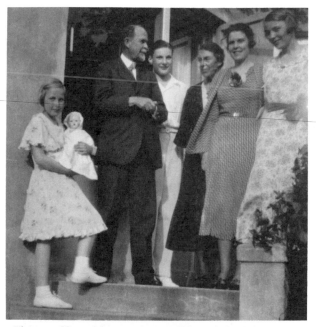

Figure 118. Thomas Hunt Morgan (second from left), Mrs. Morgan (third from right), and their daughter Isabel Morgan Mountain (second from right). The Morgans were visiting friends in Oslo on their way to Stockholm, where Dr. Morgan received the Nobel Prize for physiology and medicine. (Courtesy of Dr. Isabel Morgan Mountain.)

netic principles was *Thomas Hunt Morgan*. Morgan was a Kentuckian, and he received his higher education at the State College of Kentucky. He did postgraduate work in comparative anatomy and physiology under W. K. Brooks and H. N. Martin at Johns Hopkins, where he received his Ph.D. in 1890. From 1891 to 1904, he was Professor of Biology at Bryn Mawr College, and then he went to Columbia University as Professor of Experimental Zoology and remained there until 1928. From the latter year until his death in 1945 he was Director of the William G. Kerckhoff Laboratories of Biological Sciences at the California Institute of Technology. Though he had written on the subjects of *Regeneration* (1901) and *Evolution and Adaptation* (1903), his extensive experiments in the field of genetics did not get under way until 1909. It was in that year that Morgan, following a suggestion made by Professor W. E. Castle of Harvard, began to work with the fruit fly, *Drosophila melanogaster*. The virtues of this insect for experiments in heredity are manifold: it thrives in a laboratory environment; males and females can be distinguished from each other easily; the female lays about 1000 eggs; a new generation is produced every twelfth day, making some 30 generations in a year; and there are only four pairs of chromosomes, which simplifies the role that they play in the genetic process. Working with *Drosophila,* Morgan found that a vast amount of hereditary data could be accumulated in a short time. In his early experiments he exposed the flies, in all developmental stages, to a great variety of abnormal conditions, hoping to produce mutations which would lead to the development of new species.

Finally, in the spring of 1910, a *mutant* appeared in a pedigreed strain of flies. This mutant, a male, instead of having the normal red eyes of *Drosophila,* turned up with white eyes. This enabled Morgan to cross the white-eyed fly with a red-eyed fly in the way that Mendel had crossed tall plants with short plants. In these experiments Morgan found that there were no white-eyed females but that the female offspring of white-eyed males were carriers of the white-eyed trait, since their male offspring had white eyes. Morgan quickly recognized that white-eyedness in *Drosophila* is a sex-linked character similar to colorblindness and hemophilia in human beings. In his long series of experiments, Morgan encountered a number of other mutations, some of which were sex-linked and some which were not. He discovered that some of the characters which were not sex-linked had a tendency to be linked to each other and to appear together in the offspring (e.g., white eyes with yellow wings). This was also a case of linkage, but not to sex.

When Morgan first went to Columbia University in 1904, he came under the influence of the cytologist Edmund Beecher Wilson, who strongly supported the idea that chromosomes are the basis of heredity. It was known by that time that every species has its own characteristic number of chromosomes. Just before a cell divides to form two new cells, the chromosomes go through a series of complex steps during which each chromosome splits lengthwise, thus duplicating itself. At the time of cell division one half of each of the original chromosomes goes to each daughter cell so that every cell continues to have the number of chromosomes characteristic for the species (46 in human cells). The chromosomes are arranged in pairs; for example, there are 23 pairs in human cells and 4 in *Drosophila* cells. The process of cell division is quite different in the sex cells: both the egg and

564

the sperm go through a preliminary process of maturation in which the members of each pair of chromosomes come together and twist around each other, making one body. They then split down the middle, and the entire cell divides. Each mature egg and sperm, therefore, has half the number of chromosomes characteristic of the species; for example, in the human egg and sperm there are 23 rather than 46 chromosomes. When the mature egg and sperm unite, the new cell formed by their union contains 46 chromosomes, of which one half are contributed by each parent.

This chromosome story is important for understanding Morgan's explanation of linkage. Morgan's *Drosophila* had four pairs of chromosomes — three large ones and one so small that it appeared as two dots under the microscope. This tiny pair had been named the "m" chromosome. Morgan decided that the three pairs of large chromosomes could account for the three linkage groups that he had observed. Any new mutant that appeared must have a mutant character associated with one of the three major pairs of chromosomes. This did not explain the function of the "m" chromosome. In 1914, Hermann Muller, one of Morgan's students, discovered a fly with a new type of wing. This "bent wing" seemed to be inherited by itself. Finally it was concluded that the bent-wing character belonged to the "m" chromosome, and since a function could now be assigned to it, it was renamed, chromosome 4. Then Morgan and Muller found an eyeless mutant as well as one with no bristles on its chest. The bent-wing fly was bred with the two newly discovered mutants. The results showed that both new characters could be linked to the bent-wing and not to any others. They were then faced with the question of how the four groups of factors were represented in the chromosomes. The word *factor* as used at that time referred to a particular character: the factor for red eye, or curved wing, or reduplicated legs. Morgan decided to adopt, in place of the word *factor,* the word *gene,* which comes from the Greek word meaning race and which had been used loosely by biologists for a number of years to signify each chromosome factor.

Later an undergraduate student named Sturtevant proposed that the genes must be arranged in a particular order, a suggestion which fitted in well with the linkage theory. Subsequent events appeared to indicate that something happened at the time of maturation of the sex cells which made whole blocks of genes from one chromosome shift to the other in the pair. Morgan postulated that in the twisting, sections of the chromosomes are broken off and become rearranged, a chromosome exchanging parts with its counterpart. This process was named *crossing-over* by Morgan. Later studies showed that factors that are easily separated during crossing-over must be far apart on the chromosome, and those that are only rarely separated must be close together.

By this time it had become apparent that each chromosome is made up of a series of genes strung together somewhat like the pearls of a necklace. After thousands of experiments involving the crossing-over of many different mutants, Morgan was able to construct a "chromosome map" indicating the location in the "necklace" of the genes responsible for certain traits.

Morgan's brilliant experiments established the chromosomes as the repository of the hereditary material that is passed on from cell to cell, from parent to offspring, from generation to generation. Chromosomes were easy

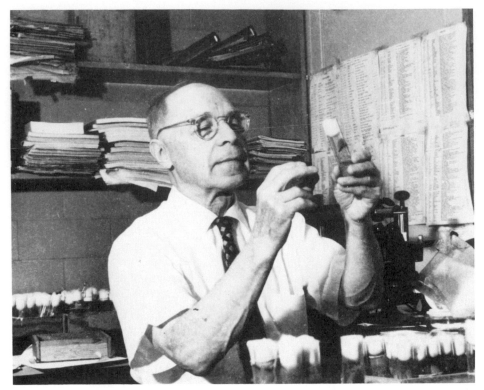

Figure 119. Hermann Joseph Muller (Courtesy of Dr. Walter J. Daly.)

to count, to stain for microscopic study, and to describe, but the genes, which Morgan considered to be the basic units of heredity, were not. The intricate maps of gene positions in the chromosomes were based on indirect evidence—the appearance of mutations either as single or linked characters or traits. What caused the mutations that Morgan and many others had observed? The answer to this question came from Morgan's most distinguished pupil, *Hermann Joseph Muller.*

MUTATIONS PRODUCED BY RADIATION The study of mutants had been limited to spontaneous mutations, which were quite rare—Morgan's specimens having produced in 17 years only 400 mutants among 20 million flies. Muller knew that mutations frequently involved only a single gene so that the change occurred at only one locus or point on the chromosome. It occurred to him that since the gene is ultramicroscopic, perhaps an atomic event would disturb it. He decided to try X-rays, for he conceived that they might produce a sharp hit on a gene, which would bring about a mutagenic effect. It was like "shooting at an atom with a bullet the size of an electron."

He began these experiments in 1926, using fruit flies whose genetic history was well known so that he was aware of the combinations of genes in their cells. If the anticipated combinations of traits did not show up after the X-ray exposure, it would mean that a mutation had resulted from a lethal gene. He could then trace the mutation by the altered trait to its position on the chromosome.

Muller obtained by half an hour's radiation exposure more than one hundred times as many mutations in one generation as would have occurred spontaneously. The mutants were as bizarre as they were numerous, occurring point-wise and randomly in one gene at a time. In addition, the X-rays produced rearrangements of parts of the chromosomes. Breakages in the chromosomes could be seen under the microscope. The broken ends joined together, but their order was different than before. Some of the breaks were far apart, others were close together, each break being caused by an independent hit. Thus, these artificially induced mutations resembled the natural ones, the only difference between them being a speeding-up of their occurrence. Muller soon recognized that the rays emitted by atomic fission are capable of causing mutations that could be passed on for generations to come. He advanced the concepts that genes constitute the basis of life and that mutations are a force in evolution, which may be caused by minute amounts of natural radiation from cosmic and other rays to which all earthbound living things are constantly exposed (Riedman and Gustafson, 1963).

Morgan's work established the chromosomes as the bearers of hereditary traits. For this work he was awarded the Nobel Prize in physiology and medicine in 1933, the first such award to be made to a native-born citizen of the United States. Muller then discovered that X-rays can produce mutations which bring about biological changes in a species. For this discovery he received the Nobel Prize in 1946.

BIOCHEMICAL GENETICS

Classical genetics is concerned with the way in which organisms receive genes from their parents and transmit them to their offspring. The study of the physical and chemical characteristics of genes has come to be known as *biochemical genetics*.

In 1869 Friedrich Miescher found a substance in the nuclei of white blood cells, which he called "nuclein." In 1884 Oscar Hertwig published in Germany a paper in which he stated, "I believe that I have at least made it highly probable that the nuclein is the substance that is responsible not only for fertilization but also for the transmission of hereditary characteristics" (Mirsky, 1968). Hertwig was close to the mark. We know now that nuclein is DNA, the genetic molecule of the genes, which was not actually identified until 1942.

In 1900 Archibald Garrod of Great Britain became interested in certain human diseases which he called "inborn errors of metabolism." Garrod investigated an inborn error called alcaptonuria. In this abnormality the individual is unable to metabolize alcapton, which chemically is known as 2,5-dihydroxyphenylacetic acid. Affected persons cannot break the benzene

567

ring of this molecule, and as a result they excrete alcapton in the urine. This substance turns black on exposure to air, and the disease is referred to as "black urine disease." Garrod recognized the biochemical nature of this disease, and after consultation with the British geneticist Bateson he concluded that the disease is inherited as a simple Mendelian recessive. He further concluded that the mutant gene must be modified in such a way that an enzyme responsible for the breaking-up of the alcapton benzene ring is absent or inactive. Thus, Garrod was the originator of the concept that a gene controls a chemical reaction through an enzyme as an intermediary—a major landmark in biochemical genetics.

Although Garrod published his classical book on *Inborn Errors of Metabolism* in 1909, over 30 years passed before geneticists recognized this interrelation between a gene, an enzyme, and a chemical reaction. Like Mendel, Garrod was ahead of his time by a third of a century. In 1923, when the second edition of his book was published, nobody knew the chemical nature of enzymes. However, even after the enzyme urease was isolated in crystalline form in 1926 by James B. Sumner of Cornell University (for which he received the Nobel Prize in chemistry in 1946) and shown to be a protein, biochemists were still skeptical, and another 10 years were to elapse before there was general agreement that all enzymes either are or contain proteins and that they act as specific catalysts by virtue of their protein components.

Garrod further surmised that alcapton comes from the amino acid phenylalanine, which is a component of our food. Some phenylalanine molecules are oxidized to tyrosine and then, through a series of reactions, to alcapton, finally ending up as carbon dioxide and water. When the metabolism of alcapton is blocked, it is excreted in the urine. Garrod found that if alcaptonuric patients were fed precursors of alcapton, such as phenylalanine or tyrosine, the excretion of alcapton was increased. In this way he identified a number of precursors of alcapton. This type of experiment has proved to be a valuable biochemical method for identifying metabolic pathways.

It was approximately 50 years after Garrod proposed his hypothesis that it was fully verified through the resolution into six enzymatically catalyzed steps of phenylalanine-tyrosine metabolism via the homogentisic acid pathway and by the demonstration that homogentisic oxidase is lacking in the liver of the alcaptonuric individual. La Du, in 1958, confirmed Garrod's prediction of this enzyme deficiency. However, the first enzyme deficiency shown to be responsible for an inborn error of metabolism was that of hepatic glucose-6-phosphatase in a glycogen storage disease. This discovery was made by Carl F. and Gerty Cori of Washington University, St. Louis, in 1952. Since these early observations, there has been a logarithmic increase in the discovery of enzymatic defects in inborn errors of metabolism.

The delay in recognizing the significance of Garrod's discoveries was due in part to the overriding attention given to nutritional and infectious diseases at that time. Garrod offered, as justification for his study of rare diseases, a quotation from William Harvey (1657): "Nature is nowhere accustomed more openly to display her secret mysteries than in cases where she shows traces of her workings apart from the beaten path; nor is there any better way to advance the proper practice of medicine than to give our minds to the discovery of the usual law of Nature by careful investigation of cases of rarer forms of disease. For it has been found, in almost all things, that what they contain of useful or applicable nature is hardly perceived unless we are deprived of them or they become deranged in some way." As Bateson put it: "Treasure your exceptions!"

In 1935, *George W. Beadle,* who had just completed a fellowship at the California Institute of Technology, went to Paris to work in Boris Ephrussi's laboratory, where he found that tissue culture techniques were being used, and he set out to perfect his performance of this technique. In those days this was a difficult task, involving work under strictly aseptic conditions, since the antibiotics had not yet been discovered. After much discouragement in working with *Drosophila,* workers in Ephrussi's laboratory ultimately produced a fly that had three eyes, and they knew that they had succeeded in transplanting an eyebud. They then began to look into the transmission of eye color by their transplantation technique. In the end, they found two substances that worked in tandem. The first was converted into the second, which in turn was converted into the pigment. They identified two genes, vermilion and cinnabar, that blocked two successive reactions. They could use one mutant type, cinnebar, to accumulate the first substance in much the same way that Garrod used alcaptonurics to ac-

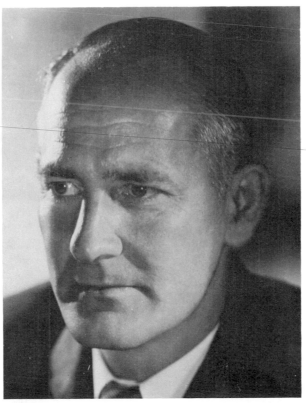

Figure 120. George W. Beadle. (National Library of Medicine, Bethesda, Maryland.)

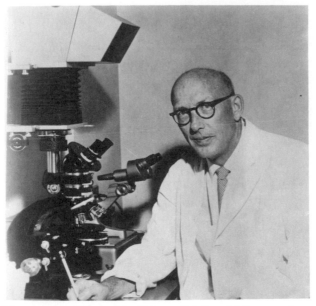

Figure 121. Edward L. Tatum. (National Library of Medicine, Bethesda, Maryland.)

cumulate and excrete alcapton. They had thus uncovered a sequence of two successive reactions controlled by genes. Then they investigated all the eye color mutants known in *Drosophila* and found that no other color gene of the 26 then available had anything to do with these two reactions. From this work they advanced the hypothesis that each gene has but a single function. Thus was originated the one gene—one enzyme concept, later to become the one gene—one protein hypothesis.

Working later with *E. L. Tatum* at Stanford University, Beadle reasoned that if the primary function of a gene is to control a particular chemical reaction, one might begin with known chemical reactions and look for the genes that control them. They searched for an organism whose chemical reactions were well known, in which they could then induce mutations that would block specific identifiable reactions. They finally hit upon the idea of using the bread mold, *Neurospora*. Back in 1928 Dodge and Shear, then at the U.S. Department of Agriculture, had worked out the life cycle of this organism, and Dodge had insisted that *Neurospora* was a more favorable organism for the study of genetics than was *Drosophila*.

Beadle and Tatum found that *Neurospora* would grow on a synthetic medium containing inorganic salts, a source of carbon and energy, and the vitamin *biotin*. From these ingredients the organism could synthesize for itself the other constituents needed for growth. The investigators first induced mutations at random in *Neurospora* with ultraviolet or X-rays. They found that some of the mutants were unable to grow on the synthetic medium, because they lacked the ability to induce certain of the chemical transformations necessary for growth. For example, one mutant could not synthesize vitamin B_6; another could not synthesize vitamin B_1. However, when the deficient vitamins were supplied in the medium, the growth of

570

the mutant was resumed. In the many mutants that were produced, Beadle and Tatum were able to identify a variety of specific chemical disabilities. Their technique was such that they could determine whether or not a single mutant gene was involved. Thus, they rediscovered what Garrod had found 38 years earlier. It is interesting that they did not know of Garrod's findings, because "we had not done our library work" (this in spite of the fact that the two editions of his book, *Inborn Errors of Metabolism,* were not rare or difficult to find). The essential difference was that geneticists and biochemists were, by that time (1941), prepared to accept Garrod's hypothesis, which had not been the case four decades earlier.

The basic concepts that had evolved up to this time and that were elegantly demonstrated by the work of Beadle and Tatum were (1) that all biochemical processes in all organisms are under genetic control; (2) that these overall biochemical processes are resolvable into a series of individual stepwise reactions; and (3) that each single reaction is controlled in a primary fashion by a single gene—a one-to-one correspondence of gene and biochemical reaction exists. In other words, each gene controls the production, function, and specificity of a particular enzyme. It follows that the primary effect of gene mutation may be as simple as the substitution of one amino acid for another, which may lead to profound secondary changes in protein structure and properties. In microbiology, the roles of mutation and selection in evolution are now better understood through the use of bacterial cultures of mutant strains.

In more immediate and practical ways, mutation proved to be of primary importance in the improvement of yields of important antibiotics, the classic example being penicillin, the yield of which went up from around 40 units per ml. of culture shortly after its discovery by Fleming to approximately 4000 units as the result of a long series of successive experimentally induced mutational steps. On the other hand, the mutational origin of antibiotic-resistant micro-organisms is of great medical significance. The therapeutic use of massive doses of antibiotics to reduce the numbers of bacteria which by mutation might develop resistance is a direct consequence of the application of genetic concepts. As important examples of the application of these same concepts to mammalian cells, one may cite the probable mutational origin of resistance to chemotherapuetic agents in leukemic cells, and in the field of cancer research it seems probable that neoplastic changes are directly correlated with changes in the biochemistry of the cell.

SEXUAL RECOMBINATION IN BACTERIA   After Tatum went to Yale in 1945, a medical student, *Joshua Lederberg,* was working in his laboratory and had just completed his second year at Columbia's College of Physicians and Surgeons. His intention was to spend the summer months only in Tatum's laboratory, but he never returned to medical school. He began his work on *Escherichia coli* which inhabit the intestine of man. Bacteria are among the lowest of living forms and are known to reproduce by simple division.

571

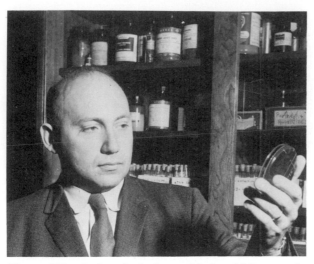

Figure 122. Joshua Lederberg. (National Library of Medicine, Bethesda, Maryland.)

Tatum and Lederberg were able to show that certain strains of *E. coli* could reproduce by a form of "genetic recombination" that resembles sexual reproduction. Within the year they had found that bacteria possess a mechanism for the sexual union of two organisms with the exchange of genetic material. In addition, by "mating" two different strains of bacteria they produced a third strain having the characteristics of both parent cells. In 1948 Lederberg went to the University of Wisconsin, where he became a full professor at the age of 29. In 1957 he organized a Department of Medical Genetics, of which he was the first chairman. For the next decade he continued to work on bacteria. He demonstrated that either an entire complement of chromosomes may be transferred from one bacterial cell to another, or only fragments of hereditary material may be transferred.

The *E. coli* organism with which Lederberg was working is often invaded by viruses. The virus pre-empts the metabolic machinery of the bacterial cell, taking it over for its own growth. The bacterium is destroyed, and several hundred virus particles emerge from the ruptured cell and go to another cell to repeat the process of bacterial destruction. After penetrating one cell, the virus may carry this cell's hereditary material to another bacterium. If the bacterial cell survives this invasion, it ends up as a new bacterial strain. Thus, Lederberg was able to produce strains with a new "heredity," or more correctly, bacteria which lost their resemblance to the parents from which they originated. He was also able to alter the virulence of bacteria by exposing them to antibiotics. Lederberg produced bacteria resistant to streptomycin and paired them with penicillin-resistant strains. The new strain, combining both traits, was resistant to both drugs. If bacteria could be made more virulent, it seemed probable that they also could be weakened by the process of genetic transference, with possibly profound effects in the control of disease-producing organisms. In addition, the basic idea that heredity can be changed gave promise of a clearer understanding of other diseases, such as cancer (Riedman and Gustafson, 1963). In 1958, Joshua Lederberg shared the Nobel Prize with Tatum and Beadle.

BACTERIOPHAGE   Viruses, as well as bacteria, have genes, and some of the most productive genetic studies have been carried out on a virus called bacteriophage (or phage, for short). In the late 1920s, Emory Ellis, at the California Institute of Technology, began a series of studies on a bacteriophage which infects the common colon bacillus. This work went slowly at first because Ellis was engaged primarily in cancer research, so he did his work on phage in his spare time. However, things began to move more rapidly in 1937, when Ellis was joined by *Max Delbruck*. Delbruck was born in Germany in 1906, and he received his Ph.D. in physics from the University of Göttingen in 1930. In 1931, he worked in the physics laboratory of Niels Bohr in Copenhagen. During the next few years his interest shifted from physics to genetics, and to gain experience in genetic research he went to the California Institute of Technology in 1937, on a Rockefeller Foundation fellowship, to work in Morgan's Department of Genetics, which was then at the peak of its fame. The collaboration of Ellis and Delbruck was extraordinarily fruitful. They had soon worked out the important features of the life cycle of bacteriophage. They found that about a half-hour after entering the colon bacillus, the parental phage multiplied to yield several hundred progeny. Delbruck realized that

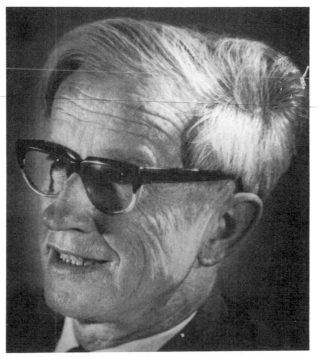

Figure 123.   Max Delbruck. (National Library of Medicine, Bethesda, Maryland.)

573

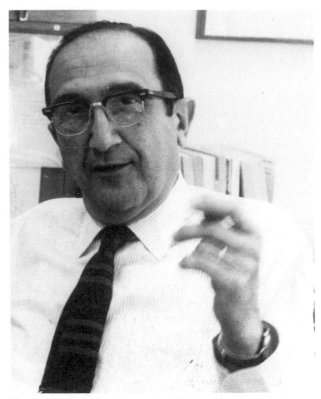

Figure 124. Salvador Luria. (National Library of Medicine, Bethesda, Maryland.)

the self-replication of the phage in the bacterial cell offered an ideal experimental system for genetic studies. Although he moved to Vanderbilt University in 1940, and while there held a position as Instructor in Physics, he did not give up his work on bacteriophage and returned to the California Institute of Technology in 1945 to continue his research there.

In 1940 at a meeting of the American Physical Society in Philadelphia Delbruck met *Salvador Luria,* a young Italian who had received his M.D. degree from the University of Turin in 1935 and had just arrived in the United States, a refugee from war-torn Europe. It soon became apparent that they both had an interest in the same fundamental problem, namely, the enigma of self-replication, and they agreed to work toward a common goal. From 1940 to 1942 Luria held a position on the faculty of Columbia University. At the same time Thomas F. Anderson, who had received his Ph.D. in Chemistry from the California Institute of Technology, was a National Research Council fellow in the laboratories of the Radio Corporation of America, where an effort was being made to develop a practical electron microscope. In collaboration with Anderson, Luria obtained an electron micrograph in 1942 of bacteriophage particles, which showed that the virus consists of a round head and a thin tail. A similar picture had been obtained the year before by E. A. F. Ruska, a German electrical engineer who had done some of the early work on the development of the electron micro-

574

scope. In 1943 Luria and Delbruck published a joint paper, which gave birth to the science of bacterial genetics by showing that the appearance of phage-resistant variants in cultures of phage-sensitive bacteria represents the selection of spontaneous bacterial mutants.

While this work was in progress, Alfred E. Mirsky, an American biochemist who had graduated from Harvard College and had received his Ph.D. from Cambridge University in England, and his co-workers at the Rockefeller Institute had been able to separate chromosomes from other cellular material and had shown that they were made up largely of deoxyribonucleic acid. At about this same time Avery and his associates at the Rockefeller Institute were carrying out their work on the "transforming substance" (described in Chapter 12), which proved also to be deoxyribonucleic acid (DNA).

By 1950 T. F. Anderson had shown that the head of the phage which he and Luria had photographed in 1942 was composed primarily of DNA stuffed into a capsule of protein and that when the phage attacks a bacterial cell, it attaches itself by the tip of its tail to the surface of its victim.

Another important worker in the field of phage research was *Alfred D. Hershey*. Hershey received his Ph.D. from Michigan State College in 1934, and from 1934 to 1950 he was on the faculty at Washington University, St. Louis. There he came under the influence of J. Bronfenbrenner, one of the first American bacteriologists to take up the study of phage. In 1945 both Hershey and Luria demonstrated the occurrence of spontaneous phage mu-

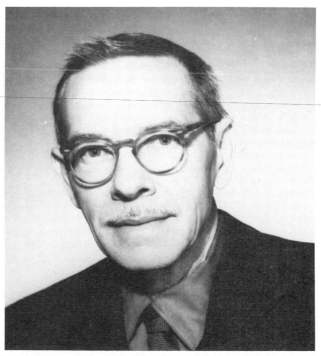

Figure 125. Alfred D. Hershey. (National Library of Medicine, Bethesda, Maryland.)

tants, and the following year Delbruck and Hershey independently discovered the existence of genetic recombination in phage.

In 1950 Hershey moved to Cold Spring Harbor, New York, where he became a member of the Department of Genetics of the Carnegie Institution. Working there with Martha Chase, in the early 1950s he performed several fascinating and crucial experiments. Anderson had shown that phage consists mainly of DNA and that the shell-like covering and tail are made up of protein. DNA contains phosphorus but no sulfur; protein contains sulfur but no phosphorus. Hershey and Chase therefore decided that it would be informative to tag bacteriophage with radioactive sulfur and radioactive phosphorus. The phage was then mixed with bacteria, and after time had been allowed for the phage to attach itself to the bacteria, the mixture was placed in a kitchen blender. The activity of the blender sheared away what remained of the phage from the bacteria, and the two were then separated in a centrifuge. Measurements of radioactivity revealed that virtually all of the radioactive phosphorus had entered the bacteria and that very little of the sulfur had done so. In other words, the phage virus had injected its DNA into the bacterial cell, but the covering and tail of the phage had not entered the bacterium. Since the injected material is able to produce a new generation of phage particles, and since viruses have genes, and genes must be transmitted to the new generation, it was concluded that the genes must be DNA and that DNA must carry the specifications for making new viruses. Thus, DNA is the genetic material—the basis of life.

It was only after the Hershey-Chase experiments had been reported that scientists began to realize the significance of the work carried out eight years before by Avery and his associates; that DNA could transform one type of pneumococcus into another type.

The Nobel Prize in physiology and medicine for 1969 was awarded jointly to Max Delbruck, Salvador Luria, and Alfred Hershey. These three men had begun their careers in different countries and in different scientific disciplines: Delbruck in Germany as a physicist; Luria in Italy as a physician; and Hershey in the United States as a chemist. Partly as a result of the war, they came closer together geographically, and as a result of their common interest in the self-replication of viruses they became friends and collaborators, although they all worked in different laboratories and in quite different research environments. Their work marked the transition from classical Mendelian genetics to the present-day "molecular biology." A better understanding of how each of the three men and their friends and colleagues contributed to this development can be obtained from the collection of autobiographical essays entitled *Phage and the Origin of Molecular Biology* (1966).

THE MOLECULAR STRUCTURE OF DNA

The discovery of the molecular structure of DNA, the substance that carries the information for heredity, had a tremendous impact upon virtually all of the scientific disciplines in the life sciences. The early study of DNA had revealed that it is an extremely long but exceedingly thin molecule. It was also known that six types of molecular units are included in its structure: sugar, phosphate, and four nucleotide bases—adenine, thymine, guanine, and cytosine. Studies had indicated that these relatively simple chemical units are repeated many times in the total structure of the DNA molecule. The units appeared to be linked together in long chains, more than a thousand times as long as they are wide. Chemical analysis disclosed that the proportions of sugar and phosphate in DNA are essentially the same in all species, but the proportion of the nucleotide bases seemed to vary widely. It was found that in any given species, the quantity of adenine (A) always equaled that of thymine (T), and the amount of guanine (G) was always the same as that of cytosine (C); and the evidence indicated that A and T somehow always were linked to each other, as were G and C. Professor M. H. F. Wilkins, working at King's College, London, found that when DNA is examined under polarized light it appears to possess the regular pattern of a crystalline substance. Using X-ray diffraction, Wilkins was then able to show that DNA from different species have roughly identical diffraction patterns, indicating some sort of universal molecular structure.

Erwin Chargaff received his Ph.D. in chemistry from the University of Vienna in 1928 and in that same year came to the United States for a two-year period as a research fellow at Yale University. He returned to the United States in 1935 and became a member of the faculty of Columbia University. It was the work of Chargaff and his colleagues, reported in 1950, which indicated that there is a DNA molecule characteristic of each species of organism. It was they who discerned that adenine and thymine are linked together in the DNA molecule and that the same is true of guanine and cytosine. The knowledge of the existence of these linkages was basic to the deciphering of the structure of the DNA molecule.

At about this time the British biologist Francis H. C. Crick at Cambridge University was beginning to work on the DNA problem, and in 1951 he was joined by the young American biologist *James D. Watson,* who just the year before had received his Ph.D. from Indiana University and had come to Cambridge to obtain additional experience in biological research.

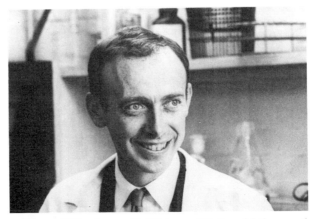

Figure 126.   James D. Watson. (National Library of Medicine, Bethesda, Maryland.)

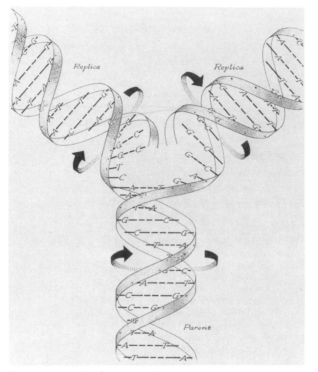

Figure 127. Replication of DNA, according to the mechanism described by Crick and Watson. (From Stent, G. S.: Molecular Biology of Bacterial Viruses. San Francisco, W. H. Freeman and Co., 1963.)

Crick and Watson believed that Wilkins's X-ray diffraction studies might indicate that the DNA molecule is helical in shape (a helix is a coiled form twisted like a corkscrew around its axis, its general contour being that of a cylinder of the same diameter throughout its length). Working on this assumption, Crick and Watson constructed a series of theoretical models of the DNA molecule. They believed that the general pattern would have to be that of two long narrow strands coiled around each other in a double helix, and that in this structure they would have to fit together the known pieces of the molecule: sugar, phosphate, and the four nucleotide bases. Their knowledge of the laws of chemistry indicated that the long narrow strands had to consist of alternating units of sugar and phosphate, but for a long time they were puzzled as to how to fit the nucleotide bases into the pattern. They tried first to hang them around the outside of the helix, but this did not work. The bases were of unequal length; adenine and guanine were long, and thymine and cytosine were short. If they hung a long cross-piece to one strand they would have to match it with a short cross-piece on the other strand, since only in this way could the bases be fitted into a helix.

This linkage of a long with a short piece would also be in accord with the previous discovery by the chemists, namely, that every A had to be linked with a T and every G with a C. Thus, cross-linked, the model of the DNA molecule resembled a twisted ladder with the long rails made of alter-

578

nating sugars and phosphates and the rungs of paired bases. With such a model, the possible variation in the total number and sequence of the bases could account for species differences in nearly two billion different kinds of living things as well as for individual differences within a species. Such a model also seemed to be in agreement with Wilkins's X-ray findings. The discovery of the ladder-like double-helical structure of the DNA molecule was announced in 1953 in a brief article by Watson and Crick in the British journal *Nature,* and at the same time Wilkins reported that the X-ray diffraction pattern was in reasonable agreement with the model.

In 1962 the Nobel Prize for physiology and medicine was awarded to Crick, Wilkins, and Watson for their elucidation of the structure of DNA. By that time Watson was Professor of Biology at Harvard University.

Since 1953 the work in many laboratories has confirmed the accuracy of the Crick-Watson model of the DNA molecule. In fact, it forms the very foundation for the present-day understanding of genetics and molecular biology.

Once the structure of the molecule had been established, the events in

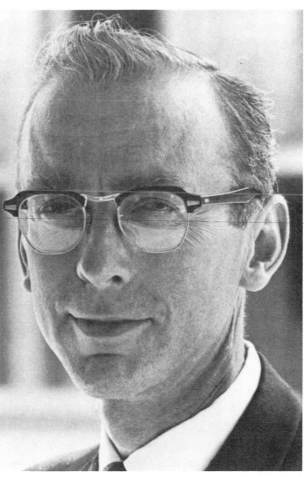

Figure 128.   Robert W. Holley. (National Library of Medicine, Bethesda, Maryland.)

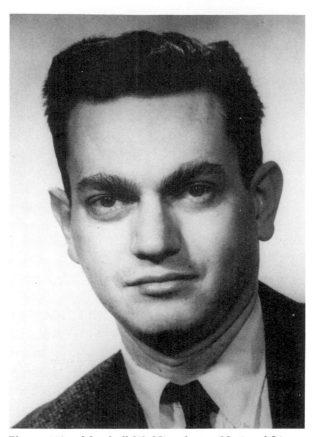

Figure 129. Marshall W. Nirenberg. (National Library of Medicine, Bethesda, Maryland.)

the genetic process began to fall into place. Briefly stated, the main features are as follows. A gene contains a molecule of DNA. From the point of view of heredity, the most important features of the molecule are the rungs of the ladder, each of which is made up of either adenine paired with thymine or guanine paired with cytosine. When a cell divides, the genes' ladder splits down the middle of all the rungs, and each half-rung on each half-ladder picks up a new half-rung from its environment in the cell, so that eventually each half-ladder will look like the old whole ladder. As a result, both of the new cells have a complete ladder resembling that of the parent cell. The number and order of the rungs of the ladder dictate the type of protein that will be formed within the cell. The message, locked in the sequence of the rungs, is read by the complicated system of ribonucleic acids (RNA molecules). The RNA receives its message as it would from a template, and the transcribed message is carried to the ribosomes in the cytoplasm of the cell. The ribosomes then synthesize a protein according to the specifications dictated by the DNA and transmitted by the RNA. In the composition of the new protein each different amino acid is specified by one sequence of three rungs in the original DNA ladder, and the arrangement of the amino acids is also dictated in the message carried by the RNA. It therefore follows that if a mutation has changed a single rung in the ladder, an abnormal protein is formed.

Many research workers were involved in working out the details of the genetic code contained in the DNA molecule and transmitted by the RNA messenger (mRNA). In 1965 three Frenchmen, François Jacob, André Lwoff, and Jacques Monod, of the Pasteur Institute in Paris, won a Nobel Prize for the part that they played in the discovery of the messenger role of RNA. In 1968 three American research workers received a Nobel Prize for "their interpretation of the genetic code and its function in protein synthesis." The work that these three scientists performed was carried on in different laboratories. *Robert W. Holley,* whose studies were performed at the United States Plant, Soil, and Nutrition Laboratory at Cornell University, determined the chemical structure of the RNA molecule responsible for translating the message in order to select specific amino acids. *Marshall W. Nirenberg* of the National Institutes of Health deciphered the "coded messages that DNA transmits to RNA which in turn prescribes the manufacture of new proteins." *Har Gobind Khorana* of the University of Wisconsin proved that the genetic code is made up of "triplets, that the triplets do not overlap, and that they are read in sequences without gaps between them."

Prior to this, two other American workers shared a Nobel Prize in 1959 for the artificial synthesis of DNA and RNA. One of the workers, *Severo Ochoa,* was born in Spain and received his M.D. degree from the University

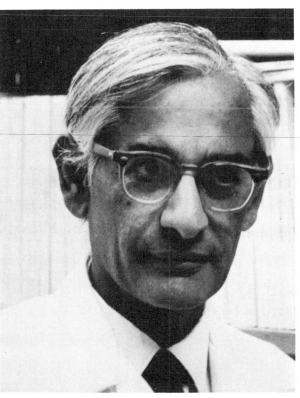

Figure 130. H. G. Khorana.

581

of Madrid in 1929. He came to the United States in 1941, and after spending a year at the Washington University School of Medicine, St. Louis, he went to the New York University College of Medicine. There he advanced to the chairmanship of the Pharmacology Department in 1946 and the chairmanship of the Biochemistry Department in 1954. Ochoa obtained an enzyme from the bacterium that turns alcohol into acetic acid. With this enzyme he and his associates were able to synthesize RNA from the four constituent nucleotides. When these were put together in a test tube with the enzyme, all four types positioned themselves to form the pattern of RNA. This synthetic product was indistinguishable from natural RNA by all the tests that could be applied.

The other American scientist who shared the 1959 prize, *Arthur Kornberg,* received his M.D. degree from the University of Rochester Medical School in 1941. He went to work at the National Institute of Health the following year. In 1946, he did postgraduate work at New York University under Professor Ochoa and then returned to the National Institute of Health, where he became head of the Enzyme and Metabolism Section in 1947. In 1952 he became head of the Microbiology Department of the Washington University Medical School, St. Louis, and in 1959 he moved to the West Coast to become executive head of the Stanford University Medical School Biochemistry Department. Kornberg had been looking for an enzyme that could be used to build DNA from individual units. In 1949 he reported that he had obtained from *E. coli* an enzyme with which thymine

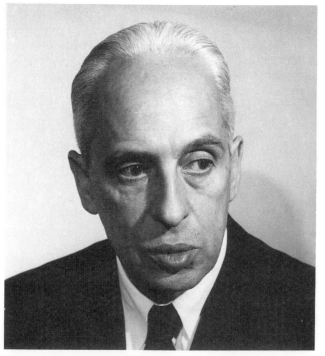

Figure 131.   Severo Ochoa. (Photo by William R. Simmons, November 16, 1959. Courtesy of Dr. Saul J. Farber.)

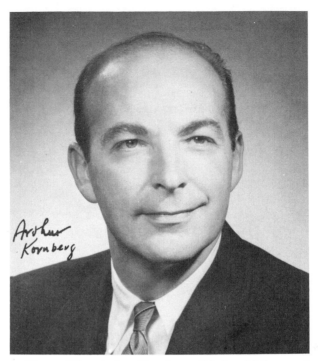

Figure 132. Arthur Kornberg, (National Library of Medicine, Bethesda, Maryland.)

could be incorporated into a molecule having some of the properties of a DNA fragment. Finally, two years later he achieved his objective: he mixed together the template nucleotide forms of the four bases (adenine, cytosine, thymine, and guanine), the purified enzyme, and a minute amount of DNA to act as a "starter." With these ingredients he was able to synthesize DNA in a test tube.

The process of synthesis was carried one step further by Khorana (recipient of the 1968 Nobel Prize), when he and his associates at the University of Wisconsin synthesized the first artificial gene—a 77-nucleotide gene that codes for the production of transfer RNA (tRNA) for the amino acid alanine. This remarkable feat was accomplished in 1970, and in 1973 Khorana and his group synthesized another gene, this time a 126-unit DNA fragment that codes for the production of the transfer RNA for the amino acid tyrosine.

To state the accomplishments of Nirenberg and Khorana in somewhat simpler language, Nirenberg synthesized a transfer RNA containing only uracil (thymine, mentioned earlier, is 5-methyl uracil). This synthetic RNA stimulated the production of a polypeptide chain consisting exclusively of the amino acid phenylalanine. This was the first item in the genetic code dictionary: UUU = phenylalanine. Khorana developed a method to synthesize long RNA chains in which the sequence of bases was known with certainty. He and his associates discovered that an RNA-like molecule containing alternating triplets of CUC (cytosine-uracil-cytosine) and UCU directs

583

the synthesis of a polypeptide in which the amino acid leucine alternates with the amino acid serine. Thus, CUC is a code word for leucine and UCU a code word for serine.

The synthesis of genes with specific molecular effects raised hope that the day might not be far off when scientists could effect a biochemical cure for genetic defects. In recent years the news media have taken hold of this subject to paint a variety of pictures, some pleasing, others frightening, of a future race produced by the use of artificial genes. Professionals outside of biology and medicine have become interested in these issues, and theologians have joined biologists, physicians, and geneticists in discussing the current scene and how to approach the future. The subject of their discussions is now known as bioethics.

THE CONCEPT OF MOLECULAR DISEASE

George W. Beadle left Stanford University to take over Morgan's position as chairman of the Department of Biology at the California Institute of Technology in 1941. One of Beadle's colleagues in his new position was the physical chemist *Linus Pauling*. Through a series of interesting coincidences Pauling was led to work on the disease sickle cell anemia. This disease is frequently encountered among black patients at the Johns Hopkins Hospital. While still a medical student, Irving J. Sherman, who graduated from the Johns Hopkins Medical School in 1940, had done some experiments on the blood of sickle-cell patients. He noticed that as the red blood cells changed from their normal round appearance to the sickle shape characteristic of the disease they became birefringent (doubly refractive). Though he could not explain why this change came about, his observation attracted the attention of William B. Castle, the Harvard hematologist who had done such important work on pernicious anemia. During World War II, Castle happened to be on a committee that included Linus Pauling in its membership. While Castle and Pauling were traveling

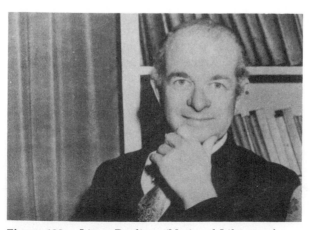

Figure 133. Linus Pauling. (National Library of Medicine, Bethesda, Maryland.)

584

together by train on their way to a meeting, Castle told his companion about Sherman's observations and other related findings which had led him to suspect that there might be a basic abnormality in the sickle-cell hemoglobin molecule. Pauling, with his background in protein chemistry, quickly realized the potential significance of this observation, and when he returned to his laboratory he began a study of sickle-cell hemoglobins.

In 1949 Pauling and his co-workers, Itano, Singer, and Wells, reported that sickle-hemoglobin is electrophoretically different, and therefore chemically different, from normal hemoglobin. In that same year James V.G. Neel reported from the University of Michigan that sickle cell disease is inherited in simple Mendelian fashion, the heterozygote possessing both sickle-hemoglobin and normal hemoglobin and the homozygote having the disease. Here then was a human "molecular disease" arising from a genetically altered molecule, a reminder of Garrod's conception of the "absent enzyme" in the hereditary diseases characterized by inborn errors of metabolism.

The work of C. C. W. Hirs, W. H. Stein, and S. Moore (1954) on ribonuclease, together with the brilliant studies of Frederick Sanger and his associates (1957), who fingerprinted the insulin molecule until its full sequence of amino acid residues had been deciphered, paved the way for the work of Vernon M. Ingram (1957) on the nature of the genetic changes introduced in the hemoglobin molecule by the mutant sickle-hemoglobin gene. After it had been shown that the hemoglobin molecule actually consists of four loosely combined polypeptide chains, the one gene–one protein hypothesis became a one gene–one polypeptide hypothesis. Ingram showed that only one of the two kinds of polypeptide chains (alpha and beta) in the hemoglobin molecule is modified by the sickle-cell hemoglobin mutant and that both identical (beta) chains are correspondingly modified. Ingram's great discovery was that only a single amino acid residue in the entire polypeptide is replaced as a consequence of the mutation. This discovery led to the conclusion that, as predicted from the Watson-Crick model of the DNA molecule, the sequence of nucleotides in the DNA molecule specifies the sequence of amino acids in the polypeptide. It thus became possible for the first time in the history of science for geneticists, biochemists, and biophysicists to discuss basic problems of biology in the common language of molecular structure, and this language was soon to become of practical importance for the clinical scientist and the practicing physician.

The hemoglobinopathies (diseases caused by defects in the hemoglobin molecule) are illustrative of the simply inherited disorders. As Victor A. McKusick has pointed out, a course in medical genetics could be taught by illustrating principles with examples drawn exclusively from the hemoglobins. Ingram's fundamental studies in this field began when he was at Cambridge University, but in 1959 he came to the United States to become a member of the faculty of the Massachusetts Institute of Technology, where he became Professor of Biochemistry in 1961. His early work in this field is described in two monographs, which appeared in 1961 and 1963. Since his original discovery of the molecular defect in sickle-hemoglobin, the continuing electrophoretic analysis of human hemoglobins has provided many additional examples of molecular variation. Indeed, the number of such variations is now so great that the Western alphabet does not contain

585

enough letters to designate them. Rhinesmith, Schroeder, and Pauling, in 1959, established that the human hemoglobin molecule contains two each of two types of polypeptide chains, designated alpha and beta. Subsequently, it was found by Vinograd, Hutchinson, and Schroeder that the sickle-cell defect occurs in a beta chain. Then studies by Itano and Singer, Itano and Robinson, and Smith and Torbert combined to show that a single gene controls the formation of a single kind of polypeptide chain. A corollary of this conclusion is that a protein molecule such as the hemoglobin molecule, which is composed of several different types of polypeptide chains, is controlled by several genetic loci. In the study of hemoglobin and other proteins, the development of starch gel electrophoresis by Oliver Smithies has been of considerable importance to human genetics in providing detection of previously unknown inherited protein variations.

At this point it might be helpful to cite several examples of inherited diseases involving abnormal hemoglobin. Sickle cell anemia is a lifelong disease that is found almost exclusively in black people. Its incidence is about 1 in every 600 blacks. It is therefore seen fairly frequently in the hospitals of cities with a large black population. The anemia, which is of the hemolytic type, may be quite severe, and it is often accompanied by a variety of debilitating symptoms. In spite of this, the disease went unrecognized until 1908, when a Jamaican Negro with anemia entered the Presbyterian Hospital in Chicago. On examining the blood of this patient, James B. Herrick, one of the country's outstanding clinicians, noted that many of the red blood cells had bizarre shapes, some of them resembling sickles. Dr. Herrick was fearful that the shape of the cells might be due to some sort of artefact, and being a rather conservative gentleman he was hesitant about claiming credit for the discovery of a new disease. It was only after examining the blood many times that he convinced himself that the shape of the cells is characteristic of the condition, and finally in 1910 he published the first paper describing sickle cell anemia. It is now known that this disease is the result of the homozygous inheritance of hemoglobin S. Hemoglobin S results from the substitution of valine for glutamic acid in position 6 of the beta chain of hemoglobin. In the heterozygous condition, SA (hemoglobin S combined with normal hemoglobin), significant anemia does not occur, but the presence of hemoglobin S in the blood can be detected by appropriate tests. This condition is known as sickle cell trait. If two persons with the sickle cell trait procreate, they will produce on the average one normal child, one with sickle cell anemia, and two with the sickle cell trait.

Among the other diseases characterized by defective hemoglobin is hemoglobin C disease. This disease, a mild form of hemolytic anemia, occurs also in the homozygous state only and not in the heterozygous. The type of inheritance is the same as that for sickle cell anemia. If a man who has the hemoglobin C trait, AC, has children by a woman with the sickle cell trait, AS, on the average their children will be AA, AS, AC, CS. Of these, none will be anemic except the CS individual. In the latter case there will be a relatively severe hemolytic anemia, usually more severe than that which is encountered in hemoglobin C disease but less severe than that encountered in sickle cell anemia.

In addition to the genetic defects that may be revealed by examination of the blood, there are others that may be recognized by growing the cells of the individual in tissue culture. In the cultured cells it may be possible to recognize specific enzyme deficiencies; for example, in cultures of fibroblasts it is possible to demonstrate deficiency of the enzyme P-gal-transferase in the disease known as galactosemia, and a deficiency of cystathionine synthetase in the condition known as homocystinuria.

THE Rh SYSTEM Another type of medical problem arises not from genetic defects but from genetic differences between individuals. It has long been known that organs transplanted from one animal to another are rejected by the recipient and that when blood is injected from one animal into another it causes a violent and frequently fatal reaction. The incompatibility is noted not only between animals of different species but also between individuals of the same species. It was these individual differences that made blood transfusion such a hazardous undertaking until Landsteiner discovered the ABO blood groups.

Few discoveries in the field of genetics have had as much practical importance to medicine as the almost casual observation in 1939 by Levine and Stetson of an unusual case of intragroup agglutination. In this note the consequences of immunization of a mother by a heterozygous, antigenically distinct fetus are clearly set out. Then in a classic paper Landsteiner and Wiener independently provided a superb description of the serology and inheritance of the Rh system. In these two papers, two quite different means of observation—one purely clinical and the other, in its inception at least, purely experimental—converged on the same problem.

This Rh grouping, as it is called, has an important place in the technique of blood transfusion. It has been shown that the Rh factor is responsible for hemolytic disease in the newborn, and for this reason special precautions were soon introduced in transfusing women patients of childbearing age. During World War II transfusion became a common practice in obstetrics, and the discovery of the Rh factor came just in time to prevent disastrous consequences as a result of transfusion with blood, which from the aspect of this factor, was incompatible. Routine determination of the Rh blood grouping in all females led to a marked reduction in the transfusion of young Rh negative females with Rh positive blood. This measure was intended to prevent Rh immunization.

In 1960 Finn had been studying the role of ABO incompatibility between mother and fetus in protecting against Rh immunization. He speculated that the protection conferred by naturally occurring maternal anti-A and anti-B antibody might be mimicked by injection of anti-D antibodies.

Soon after the discovery of the Rh blood groups, it was realized that of the Rh negative women who have Rh positive mates, only a small proportion become immunized and have children affected by the hemolytic disease. The Rh antigen, D, has been demonstrated on red cells only, and it seemed certain that women became immunized because whole Rh positive fetal red cells crossed the placenta and entered the maternal circulation. There was much evidence that the protection afforded by ABO incompatibility was due to the mother's anti-A and anti-B antibodies. The mecha-

587

nism may be removal of Rh positive fetal cells of groups A and B from her circulation before they have had time to immunize her.

Rh hemolytic disease is very rare among firstborn, and it has been demonstrated that in families in which a case of hemolytic disease occurs, there is nearly always a preceding ABO-compatible Rh positive baby (the immunizing fetus).

Massive transplacental hemorrhage from the fetal into the maternal circulation was first postulated by Wiener in 1948, and six years later Chown proved by means of differential agglutination and tests for fetal hemoglobin that it had taken place. Neither of these techniques is sufficiently sensitive to detect the small amounts of fetal blood that are responsible for many cases of Rh immunization. A more sensitive method to demonstrate fetal red cells in the blood of women after delivery based on the principle of differential elution of adult and fetal hemoglobin has been developed. Cohen and his co-workers tested 622 women soon after delivery of an ABO-compatible baby and found fetal cells in 303 (49 per cent). It was determined by Know, Murray, and Walker that Rh immunization is particularly likely to follow a difficult delivery. Jandl, Jones, and Castle showed in 1957 that red cells fully coated with incomplete anti-D *in vitro* are rapidly removed from the circulation by the spleen and that the proportion of cells destroyed depends on the completeness of the coating. Thus by 1960 the time was right for undertaking research to develop a method of preventing Rh immunization.

John G. Gorman, Vincent J. Freda, and William Pollack started work on experimental prevention of Rh hemolytic disease in 1961 independently of a group in Liverpool, England, but they were not seeking ways and means of eliminating fetal cells. They tried to put to practical use the 1909 finding of Theobald Smith that a mixture of diphtheria toxin and antitoxin with antibody excess does not immunize when injected. Later it had been shown that if specific antibody is given passively to an individual, subsequent injections of antigen completely fail to immunize, provided there is a state of antibody excess at all times. Because of this, in the early New York experiments with male Rh negative volunteers, the antibody injection was given before the Rh positive cells were injected. Though this concept of the New York workers differed in detail from that which motivated the Liverpool research, there is no essential difference. The injection of anti-D to clear Rh positive fetal cells from the circulation is probably merely a practical application of the "antibody excess and antigen" with which Gorman and co-workers were concerned.

During a period of several years, a number of experiments were carried out in Liverpool, Baltimore, New York, and Freiberg, in which attempts were made to prevent the development of antibodies in Rh negative male volunteers into whom Rh positive blood was injected. These and other experiments ultimately demonstrated that protection is possible in the male. Further support for this concept came from the first experiment of Gorman, Freda, and Pollack. Four volunteers were given five milliliters of gamma globulin intramuscularly before two milliliters of Rh positive blood was injected intravenously, and none of the volunteers developed an immune antibody. The importance of the work of Gorman, Freda, and Pollack was their introduction of anti-D gamma globulin instead of whole plasma to prevent immunization, thus eliminating the danger of serum hepatitis from this technique. The next step was to demonstrate that it is possible to clear Rh positive fetal blood from Rh negative women, which was easily accomplished. These experiments illustrate a successful therapeutic endeavor in a genetically based disease.

TRANSPLANTATION OF THE KIDNEY   In the past 20 years there has been a vast amount of experimental and clinical work carried out on the transplantation of kidneys. A necessary prelude for a successful program of renal transplantation was the development of an artificial kidney. There is frequently a long delay before a transplantation can be effected, and during this interval an artificial kidney helps to get the patient into the best possible condition for the operation and allows time for the search for an appropriate donor.

The first successful application of the technique of renal dialysis (the activity performed by the artificial kidney) to living animals was made by John J. Abel, L. G. Rowntree, and B. B. Turner of the Johns Hopkins Medical School in 1913. They passed the blood of dogs through a branching network of collodion tubes immersed in a bath and showed that toxic amounts of acetylsalicylic acid (aspirin) could be rinsed out of the blood. Their prediction that an artificial kidney (a term they used for the first time) would one day be used to treat acute renal failure in human beings has been amply demonstrated.

One of the problems that they had to solve in their experiments was to prevent the blood from clotting while it flowed through the artificial vessels. Abel used the leech, which was known to secrete an anti-clotting factor called *hirudin* as it sucked blood. They ground up the heads of thousands of leeches to obtain enough hirudin to keep the dog's blood from clotting in the collodion tubing. As an experiment Abel's attempt was quite successful, but the apparatus and the technique were at that stage not suited to use in human patients. The two major problems were to obtain (1) a more convenient and plentiful material for making the permeable membrane, which would hold back the protein and the cells of the blood while allowing dissolved substances to pass through and (2) a more readily available anticoagulant. In time, satisfactory answers were found to both of these problems: suitable semipermeable membranes can be made from cellophane, and a suitable anticoagulant is heparin, the material mentioned when we were describing George Minot's work in Howell's laboratory (Chap. 12).

With these techniques available, a Dutch physician who has now been a resident of the United States for many years, Willem J. Kolff, developed the prototype of the present artificial kidney in 1945 and with it treated patients suffering from uremia, the fatal condition that results from kidney failure. The pioneers in the use of the artificial kidney in this country were John P. Merrill and his group, who began their work in 1947 at the Peter Bent Brigham Hospital in Boston, using a modification of the Kolff kidney devised by Karl Walter, a surgeon-engineer at that hospital. This type of kidney is still the simplest and most effective. In it the blood passes through a cellophane tube wound around a wire-mesh drum. As the drum rotates, the blood is carried along the tube through the dialyzing bath in which the drum is immersed. Substances such as urea and sugar, which are dissolved in the blood plasma, pass through the membrane into the bath. During the early years, the artificial kidney could be used only in hospitals where the patients were under close supervision by doctors and nurses. In recent years a simpler apparatus has been designed which can be used in the patient's home.

In the usual case the patient is hooked up to the artificial kidney only intermittently: a number of hours for each of two or three days a week, and this may go on for years. Such repetitive dialyses presented a surgical problem because the tubes that carry the blood to and from the apparatus must be inserted repeatedly into the patient's artery and vein, since the blood from the artery must flow through the apparatus and back to one of the patient's veins. Belding H. Scribner of the University of Washington devised a technique that made frequent operations unnecessary. He put two lengths of plastic tubing into the blood vessels of the arm, one in the artery and the other in the vein, and left them there. Most of the time they are connected by a short, semicircular shunt. Blood flows from the artery to the vein through the shunt. When it is time for a dialysis treatment, the shunt is removed and the two implanted tubes are connected to the apparatus.

As the years have passed, many other improvements have been made in the technique of renal dialysis, and it can now be used conveniently on a large scale over a long period of time. In addition to its use in the treatment of patients with renal failure and in the removal of various toxic substances from the blood, the artificial kidney has made possible a wide range of investigations, and much basic information of importance has been accumulated.

In 1908 Alexis Carrel transplanted kidneys in both dogs and cats. There is some uncertainty about how long these animals survived, but probably it was not for more than a few days to a week or two. At any rate, Carrel demonstrated that transplantation in these animals is surgically feasible, and he observed what has frequently been observed since then; that when the animals died, the transplanted kidneys were infiltrated with white blood cells. In 1923 C. S. Williamson of the Mayo Clinic attributed the infiltration of the grafted kidney to a "biological incompatibility" between donor and recipient.

Several unsuccessful attempts at renal transplantation in man using kidneys obtained from fresh cadavers were carried out in the years 1936 to 1951. In 1952 and 1955, Hume and co-workers reported on experiences with nine clinical cadaver transplants performed in 1951 to 1953, among which were the first transplants to achieve function adequate to maintain the life of the recipient up to, in one instance, as long as six months. The pioneer work in this country was done at the Peter Bent Brigham Hospital in Boston. In 1955 John P. Merrill, in collaboration with David M. Hume, Benjamin F. Miller, and George W. Thorn, reported his experience in nine cases in which renal transplantation had been attempted. All of the patients were terminally ill and required treatment with an artificial kidney. In eight cases the transplanted kidney came from a patient who had died of heart disease. The kidney was not placed in the normal location but was inserted into a pocket that had been fashioned in the skin of the thigh. The blood vessels of the kidney were connected with vessels in the thigh, and the urine was allowed to drain to the outside through an opening in the skin. Four of the nine transplanted kidneys functioned, and two did so well that the patients had some relief of symptoms.

In 1953 Dr. Merrill happened to be in Paris, and while there he saw a renal transplantation performed which was later reported by Michon and others. In this case the recipient was a young man, and the donor of the kidney was the young man's mother. This was the first transplantation in which the kidney came from a living donor. The immediate results were gratifying. The kidney began to form urine and functioned well for three weeks. On the twenty-first day after transplantation, blood appeared in the urine, and the kidney soon stopped functioning. This kidney on microscopic examination showed the same changes that Merrill and his associates had seen in kidneys transplanted from one dog to another.

As a result of the increasing transplantation of organs, the study of histocompatibility by tissue typing and tissue matching has become of practical importance. Transfusion is a form of tissue transplantation, and in general the rules of histocompatibility involved in transplantation of kidneys and other organs are the same as those for blood groups. In addition to the ABO locus, the important histocompatibility locus in man is that which is called HL-A because it is studied by means of antisera which are used for typing human leukocytes (the A means that this was the first human leukocyte locus to be designated). The HL-A locus may in fact be a region with two main loci (called LA and 4), closely situated on the same chromosome and each with a large number of alleles. This means that the two parents are likely to have between them four different combinations, e.g., AB in the father and CD in the mother. It follows that tissue compatibility is more likely between siblings than between parent and child. For example, if the parents are AB and CD, the offspring will be AC, AD, BC, and BD in equal proportions. Any child will therefore have a 25 per cent chance of being compatible with a given sibling but, in this example, no chance of compatibility with either parent. Because of the large number of different HL-A combinations, the proportion of unrelated individuals who are compatible is a very small value, but the proportion of compatibility of siblings is never less than 25 per cent on the average. From a genetic point of view, the ideal situation would be presented by identical twins, in whom one could expect the ABO, the HL-A, and other factors to be compatible.

In 1954, David Miller, a young physician working at the U.S. Public Health Service Hospital in Boston, had a 24-year-old male patient who was dying of renal failure. This patient had an identical twin who was in good health. Knowing that biological incompatibility was the reason that transplantation of tissues generally failed, Miller thought that if the two young men were truly identical twins, their tissues might not be biologically incompatible. He knew that there were reports of successful skin transplants between identical twins. Miller referred his patient to the group at the Peter Bent Brigham Hospital. There a number of tests were carried out to verify the fact that the two brothers were indeed identical twins. The most decisive of these tests was a successful skin graft from the healthy to the sick twin. While the tests were in progress, the patient was kept in rela-

591

tively good condition by the use of an artificial kidney. However, toward the end of 1954, his blood pressure rose and his condition deteriorated rapidly; it was therefore decided to proceed with renal transplantation. A normal kidney was removed from the donor twin by J. Hartwell Harrison, and it was transplanted into the sick twin by Joseph E. Murray. In this instance the kidney, instead of being transplanted into the thigh, was placed in the hollow of the pelvis, and the ureter was implanted directly into the bladder so that the urine would follow a normal course rather than being drained to the outside. The patient's uremia cleared up rapidly, and his blood pressure fell toward normal. Six weeks after the transplantation, the patient's own diseased kidneys were removed, and after this operation the blood pressure fell to the normal range and remained there. The transplanted kidney continued to function normally, and during the next several months the patient gained weight and returned to a normal state of health (Merrill et al., 1955).

Many valuable lessons were learned from this highly successful experience: that when genetic barriers are removed, homotransplantation of the kidney in man is at least a technically feasible procedure; that the kidney is not seriously damaged by a relatively prolonged period without circulation — in this instance the kidney was without circulation for one hour and twenty minutes while it was being transferred from the donor to the recipient; that when hypertension is associated with disease of the kidneys, it may be cured when the diseased kidneys are surgically removed. Within a relatively few years other renal transplants had been performed between identical twins, and the highly successful results fully confirmed the experience of the group at the Peter Bent Brigham Hospital.

P. B. Medawar's experiments with skin grafts in the mid-1940s had demonstrated that an animal's rejection of transplanted tissue is of the nature of an immunological reaction: the fight of antibodies against an intruding antigen. The first clue that ways might be devised to circumvent the formidable immunological barriers to transplantation came from the finding by R. E. Billingham, L. Brent, and Medawar in 1957. In experiments with a variety of animals, they found that the immune status of an animal does not become fixed until after birth, and that if a donor antigen were injected into a potential recipient *in utero,* the recipient after birth would accept a transplant from the donor of the antigen. The transplant not only would be accepted without reaction but also would last for the life of the recipient. The same research workers also developed a method for inducing tolerance in adult rats and mice. The animal's entire body was exposed to X-rays in a dose sufficient to cause death. However, death can be prevented in such an animal if it is given an infusion of cells obtained from the bone marrow or spleen of another animal. After this, the rat or mouse will accept and tolerate a transplant from the donor of the cells that saved its life. This method of inducing tolerance is very satisfactory for the mouse or rat, because their small size will permit a relatively uniform total body radiation; but it is difficult to accomplish in the dog and even more difficult to accomplish in man. Nevertheless, somewhat similar results could be obtained by combining sublethal radiation with a chemical immunosuppressive agent (i.e., an agent that suppresses the antibody reaction). The early work with combinations of radiation and chemical agents led to longer survival of renal transplants in both dogs and man, and although the vast majority of these

592

transplants were ultimately unsuccessful, several patients survived for a relatively long period.

The much greater success of renal transplants in recent years has resulted largely from the development of better methods of immunosuppression. These methods date back to the work of Schwartz and Dameshek in 1959. These workers found that when 6-mercaptopurine (6-MP) was administered to a rabbit, the animal became tolerant to a protein antigen, although this tolerance was not permanent. Meeker and co-workers then showed that 6-MP would make possible prolonged survival of skin homografts. Shortly thereafter, Roy Y. Calne and co-workers showed that the survival of renal homografts in dogs could be prolonged by the use of 6-MP and also by means of its analogue, azathioprine (Imuran).

The experimental work demonstrating that it is possible to suppress the damaging effect of the immune reaction to transplanted tissues gave new impetus to work on renal transplantation. Transplant teams made up of experts in surgery, renal dialysis, radiology, nephrology, immunosuppression, and other special fields were formed all over the world. Between 1951 and the end of 1972 almost 13,000 renal transplants had been performed. Sixty-three per cent of the transplanted kidneys were obtained from cadavers and the remainder from living donors including identical twins, siblings, parents, more distant relatives, and occasionally friends.

The 12th Report of the Human Renal Transplant Registry, which reports the experience through 1974, contains much statistical information concerning the success of transplants. A total of 16,444 transplants had been registered by 288 institutions, 164 of them in the United States. Data are given for transplants from different types of donors into recipients with various types of renal disease. The statistics show that there was a steady improvement in the results up to about 1968 but that since then there has been little improvement. If we consider only first transplants (excluding retransplants) made in 1970, the patients surviving with functional kidneys at the end of four years were as follows: (1) 70 per cent of 266 when the donor was a sibling; (2) 57 per cent of 261 when the donor was a parent; (3) 41 per cent of 1147 when the donor was a cadaver. In some of the cases in which the first transplants failed, a second or subsequent transplant succeeded, so that the chances of ending up with a functional transplant were somewhat better than the foregoing figures might indicate. The statistics also show that when there is a good HL-A tissue match, the chance of success is increased. For example, with cadaver transplants the three-year graft survival rate was only about 30 per cent when there was no match but about 45 per cent when there was a good match.

In spite of the great improvement in the results of renal transplantation, the physicians and surgeons carrying out this type of work were still faced with the need to answer the question: Should the patient remain on renal dialysis or should he undergo transplantation? The information obtained, at least up to 1974, indicates that patient survival is significantly better in recipients of transplants from living related donors; whereas the results obtained by dialysis are better than those obtained with grafts of cadaver kidneys. One great advantage of a successful renal transplant is that the patient no longer has to spend many hours each week hooked up to an artificial kidney; he can therefore lead a more independent life. The immune reaction is

593

still the factor that makes many transplantations unsuccessful. To reduce the influence of this factor, a search is constantly going on to find better methods of tissue matching and better immunosuppressive agents.

The treatment of end-stage renal disease presents financial and moral problems that are not easily solved. Only people of well above average means can individually meet the cost of either renal dialysis or transplantation. The expense, therefore, must be borne, or at least shared, by government or insurance or some other third party. If every patient with end-stage renal disease were to be treated by one method or the other, the cost could scarcely be met by all parties combined. The cost factors and the relative scarcity of suitable kidney donors have made it necessary to choose between those patients whose lives should be saved and those who should be allowed to die of their disease. In some areas, the job of making this onerous decision has been placed in the hands of committees of citizens, including doctors, clergymen, and other responsible members of the community. Regardless of the way that the decision is made, priority is usually given to relatively young individuals who are performing effectively in the community or home and who have the emotional stability needed to contend with all the unpleasant and difficult problems that attend either dialysis or transplantation.

Other organs as well as kidneys have been transplanted, but the work with the kidneys has been far more extensive and more successful. Cardiac transplantation has attracted much attention in the press, and these operations are certainly dramatic *tours de force* in surgical technique and teamwork. The first technically successful cardiac transplantation was performed in South Africa in 1967 by Christiaan N. Barnard and a team of 30 surgeons, anesthesiologists, nurses, and technicians. Barnard's patient did surprisingly well for about two weeks but died of pneumonia on the eighteenth postoperative day. Between 1967 and 1974, 263 human cardiac transplant operations were performed by 64 teams in 22 countries. The cardiac surgery team at the Stanford University Medical Center has been particularly active in this field. In 1974, 15 cardiac transplants were performed at Stanford, and only 12 were performed elsewhere. The survival rate at Stanford for their entire series of 82 transplants was 48 per cent at the end of one year and 25 per cent at the end of three years (Rider and others, 1975).

Liver transplantation has also been performed but without very encouraging results, though in a recent case a child survived for one year after receiving a fetal liver transplant (Keightley and others, 1975). Bone marrow transplantation has been performed with variable degrees of success. E. D. Thomas and his colleagues have been pioneers in this field, first at The Mary Imogene Bassett Hospital, Cooperstown, New York, and more recently at the Medical School of the University of Washington, Seattle (Thomas and others, 1975). Much work has also been done in an effort to transplant the cells of the islands of Langerhans into patients with diabetes to enable them to produce their own insulin without having to rely on exogenous sources for a supply of this hormone. A brief review of this subject, with references to current work, appeared recently in the *Lancet* (November 8, 1975, p. 909).

In all of these organ and tissue transplants, the major problem is that of inducing the recipient to accept genetically incompatible tissue without arousing a stormy and often disastrous reaction. The immunosuppressive agents now available will usually suppress or moderate the more injurious reactions, but more effective agents are urgently needed.

FETAL GENETICS AND GENETIC ENGINEERING

Much of our knowledge of human chromosomes has been acquired during the past 20 years. For a long time it was believed that the number of chromosomes in man is 48. In 1956, Tjio and Levan demonstrated that the human chromosomal complement is in fact 46. Methods have been developed for spreading out the chromosomes in a human cell so that they can be arranged in pairs and counted, and individual chromosomes can be identified. This technique has made it possible to assign numbers to all of the chromosomes and to distinguish the X chromosome of the female and the Y chromosome of the male. As a result it has become possible to identify chromosomal abnormalities with particular human diseases. For example, Lejeune in France discovered that the cells of children with Down's syndrome (mongoloid idiocy) have an extra chromosome, the total number being 47 rather than 46; and two other serious affections of infants have been found to be associated with alterations in the complement of the sex chromosomes by their staining characteristics and their fluorescence.

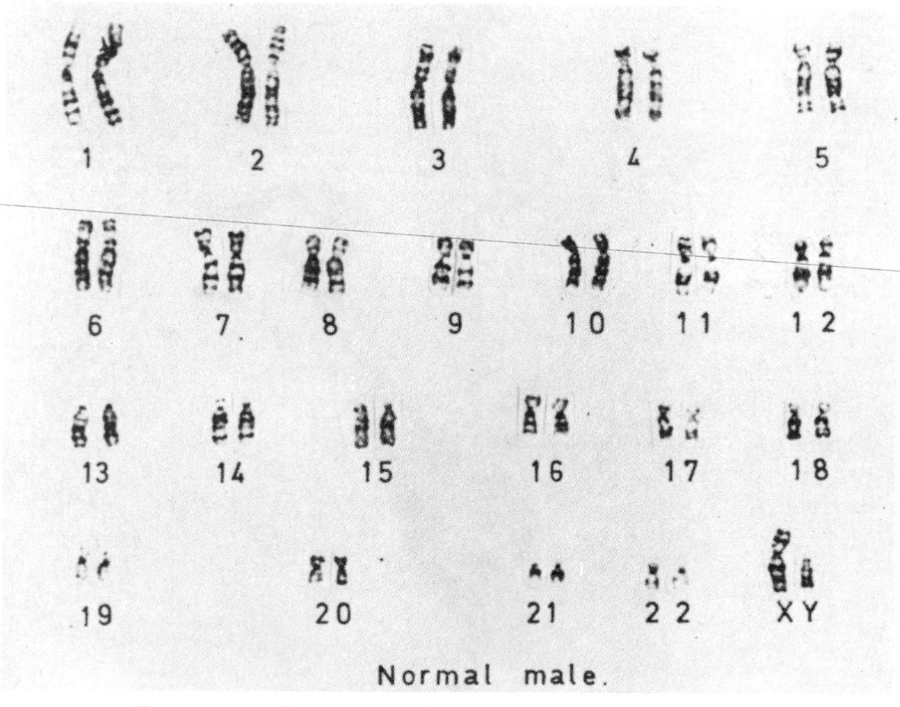

Normal male.

Figure 134. Karyotype of normal male stained with Giemsa after treatment with trypsin. (From Hirschhorn, K. C.: Chromosome identification. Ann. Rev. Med. *24*:1973. Copyright © 1973 Annual Reviews, Inc. All rights reserved.)

Murray Barr discovered in 1949 (Barr and Bertram) that cells from female subjects can be distinguished from those of male subjects by the fact that the former contain a chromatin mass, which has come to be known as the "Barr body." This has been a very useful tag in some lines of genetic research.

These chromosomal abnormalities and the developmental defects associated with them are quite apart from the 1500 human diseases caused by defects in the content or the expression of the genetic information in DNA. It has been estimated that more than 25 per cent of children admitted to hospitals have illnesses with a major genetic component. As a result of new techniques of biochemistry and cell biology, much has been learned about the biochemical mechanisms that lead from a genetic defect to clinical disease. Cells from patients can be grown and studied by tissue culture methods, and these cells often continue to express the abnormal function of a mutant gene. A major application of this technique undergoing active study at present is prenatal genetic diagnosis.

Amniocentesis was tried in 1930 by three Michigan radiologists, Thomas O. Menees, J. Dwayne Miller, and Leland B. Holly, who devised a technique for injecting radiopaque solutions into the gravid uterus. Few other reports appeared until 1952, when Douglas C. Bevis of England inserted a needle through the abdominal wall and into the uterus to extract

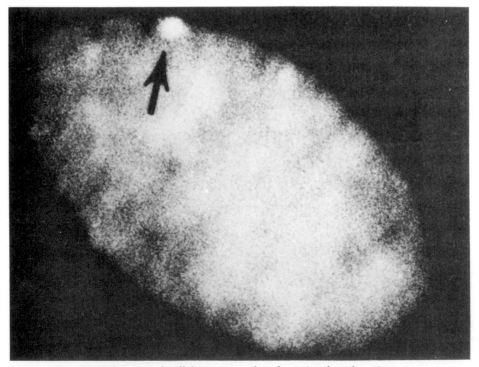

Figure 135. Buccal mucosal cell from normal male stained with quinacrine and photographed with fluorescent microscope. Arrow points to fluorescent Y body at periphery of nucleus. (From Hirschhorn, K. C.: Chromosome identification. Ann. Rev. Med. *24:* 1973. Copyright © 1973 Annual Reviews, Inc. All rights reserved.)

amniotic fluid and analyzed it to predict hemolytic disease in newborn infants. Five years later, Walker aspirated amniotic fluid and analyzed it spectrophotometrically. He reported that he could predict accurately the occurrence and severity of erythroblastosis fetalis in nearly 95 per cent of cases. More recently, amniocentesis has been used in the early part of the second trimester in order to carry out analyses on both the amniotic fluid and the cells contained in it. Cultivation of the amniotic fluid cells is required for chromosome analysis and for the identification of enzymes and other biochemicals.

Since amniotic fluid cells are mostly fetal in origin, investigators have used them for detecting the kinds of genetic disease that are caused by mutations on the X chromosome and therefore affect only males. The best known of the X-linked diseases is the bleeding disorder hemophilia. Predictions can also be made of the genetic constitution of the fetus in the case of diseases associated with an abnormal number of chromosomes or an abnormal arrangement of chromosomes. For instance, the extra chromosome found in Down's syndrome can be detected in this way.

Special types of procedures have been developed for identifying certain genetic defects in cultured amniotic fluid cells. The Lesch-Nyhan syndrome, a disease of male infants that is characterized by mental retardation and severe neurological disorders, is due to a defective gene on one of the X chromosomes of the healthy mother. The normal gene at this locus carries an enzyme which is required for the normal function of some of the cells of the brain. To determine whether a male fetus carries a defective gene at this locus, amniotic cells in tissue culture can be labeled with radioactive hypoxanthine and then exposed to X-ray film. Normal cells appear densely labeled with this radioactive material, whereas cells from a Lesch-Nyhan infant will remain free of radioactivity.

A number of other ingenious methods have been developed for diagnosing different types of serious abnormalities early in pregnancy. On the basis of these findings, parents can be advised about whether or not to interrupt the pregnancy by abortion at an early period. When pregnancies that are sure to result in the production of distressingly abnormal offspring can be aborted, it saves the parents from a great amount of emotional trauma. Furthermore, it has been calculated that large dollar economies could be effected if states provided free prenatal screening to all pregnant women over the age of 35 and to others who have a genetic background that indicates the presence of a high risk. The risk of a chromosomal defect is known to be much higher in women who are over 35 years old at the time of pregnancy. A "partial" experiment along these lines has been under way in Massachusetts since 1969, in which the state has funded cell culture and chromosome studies performed by the genetics laboratory of the Eunice Kennedy Shriver Center at Waltham.

Prenatal diagnosis of hereditary disorders is now an established part of routine antenatal care in many medical centers. It is obviously important, since each year in the United States there are more than 20,000 live births in which the infant has a chromosomal abnormality. There are also the many genetic abnormalities, some of which may not give rise to clinical disorders until the infant has become an old man or woman.

In addition to the genetic defects that can be discovered and dealt with

597

early in pregnancy, there are those which can be discovered and dealt with early in infancy. Enzyme and transport defects account for the majority of these diseases, and they are potentially amenable to dietary therapy. In the treatment of enzyme defects, the diet can be altered to reduce substrate or its precursors, add product or its derivatives, add cofactor, or add a substance that will reduce excessive enzyme activity.

The most dramatic instance of the dietary management of a genetic defect is in the case of phenylketonuria (PKU). In this disease the amino acid phenylalanine and some of its metabolites accumulate because of a defect in the hydroxylation of phenylalanine to tyrosine. Numerous experimental studies suggest that phenylalanine and its metabolites produce deleterious effects on brain metabolism. At present a casein hydrolysate is available, which although it contains almost no phenylalanine, contains adequate amounts of tyrosine, which can be used in the dietary management of infants with the PKU defect. Newborn infants are now screened for this defect by chemical tests. When the tests are positive, the infant is started on the special diet. If the diet is started early, little difficulty is encountered in maintaining a low blood phenylalanine level. The diet eliminates or greatly reduces the degree of mental retardation. Just how long the diet needs to be continued is still undetermined. Some preliminary information indicates that if the low phenylalanine diet is discontinued after the age of 4 years, there may be some temporary deterioration of behavior, but this has not been associated with a reduction of the child's I.Q.

Not all inborn errors become manifest before birth or even immediately after birth. Those involving enzymes that are not required by the fetus will not interfere with intrauterine development, and they may or may not be amenable to postnatal therapy. If the defect involves an enzyme that is required for the digestion of a nutrient, therapeutic success will depend upon whether the enzyme can be supplied from an exogenous source and, if not, whether an alternate nutrient can be provided. Both of these approaches have been employed successfully in treating disaccharidase and trypsinogen deficiencies. If the inborn error involves the metabolism of an essential nutrient for which there is no substitute, successful therapy, though less likely, is still possible provided that the requirements for the nutrient can be met by limiting it to a concentration low enough to avoid toxicity (e.g., PKU).

We still have much to learn about molecular variations and the nature and effect of the inborn errors of metabolism. The rarity of most of these diseases would seem not to warrant the time and effort devoted to their further study were it not for the human misery that they so often entail.

The extent to which genetic research has revolutionized science during the past quarter of a century is indicated by the number of Nobel Prizes awarded in this field. Many of these prizes have been won by, or shared by Americans, and the research still goes on at a dazzling pace. In 1973, Chang and Cohen at Stanford University and Boyer and Helling at the University of California (San Francisco) reported the construction in a test tube of biologically functional DNA molecules that combined genetic information from two sources. They made the molecules by splicing together segments of two different plasmids (plasmids are bits of DNA that exist apart from the chromosome in some bacteria) found in the colon bacillus and then insert-

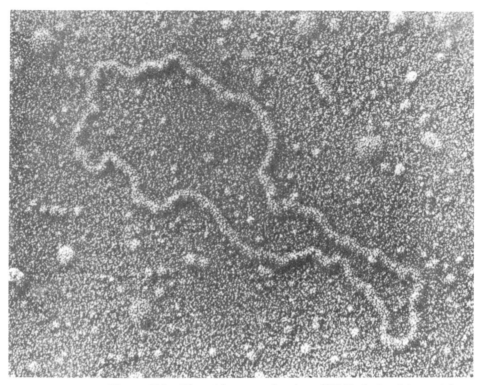

Figure 136. Plasmids are molecules of DNA that exist apart from the chromosome in a bacterium and replicate on their own. Here plasmid p SC 101 is shadowed with platinum-palladium and enlarged 230,000 diameters by electron microscopy. (From Cohen, S. N.: The manipulation of genes. Sci. Am., July, 1975, p. 24. Copyright © 1975 by Scientific American, Inc. All rights reserved.)

ing the composite DNA into *E. coli* cells, where it replicated itself and expressed the genetic information of both parent plasmids. They called these composite molecules "DNA chimeras" because they were conceptually similar to the mythological chimera (a creature with the head of a lion, the body of a goat, and the tail of a serpent). This type of procedure, which has the potential for creating a wide variety of genetic combinations, is now referred to as genetic engineering.

The scope of the technique for making chimeras continues to be broadened (Cohen, 1975). Gene manipulation opens the prospect of constructing bacterial cells that will synthesize a variety of biologically produced substances such as antibiotics and hormones or enzymes that can convert sunlight directly into food substances or useable energy. It may also provide a basis for introducing genetic information into plant or animal cells. However, such construction of novel gene combinations may give rise to serious biological hazards, and the scientific community has been cautioned against research involving genetic manipulations that might endanger the public. In 1974, the National Academy of Sciences asked Paul Berg to form an advisory committee that would consider this issue. In a report released in July, 1974, and in a letter addressed to leading professional journals, the members of the Committee expressed their concern "about the possible unfortunate consequences of indiscriminate application" of gene manipulation and formally requested all research workers to join in voluntarily deferring experiments that might lead to the creation of new organisms containing combinations of toxin-producing capabilities or of antibody-resistant genes, as well as experiments involving the introduction of DNA from tumor viruses and other animal viruses into bacteria. The committee noted that such recombinant molecules might increase the incidence of cancer and other diseases.

As pointed out by Motulsky (1974), the public media in the last few years have been filled with articles about research in molecular biology and genetics. As a result, DNA has become almost a household word. The media outdo each other in presenting lurid stories, which have aroused concern about artificial fertilization, human-primate chimeras, creation of humans according to genetic specifications, and other far-fetched consequences of the new biology. Unfortunately, but unavoidably, current research into the prevention and treatment of genetic diseases does raise ethical issues, but the real issues are quite different from the sensational ones so frequently exploited by the public press.

26

Immunology

Nothing is more satisfying for the mind than to be able to follow a discovery from its very origin up to its latest development.

(Louis Pasteur)

It has been known for centuries that a single attack of the common childhood diseases and of certain other infectious diseases renders an individual immune to subsequent attacks. This principle was first put to practical use in the early part of the eighteenth century, when it was discovered (in Turkey) that if material obtained from the pustules of a person ill with smallpox were rubbed into the skin of a healthy individual, the latter would usually develop a mild form of smallpox and would then be immune to further attacks. Unfortunately, the induced disease was not always mild; occasionally it was fatal. This method of inducing immunity was employed during a smallpox epidemic in Boston in 1721 by Dr. Zabdiel Boylston, who courageously inoculated his son and two Negro slaves. He was so pleased with the results that before the epidemic was over he had inoculated 280 persons, of whom 6 died. This was far below the mortality rate—about 15 per cent—for those who acquired the disease naturally. Nevertheless, Boylston's good work aroused a storm of protest (he was actually threatened with hanging) because the prople considered it wicked and contrary to the will of God to produce the disease deliberately (Fitz, 1911).

If one excludes these fumbling attempts at smallpox inoculations and Jenner's discovery of vaccination at the end of the eighteenth century, the science of immunology is no more than 100 years old. The year of its birth was 1881, when Pasteur discovered that he could modify the anthrax bacillus so that it would produce immunity without producing disease. Today this practical aspect of immunology—the prevention of disease—is only one facet of a very broad subject, which includes study of antigen-antibody reactions, humoral immunity, tissue immunity, transplantation immunity, tumor immunity, autoimmunity, the role of complement and

601

phagocytes, and various serologic tests and skin tests for the diagnosis of disease.

Immunochemistry, a basic area within immunology, began to emerge in the early years of the twentieth century. This new discipline was dominated for several decades by Landsteiner and his associate, the chemist Michael Heidelberger, and their students, who concentrated on the quantitative aspects of antigen-antibody reactions. Another area of immunology of more recent origin is immunobiology, which is concerned with allergy and hypersensitivity, immune tolerance, autoimmune disease, and related subjects.

In the past two decades the great increase in our knowledge of immunology has created what is sometimes called the "new immunology" (Medawar, 1974). The "old immunology" was relatively simple, concerning itself with antitoxins, skin tests, complement, and agents of defense against infections, such as agglutinins, precipitins, and lysins. In contrast, the "new immunology" concerns itself with the biology of self-recognition, the molecular basis of specificity, and the nature of information-transfer in biological systems. To use Medawar's (1974) characterization: "The new immunology can be described as the immunology that grew up in the full recognition of the fundamental principle of molecular biology that the information that specifies the structure of a protein or other macromolecule can issue only from nucleic acid." Medawar points out that formerly it was believed that certain information resided in the antigen molecule itself, as if the antigen taught the antibody-forming cell how to make an antibody complementary to it. Now it is generally conceded that antibody of a particular specificity is formed because an antigen "releases," "induces," or "activates" an antibody-forming cell in which that reaction capability already exists.

The "old immunology" achieved many important practical accomplishments such as vaccination, development of antitoxins, and the prophylactic use of toxoids. The "new immunology" has yet to establish itself in terms of practical discoveries of equal importance (Medawar, 1973).

"THE OLD IMMUNOLOGY"

In the 1790s the English physician Edward Jenner decided to put an old wives' tale to an experimental test. The gossip among the local farmers was that dairymaids who developed the blebs of cowpox on their hands never contracted smallpox. Between 1796 and 1798 Jenner inoculated 23 people with material obtained from cowpox sores and then demonstrated that the inoculated individuals were immune to smallpox. In present-day terms his experiments were not well controlled, but his conclusions were correct: inoculation with cowpox renders an individual immune to smallpox. Many decades later, Pasteur coined the term "vaccination" for such procedures to honor Jenner's important discovery (Latin *vacca* = cow).

Pasteur was the first to realize that a disease-producing micro-organism could be weakened so that it would not produce disease but retained its power to produce immunity (see Chapter 12). In 1881 he succeeded in preventing anthrax by inoculations with an attenuated anthrax bacillus. Then in 1885, employing the same principle, he demonstrated that it was possible to prevent the development of rabies in a man who had been bitten by a rabid dog.

CELLULAR
AND HUMORAL
IMMUNITY

In 1882 a young Russian zoologist, Elie Metchnikoff, took his family to Sicily so that they could enjoy a seaside vacation while he had an opportunity to study his favorite animals, aquatic invertebrates. "One day, as the family was at the circus to see some trained apes, I remained home along with my microscope and I was observing the activity of the motile cells of a transparent starfish larva, when a new thought suddenly dawned on me. It occurred to me that similar cells must function to protect the organism against harmful intruders." To test this new thought, Metchnikoff obtained some rose thorns from the garden and "introduced them under the skin of some beautiful starfish larvae which were as transparent as water." The following day he found, as he had hoped, that each thorn was surrounded by motile cells to defend the larvae against this invading foreign body. "This experiment was the basis of the phagocytic theory, to which I devoted the next 25 years of my life" (Lechevalier and Solotorovsky, 1974).

Metchnikoff named the cells that defended the body against invading agents *phagocytes* (cells that eat) because he observed that when the invading agent was small enough, it was ingested by the phagocytes. The experiments in which he clearly demonstrated how phagocytes defend the body against micro-organisms were carried out in 1883–84 using a transparent insect, the water-flea, *Daphnia*. This insect is subject to a disease caused by a fungus. Metchnikoff was able to observe and to describe in detail the battle that was waged between the invading fungus and the defending phagocytic blood cells of *Daphnia*. The battle was usually won by the phagocytes.

Metchnikoff believed that phagocytosis of invading micro-organisms is the way in which the body defends itself against disease. His hypothesis was challenged, but in time phagocytosis was recognized as one, though not the only one, of the body's defensive mechanisms.

While Metchnikoff was carrying out his early experiments on phagocytosis, a young American, *George H. F. Nuttall,* was working toward his Ph.D. at Göttingen. In 1888 Nuttall reported experiments in which he had demonstrated that the noncellular portion of blood is capable of killing bacteria but that this bactericidal property is lost if the blood is heated to 55° C (131°F). In concluding his report Nuttall said, "Metchnikoff's position that destruction of bacilli in the living body is due solely to phagocytosis, could not be confirmed."

Nuttall's discovery of the bactericidal properties of blood established the base for understanding of the humoral aspects of immunity, and Metchnikoff's work on phagocytosis established the base for the cellular aspects.

603

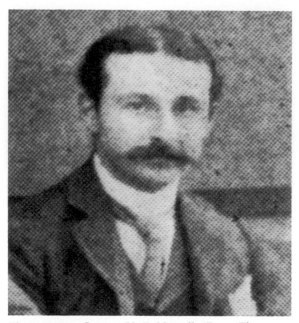

Figure 137. George H. F. Nuttall. (From The Archives Office, the Johns Hopkins Medical Institutions.)

VACCINES AND
ANTITOXINS

The diphtheria bacillus, *Corynebacterium diphtheriae,* was discovered in 1883 by Edwin Klebs, and its causal relationship to diphtheria was established by Friedrich Löffler the following year. In 1889 Emile Roux and Alexandre Yersin, working at the Pasteur Institute, reported that when diphtheria bacilli were grown in a culture medium, a toxin was produced which when injected into animals in infinitesimal doses elicited many of the characteristic features of diphtheria, followed by the death of the animal. Roux found that when he gave a very small dose of the toxin to a large animal (horse) and then injected it in gradually increasing amounts over a period of weeks, the animal developed an immunity and could tolerate enormous doses of the diphtheria toxin without displaying any symptoms. Two years later, Emil von Behring and Shibasaburo Kitasato at Koch's Institute demonstrated that the serum of a horse immunized against diphtheria toxin could be used in other animals to protect them from the effects of a lethal amount of toxin. The first human subject to be treated with the antitoxin developed in a horse was a child who was given the serum in a Berlin clinic on Christmas night, 1891.

Diphtheria antitoxin from horses began to be produced commercially under Behring's direction in 1892. The horse makes an ideal antitoxin factory: when appropriately treated with injections of antigen (toxin), it manufactures large quantities of antibody, and production of the latter may continue over a period of years. Horses grow old in such service, yielding up crop after crop of antibody. Other animals have been used for antibody production, including cattle, sheep, and even smaller animals such as rab-

604

bits, but the horse has been the most satisfactory and the most productive source.

By 1895 diphtheria antitoxin was being produced on a grand scale and was available worldwide. After the introduction of antitoxin there was an abrupt and sharp decline in the death rate from diphtheria. In the city of Baltimore, for example, the average annual diphtheria death rate, which had been more than 100 per 100,000 population during the period 1850 to 1890, fell to about 12 per 100,000 during the period 1900 to 1920.

The success with diphtheria antitoxin aroused hope of similar success in other diseases, and Behring and Kitasato quickly developed a tetanus antitoxin, which was widely used to prevent the development of tetanus following certain types of wounds. Almost all other infectious diseases proved not to be amenable to this type of therapy. However, Albert Calmette at the Pasteur Institute developed antivenins that were highly successful in preventing the toxic effects of snake bites.

NEUTRALIZATION
AND SIDE-CHAINS

In 1892 George M. Sternberg, then a lieutenant-colonel in the United States Army, infected a cow with cowpox virus and then estimated the amount of specific antibody formation by determining the amount of the cow's serum that was required to neutralize the virus. Since then this "neutralization method" has been used in various ways: evaluating and standardizing antisera; diagnosing viral infections; assessing degrees of immunity and measuring the immune response; distinguishing antigenic similarities and dissimilarities; and conducting retrospective epidemiological surveys.

Another quantitative method was introduced into immunological studies in 1897 by Paul Ehrlich. He proposed the concept of the "minimal lethal dose" as a standard measurement for toxins (i.e., the minimal amount of toxin that will cause death within four days in a guinea pig weighing 250 grams). Ehrlich's paper contained other very important principles and methods and is one of the classics of immunological science. It was in this paper that he gave the first description of his famous side-chain theory, which states that a molecule of protoplasm consists of a central core-group with a number of side-chains or receptors that have a combining affinity for food molecules and for toxins. When a toxin molecule becomes anchored to one of these receptors, the cell becomes poisoned. The receptor with its anchored toxin is then cast off into the bloodstream and is replaced by a new one. In certain circumstances, the production of new receptors is greatly in excess of requirements, and the blood is flooded with free receptors, which become anchored to toxin molecules before the latter can affect the cell. This is the bare skeleton of the famous theory that was progressively modified by Ehrlich to meet criticisms (Singer and Underwood, 1962).

COMPLEMENT

The bodies of animals or humans killed by the bite of a rattlesnake decompose with unusual rapidity. In 1893 Charles B. Ewing, a U.S. Army surgeon working in the pathology laboratory of the Johns Hopkins Medical School, began a study of this phenomenon. Rabbits were injected with rattlesnake venom, and their blood was cultured at intervals for bacteria. The blood of control rabbits, which had not been injected with venom, was cultured at the same intervals. After 24 hours the blood cultures of the venomized rabbits contained innumerable bacteria whereas those of the control rabbits contained none.

Ewing's explanation of these findings was that the venomized blood had lost all power of resisting the invasion and multiplication of certain bacteria and that the blood had been invaded by the putrefactive bacteria which are normally present in the intestines; this accounted for the rapid decomposition of the body. Ewing's discovery of the action of rattlesnake venom upon the bactericidal power of the blood anticipated the discovery of complement by Jules Bordet and Paul Ehrlich in 1899. Bordet and Ehrlich suggested the name "complement" because this substance completes the antibody's immune response. More than a decade later (1912), Simon Flexner and Hideyo Noguchi at the Rockefeller Institute determined that the manner of destruction of the blood's bactericidal property consists in the fixation of the serum complement by the snake venom. As a result, complement is not available to assist in the destruction of bacteria.

IMMUNOCHEMISTRY   The first major contribution of immunochemistry came from the study of *haptens* (Greek *haptein* = to grasp), a word coined by Landsteiner in 1921. Haptens are small chemical fragments which, when attached to already existing antigens, confer upon them a new specificity. Landsteiner pursued the subject of chemically modified antigens and haptens for more than 25 years.

An *antigen* is a substance which, when introduced into the blood or tissues, incites the formation of *antibody*. For many years only proteins were recognized as antigens. The meager knowledge of the chemistry of physiologically active proteins limited progress in immunochemistry. Nonprotein antigens first came to light during the course of experiments, conducted at the Rockefeller Institute, concerning the pneumococcus. In 1917 Dochez and Avery observed that a specific soluble substance appeared in the culture fluid in which pneumococci were actively growing. Precipitin tests indicated that each type of pneumococcus had its own particular type of *soluble substance*. Avery persuaded Michael Heidelberger to join in the work to identify this substance. The study began by demonstrating that it was a carbohydrate, a polysaccharide. Polysaccharides, having no nitrogen and a relatively simple chemical structure, lend themselves more readily than proteins to the development of quantitative immunochemical methods. Heidelberger and his associates devised techniques that allowed them to determine by weight the amount of antibodies present in a given serum. The study of the nature of antigens led the immunochemists to use specific immune sera in the determination of the chemical structure of antigens.

After Heidelberger and Kendall had demonstrated that analytical chemical techniques could be applied to the precipitin reaction, chemical procedures were applied to other serological reactions. E. A. Kabat, one of Heidelberger's students, applied quantitative techniques to the agglutination reaction. While doing postgraduate research in Sweden, Kabat conclu-

606

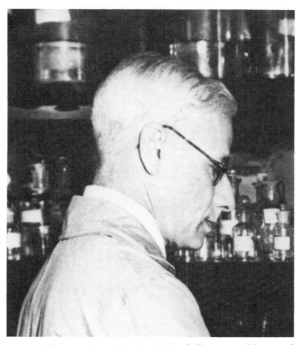

Figure 138. Michael Heidelberger. (National Library of Medicine, Bethesda, Maryland.)

sively identified antibodies as being in the gamma globulin fraction of the serum. This he determined by the use of the analytical ultracentrifuge that had just been developed in Sweden.

ANAPHYLAXIS AND HYPERSENSITIVITY
While antigen-antibody reactions protect the individual against the harmful effects of bacteria, other reactions to antigen have a destructive rather than a protective effect. Early in the twentieth century, Theobald Smith noted that guinea pigs used for the testing of diphtheria antitoxin became acutely ill if the test injections were separated by an interval of more than two weeks. These animals had become "hypersensitive" to the antitoxic serum. This phenomenon was investigated by Richard Otto in Germany in 1905; he demonstrated that it was not the antitoxin which produced the destructive reaction but the horse serum in which the antitoxin was contained. The reaction could be produced by horse serum that contained no antitoxin, but it did not take place unless there had been an interval of more than 10 days between successive injections; large doses of the serum could be given at short intervals without producing any ill effect. The following year Milton J. Rosenau and John F. Anderson at the Hygienic

607

Laboratory of the U. S. Public Health Service proved that the reaction was species-specific: a guinea pig which had been injected with horse serum became hypersensitive to horse serum only and not to the serum of other animals. Further, they demonstrated that an extremely minute amount of serum was sufficient to produce hypersensitivity. With the increasing use of horse serum in the form of diphtheria and tetanus antitoxins, more and more people became hypersensitive to horse serum and, when they received a second injection more than 10 days after the first, developed a brief illness known as serum sickness.

The tuberculin reaction, which was discussed in Chapter 12, is an example of a hypersensitivity reaction. In his original experiments with tuberculin in 1891, Koch found that the injection of tuberculin into a normal guinea pig produced practically no reaction, whereas the injection of a minute amount into a guinea pig which had been given a tuberculous infection two months previously resulted in a severe reaction. Since people who have tuberculosis are hypersensitive to tuberculin, the tuberculin skin test has been used for many decades to determine whether an individual has, or has had, a tuberculous infection. The typical positive tuberculin skin reaction does not appear for at least several hours and usually does not reach its peak for 24 hours. This delay reflects the fact that the tuberculin type of hypersensitivity, unlike the hypersensitivity to horse serum, is not mediated by an antigen-antibody complex but is the result of a reaction between sensitized cells and antigen. Hypersensitivity to tuberculin cannot be transferred from one animal to another by injection of serum, but it can be transferred by "sensitized lymphocytes."

The first widely used tuberculin skin test was devised by Clemens von Pirquet (see Chapter 11). In making this test a drop of Koch's *old tuberculin* was placed on the skin, and the skin under the drop was scratched with a needle. With the von Pirquet test it was impossible to control the amount of tuberculin that was introduced, so in 1910 Charles Mantoux devised an intracutaneous test in which a precise amount of tuberculin could be injected into the skin. Mantoux's method is the one usually employed today. It has undergone some modifications over the years, and a purified protein derivative of tuberculin (PPD) is usually substituted for the old tuberculin of Koch.

The term *anaphylaxis* (Greek *ana* = backward; Greek *phulassis* = protection) was coined in 1902 by Charles Richet, Professor of Physiology in Paris. Richet observed this condition in dogs which tolerated initial injections of an extract made from sea anemones and mussels but reacted adversely to later injections of the same extract. Countless studies carried out since then have shown that a similar condition can be induced with injections of a variety of foreign substances in many mammalian species. The research on this subject has led to the concept of a system activated by the union of antigen with a special type of antibody. This antibody becomes attached to a specific cell-membrane receptor, and excitation of the receptor results from union of the antibody with antigen. The end result is the release from the cell of materials such as histamine, serotonin, and kinin-forming enzymes. There is no general requirement for complement in this reaction. As we shall see, many years of painstaking research were necessary to arrive at an understanding of this complex subject.

ALLERGY AND
ALLERGIC DISEASES

Hay fever and asthma are well-known examples of allergic diseases. There are records of asthma in ancient history, and hay fever, first known as "summer catarrh," has been recognized for at least three centuries and was identified in the United States in 1872 by Morrill Wyman (see Chapter 8). The significance of these diseases was first pointed out in 1903 in a letter written to the Academy of Sciences in Vienna by von Pirquet and his associate Bela Schick. In this letter, agents capable of inducing the allergic state were designated as antigens or allergens. The authors of the letter stated that after the initial contact with an allergen such as a bacterium or foreign protein, there was a specific alteration of the reactivity of the organism to subsequent contact with the allergen. The specificity of the allergic state was ascribed to the formation of antibodies. Von Pirquet and Schick set forth their view that the anaphylactic state, with its dramatic immediate reaction to the antigen, and the immune state, with no reaction to the antigen, are different expressions of the allergic state. They wrote: "Allergy is not identical with hypersensitivity but shall unite the big complex which we today characterize as immunological phenomena; the term 'immunity' as a part of this concept, shall be limited to processes in which the organism acquired a complete unresponsiveness." Von Pirquet and Schick also reached the conclusion that although the antigen is neutralized by its reaction with its antibody, the antigen-antibody complexes can induce cellular lesions, the sum of which may result in systemic syndromes, such as anaphylactic shock or serum sickness (Samter, 1969).

If the von Pirquet–Schick hypothesis were correct, it should be possible to transfer passively the allergic reactivity from an allergic to a nonallergic individual by injecting the latter with the serum of the former. That such a "reaginic" antibody is in fact present in the serum of allergic patients was first proved by Prausnitz, who passively sensitized himself to fish by an intracutaneous injection of the serum of his colleague Kustner, who had an allergic sensitivity to fish. The Prausnitz-Kustner (or P-K) reaction has been used extensively in studies of allergy.

Americans have made important contributions to the study and treatment of allergic states. In 1900 Solomon Solis-Cohn of the Jefferson Medical College introduced the use of "adrenal substance" (epinephrine) for the treatment of hay fever, asthma, and urticaria (hives). This became the standard treatment for severe forms of allergy.

It was shown in 1910 by John Auer and Paul A. Lewis at the Rockefeller Institute that in true anaphylaxis in guinea pigs, death is due to asphyxia caused by a tetanic contraction of the bronchial muscles, preventing any air from entering the lungs. In the same year Samuel J. Meltzer, also at the Rockefeller Institute, suggested that the mechanism of production of an attack of bronchial asthma in human subjects was similar to the anaphylactic attack in guinea pigs and that bronchial asthma of this type should therefore be included among the allergic diseases.

The attention of Oscar M. Schloss of Cornell Medical College was attracted to allergy when he conceived the idea that a scratch test similar to von Pirquet's tuberculin test might be utilized to determine the substances to which an allergic individual is sensitive. In 1912 Schloss established the fact that the scratch test yields significant information in the diagnostic study of allergic patients.

In 1915 the intracutaneous test was introduced by Robert A. Cooke. This method of testing for sensitivity is superior to the scratch test, since it allows the physician to control the dose of the allergen. Cooke's interest in allergy dated from his childhood, when he suffered periodic attacks of asthma. He graduated from the Columbia College of Physicians and Surgeons in 1904. In 1910, while he was working at the Bellevue Hospital, one of his duties was to ride in the ambulance, and on each ambulance trip he developed a sharp attack of asthma. He realized then that he had "horse asthma" (sensitivity to horse emanations), which was not uncommon in those days. At that point he recalled that during his internship, a prophylactic injection of diphtheria antitoxin (horse serum) had caused a nearly fatal reaction (Rackemann, 1961). Cooke had a small laboratory in the old New York Hospital on East 16th Street, where he and his associates did some of the early basic work in clinical allergy. They extracted protein from pollen to use for skin tests, and they established the protein nitrogen unit for the standardization of extracts.

In 1911 Leonard Noon introduced the method of testing individuals for pollen sensitivity by the instillation of a pollen extract into the conjunctival sac of the eye. Noon's method was of interest and is still used occasionally under special circumstances, but Cooke's intracutaneous method, which was introduced in 1915, was preferred by most workers in this field. Following a lead of Noon's, Cooke also developed the method of desensitization that has been in common use for many years, and with M. E. Loveless he demonstrated the development of "blocking antibody" after desensitization. Most important was Cooke's recognition of the role of heredity not only in hay fever, urticaria, and bronchial asthma, but also in acute gastroenteritis following the ingestion of certain foods. In a paper written jointly with Albert VanderVeer, Jr., Cooke made the following significant comment: "The results of a clinical study compel us to conclude that sensitized individuals transmit to their offspring not their own specific sensitization but an unusual capacity for developing bioplastic reactivities to any foreign proteins" (Cooke and VanderVeer, 1916).

An important event of the 1920s was the introduction into Western medicine of a drug that had been used in China for 5000 years. *Ephedrine* is the active principle of the ancient Chinese drug *ma huang;* its pharmacological effects were investigated for the first time during the 1920s by K. K. Chen (who later became Director of Pharmacologic Research of the Eli Lilly Company) and C. F. Schmidt (who later became Professor of Pharmacology at the University of Pennsylvania). Ephedrine has an action similar to that of epinephrine. It is less powerful but has a more lasting effect, and it has an advantage over epinephrine in that it can be given by mouth.

"THE NEW IMMUNOLOGY"

If one had to set a year for the start of the new immunology, it would probably be 1949. Prior to that time the theory which had held sway was that the pattern of an antibody was shaped by the antigen that called it forth; the antigen molecule acting as a template at the site of production in the antibody-forming cell. F. M. Burnet and F. Fenner (1949), in Australia, pointed out that there was something lacking in this theory, since it did not account for the fact that only foreign antigens elicit a positive immune response. The cellular machinery responsible for antibody production must be able to recognize "self"; otherwise it would produce antibodies reactive against the individual's own antigens. R. E. Billingham, L. Brent, and P. B. Medawar (1953), in England, provided evidence to indicate that this tolerance of one's own antigen is acquired before birth; when foreign cells were injected into a mouse before birth, the mouse in later life would accept skin grafts from the donor of the foreign cells without any sign of the usual rejection-reaction. Medawar pointed out that acquired tolerance of a similar type occurs naturally in twin cattle. Even when the twins arise from different eggs and are genetically dissimilar, there is a mingling of their blood cells through vascular communications in the placenta. In consequence, a mutual tolerance of each other's cells emerges and continues into adult life.

These and other observations led Burnet in 1959 to discard the template theory of specific antibody production and to substitute for it his "clonal" theory. He proposed that individual lymphocytes are conditioned in some manner to respond to a single antigenic stimulus by the production of the appropriate antibody. The stimulation also leads to proliferation of the cells which respond to the antigen, thus forming a "clone" of cells that are all engaged in the production of a single specific antibody. The formation of the antibody protein, according to Burnet's theory, is determined not by the antigen's template but by the coding sequences in the DNA of the cell which responds to the antigen. When the clone is formed, all of the cells have the same genetic endowment and produce identical antibody molecules. Tolerance to the body's own antigens can be explained as a suppression of clonal proliferation. The clonal selection theory of antibody formation has frequently been challenged, but it has held its ground over the years. One of its most important aspects is that it postulates an essentially genetic basis for the specificity of immune reactions (Holborow, 1973).

IMMUNOGLOBULINS AND ANTIBODIES   In 1937 the Swedish biochemist Arne Tiselius determined by electrophoresis that the antibody-active proteins of the blood serum are globulins and that they are among the gamma globulins that move very slowly in the electrophoretic field. The globulins involved in immune reactions have been designated immunoglobulins. These proteins are not homogeneous but vary in molecular size, molecular weight, electrophoretic migration, and in other respects. Following a recommendation of the World Health Organization (WHO), the immunoglobulins are designated by the symbol Ig. This symbol is followed by a capital letter indicating the antigenic class (see Table 7).

Antibodies belong to the family of immunoglobulins. Gerald Edelman, working at the Rockefeller Institute in 1959, found that antibody molecules are composed of polypeptide chains (chains of amino acids hooked together) of more than one kind, which could be separated from one an-

611

TABLE 7. MOLECULAR WEIGHTS AND RANGE OF NORMAL
SERUM LEVELS OF IMMUNOGLOBULINS*

Class	Molecular Weight	Serum Level *mg. per 100 ml.*
IgG	150,000	300–1600
IgM	900,000	50–200
IgA	160,000	140–420
IgD	185,000	0– 40
IgE	200,000	<0.01

*Adapted from Holborow, 1973.

other by chemical means. One chain is longer and has a higher molecular weight than the other; hence one is designated the heavy chain and the other the light chain. Subsequent research has disclosed that each antibody molecule is composed of two heavy and two light polypeptide chains. The light chains can be either of two types, kappa or lambda, although in any one molecule both light chains are always of the same type. There are five types of heavy chains, which determine the immunoglobulin class of the antibody. Table 7 shows the symbols assigned to each of these classes by the World Health Organization, their molecular weight, and the upper and lower limits of the amounts usually found in normal serum. In addition, some of the five classes shown in the table have several subclasses.

Each heavy and light chain can be subdivided into domains on the basis of the amino acid sequence. A light chain has two such domains, one variable and one constant. The amino acid sequence of the variable domain differs for each antibody, whereas that of the constant domain is the same for all chains of the same type. An IgG heavy chain has one variable domain and three constant domains. The variable domain confers specificity on the antibody molecule and provides two binding sites for the antigen, one from a light and one from a heavy chain.

The characteristics of the antibody molecule are determined by genetic events in the cell that synthesizes it, and the diversity of immunoglobulins reflects the remarkable genetic diversity of the cells. Each cell is limited to the production of antibody of a single class or subclass.

When most proteins are formed, a single gene encodes all the information for the synthesis of a single polypeptide chain. That this is not the case in the synthesis of the immunoglobulins was first pointed out by W. J. Dreyer and J. C. Bennett of the California Institute of Technology. Studies of heredity and of the amino acid sequences of immunoglobulins both suggested that the constant and the variable regions of each polypeptide chain are specified by different genes and that there are probably three distinct families of structural genes for antibody molecules.

Analysis of the structure of antibodies has taken place largely in the 1960s. A few years after Edelman reported his early work on polypeptide chains, R. R. Porter of Oxford University demonstrated that the IgG molecule could be split into three pieces by the action of the proteolytic enzyme *papain*. Two of the pieces, which he termed *Fab* (fragment, antigen binding), were identical and would still combine with antigen. The third, *Fc* (fragment crystalline), was different; it would not combine with antigen but was readily crystallized (Holborow, 1973).

Unlike other proteins whose structure had been determined previously, antibody molecules were known to be heterogeneous—no single sequence of amino acids could represent the polypeptide chains. Studies to determine exactly how antibodies bound to various antigens differ from one another were aided greatly by the availability of antibody proteins made by tumors of plasma cells, myeloma proteins. The story of these proteins goes back more than 100 years; in 1847 Henry Bence Jones of London published a paper on "A new substance occurring in the urine of a patient with Mollities Ossium" (osteomalacia). The new substance described in that paper became known as Bence Jones protein, and for a long time the finding of this substance in the urine was the best diagnostic sign of plasma cell tumors (myelomas). With the development of newer techniques, it was recognized that this protein is an immunoglobulin.

Edelman's discovery that immunoglobulins contain multiple polypeptide chains suggested that Bence Jones proteins are homogeneous light chains of the myeloma protein made by the plasma cells of the tumor but not incorporated into whole molecules. This hypothesis was confirmed in 1962 by Joseph Gally and Edelman who, realizing that different Bence Jones proteins have different amino acid compositions, compared their properties with those of light chains of antibodies. These comparisons were instrumental in suggesting that antibodies with different antigen specificities differ from one another in the sequence of amino acids of which they are composed. From the first reports of partial sequence determinations by Norbert Hilschmann and Lyman Craig of the Rockefeller University (formerly Rockefeller Institute) in 1965, it became clear that these proteins have a unique structure. Concurrent studies in several laboratories suggested that the heavy chains of myeloma proteins also have variable and constant regions. The homogeneity of the constant region enabled Robert Hill and his associates at Duke University to determine the amino acid sequence of the Fc fragment of rabbit immunoglobulin.

Edelman and his colleagues at Rockefeller University then decided to determine the complete amino acid sequence of the whole immunoglobulin molecule. This molecule is about 25 times as large as the insulin molecule, in which the sequence of amino acids previously had been determined. If the immunoglobulin molecule, its chains and its fragments could be broken into small pieces about the size of insulin, it might be possible to use standard techniques for determining amino acid sequence. To accomplish this, Edelman decided to use a method that had been devised by Gross and Witkop of the National Institutes of Health. This method made use of cyanogen bromide, a reagent that selectively cleaves polypeptide chains at the positions occupied by the sulfur-containing amino acid methionine. Employing this technique, each piece was then separated from the others by chromatography; a key procedure in these separations was molecular sieving on Sephadex, a technique developed largely by Porath at the University of Uppsala, Sweden, which accelerated the thousands of separations that had to be carried out.

After the pieces had been separated, the next step was to determine the order in which they occur in the chain. This was done by cleaving the origi-

613

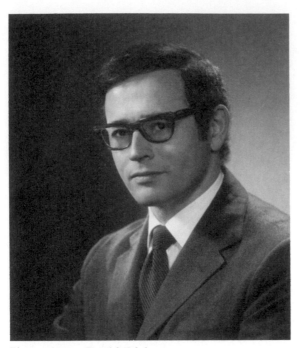

Figure 139.   Gerald Edelman.

nal chains; this time, not with cyanogen, but with enzymes that attack polypeptides at other specific sites. By comparing the two kinds of fragments, it became possible to determine which ends of the cyanogen bromide fragments butted up against one another. Many others participated importantly in work of this type, including H. D. Nial and P. Edman, C. Milstein, Frank W. Putnam, and Lee Hood. Thus within a few years it became possible to combine all of this information to reveal the structure of IgG; it is a tetrapeptide, and all five classes of immunoglobulins have a similar structure (Edelman, 1973). For their work in elucidating the structure of antibodies, Edelman and Porter were awarded the Nobel Prize in physiology and medicine in 1972.

Recent work has demonstrated the three-dimensional structure of four different antibodies from two species, worked out principally by X-ray crystallography. Studies have been carried out on human Bence Jones proteins by two groups of workers: (1) Allan Edmundson, Marianne Schiffer, and Kathryn Ely of the Argonne National Laboratory and Harold Deutsch of the University of Wisconsin; (2) Robert Huber and his colleagues at the Max Planck Biochemical Institute in Munich, Germany. Similar work has been carried out on the Fab fragment of the antibody molecule that binds the corresponding antigen by (1) Roberto Poljak and L. M. Alzel of the Johns Hopkins School of Medicine, on a Fab fragment obtained from the blood of a patient with multiple myeloma, and (2) David Davies, Eduardo Padlan, and David Segal in England, on the antibody produced by a plasma cell tumor of mice. As a result of these investigations, the backbone of the polypeptide chain could be traced, and some side-chains of the large amino acids could be identified, but each atom could not be distinguished. It therefore became necessary to determine the amino acid sequences of the proteins in order to interpret the X-ray data and to build molecular models. This was done at the National Institutes of Health by Michael Potter and Stuart Rudikoff. All of these investigators found essentially the same folding pattern in each region of the four antibody components that they were studying.

In the past few years it has been established that six to seven noncontiguous short sectors within the variable domains (three on immunoglobulin light chains and three to four on heavy chains) have unusually variable amino acid sequences; these highly variable sectors determine the shape of the antigen-binding site, constitute its boundaries, and establish its functional specificity. In this way nature accomplishes the amazing structural diversity of antibodies to meet all situations that may be encountered in the lifetime of a given individual. Genetic research in this area is still at a relatively primitive stage, but genes that code for the constant domains of immunoglobulins have been identified by serological tests for heritable immunoglobulin markers (allotypes). More recently, it has been discovered that there are genes that code for variable domains, a fact established by serological tests for the individually distinctive elements of variable domains (idiotypes). It has been shown that allotypes and idiotypes are genetically linked, a fact that is in agreement with other evidence that there are two separate genes, one for the constant and one for the variable domain, which cooperate in specifying a complete immunoglobulin chain. There is another special feature of immunoglobulin genetics, notably allelic exclusion: the expression in a heterologous cell of one or another allele, not both. The mechanism of this process is still not understood, but the result is a necessary one to insure that individual cells can produce antibodies of a single specificity only.

THE CELLS AND TISSUES OF THE IMMUNE SYSTEM

In 1936 Arnold R. Rich wrote of the lymphocyte: "Ignorance of the function of this cell is one of the most disgraceful gaps in our medical knowledge." Since that time a vast amount of information has been gathered concerning the tissues and cells involved in immune reactions. The lymphocyte has emerged as the most important component of the immune system, and in studying the lymphocyte, a great deal was also learned about the part played by the thymus, the bone marrow, the lymph nodes, and other lymphocytic tissues in relation to the lymphocyte.

There are two prongs of the immune apparatus, which perform different but related activities: (1) the cell-mediated immune response, which combats fungi and viruses and which initiates the rejection of tumors and foreign tissues such as transplanted organs; (2) humoral immunity, which is effective against bacterial infections and viral reinfections. Although these two mechanisms have elements of cooperation between them, they are quite distinct. The effective elements in the immune system reside in two populations of cells, both native to lymphoid tissue but also found in the circulating blood and in other parts of the body. Each cell in these two pop-

615

ulations has the capacity to recognize a specific antigen determinant, one of the chemical groupings by which biological substances such as proteins communicate their identity (Cooper and Lawton, 1974).

Recognition of the importance of the lymphocyte in immunology was largely due to the work of W. E. Ehrich of the University of Pennsylvania Medical School and M. W. Chase of the Rockefeller Institute, who with their associates clearly demonstrated (1945) its role in immunological reactions. Chase and his co-workers demonstrated that certain immune reactions could be transferred from one animal to another by the exchange of lymphocytes, whereas others could be transmitted by the blood serum only. The transference of bacterial immunity by the antibodies contained in the gamma globulin portion of serum was already well known, but this was the first indication that lymphocytes played a role in the immune process.

A major advance in the study of lymphocyte physiology came in 1960 when Peter C. Nowell, at the University of Pennsylvania, discovered that the small lymphocyte was not an endstage cell, as had been previously thought, but could proliferate and take on new functions when appropriately stimulated (Mills and Cooperband, 1971).

All evidence at present points to the concept that antibodies are formed by lymphocytes under the stimulation of antigen. A specific cell is responsive to a specific antigen. The responding cell proliferates, clones are formed, and antibody is produced and released. The evidence appears to bear out Burnet's original hypothesis that each lymphocyte engaged in antibody production is genetically equipped to produce only a single specific antibody.

Prior to the 1960s the function of the thymus was no less obscure than that of the lymphocyte. The thymus was often classed as one of the endocrine glands, though no one had been able to assign to it a specific physiological role. It was known that removal of the thymus in adult animals, from mice to humans, has no appreciable effect. Then in 1961, Jacques F. A. P. Miller of London, and Robert A. Good and his colleagues at the University of Minnesota reported almost simultaneously their results on the removal of the thymus in newborn mice and rabbits. Miller found that when the thymus was removed from mice within a few hours after birth, the animals failed to achieve the usual population of lymphocytes in both the blood and the lymphoid tissues. The reduction in the number of lymphocytes was accompanied by evidence of immunological deficiency; when the mice were six weeks old they failed to reject allogeneic (genetically incompatible) skin grafts, as normal mice did, and a second skin graft from the same donor failed to produce the usually enhanced rejection-reaction. Before three months had elapsed, most of the thymectomized mice had died of a wasting disease with some sort of terminal viral infection.

Miller found that the unfavorable effects of thymectomy were averted by transplanting subcutaneously either syngeneic (genetically compatible) or allogeneic normal thymus tissue. The mice did not reject the allogeneic graft because of their immunological deficiency, and when the graft had taken root and had overcome the deficiency, the mouse would accept a subsequent tissue graft from the same allogeneic donor. A normal immunological state could also be achieved by the injection of cells from the lymph nodes or spleen of normal mice. Under these circumstances the re-

616

turn of immunological function is due to the donated supply of immuno-logically competent cells. The thymus *graft* works in a different way. It re-stores function by conferring immunological competence on the host's own primitive lymphoid cells.

Osoba and Miller (1963), in trying to find out how a transplanted thymus could affect distant tissues, performed some experiments in which thymus implants were placed in sealed millipore-membrane diffusion chambers in the peritoneal cavity of young mice thymectomized at birth. Although cells could neither enter nor leave these chambers, the thymus implants restored immunological function in the mice so that they were able to reject allogeneic skin grafts. When the chamber was opened it was found to contain viable epithelial cells; it seemed likely that these cells had elaborated a humoral factor which escaped from the chamber, entered the circulation, and restored immune function (Holborow, 1973). In line with these findings, Allan Goldstein and Abraham White at Albert Einstein Medical College, in 1966, isolated from thymus tissue a polypeptide, *thymosin,* which could substitute at least partially for a functional thymus gland. They reported that when this substance was administered to mice which had been thymectomized immediately after birth, cell-mediated im-munity was partially restored and the incidence of wasting disease and death was reduced.

Miller's observations on the effect of thymectomy in newborn animals have been confirmed and elaborated by many investigators, and they have served to focus attention upon the important role that the thymus plays in the development of the immune system. Not all animal species respond to thymectomy in the same manner as mice, but it has become evident that much of the information gathered in the mouse is applicable to other species, including humans.

At the present time it is believed that the thymus performs its great and indispensable task near or shortly after the birth of an animal. During that brief period, it endows certain cells with "immunological competence." Once endowed, the cells pass along their immunological competence from one generation of cells to the next, for the life of the animal, without need-ing further assistance from the thymus. The lymphocytes and their progeni-tors and offspring are the cells that carry forward the competence.

Having performed its essential neonatal task, the thymus is no longer an indispensable organ. The lymphocytes retain their ability to react to an-tigens even after the thymus has been removed. Nevertheless, as long as it is present, the thymus continues to play a role in the animal's immunologi-cal activities. It produces a special class of lymphocytes (T-cells) whose function will be described later.

The prong of the immune apparatus that is lacking in animals deprived of the thymus at birth is the cell-mediated type of immunity. Miller's mice had a severe deficiency of this type, recognized by their inability to reject grafts of skin and other tissues from unrelated mice. Although cell-mediated immunity is deficient, these animals have an abundance of the plasma cells that produce humoral antibodies, and they display a vigorous antibody response to certain antigens.

A new light was thrown on the humoral prong of the immune appara-tus when Bruce Glick, who was then a graduate student at Ohio State Uni-

617

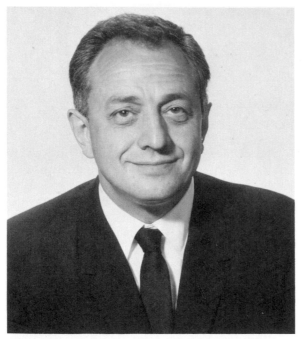

Figure 140. Robert A. Good. (From Samter, M.:
Excerpts from Classics in Allergy. Columbus,
Ohio, Ross Laboratories, 1969.)

versity, made an important discovery. Glick and his associates found that
the development of humoral immunity in chickens could be markedly impaired by the removal, shortly after hatching, of a lymphoid organ called
the bursa of Fabricius. This small pouch of lymph tissue is found only in
birds. The cell-mediated immune response of bursectomized birds is unimpaired, but N. L. Warner and A. Szenberg (1964) in Australia found that
when the thymus was removed in chickens at hatching, they developed the
same type of cell-mediated immune deficiency as was observed in Miller's
mice. They concluded that in birds the thymus and the bursa exert different
influences on immunological development. This was the first suggestion of
a basic division of the immune system into two components.

A new approach was worked out by Robert A. Good, R. D. Peterson,
and M. D. Cooper of the University of Minnesota in 1965. Either the
thymus or the bursa was surgically removed from newly hatched chicks.
Then, in order to destroy any cells influenced earlier by these organs, the
chicks were exposed to X-rays. After they had recovered from the radiation,
the structure and function of their immune systems were examined. It was
found that the effects of thymectomy and irradiation on the immune system
were remarkably similar to those of thymectomy alone in mice: the treated
birds were runty and deficient in lymphocytes, and all cell-mediated immune functions were suppressed. Birds subjected to bursectomy and

irradiation, on the other hand, had plenty of lymphocytes and normal cell-mediated responses but lacked plasma cells and humoral antibodies.

By 1965 it was possible to construct a model of the development of the immune system in chickens and mice, based on the differentiation of cells into thymic and bursal lines. This model stated that immunodeficiency diseases could be viewed as the consequence of defects in stem cells (the primitive cells from which both kinds of lymphocytes and other blood cells are descended) or of the failure of the lymphocytes to develop along one or the other pathway.

Evidence that the model could be extended to the human immune system came to light when a Temple University pediatrician, Angelo M. DiGeorge, discovered that children born without a thymus are deficient in lymphocytes and lack cell-mediated immune functions. Plasma cells and circulating humoral antibodies are present in such children, indicating that in humans the cells which produce humoral antibodies do not originate in the thymus.

The model of two distinct lines of lymphoid cells gave new insight into the behavior of the immune system. However, there were certain observations which at that stage were unexplained, including the fact that in mice and chickens deprived of a thymus, the humoral prong of the immune system is apparently insensitive to certain antigens even though plasma cells and antibodies are present. There appeared to be a need for cooperation between the thymic cells and the bursal cells in order to have a complete immune system. That such cooperation does exist was discovered through ingenious experiments performed in widely separated laboratories: Henry Claman, E. A. Chaperon, and R. F. Triplet at the Colorado School of Medicine; A. J. S. Davies at the Chester Beaty Research Institute in England; and Graham F. Mitchell and Jacques Miller, then working in Australia. The research in these laboratories led to the conclusion that in the presence of antigen, lymphocytes produced by the thymus (T-cells) promote the transformation of lymphocytes derived from the bone marrow (B-cells) into the plasma cells that synthesize and secrete antibodies (Cooper and Lawton, 1974).

This model of a dual lymphocyte population has dominated immunological research during the past decade. All of the basic elements of the theory have been demonstrated repeatedly by experimentation. The elucidation of the mechanisms by which lymphoid cells diversify and through which the two classes interact has been the subject of extensive study.

The present concept is that during intrauterine life and in the neonatal period, two systems of lymphocytic cells develop. Cells migrate from the bone marrow or other hematopoietic centers either to the thymus for differentiation, proliferation, and eventual dispersal as T-cells, or to other locations (presumably equivalent to the bursa of Fabricius in birds), to differentiate and become dispersed as B-cells. The site or sites of production of B-cells in humans is not known with certainty. B-cells are identifiable in the periphery as having easily detectable immunoglobulin on the surface, whereas T-cells have little or no immunoglobulin but have a specific surface antigen known in the mouse as *theta*.

Antigen-induction of antibody formation requires both T and B cells. T-cells regulate the responses of B-cells, which are converted into plasma

619

cells and become the actual antibody producers. Certain T-cells have the ability to enhance the differentiation of B-cells; others have the ability to suppress it. Still other T-cells, known as effector T-cells, promote and take part in cell-mediated immune reactions. These functionally diverse T-cells may be distinguished by cell surface "differentiation" antigens. Binding of antigen to either type of lymphocyte triggers transformation of the cell from a resting to an actively proliferating "blast" cell. Furthermore, the transformed T-cell secretes a variety of substances called lymphokines that act on certain other cells, stimulating or suppressing B-cell responses to antigen, or causing macrophages to differentiate into large, highly phagocytic "activated" cells, and possibly regulating the conversion of other T-cells into effectors of cell-mediated immune responses. Like hormones, the lymphokines are produced by one set of cells and have their effect on another set. However, the area over which these mediators act is restricted to specific types of cells that are close by and possibly even in contact with the secreting T-cells. Little is known about the chemistry of lymphokines.

GENETIC CONTROL
OF THE
ANTIBODY RESPONSE

Both the B and the T cells must be "precommitted, in the sense that they must exist prior to the organism's encounter with the antigen, and must have been genetically programmed to react with specific antigens that stimulate them to proliferate" (McDevitt, 1973). Since specific cells are programmed to respond to specific antigens, and since there are an enormous number of different antigens, an enormous number of genes are required to provide the appropriate control mechanism. It is therefore not surprising that the genetics of immunity has turned out to be a very difficult topic.

A few years ago Paul H. Maurer at Jefferson Medical College observed that when simple polypeptides, containing only two or three amino acids, were employed as antigens, an immune response resulted in only about 40 per cent of tested animals. This observation gave Baruj Benacerraf at the National Institutes of Health the idea of hooking the hapten onto poly-L-lysine (PLL) which was then injected into outbred guinea pigs. Some of the animals were immune responders, but others were absolute nonresponders. When he bred two responders, about 80 to 90 per cent of the offspring were responders. When he bred two nonresponders, the offspring were 100 per cent nonresponsive. These results indicated that response was dependent on a single gene inherited as an autosomal dominant. Perhaps the most significant finding was that the response to PLL was independent of the hapten conjugated with it. Thus these experiments demonstrated that responder and nonresponder animals could be differentiated in terms of the capacity to manifest reactions thought to be pure T-cell functions, indicating that the genetic defect in the nonresponder affects T-cell functions (McDevitt, 1973). Subsequent experiments seemed to imply that there are two distinct systems of antigen recognition. Antibodies recognize antigens by virtue of having heavy and light chains through which they develop combining sites for particular antigens. B-cells appear to recognize antigens via

620

antibodies on their surfaces. This is still an active area of research and will remain so until we learn how to isolate the specific gene product.

> *One can postulate that the immune response (Ir) genes control a set of recognition units or receptors for antigens that are found only on T-cells and are the T-cell receptors; they are likely to be either a heavy chain class found only on T-cells and not circulating, or a different way of recognizing foreignness on a still to be elucidated molecular basis. This view of the Ir gene product can then be fitted to the accepted view of the cellular interactions that take place when a foreign antigen is presented to the organism, as follows: the bone marrow "sees" an antigen in the form of the particular antigenic determinant complementary to its particular surface immunoglobulin. . . . At the same time a T-cell, perhaps through close proximity to the B-cell or through secretion of a molecule that attaches to another cell (a macrophage), recognizes another part of the same antigen—another determinant.*

This dual recognition (described by McDevitt, 1973) having taken place, a signal is passed from T to B cells, perhaps chemically, that incites the B-cells to produce antibody or switches them to make IgG rather than IgM antibodies. The basic point seems to be the simultaneous recognition of the haptenic determinant by the B-cell and of the carrier determinant by the T-cell.

In the 1930s, Gorer and Snell in England found that there were no barriers to transplantation of tissue within an inbred strain but that rejection of tissue was universal upon transplantation between strains. Studies revealed that there are several genes, located on different chromosomes, that code for cell-surface transplantation antigens. It was later found that these transplantation antigens are in a linkage group in which one finds a number of genes that code for cell-surface proteins. Such linkage groups are identified by the high frequency with which the genes involved are found to segregate together in crossbreeding studies of inbred strains. It became known that the major barrier to tissue grafts—the cause of rejection of skin allografts within 12 to 14 days of transplantation—is a set of antigens coded for the ninth mouse linkage group. These H-2 genes (so called because they happen to be on the second histocompatibility locus to be studied) appeared to be not at a single-point locus but rather to involve many genes spread over a considerable chromosome length. Knowledge of the H-2 region is of importance because of the localization of the Ir genes in the same region and the linkage between the two systems. Establishing the linkage between Ir and H-2 was possible because Ir happened to be linked with an extremely well-studied chromosome region. This Ir—H-2 linkage has greatly facilitated the precise mapping on the chromosome of many of the 30 specific Ir genes that have been identified (McDevitt, 1973).

Lieberman found that there is a recombination between two genes among the relatively small number of antigens known to be under this type of genetic control, and this suggests that a linear array of genes controls the recognition of different foreign antigens. At the cellular level, such genes are probably expressed as receptor sites on the T-cell. If the individual is a high responder to the antigen, the cell will recognize the carrier determinant on the antigen because of a close complementarity between receptor and antigenic determinant. In the low responder, the gene presumably still codes for a receptor on the T-cell, but this receptor is deficient in its complementarity for the carrier determinant, although it may have great efficiency in recognizing other antigens (McDevitt, 1973).

What has emerged is a picture of a large chromosome region containing hundreds to thousands of genes that have arisen together in evolution and remain together; most of them seem to code for a series of structurally and possibly functionally related molecules on the cell surface. Such a system of cell recognition and cell-to-cell interaction would serve the organism both in protection against foreignness and in identification of cell components. Clinically such a system has important implications, including a possible role for genetically determined defects of the Ir system in the etiology of both autoimmune and malignant disease. In humans, associations have been shown between Hodgkin's disease and a number of cross-reacting HL-A types. Cross-reacting types also have been found in some cases of systemic lupus erythematosus and ankylosing spondylitis. Such associations, however, are not absolute, although they do have statistical significance. Recently, evidence has been obtained for the existence of H-linked Ir genes in humans. B. B. Levine at New York University has shown a close correlation between one HL-A chromosome and the IgE-antibody response to ragweed allergen E and clinical symptoms of ragweed hay fever. Other associations have been detected, including that between HL-A antigen 8 and gluten-sensitive enteropathy, and between HL-A 13 and psoriasis. Thus, if the gastroenterologist knows that a patient who has a malabsorption syndrome is HL-A 13, he will recognize that a gluten-sensitive enteropathy is highly likely (McDevitt, 1973).

The markers that determine biological individuality serve as tools for studying the intimate functions of the cell. As this knowledge increases, it should allow practical progress in improving our ability to transplant human organs and to deal with the problems of disease relating to these immunological mechanisms (Reisfeld and Kahan, 1972). P. C. Doherty and R. M. Zinkernagel (1975) of the Australian National University have introduced the following hypothesis regarding the biological role of the major histocompatibility antigens:

A central function of the major histocompatibility (H) antigens may be to signal changes in self to the immune system. Virus-induced modification of strong transplantation antigens apparently results in recognition by thymus-derived lymphocytes (T-cells), with subsequent clonal expansion and immune elimination of cells bearing non-self determinants. The extreme genetic polymorphism found in the major H antigen systems of higher vertebrates may reflect evolutionary pressure exerted by this immunological surveillance mechanism.

HUMAN REAGINIC
ANTIBODIES

Arthur F. Coca, of the faculty of the Cornell University Medical College, one of the early specialists in the field of allergy, coined the term *atopy* to designate a clinical form of hypersensitivity which he believed was peculiar to human beings and was subject to hereditary influence. Atopic individuals have in their blood an antibody that has been designated *atopic reagin.* The presence of reaginic antibody in the serum of an atopic individual was first demonstrated by Prausnitz when he transferred to his own skin the fish-hypersensitivity of his partner Kustner. This demonstration was almost immediately put to clinical use for the diagnosis of atopic hypersensitivity in patients; but for the next 50 years the nature of reaginic antibodies remained a mystery. Then J. F. Heremans and his associates in Belgium reported that the IgA globulin fraction of an atopic patient's serum contained reaginic antibodies, and they suggested that the antibodies belonged to the IgA class. Some findings were not explained by this hypothesis, and the possibility was considered that reaginic activity in the gamma globulin fraction might be due to contamination with a small amount of an unknown immunoglobulin. Studies by Kimishige Ishizaka and his coworkers in Denver identified a new and unique immunoglobulin, IgE, as the carrier of reaginic activity. Soon S. G. O. Johansson and H. Bennich, and Ogawa and Kochwa found patients with myeloma tumors in which the plasma cells secreted IgE. It was then shown that some patients with atopic asthma or hay fever, as well as some patients with parasitic diseases, have higher than normal concentrations of IgE (Ishizaka, 1970). Of immediate clinical use was the discovery that allergen-specific IgE levels correlate well with skin sensitivity and the severity of the allergic disease. These correlations permit the clinician not only to predict the severity of the disease but also to determine whether or not a sensitivity is actually linked with the suspected allergen.

The histamine release test, originally developed by L. M. Lichtenstein and A. G. Osler, at the Johns Hopkins Medical School, has recently been automated through the work of R. P. Siranganian and A. G. Osler of the Public Health Research Institute of New York City, so that one can now test for multiple allergens in a short time with a single sample of blood. The radioallergosorbent test (RAST) and other new procedures have helped researchers to gain further insight into the immunotherapy of allergic disease, and the time-honored method of desensitization introduced by Noon in 1911 is now being restudied.

Thus the identification of IgE as the immunoglobulin class responsible for reagin hypersensitivity has profoundly influenced research on the pathogenesis of immediate hypersensitivity diseases. This influence has expressed itself in the first instance in the scientific systematization of our knowledge of underlying mechanisms and secondly in an improvement of diagnostic techniques available to the clinical allergist. That it will also result in improved and specific therapy seems inevitable (Norman, 1975).

CHEMICAL MEDIATORS OF HYPERSENSITIVITY   To IgE one must add, as participants in sensitivity responses to allergens, the basophils and mast cells and the many chemical mediators they secrete. In the early 1940s, G. Katz and S. Cohen, at the Tulane University School of Medicine, observed that histamine was released when whole blood from an allergic individual was incubated *in vitro* with the specific allergen to which the individual was hypersensitive. Lichtenstein and Osler demonstrated that this reaction comes from leukocytes, and subsequently Ishizaka and co-workers identified the cells that participate in the reaction

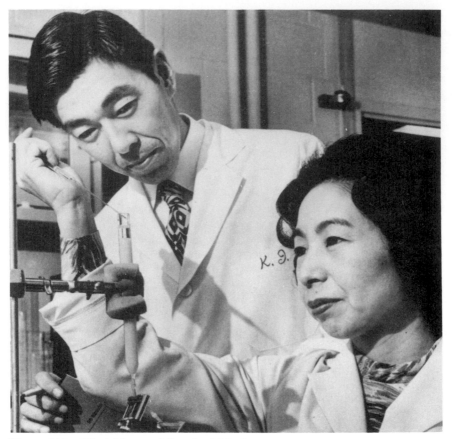

Figure 141. Kimishige and Teruko Ishizaka.

as basophils. The other type of cell associated with histamine release is the mast cell, which is functionally similar to the basophil but is tissue-bound rather than in the circulating blood. Mast cells are most numerous in the linings of the respiratory and gastrointestinal tracts and under the skin. These are also the main sites of lymphoid cells that form IgE and the main loci for various kinds of IgE-mediated allergic reactions. In human beings, both basophils and mast cells are able to secrete histamine, slow-reacting substance (SRS-A), and eosinophil chemotactic factor (ECG-A) during allergic reactions. There is evidence for other chemical mediators such as serotonin and heparin, and H. H. Newball, Lichtenstein, and R. C. Talamo at Johns Hopkins have discovered that human basophils and probably mast cells from the lung liberate a kallikrein-like enzyme that serves to activate bradykinin.

Lichtenstein and S. Margolis showed that drugs that activate intracellular cyclic AMP (cAMP) inhibit histamine release, which is opposite to the usual stimulatory role of cAMP. Lichtenstein, H. R. Bourne, and E. Gillespie have added evidence that drug inhibition of histamine release is closely related to actual changes in the intracellular concentration of cAMP. Of particular interest is the discovery that the drugs that are cAMP activators are

624

the very drugs that we have been using effectively for years in the treatment of allergies, especially allergic asthma. Epinephrine and beta-adrenergic agents such as isoproterenol act through adenylate cyclase to raise cAMP. Similarly, theophylline raises intracellular cAMP by inhibiting its degradation to phosphodiesterase. In addition, prostaglandin E raises cAMP and lowers histamine release.

SECRETORY GAMMA
GLOBULIN ANTIBODIES
As early as 1919 Alexander Besredka, a Russian bacteriologist and immunologist who became Director of the Pasteur Institute in Paris, postulated that local immunity could be established independently of systemic immunity. A number of older reports suggested that susceptibility to infections and resistance following immunization were not always directly related to the amount of antibody in the serum. Moreover, several investigators had found that the mucoantibodies in the secretions that bathe the respiratory and gastrointestinal tracts could be more closely correlated with resistance to infections than could the antibodies in the serum. After the immunoglobulin classes in the serum had been identified, Thomas B. Tomasi, Jr., of the State University of New York at Buffalo, and his colleagues, in 1965, described an immune system common to certain external secretions. This system, which is involved in the local production of a distinctive type of antibody, acts quite independently of the system responsible for the production of circulating antibodies; and it is now known to play a significant role in the body's defense against allergens and microorganisms. It has been demonstrated in the respiratory and gastrointestinal tracts (Samter, 1969).

Tomasi's work disclosed that the antibodies of the secretory system are predominantly of the IgA class, apparently synthesized locally by plasma cells in the secretory organ. Since then it has been found that many patients with isolated IgA deficiency are prone to repeated infections, and it has been suggested that this susceptibility is a result of a defect in antibody production by the mucosa. In these patients there is a selective absence of IgA from both the serum and the secretions.

ANTIBODIES IN
PERNICIOUS ANEMIA
In recent years it has been suggested that the development of pernicious anemia is due to the presence in the gastric juice of antibodies against intrinsic factor (IF). Such antibodies are present in the saliva and gastrointestinal secretions and could directly inhibit the IF-mediated absorption of vitamin B_{12}, particularly when only small amounts of IF are being produced because of extensive atrophic gastritis. Or perhaps IF antibodies selectively inhibit the synthesis of IF. Suppression of synthesis by antibody has been reported in other systems. There are reports of two infants born of mothers having pernicious anemia and anti-IF antibodies in their serum who were found to have no detectable IF in their gastric juice following birth. In one of these infants, IF antibodies could not be detected in the gastric juice, suggesting that the absence of IF was not due to transplacental passage of

625

maternal IF antibodies. From the point of view of diagnosis, the presence of IF antibodies in either serum or gastric juice, or both, is strong evidence of pernicious anemia (Tomasi and DeCoteau, 1970).

THE COMPLEMENT
CASCADE

The complement system has evolved into a definite pathway with 11 discrete blood proteins — C1 through C9 plus C1 subunits q, r, and s — which interact in a very intricate cascade. When antibodies link up with antigens on the cell surface of invading bacteria or on erythrocytes in hemolytic anemia, the classic complement chain reaction commences. It finishes up with the lysis of the bacterium or erythrocyte, but along the way other events take place, including the formation of ingredients involved in the inflammatory response and phagocytosis. The proteins composing the complement cascade enter the serum from widely separated areas of biosynthesis. Using cell culture techniques, Harvey R. Colton of the Boston Children's Hospital has determined the probable origin of most of these components. Some are made in the columnar epithelial cells of the large and small bowels; others are produced in spleen, liver, lymph nodes, and lung (Ruddy, 1974).

In the early 1960s Robert Nelson of the University of Miami School of Medicine found that cobra venom inactivated complement systems of guinea pigs for three to four days by paralyzing the C3 step of the complement cascade. This event took place only after C3 had combined with an intermediate serum protein. In 1966 Hans Muller-Eberhard of La Jolla, California, characterized this C3-inactivating factor from cobra venom. In 1971 I. H. Lepow of the University of Connecticut suggested that the C3 proactivator might be the same protein as factor B of the long-neglected properdin-alternate to the classic complement pathway. Lepow had been a research associate 20 years earlier in the laboratory of Louis Pillemer at Western Reserve University. Pillemer had postulated a pathway circumventing the standard pathway. What appeared important about properdin to Pillemer and his colleagues was that "it seemed to detonate the cytolytic action of complement without relying on cell-bound antibody as the fuse." The action was set off by yeast cell walls (zymosan) acting on a protein which was named properdin. Out of this research came Pillemer's theory of a nonimmunological, nonspecific resistance mechanism against infection. By 1974 the existence of this alternate pathway was accepted, and it is referred to as either the "alternative pathway" or the "properdin pathway."

Complement in Disease. Nature has a way of providing unique "experiments" which help to unravel the normal mechanisms by which the body functions. In 1967, Chester A. Alper and Fred S. Rosen studied a boy at the Children's Hospital in Boston who had a homozygous genetic deficiency of the C3B inactivator as the primary protein defect in his complement system. Thus he had no way to shut off C3 cleavage without this key inhibitor and therefore kept firing the alternative pathway. After purified C3B inactivator became available, injection of this substance restored all of this patient's complement function (Ruddy, 1974).

The hereditary form of angioedema, first described by William Osler in 1888, is characterized by recurrent acute circumscribed and transient edema

626

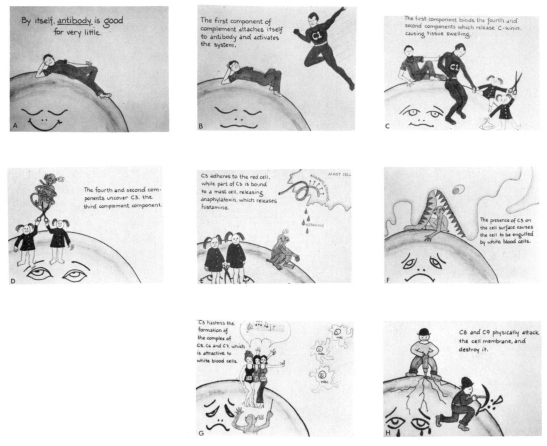

Figure 142. Killer Complement and the Great Membrane Massacre. (From Ruddy, S.: The human complement system. Med. World News, October 11, 1974. Drawing by Suzanne Koch-Weser.)

of the skin, gastrointestinal tract, and upper respiratory tree. The abnormality unique to this disease has been found to be the functional absence of the alpha-globulin inhibitor of C'-1A-esterase, which was first described by V. H. Donaldson and R. R. Evans at Western Reserve University School of Medicine in 1963. Subsequently, Rosen and his collaborators described a hereditary variant in which normal amounts of structurally altered, antigenetically intact, but nonfunctional protein was being synthesized.

There are also various acquired abnormalities of the complement system. In systemic lupus erythematosus (SLE), there is complement fixation by circulating or trapped complexes. There is a close correlation between serum levels of whole complement and the degree of activity of nephritis in this disease. The low levels of whole serum complement are believed to be due to immune complexes forming in the circulation between DNA and antibodies to DNA. This interaction is known to fix complement. DNA has been localized on the glomerular basement membrane in the same locality as gamma globulin and complement (Koffler et al., 1967). Low levels of

627

whole serum complement have also been well documented in patients with glomerular nephritis.

The serum level of C4 is a highly sensitive indicator of clinical activity in SLE, suggesting that activation of the classic pathway is implicated. Recent findings that factor B of the properdin bypass is also frequently depressed in SLE has led to the view that activation of the complement system in SLE is mainly due to triggering of the classic pathway by circulating immune complexes, with amplification of the cascade by the C3B feedback loop of the alternative pathway during intense clinical flare-ups.

Patients with subacute bacterial endocarditis occasionally have renal disease, generally considered to be a focal or embolic glomerulonephritis. R. C. Williams, Jr., and H. G. Kunkel, at the Rockefeller Institute in 1962, first demonstrated that patients with subacute bacterial endocarditis and renal disease had reduced levels of whole serum complement and C'3, whereas patients with subacute bacterial endocarditis without renal disease had either normal or elevated complex levels. The low complement levels may reflect complement fixation by antibodies and bacterial antigens forming immune complexes and initiating the nephritis (Schur and Austen, 1968).

K. F. Austen and P. S. Russell of the Harvard Medical School, in 1966, presented evidence that the measurement of C'2 offers an immunochemical method of assessing the threat of renal allograft rejection in man. In seven patients experiencing rejection, the C'2 titer fell to less than one-half the preoperative level.

R. L. Kassel and L. J. Old at the Sloan-Kettering Institute in 1974 observed that the AKR mouse strain, which is associated with an 85 per cent incidence of spontaneous lymphoma, lacks C5 genetically. They infused normal non-AKR mouse serum into lymphomatous AKR mice, and the lymphomas decreased considerably in size. Robert Nelson, Jr., has postulated that certain cancer cells produce material that destroys certain complement components, thus shielding the tumor from cytolytic attack by the classic complement pathway. He has described a material produced by a line of human tumor cells that blocks the uptake of C' by antibody and thus fractures the entire complement cascade. Nelson has suggested that complement manipulation may be a means of circumventing transplantation rejection.

In patients with recurrent pyogenic infections, once agammaglobulinemia and phagocyte malfunction have been ruled out, a defective complement system should be considered. If the patient's serum will not sustain lysis of antibody-coated sheep erythrocytes, a deficient complement activity in the classic or alternative pathway or in one of the dependent activators of inhibitors is possible (Schur and Austen, 1968).

CLINICAL
IMPLICATIONS
OF IMMUNOLOGY

Clinicians have made important contributions to the understanding of immune mechanisms, and they have also derived benefit from the contributions that immunological research has made to diagnosis and treatment. Many examples have already been cited of this two-way relationship. It may be recalled that DiGeorge's discovery that children born without a thymus are deficient in lymphocytes and lack cell-mediated immune functions served to relate previous observations on experimental animals to human disease. One of the earliest observations (1952) revealing the functional duality of the immune system in humans was made by Ogden Bruton, a pediatrician at the Walter Reed Army Medical Center. Bruton identified an impairment of humoral immunity in a young boy afflicted with multiple bacterial infections. The disease was characterized by a lack of plasma cells and a consequent inability to make antibodies. Lymphocytes of the cell-mediated prong of the immune system were normal, so the boy could resist viral and fungal infections. Subsequently, the opposite (DiGeorge) pattern of immunodeficiency was observed. Individuals with this condition are vulnerable to viral and fungal infections, and they have fewer than the normal number of lymphocytes, but they have abundant plasma cells and produce humoral antibodies. Children who are born with neither system of immunity lack both lymphocytes and plasma cells, and they die quickly of infection.

The multitude of developments in the "new immunology" soon focused attention on the immunological mechanisms by which tissue injury is produced in disease. Immune mechanisms have now been implicated in a wide variety of clinical disorders, including pernicious anemia, Grave's disease, glomerulonephritis, pemphigus, myasthenia gravis, ulcerative colitis, and rheumatoid arthritis, among others. However, the identification of a specific etiological role for the immunological process in these diseases is difficult.

A dramatic change in the methods of immunological study became available in 1941, when *Albert H. Coons* at Harvard perfected the identification of globulins by means of fluorescent labels. This technique, *immunofluorescence,* has contributed immeasurably to our understanding of the interaction of antigen and antibody both *in vitro* and *in vivo* (Samter, 1969; Miller, 1975).

Coons based his technique on earlier studies by Marrack with the use of azo dyes. Coons's method, which today is regarded as relatively simple, originally was considered to be so difficult that almost ten years elapsed before it came into general use. We now capitalize on the high degree of specificity with which antibodies pick up recognizable markers. In recent years, ferritin-coupling has been developed so that the method can be extended to electron microscopy, and ultrastructural localization of particular antigens has become possible. Many other technical advances have been made in this field.

The study and clinical management of kidney disease have been enhanced by the use of immunofluorescent microscopy of renal biopsies. The fact that circulating serum complement levels drop in poststreptococcal acute glomerulonephritis has been known for 60 years; but now it is realized that the profile of the various complement proteins correlates well with the clinical course of the disease. C4 and C2 are depressed while complement and presumed immune complexes can be seen together, scattered along the capillary walls and glomerular basement membrane as lumpy granular deposits. At this stage, acute glomerulonephritis resembles SLE nephritis, which displays similar granular deposits of undoubted immune complexes (DNA-antiDNA).

The practical application of these new findings in experimental models

629

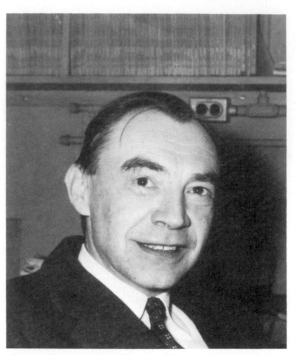

Figure 143. Albert Coons. (National Library of Medicine, Bethesda, Maryland.)

to the study of specific human pathology, particularly in the field of complement and its relationship to glomerular alterations, have been made possible by the development of pure components of the complement system, the production of unispecific antibody, and the preparation of active fluoresceinated and other immunocytochemical reagents. Thus the development of immunofluorescent technology has permitted correlation between experimental immune-complex disease and human counterparts. Advances in research on inflammation, complement, and kinins have provided information about humoral mediation and the mechanism of actual tissue damage.

IMMUNE COMPLEXES One of the important contributors to the understanding of immune-complex disease has been Frank J. Dixon, Jr., a pathologist whose work has been carried on successively at Harvard (1946–48), Washington University, St. Louis (1948–50), the University of Pittsburgh (1950–61), and the Scripps Clinic and Research Foundation, La Jolla, California. Dixon and his associates clarified the pathogenesis of serum sickness and the role of antigen-antibody complexes in disease. They succeeded in passively transferring acute glomerulonephritis to monkeys by means of antibodies derived from human glomerular basement membranes. "These researches have led to the concept that the antigen-antibody complexes themselves may be the pathogenic agent; that is, the interaction between antigen and antibody may form a

630

macromolecular complex which, if soluble, can circulate in the host and upon further reaction with serum factors or cells, can act as an inflammatory stimulus and injure any tissue in which it is deposited."

In Dixon's laboratory, using a combination of isotopically labeled antigens and the fluorescent antibody technique in the study of experimental serum sickness, it was possible to demonstrate soluble antigen-antibody complexes in the circulation during the disease, and further to demonstrate the localization of antigen and, presumably, of antibody at the specific site of the lesions of the disease. The deposition of complex itself in a sequestered site appears capable of interfering with the function of adjacent structures without involving phlogogenic factors (factors causing acute inflammation). In patients with glomerulonephritis and SLE, immunohistological analysis of involved glomeruli for host gamma globulin and host complement gives results comparable to those obtained in the experimental animal with complex-induced nephritis. Similarly, extraglomerular lesions in SLE, rheumatic fever, rheumatoid arthritis, and polyarteritis nodosa reveal, on examination with fluorescent antibody, a specific concentration of host gamma globulin, suggesting the participation of immune complexes in a wide variety of lesions in human disease.

EXPERIMENTAL AUTOIMMUNE DISEASE An important advance in the experimental approach to the study of immunological disease was made by Jules Freund when he noted that "adjuvants" (oil emulsions with or without killed mycobacteria) enhanced antibody production and delayed hypersensitivity responses to a variety of antigens. This technique has been utilized for the production of experimental autoimmune or autoallergic disease. The first example of this was the production of an autoallergic encephalitis by the injection of the animal's own altered nervous-system tissue by Thomas M. Rivers and Francis F. Schwentker, working in the early 1940s at the Rockefeller Institute.

Another important contributor in this area was Ernest Witebsky, a German-born physician who received his M.D. from the University of Heidelberg and immigrated to the United States in 1934; he joined the faculty of the Medical School of the State University of New York at Buffalo in 1936 and became Chief of the Department of Bacteriology and Immunology at that institution in 1941. Witebsky was responsible for setting forth "Postulates for Autoimmune Diseases," which have been compared with Koch's "Postulates for Infectious Diseases." At the time that these postulates were proposed, no experimental animal was known to exhibit spontaneously a disease similar to human autoimmune disease. Since that time strains of New Zealand mice have been discovered in which acquired hemolytic anemia as well as SLE-like lesions have occurred spontaneously (Witebsky, 1957; Samter, 1969).

T-CELLS AND B-CELLS IN DISEASE It has been clearly shown that certain disease states are associated with one or another of the two fundamental types of lymphocytes. The cells in Waldenström's macroglobulinemia and in chronic lymphocytic leukemia

631

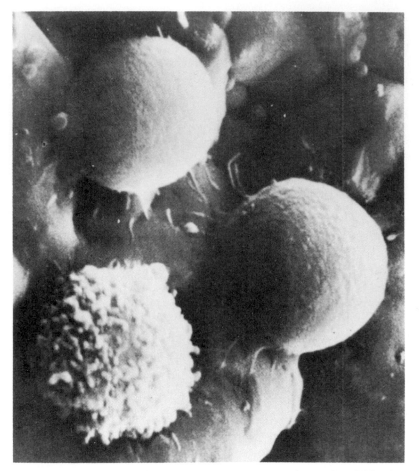

Figure 144. Scanning electron microscopic view of peripheral blood lymphocytes, showing both smooth and villous surfaces. The smoother cells are generally felt to represent T-cells, whereas B-cells show more prominent villous projections (magnification ×13,200). (From Ann. Rev. Med. *26*:183, 1975. Copyright © 1975 by Annual Reviews, Inc. All rights reserved. Photo by Aaron Polliack.)

represent proliferations of B-cells, with differences in their maturation. In Sezary's syndrome, an unusual dermatological disorder associated with lymphoid infiltrates, and in infectious mononucleosis, it would appear that the involved cells are T-cells.

It is now known that T-cells in the peripheral blood bind the erythrocytes of other species to their surfaces. By layering sheep red blood cells over a fresh frozen tissue section, Jaffe and his co-workers found that the area containing T-cells could be highlighted by the selectively bound red blood cells. Taking advantage of the fact that B-cells have receptors for the third component of complement and that erythrocytes treated with anti-erythrocyte antibody can be made to bind C3, homologous erythrocytes carrying complement could be prepared to identify B-cells in an analogous manner. The location of these cells in the tissues could then be determined by staining them with fluorescein-labeled antihuman globulin-immunoglobulin antibody. This method was used to establish the B-cell origin of a nodular lymphoma; it has also been used to study the distribution of B and T cells in normal lymph nodes. Determination of the cells involved in various disease states is still being actively investigated and has not reached a level of practical clinical applicability in most instances. Rheumatoid arthritis, systemic lupus erythematosus, and other immunologically based diseases are among those in which the lymphocyte populations are being most intensely studied (Miller, 1975).

TRANSFER FACTOR
IN THE TREATMENT
OF IMMUNE
DEFICIENCY STATES

In 1955 Sherwood Lawrence of the New York University School of Medicine, while investigating the passive transfer of cellular immunity by intact leukocytes, discovered that passive transfer could also be accomplished with dead lymphocytes. He then found that cellular immunity could be transferred by homogenates of leukocytes. In further experiments he discovered that if the leukocyte homogenate were dialyzed, it lost its activity. The "transfer factor" in the dialysate can be concentrated and can be used passively to transfer skin-test reactivity with donor specificity (Lawrence, 1955). Transfer factor is nonantigenic and contains no transplantation antigens. Therefore, under conditions in which it is effective, it is preferable to the use of whole lymphocytes or bone marrow, since these modalities carry the hazard of fatal graft-versus-host reaction in the immunologically incompetent host.

Transfer factor was given its first clinical trial in 1970 by A. S. Levin and associates, at the University of California, San Francisco, who reported its use in a patient with Wiskott-Aldrich syndrome. This is a rare inherited disease, with X-linked recessive inheritance, which manifests itself by dermatitis, bloody diarrhea, thrombocytopenic purpura, and increased susceptibility to infection. Most patients succumb in late infancy or early childhood. Most of them lack isohemagglutinins, and the level of IgA in the serum is elevated. Since the initial report by Levin and co-workers transfer factor has been employed in the treatment of other patients with Wiskott-Aldrich syndrome and has been found to be effective in about half of them. Immunologists at many research centers have become interested in the possible therapeutic benefits of transfer factor, and it is currently being tried in a number of disorders associated with defects in cellular immunity (Stites, 1970). One of the fields of exploration at the present time is the therapy of hepatitis and other infectious diseases.

SUMMARY

In the 1946 to 1976 period we have learned much about how the immune system works, sometimes to prevent or cure, sometimes to aggravate or produce disease. "Gamma globulin" is no longer considered a single entity but an array of physically and functionally distinct proteins. Lymphocytes have emerged from obscurity as the key cellular elements in the immune system, and they have been divided into two functionally different classes. The thymus has been recognized as the indispensable endower of immunological competence. We have discovered how to distinguish humoral and cellular immunity and have learned more about the part that each plays in beneficial or destructive responses. We have found out how to tag antigens and antigen-antibody complexes so that they may be identified in the tissues. A better understanding has been acquired of the role of complement and the complement cascade. Efforts to transplant organs have brought to light the graft-versus-host reaction, and immunosuppressive drugs have been developed to deal with this and similar deleterious reactions. It has been found that an individual's immune defenses can be turned against his own antigens in such a way as to impair his health and shorten his life. The possibility has arisen that such diseases as pernicious anemia, rheumatoid arthritis, SLE, and others are autoimmune in origin. And, quite surprisingly, it has been discovered that immune mechanisms sometimes abet the development of malignant tumors.

It seems safe to say that the therapeutic potentialities of the new immunology have not yet been fully realized. To date, its unique therapeutic applications have been in the management of relatively rare diseases such as the immune deficiencies of infants and children. However, it has also enabled us to deal more effectively with a broad spectrum of immunological problems, and it has provided a new and more hopeful attitude toward many diseases previously considered incurable. It seems certain that the extraordinary advances in this field, which is still a very active area of research, will have their greatest impact upon clinical medicine in the future.

27

Virology

(The foregoing dedicatory letter, addressed to C. H. Parry, M.D., was dated Berkeley, Gloucestershire, June 21st, 1798. It appeared in "An inquiry into the causes and effects of the Variolae Vaccinae, a disease discovered in some of the western counties of England, particularly Gloucestershire and known by the name of the cowpox, by Edward Jenner, M.D., F.R.S.")

A virus, as the term is understood today, is a self-replicating infectious agent small enough to pass through the fine pores of a porcelain filter.

It has been known since the early 1880s that a porcelain filter would allow water to pass through it but would not permit the passage of bacteria. In 1884 Charles Chamberland, one of Pasteur's research associates, advocated the use of this type of filter to obtain pure drinking water. He said that since water was considered to be "one of the principal agents in the propagation of diseases," it seemed important to have "a filter capable of removing from water all of the microbes that it contains." He continues (Lechevalier and Solotorovsky, 1974):

> *I have been able to do just that by filtration through a porous vase of porcelain, a method of filtration used in the laboratory of M. Pasteur for the separation of microbes from their culture medium. I have noted that even the most impure water, filtered through these vases, was deprived of microbes and germs.*
>
> *. . . . Under a water pressure of about 2 atmospheres, as found in M. Pasteur's laboratory, one obtains with a single porous tube or filtering candle of 0.20 m. of length by 0.025 m. of diameter, about 20 liters of water a day. This seems to me sufficient for the ordinary consumption of a family.*

Eight years after the publication of Chamberland's paper, a young Russian scientist, Dmitri Ivanovski, while studying diseases of plants, found that the sap of leaves attacked by mosaic disease retained its infectious properties "even after filtration through the candle filters of Chamberland" (Lechevalier and Solotorovsky, 1974).

Ivanovski was the first to discover that a disease-producing agent—the virus which produces mosaic disease of tobacco plants—is capable of passing through a porcelain filter.

For many years, viruses were known more for what they did than for what they were. They were too small to be seen by the best laboratory microscopes, and their physical features were unknown until the electron microscope was invented. The first filterable virus to be photographed (1939) was the tobacco mosaic virus which had aroused Ivanovski's interest a half-century earlier. Then in 1942, using the first American electron microscope, which had just been assembled in the RCA laboratories, Luria and Anderson obtained a photograph of a virus that attacks bacteria (see Chapter 26).

EARLY VIRUS RESEARCH

Fifty years ago the science of virology was in its infancy. Viruses were then regarded as minute intracellular parasites differing from larger parasites only by their capacity to pass through filters that held back bacteria. The *medical* virologist performed experiments on a few animals (chiefly monkeys and rabbits) as well as on human subjects; his filters were of nonuniform porosities; and he used some immunological techniques for identifying the small number of viruses then known. In 1925 only 10 human diseases were known to be caused by viruses. During the past 50 years, hundreds of new viruses pathogenic for human beings have been discovered. These viruses produce a broad spectrum of diseases (Sabin, 1965).

In virology, as in other fields of scientific endeavor, new methods brought new knowledge. The introduction of new animal hosts and tissue-culture systems for the propagation of viruses and the development of techniques for recognizing their presence were responsible for the continuing discovery of new viruses. In the beginning, larger animals such as ferrets, horses, and guinea pigs were used to isolate certain viruses, but more rapid progress was made when techniques were devised for transmission of viral diseases to mice and embryonated chicken eggs.

636

In recent years virology has become one of the most dynamic of biological sciences. Although it is still concerned with the understanding, control, and cure of disease, it has also become involved in exploring the fundamental processes of life. Viruses offer a type of genetic material suitable for quantitative study and analysis; they provide excellent models for examining the intimate function of cells and the mechanisms of heredity (Sabin, 1965).

MILESTONES IN THE DEVELOPMENT OF VIROLOGY

In the same year in which Ivanovski found that the tobacco mosaic virus was filterable (1892), George M. Sternberg made the first important American contribution to virology. In a paper read before the Association of American Physicians, Sternberg reported experiments demonstrating the formation of a specific antibody following infection with the virus of cowpox, and he noted that the blood serum from an animal which had been rendered immune would neutralize the virus (see Chap. 26). The neutralization test introduced by Sternberg has become a mainstay of virus serology.

In 1898 Friedrich Löffler and Paul Frosch, in Germany, discovered that the agent causing foot-and-mouth disease in cattle would pass through a filter, thus proving for the first time that a mammalian disease was due to a filterable virus.

The first proof that a disease of man could be caused by a filterable agent came from the work of Walter Reed and the Yellow Fever Commission, which was reported in 1902 (see Chap. 12). These classic studies proved not only that yellow fever is due to a filterable virus but also that it is transmitted by a particular species of mosquito. The earlier work by Smith and Kilborne (1893) had shown that an insect transmits Texas fever of cattle. The findings of these two research groups focused attention upon the possible role of insects in the dissemination of infectious diseases of both animals and plants.

The first indication that a virus was involved in the production and transmission of a malignant disease came in 1908 when V. Ellerman and O. Bang found that a form of leukemia which occurs in chickens could be transmitted from one fowl to another by an agent that passed through a porcelain filter. The work in this area took a giant step forward in 1911 when Peyton Rous of the Rockefeller Institute reported the discovery of a malignant tumor, a sarcoma of chickens, which could be transmitted from one fowl to another by a cell-free, bacteria-free extract of the tumor which had been passed through a porcelain filter. Rous believed that the causative agent of the tumor was a filterable virus. Later in the same year, Rous and Murphy demonstrated that the cells of the chicken sarcoma, or filtered extracts of the tumor, induced tumors or lesions on the chorioallantoic membrane of an embryonated chicken egg. (In spite of this demonstration, the potential value of the chick embryo in virus research was not recognized until two decades later.) These pioneer studies by Rous, although slow to be appreciated, are now classed among the major advances in the development of our knowledge of virology.

637

In 1913 Edna Steinhardt, C. Israel, and R. A. Lambert of Columbia University were the first to report an effort to propagate a virus in tissue culture. They first tried to grow the virus of rabies, but when this was unsuccessful they turned to the virus of cowpox, employing cell cultures of the hanging-drop type first used by Ross G. Harrison. Though they believed that they had demonstrated multiplication of the virus in the cell cultures, there is some doubt about this, though it is clear that they were able to retrieve a living virus from the cultures after as much as 34 days' incubation.

Frederick W. Twort, a British plant pathologist working at Brown Institute, London, had been impressed by the fact that viruses were recognized only by the diseases which they produced; and whereas many of the known bacteria were not disease-producers, no filterable virus of this type had been recognized. Twort therefore embarked (1915) on a series of experiments in which he inoculated, on several hundred types of artificial media, stagnant water and extracts of dung, grass, hay, and straw, all of which had been passed through a porcelain filter, hoping to find a new virus. He did, indeed, find a virus of an entirely new and unanticipated variety. He recognized it by its effect upon colonies of bacteria that happened to be growing on the surface of the culture medium. It appeared to be able to dissolve and inactivate the bacterial colonies (Lechevalier and Solotorovsky, 1974).

Twort's experiments attracted little attention until his bacteriolytic agent was "rediscovered" in 1917 by Felix D'Herelle, a Canadian who received his M.D. degree in Montreal but spent his professional life as a bacteriologist in other countries, including 12 years (1909–1921) at the Pasteur Institute in Paris. D'Herelle obtained his virus from the stools of patients recovering from bacillary dysentery and after passing it through a filter found that it would destroy dysentery bacilli. He considered this agent to be "a true microbe of immunity," and characterized it as "an obligate bacteriophage." As it turned out, this bacteriophage ("eater of bacteria") proved not to be a "true microbe of immunity," and its subsequent history was a great disappointment to D'Herelle and others who expected it to be useful in the prevention and cure of human disease. Although it has found little use as a therapeutic agent, in many other respects, notably in the field of genetics, bacteriophage has turned out to be one of the most valuable viruses ever discovered (Lechevalier and Solotorovsky, 1974).

DEVELOPMENT OF TECHNIQUES FOR THE STUDY OF VIRUSES

Bacteria can be grown in laboratory glassware on simple mixtures of sterilized nutrients. Viruses, in contrast, multiply only in the living cells of a susceptible host. For research on the viruses causing human disease, the scientist must find a convenient animal whose cells are susceptible to infection by the virus under study. In addition, the experimental host must show some manifestation which permits the virologist to know when it is infected. It is also desirable to have some method to determine the amount of virus present.

At the end of World War I, the methods for virus research were relatively simple. It had become possible to determine the size of a virus by passing it through graded collodion membranes with pores of known diameter. Virus studies had also been helped by the recognition in the cells of virus-infected tissues of small round, oval, or irregularly shaped particles which were called "inclusion bodies." The viruses of herpes simplex (fever blisters and cold sores), vaccinia (cowpox), rabies (hydrophobia), and a few other diseases were studied by inoculation into the brain of rabbits. A few viruses had been grown in tissue culture. However, many viruses could be recognized only by the disease they produced in their natural hosts. The mouse was not yet being utilized as an experimental animal for the study of viruses.

Webster and Fite in 1933 succeeded in transmitting the virus of St. Louis encephalitis by inoculating it into the brain of mice—the first of the insect-borne encephalitis viruses to be subjected to detailed study. Two years before this, Alice M. Woodruff and Ernest W. Goodpasture of Vanderbilt University had adapted to virology the technique (used 20 years previously by Rous) of cultivation in fertile hens' eggs. It was found that most viruses would grow when inoculated into the chorioallantoic membrane, or into the amniotic, allantoic, or yolk-containing cavities, or into the body of the chick embryo. Woodruff and Goodpasture demonstrated that fowlpox virus forms distinct lesions on the chorioallantoic membrane characteristic of this disease. The chick embryo as an experimental tool in virus research has many advantages: availability, low cost, absence of viral antibodies, relative freedom from latent viruses, and a variety of extraembryonic cell layers, which enhance its susceptibility to many viral agents. Important results of the use of the chick embryo have been the detection and isolation of many viruses, development of a quantitative method for measuring virus infectivity, and the production of virus antigens and vaccines.

George K. Hirst at the Rockefeller Institute discovered in 1941 that allantoic fluid containing influenza virus in high titer would agglutinate the red blood cells of chickens. This discovery came as a lucky accident when Hirst was examining virus-infected chick embryos. Some infected fluid was inadvertently mixed with chicken blood. Hirst noticed that the blood cells collected into coarse clumps. It is the mark of a first-class investigator to recognize the implications of an unexpected occurrence. This fortuitous observation enabled Hirst to devise a highly useful quantitative test for the influenza virus.

THOMAS M. RIVERS AND THE ROCKEFELLER INSTITUTE

In the 1930s and for several decades thereafter, the Rockefeller Institute was one of the most active centers of viral research in the world, and *Thomas M. Rivers* was responsible for much of the work there. After graduation from the Johns Hopkins Medical School in 1915, Rivers took an internship in medicine and then became an Assistant Resident in Pediatrics under Professor John Howland. It was Rivers's declared intention at that time to return to his home state to become "the best damned pediatrician in Georgia." This might have been the case had it not been for World War I. Early in 1918 Rivers was commissioned in the United States Army Medical Corps and was assigned to the Army Pneumonia Board, headed by Rufus

639

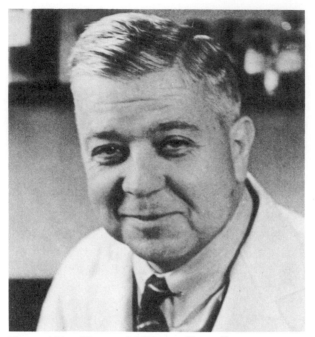

Figure 145. Thomas M. Rivers. (From Corner,
George W.: A History of the Rockefeller Institute.
New York, The Rockefeller Institute Press, 1964.)

Cole. As a result of this assignment, he spent most of his time in the Army investigating respiratory diseases, including the great epidemic of influenza. When the war ended he became a co-author of a book entitled *Epidemic Respiratory Disease*. As a result of new interests aroused by his wartime experience, Rivers returned to the Hopkins Medical School in 1919 to become a member of the Department of Bacteriology (Horsfall, 1963).

In 1922 Rivers was invited by his former chief in the Army, Rufus Cole, to join the staff of the Hospital of the Rockefeller Institute with the assignment to study virus diseases. He accepted this offer and was given charge of the Infectious Disease Ward of the Rockefeller Hospital. Virology was not then an organized branch of medical research, and for the most part Rivers had to plow virgin soil. Because of his background in pediatrics, he first became interested in chickenpox. For this work he used rabbits, inoculating the infectious material into the testicles. Other viruses had been propagated in this manner, and Rivers wanted to adapt the chickenpox virus to the rabbit as the initial step in the preparation of a vaccine for human use. After four or five passages from one rabbit to another, the rabbits developed signs of infection. Rivers thought that the infection was due to the chickenpox virus, but when immunological tests with human serum were made, it was found that the rabbit infection was due to another virus. At the same time his colleagues, C. P. Miller, Jr., Christopher Andrews, and Homer Swift, while attempting to transmit rheumatic fever to rabbits in the same manner, encountered an infection which Rivers recognized as being identical to the one in his rabbits. Both groups had isolated a hitherto unknown

640

virus that occurs in healthy rabbits. These experiments had an important influence on virus research, since they drew attention to the existence of unexpected (latent) viruses in experimental animals and emphasized the danger of confusion between the true virus of a disease and others incidentally present in the test animal.

In 1926 Rivers organized a symposium on viruses for the Society of American Bacteriologists and presented a paper in which he clearly distinguished viruses from bacteria. This paper was influential in establishing virology as a separate discipline. Two years later he published a classic paper on "Some general aspects of pathological conditions caused by filterable viruses," and in the same year his book, *Filterable Viruses,* appeared, containing almost all that was known at that time about this subject. Prior to 1928 the literature of virology was scattered through bacteriological publications or summarized in brief chapters of textbooks of bacteriology and preventive medicine such as Hans Zinsser's *Infection and Immunity* and Edward Rosenau's *Public Hygiene and Preventive Medicine.*

Rivers's *Filterable Viruses* was the first textbook devoted exclusively to virus diseases to be published in this country. The book was unique in at least two respects: it was a cooperative venture; the participants included such pioneer investigators of virus diseases as Harold Amoss, Peter Olitsky, Ernest Goodpasture, Rudolf Glaser, Louis Kunkel, and Jacques Bronfenbrenner; (2) it included information not only about animal viruses but also about plant, insect, and bacterial viruses. In an introductory chapter, Rivers for the second time clearly differentiated viruses from bacteria, stating that viruses, unlike bacteria, are obligate parasites that can live and multiply only in the presence of a living susceptible cell (Benison, 1972; Corner, 1964). A larger, widely used textbook, *Viral and Rickettsial Infections of Man,* which Rivers began to prepare shortly after World War II and which he edited single-handedly, first appeared in 1948. Subsequent editions appeared in 1952 and 1959.

The use of cell cultures as hosts for the propagation of viruses had been undertaken in Alexis Carrel's laboratory, the first virus thus cultivated being that of the Rous chicken sarcoma. In 1925 Frederick Parker, Jr., and R. N. Nye of Boston succeeded in growing vaccinia virus in small hanging-drop cultures, and two years later Rivers decided to try to produce smallpox vaccine in quantity in the laboratory rather than in calves. To accomplish this he placed vaccinia virus in flasks of culture fluid containing fragments of living tissue. Subsequently, this method was simplified by suspending the fragments of tissue in flasks of Tyrode's solution, containing only the necessary salts and a buffer substance to keep the mixture at the proper pH. This method has been widely used since that time for the cultivation of many viruses and rickettsiae. The vaccinia virus produced by Rivers and his co-workers was used successfully for the vaccination of children, but eventually it became too attenuated to afford complete protection against smallpox. This work is of historical importance because it was the first time that a virus for human use was grown in cell culture.

During the period in which Rivers was working on vaccinia virus, he was also answering some fundamental questions about viruses in general. He had convinced himself that none of the known filterable viruses would grow on culture medium except in the presence of living cells, and he was,

641

therefore, troubled by a paper written by the Director of the Institute, Simon Flexner, and Hideyo Noguchi, in which they described the cultivation of "globoid bodies," which they considered to be living particles of the poliomyelitis virus. They claimed that they had been able to cultivate this "virus" on standard bacteriological media, free from living cells. Knowing that his own experience flatly contradicted the claim of the Director of the Institute, Rivers took the manuscript in which he had stated that viruses would not grow except upon living cells first to Noguchi and then to Flexner, asking them to comment on it. After Flexner had read the paper, he observed: "This is a free country, Rivers; you must publish what you think is right" (Corner, 1964).

In 1930 Rivers and George P. Berry, then an assistant resident physician at the hospital, undertook a study of parrot fever (psittacosis), which was thought to have been introduced into the United States by South American parrots. In humans, this disease was associated with severe pneumonia, having a mortality rate of 20 per cent. In January, 1930, the Board of Health's laboratory assigned six workers to investigate the problem of psittacosis, but by March four of the workers had contracted the disease; and when the chief scientist fell ill with an unrelated illness, he interrupted the work and donated his supply of the psittacosis virus to the Rockefeller Institute. Rivers and Berry volunteered to conduct the study (Rivers and Berry, 1931), and the following year another assistant resident physician, Francis F. Schwentker, joined them (Rivers and Schwentker, 1934) Berry and Schwentker both contracted the disease and survived after severe illnesses. They succeeded in producing a typical psittacosis pneumonia in monkeys, but only by introducing the infectious material directly into the trachea. The most practical result of this dangerous work was the discovery of a quick method of diagnosing the disease by injecting the infected sputum into the body of a mouse. Many other exotic viruses were studied by Rivers and his group, with important results (Corner, 1964).

By the 1940s the Rockefeller Institute had become a world-renowned center of virological research. Its investigators dominated the field, and many virologists trained at the Institute went to other institutions, where they made fundamental contributions to their science. Rivers was the key figure in this development. He was 35 years of age when he entered the field of virology, and his career developed rapidly. In the short period of 13 years he made many basic contributions to this discipline and became an authority on a wide range of viral diseases and an accomplished laboratory worker in this field. By the age of 50 his career as an active investigator was over. During these few years an important evolution in virus research had taken place: the initial interest in virus infections in humans and animals had shifted to a fundamental concern with the structure and inner workings of viruses. Although Rivers never mastered biochemistry and biophysics, he nevertheless appreciated their importance for the future development of virology. Later in his career as a scientific administrator he employed this knowledge in organizing the Poliomyelitis Research Program sponsored by the National Foundation for Infantile Paralysis.

Until the mid-1930s, viruses were still of interest because of the pathology they created. The biochemical and biophysical techniques necessary for understanding the structure and composition of viruses were still crude. In

642

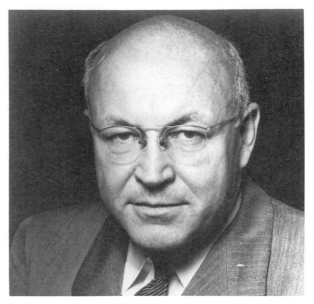

Figure 146. Wendell M. Stanley. (National Library of Medicine, Bethesda, Maryland.)

1935 *Wendell M. Stanley* succeeded in isolating and crystallizing the tobacco mosaic virus. He demonstrated that the viral crystals at high dilutions induced the typical disease on inoculation into tobacco plants and established conclusively that the crystals retained their infectious properties. This outstanding achievement provided an enormous stimulus to the biochemical approach to virus purification and to the chemical and structural analysis of virus particles (Hahon, 1964).

No discovery at the Rockefeller Institute created more worldwide interest than Stanley's accomplishment. Here was a crystalline substance able to reproduce itself in the plant, thus creating new material of its own kind. Stanley's discovery added a new dimension to the question, "What is life?" Though it was believed at first that Stanley's crystals were proteins, subsequent studies disclosed that they were *nucleoproteins*—a protein chemically combined with a nucleic acid, ribose, which had been identified by Levene at the Rockefeller Institute some two decades earlier. Thus, it became evident that the material of which viruses are made belongs to that group of substances which are vitally concerned with essential life processes and the transmission of hereditary characteristics. In 1946 Stanley shared the Nobel Prize in chemistry with John H. Northrop, also a member of the staff of the Rockefeller Institute, and James B. Sumner, Professor of Biochemistry at Cornell University. This award to Stanley, says Corner, "was a recognition not only of his successful chemical work, but also of the philosophical importance of his isolation of a cell-producing and potentially mutable agent in crystalline form—a link between living and non-living matter" (Corner, 1964).

Other valuable tools for the virologist were developed in the late 1930s. In that period Theodor Svedberg in Sweden and Ernest E. Pickels at the Rockefeller Institute perfected the ultracentrifuge; and simultaneously Arne

643

Tiselius of Uppsala, Sweden, described the electrophoretic method for separation of the proteins of body fluids. These techniques provided the means for accurately determining particle size, analyzing complex fluids, obtaining molecularly homogeneous material, and separating and analyzing proteins in a solution. The new methods made it possible to examine in depth the structure and composition of viruses. Then in 1939 Ernst A. F. Ruska and his associates in Germany, using a crude electron microscope developed at Siemen's Allgemeine Gesellschaft, succeeded in taking the first photograph of a virus. Except for the work with the electron microscope, all of these developments were the direct outcome of research programs initiated and fostered by either the Rockefeller Institute or the Rockefeller Foundation. In reality, such instruments as the ultracentrifuge, the Tiselius apparatus, and the electron microscope, so necessary for the analysis and visualization of viruses, did not become readily available to the virologist until the early 1940s.

DEVELOPMENT OF YELLOW FEVER VACCINE

In Chapter 26, brief mention was made of the work of *Max Theiler,* the South African who came to Boston in 1922 and shortly thereafter began research on the virus of yellow fever. He soon became involved in a controversy over the cause of this disease, which at that time was thought by some to be due to a virus, but Hideyo Noguchi of the Rockefeller Institute believed that he had proved that it was caused by a spirochete. Theiler demonstrated that Noguchi's organism was the cause not of yellow fever but of an unrelated disease, known now as leptospirosis. He reconfirmed the fact that yellow fever is caused by a filterable agent and was the first to show that the virus could be transmitted to mice by intracerebral inoculation. The use of mice provided a means for quantitating virus potency, and Theiler found that they could also be used as indicator hosts for measuring serum antibody levels by the virus-serum neutralization test pioneered by Sternberg (Hahon, 1964).

At about the time of Theiler's arrival in Boston, Adrian Stokes, a British physician, made the important discovery that yellow fever could be transmitted to an Indian monkey *(Macaca mulatta).* In 1928 Andrew Sellards, Theiler's chief at Harvard, found that the virus could be preserved in infected tissue and blood of the rhesus monkey by freezing, thus making it possible to transport strains of virus from human victims to the Harvard laboratories for study (Riedman and Gustafsen, 1963).

Theiler demonstrated that the virus could be maintained by serial passage from sick to normal mice. In addition, he found that rhesus monkeys became less susceptible to virulent virus which had undergone many passages in mice. The important observation was that monkeys which had been injected with the weakened virus were later found to be immune to virulent yellow fever virus obtained from another monkey. In 1929 Theiler himself suffered a mild attack of yellow fever. He demonstrated that his blood contained antibodies, showing that even a mild infection brought protection. He further demonstrated that blood serum from convalescent yellow-fever patients prevented the infection in mice which had been in-

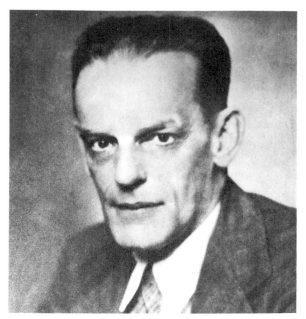

Figure 147. Max Theiler. (National Library of Medicine, Bethesda, Maryland.)

jected intracerebrally with the virus. He called this the "intracerebral mouse protection test," and it became a useful means for demonstrating whether blood serum contained antibodies to the yellow fever virus.

After eight years at Harvard, Theiler moved to New York in 1930 to join the virology group at the Rockefeller Institute. In that same year, summarizing his results up to that point in an article published in *Science,* he described how serum taken from a monkey or a human being who had recovered from yellow fever neutralized the virus whereas normal serum had no such protective action. From this point on he worked intensively to prepare a yellow fever vaccine.

Theiler's experiments had indicated clearly that successive passages of the virus through mice weakened it for monkeys but still allowed the development of protective antibodies against the disease. Utilizing this "tamed" virus, he mixed it with immune serum to make it still milder and then injected the mixture into the workers in his laboratory who had not yet come down with yellow fever. After this there were no further accidental infections among the laboratory workers.

The mouse-protection test opened the way for mapping the world's yellow-fever areas. Even in those areas in which no epidemic was in progress, if the disease had been prevalent previously, antibodies could be demonstrated in the serum of those who had had the disease.

Theiler was concerned that the strain of virus which he had been using in his laboratory, because of its attraction for brain tissue, would be dangerous to use in humans. He studied ways to culture the virus in other tissues, utilizing another virulent strain known as the Asibi virus. After three years of continuous passage through successive mouse embryo cultures, the virus was transplanted to a chick-embryo tissue culture from which the develop-

645

ing nervous tissue had been removed. In this brainless chick-embryo culture, the virus was attenuated by many serial passages. In 1936 Theiler and his associates injected this virus, now known as the 17D strain, into individuals already immune to yellow fever by virtue of having had a natural infection. Following the injection, the serum of these subjects developed a much higher titer of antibodies against the virus. Nonimmune persons receiving the attenuated virus developed very mild symptoms of yellow fever from which they quickly recovered, and their serum was later found to contain antibodies against the yellow-fever virus. A vaccine was then made from Theiler's attenuated virus and was given several years of field testing in South America.

In 1940 a special commission of the International Health Division of the Rockefeller Foundation, which had sponsored much of this work and had been impressed by the results, decided that the vaccine should be produced on a large scale. It was found that massive quantities of vaccine could be produced by growing the attenuated virus simultaneously in hundreds of chick embryos. While production was just getting under way, the United States entered World War II, and all military personnel who were scheduled to enter tropical areas where they might encounter yellow fever were given injections of the vaccine. Since then it has been used extensively and successfully in all areas where yellow fever is prevalent (Riedman and Gustafsen, 1963). Theiler received the Nobel Prize for medicine and physiology in 1951 for his work on yellow fever.

**POLIOMYELITIS
—EARLY
RESEARCH
AT THE
ROCKEFELLER
INSTITUTE**

In 1886 Mary Putnam Jacobi, Professor of Therapeutics at the Women's Medical College of New York, wrote a review of what was then known about poliomyelitis. The evidence, she said "led to the theory that all cases of acute infantile paralysis are due to a specific but still unknown infectious agent" (Paul, 1971).

In 1901 an epidemic of cerebrospinal meningitis broke out in New York City. Simon Flexner, working at the newly opened Rockefeller Institute, began an investigation of the disease, using the rhesus monkey as his experimental animal. The choice of the monkey was dictated by Flexner's conviction that such animals would have a reaction similar to that of humans. Flexner cultivated the meningococcus *in vitro* and successfully transmitted the disease to monkeys. Subsequently he produced an antiserum in horses, which prevented or modified the experimental disease. Later, antiserum proved to be equally successful in the treatment of human patients. The mortality of the disease was reduced from a high of 80 per cent to a new low of 15 per cent.

Flexner's triumph convinced him that there were no limits to what bacteriological techniques could achieve when applied to the experimental investigation of disease. As a consequence, in 1907, he happily agreed to a request from the New York Neurological Society to undertake an investigation of poliomyelitis. In view of his experience with cerebrospinal meningitis, Flexner decided to use the rhesus monkey in his poliomyelitis research.

In 1908 Karl Landsteiner, a pathologist working in Vienna, reported that he had succeeded in transferring poliomyelitis to monkeys, using an emulsion made from the spinal cord of a poliomyelitis victim. In September, 1909, Flexner transmitted poliomyelitis from human victims to monkeys and then from one monkey to another (Benison, 1972; Paul, 1971).

In his early research on poliomyelitis, Flexner worked out and described the pathology of the disease and established that it is infectious and can be passed from subject to subject by contact. However, he made several errors. As noted previously, he believed that the poliovirus could be grown on ordinary bacteriological media. Rivers and others demonstrated that this was incorrect. Flexner also believed that his studies indicated that the portal of entry and exit of the virus was through the nasal and pharyngeal mucosa. This also turned out to be inaccurate. Actually, these errors were minor in comparison with the great accomplishments of the research in Flexner's laboratory. He and P. A. Lewis were the first to produce (1910) active immunity in monkeys, but the results were unpredictable, and the technique was too hazardous to be employed in human subjects. In 1922, working with Harold L. Amoss, Flexner was able to produce a nonfatal form of experimental poliomyelitis in monkeys. They showed that these infected monkeys became immune to a subsequent inoculation with virulent virus (Corner, 1964).

During the early 1920's, Flexner recruited Peter Olitsky to devote his energies to the study of virus diseases. It was the investigation conducted by Olitsky and his associates that corrected the errors mentioned earlier. In 1930, Olitsky, in association with C. P. Rhoads and P. H. Long, published a paper which put an end to the claim by Flexner and Noguchi that poliovirus could be cultivated in the absence of living tissues. In 1939 Albert Sabin, another of Olitsky's associates, in a series of papers, presented strong evidence against Flexner's idea that the poliovirus enters the body through the nasal and pharyngeal mucosa (Benison, 1972; Paul, 1971; Corner, 1964).

THE CONQUEST OF
POLIOMYELITIS

The scientific cooperation that made possible the development of the Salk and the Sabin vaccines was due in large measure to the activities of the National Foundation for Infantile Paralysis. The cooperation grew out of continuing discussions among the poliomyelitis investigators at meetings sponsored by the Foundation, as well as from a unique program in which grantees of the Foundation agreed to exchange their research findings before publication.

The National Foundation was an outgrowth of the Warm Springs Foundation, which maintained a treatment center for poliomyelitis victims in Warm Springs, Georgia. The Warm Springs Foundation received wide publicity in the 1930s when Franklin D. Roosevelt, a victim of the disease, made frequent visits to Warm Springs for treatment. Roosevelt also assisted the Foundation in its organizing efforts. In 1934 it needed financial support, and the decision was made to solicit contributions from the public. By that time, Roosevelt had become President, and he provided the attraction for the fund-raising campaign, which was based on a series of annual balls held in various cities on Roosevelt's birthday, January 30.

The Birthday Ball Commission decided to allocate some of its funds for poliomyelitis research, and in 1935, 16 grants were made, totalling approximately $250,000. In January, 1938, President Roosevelt provided the leadership for expanding the Warm Springs Foundation into a national organization — the National Foundation for Infantile Paralysis. Its stated purpose was as follows: "To lead, direct, and unify the fight against every aspect of the killing and crippling infection of poliomyelitis." The plan was to collect small contributions from a large number of people. Basil O'Connor, Roosevelt's former law partner, became President of the Foundation. Between 1938 and 1962 the Foundation raised approximately $630 million. Most of this was spent on the medical care of poliomyelitis victims, but $69 million (11 per cent) was devoted to research (Benison, 1972; Marks and Beatty, 1973).

Thomas M. Rivers of the Rockefeller Institute was selected as Chairman of the Committee on Scientific Research of the Foundation. Out of this program ultimately came the Salk and Sabin vaccines.

The research programs supported by the President's Birthday Ball Commission had in two instances been disastrous. In part, the responsibility for these failures rested with Paul de Kruif, who as Secretary to a special Scientific Advisory Board, organized and administered the research program (Benison, 1972). In 1919 de Kruif, a bacteriologist, joined the Rockefeller Institute. In 1923 Simon Flexner dismissed him when it was discovered that de Kruif had been the author of an anonymous attack on the Institute published in *Century* magazine. Subsequently, de Kruif became a successful science writer. After leaving the Institute, he served as scientific consultant to Sinclair Lewis, who was preparing a novel about medical research, *Arrowsmith*. Lewis's description of the character of medical research and the people at the "McGurk Institute" portrayed in the novel presumably were based on de Kruif's view of his contemporaries at the Rockefeller Institute (Benison, 1972).

In his distribution of the Foundation's research funds, de Kruif allocated the major portion to William H. Park of the New York City Health Department and John Kolmer of Temple University for the development of a vaccine against poliomyelitis. Unfortunately, the vaccine developed by Park and Kolmer contained live virus, and a number of children who received this vaccine died of poliomyelitis (Benison, 1972).

In 1937, following the tragedy of the Park and Kolmer vaccine, President Roosevelt concluded that poliomyelitis could be conquered only through a broad program of scientific education and research. The organization of the National Foundation was the first step toward the realization of this goal. "It was also something more. At a time when deadly assaults had already been launched against the human spirit and life itself in Europe, the new foundation in addition stood as an affirmation of the value of conserving human life and dignity. Ordinary people everywhere recognized this quality, and quietly and emphatically made its cause their own" (Benison, 1972).

648

DEVELOPMENT
OF POLIOMYELITIS
VACCINE

Prior to 1935, many virologists, as a result of the experience with smallpox and yellow fever, believed that one could not successfully prevent a virus disease with an inactivated vaccine. In 1936, a breakthrough occurred when Peter Olitsky and his associates immunized mice against western equine encephalitis with an inactivated vaccine. In 1941, Thomas Francis, Jr., who had spent 10 years at the Rockefeller Institute and had then served at New York University as Professor of Bacteriology, went to the University of Michigan as Professor of Epidemiology. He and other investigators advanced the field of virology by developing inactivated vaccines against influenza. In 1946, Isabel Morgan (who had trained with Olitsky and was then in Baltimore with Howard A. Howe and David Bodian at Johns Hopkins) immunized monkeys against poliomyelitis with a formalinized inactivated vaccine. Morgan's work was a milestone in poliomyelitis research, since by establishing the fact that animals could be immunized against poliomyelitis with an inactivated vaccine, the question of immunizing humans in a like manner was reopened. However, instead of immediately concentrating on the development of a vaccine, the Foundation directed its efforts toward the discovery of more basic knowledge about poliovirus, especially the question of multiple strains of viruses (Benison, 1972; Paul, 1971).

In the early work on poliomyelitis, it had been assumed that there was only one type of poliovirus. In 1931, F. M. Burnet, in Australia, indicated that there was more than one strain of the virus. During the 1930s, John Paul and James Trask of Yale announced their conclusion that more than one type of poliovirus existed, and by 1940 the experience of other poliomyelitis investigators seemed to substantiate this view. In 1948–49, John Kessel of the University of Southern California and David Bodian of Johns Hopkins announced (almost simultaneously) that they had been able to identify three types of poliovirus. At that time there was some uncertainty as to whether there might be more than three types among the many strains that investigators had isolated. In 1949 the Foundation provided funds in excess of $1,250,000 to Louis Gebhard, John Kessel, Jonas Salk, and Herbert Wenner, to type all known strains of poliovirus. By 1951 these workers conclusively established that there were only three types. At about the time that the typing program was getting started (1949), *John Enders, Thomas Weller,* and *Frederick Robbins* at Harvard University reported that they had successfully cultivated poliovirus in cell cultures made up of non-nervous tissues. The manner in which this trio entered the field of poliomyelitis research was described briefly in Chapter 26.

Tissue Culture of Poliovirus. Virologists had been greatly impeded in their research because they could not make viruses grow in the ordinary media used for bacteria. They had been able to propagate them only in susceptible animals. This technique often failed because many viruses that cause human disease will not grow in any of the available laboratory animals. This handicap was overcome when Enders and his co-workers found that they could grow the poliomyelitis virus in test-tube cultures of human tissues. With this discovery, a new era in virological research had begun (Benison, 1972; Paul, 1971).

In 1937 Enders, working in the Department of Bacteriology and Im-

649

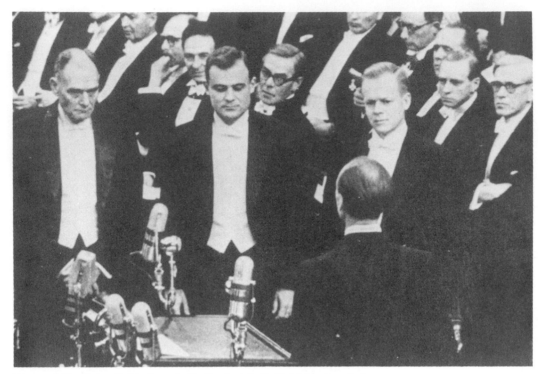

Figure 148. John F. Enders (left), Frederick C. Robbins (center),
Thomas H. Weller (right). (From Williams, Greer: Virus Hunters.
New York, Alfred A. Knopf, 1959. Photo by Black Star
Publishing Company.)

munology at the Harvard Medical School, turned from the study of bacterial
immunity to the investigation of the virus of herpes simplex. In these experiments the cell-culture method was used, with questionable results, but
Enders was convinced that this technique represented a basic tool for the
study of viruses. When he began work on poliovirus he chose, for a variety
of reasons, the roller-tube method of cell culture used by George Gey and F.
B. Bang at Johns Hopkins for the cultivation of the virus of lymphogranu-
loma venereum. By this time the advent of antibiotics had greatly facilitated
the use of cell-culture techniques (Riedman and Gustafsen, 1963).

While working with Professor Hans Zinsser on ways to grow typhus
organisms, Enders was attracted to virus research. He subsequently developed a killed-virus vaccine against mumps. His ambition was to prepare a
live vaccine from viruses tamed on chick embryo tissue, a goal which he
had the chance to pursue after World War II, when he was invited to study
infectious diseases at the Children's Hospital in Boston. It was there that he
was joined by Weller and Robbins, both of whom were receiving support
from the National Foundation for Infantile Paralysis. As recounted in
Chapter 12, while Enders, Weller, and Robbins were having morning coffee
together, Enders mentioned that he had some poliovirus in his deep-freeze.
This virus had been propagated in mouse brain tissue, but Enders
suggested that it might be possible to grow it in cultures of intestinal cells
rather than in nervous tissue. This turned out to be the case: the virus grew

well in cultures of mouse intestinal cells and also in cultures of skin, muscle, kidney, human intestinal cells, and human fetal tissues as well. That the virus could be grown in human intestinal cells was a valuable discovery, as it laid the groundwork for a later discovery by other workers, including Howe and Bodian in Baltimore; that the virus enters the body via the intestines, from which it gains access to the blood circulation and is carried to the nervous system (Riedman and Gustafsen, 1963; Benison, 1972; Paul, 1971).

In the course of this work Enders and his group made another important discovery: that the growth of the virus could be detected by using a dye that changes color as the virus grows. This obviated the need to inject the virus into animals in order to determine whether it was viable. On January 28, 1949, Enders, Weller, and Robbins reported in *Science* magazine two major achievements: (1) that poliovirus could be grown in test tubes on non-nervous tissue; and (2) that it was possible to recognize the presence of living virus without the use of a test animal. It was these two findings which made possible the successful development of poliomyelitis vaccine that was first announced six years later (Riedman and Gustafsen, 1963).

Enders and his co-workers were able to measure the neutralizing capacity of poliomyelitis antisera by determining the least amount of serum that would prevent the cytopathogenic activity of a known quantity of virus. Before this technique was developed, the isolation and typing of poliomyelitis viruses from human patients had been a time-consuming procedure that depended upon the intracerebral inoculation of monkeys. Enders was able to isolate the virus from feces or suspensions of spinal cord by adding streptomycin and penicillin to inhibit bacterial growth, followed by centrifugation to remove any contaminating bacteria. He then placed the material in cell cultures of human embryonic skin and muscle. The specific type of the virus could be determined in roller-tube cultures, using mixtures of the virus and antisera for the three known virus types. This basic method was used for the study and isolation of other viruses, and it played a major role in the development of a vaccine against measles. For their outstanding work on the poliomyelitis virus, Enders, Weller, and Robbins were awarded the Nobel Prize for medicine and physiology in 1954.

The use of tissue culture for the growth of poliovirus simplified and greatly facilitated the study of this disease. Prior to 1949, one of the chief obstacles to the experimental study of polio had been the need to employ susceptible animals, chiefly monkeys. Most of the monkeys had to be trapped in Asia, Africa, or India and transported to the United States. A laboratory in which poliomyelitis experiments were being conducted had to provide quarters for a large number of monkeys and a sizable staff to care for the animals. The work was not only expensive but also slow and cumbersome. Few institutions had the money or equipment for this type of work. The cell-culture method introduced by Enders and his associates brought about a dramatic change. Monkeys were replaced by test tubes in which the viruses were grown in cultures of tissues, and a simple, rapid test was available for detecting the presence of poliovirus and its antibodies (Benison, 1972; Riedman and Gustafsen, 1967).

Trials with Gamma Globulin. During World War II, Edwin Cohn developed a process for fractionating human blood. One of the fractions that he obtained, gamma globulin, was discovered to have the ability to prevent many infections. In 1943, shortly after Cohn's discovery, David Kramer, of the Michigan State Department of Health, demonstrated that gamma globulin protected monkeys against an intracerebral inoculation of poliovirus. Because of the war, no field trial could be organized to test whether gamma globulin had a prophylactic effect against poliomyelitis in humans (Benison, 1972; Paul, 1971).

In 1951 and again in 1952, William Hammon, with the assistance of Lewis Coriell and Joseph Stokes, Jr., and with financial support provided by the National Foundation for Infantile Paralysis, conducted a series of field trials with gamma globulin. Their results showed clearly that a small dose of gamma globulin would give children temporary protection against paralytic poliomyelitis. The significance of this discovery was quickly perceived by both Dorothy Horstmann of Yale and David Bodian of Johns Hopkins. They concluded correctly that Hammon's findings could only mean that poliovirus travels from the portal of entry (the intestinal tract) to the central nervous system via the bloodstream; and they were able to demonstrate that the virus does indeed appear in the blood early in the disease (before paralysis sets in). This indicated that even a small amount of antibody in the blood could give protection against paralytic poliomyelitis.

Two Vaccines Are Born. It will be recalled that the National Foundation for Infantile Paralysis appointed a Committee on Typing in 1949 and that after extensive study the Committee reported in 1951 that it had been able to identify only three types of poliovirus. In 1951 a Committee on Immunization was formed, and two years later a smaller Vaccine Advisory Committee was appointed. It was agreed in 1951 that an attempt should be made to develop a vaccine, but it was not known then whether it would be more profitable to work toward the development of a killed-virus vaccine or a living attenuated virus vaccine. The Foundation decided to support work along both of these lines. The work on the development of an inactivated vaccine was carried on under the direction of Jonas E. Salk, Professor of Research Bacteriology at the University of Pittsburgh, while the work on the attenuated virus was carried on under the direction of Albert B. Sabin, Professor of Research Pediatrics at the University of Cincinnati College of Medicine.

In 1952 Salk's vaccine had been thoroughly tested in animals and had reached the stage for a practical trial in human subjects. In that year, Salk inoculated 30 children at the D. T. Watson Home for Crippled Children in Leetsdale, Pennsylvania. This was a morally acceptable experiment, since the subjects had all been crippled by poliomyelitis and presumably were immune. What Salk wanted to determine was whether his inactivated vaccine would produce a rise in antibody titer. If a rise occurred, it would indicate that the vaccine had living virus in it and for this reason would be unsuitable for injection into children who had not had poliomyelitis. No rise in antibody titer occurred, and the following January, Salk inoculated 98 other subjects at the Watson Home and 63 at the Polk State School, none of whom had had poliomyelitis previously. In subsequent months he advanced the total of inoculated children to about 5000 (Paul, 1971; Benison, 1972).

652   While this work was in progress, two other investigators, Harold Cox

and Hilary Koprowski, were working on an attenuated vaccine at the Lederle Laboratories. The National Foundation was anxious to be the first to develop a successful vaccine, and since the Salk vaccine had been found to be safe in experiments with 5000 children, the Vaccine Advisory Committee recommended holding a large-scale trial of this vaccine (Benison, 1972). Thomas Francis, Jr., Chairman of the Department of Epidemiology at the University of Michigan School of Public Health was selected to conduct a nationwide field trial. The children involved were divided into two groups, one to receive an inert solution (placebo), the other the vaccine. The trial was initiated in April, 1954, using schoolchildren of the first, second, and third grades. Approximately a year was spent in evaluating the results, but by April, 1955, Francis had sufficient evidence to state unequivocally that Salk's vaccine was a success (Paul, 1971; Benison, 1972).

Sabin's effort to develop an attenuated live vaccine did not get under way until 1953. In spite of its decision to make a major effort with the Salk vaccine, the Foundation continued to support Sabin's work. Within a few years, Sabin had developed an attenuated vaccine that could be administered orally. Such a vaccine offered certain advantages. The Salk vaccine did not prevent virus from multiplying in the intestinal tract. This meant that the virus could still be transferred from person to person even in a population free of the disease; and if immunity lapsed in that population, the virus would be there to start a new epidemic. In contrast, live virus taken orally does immunize the intestinal tract just as do natural infections. Nevertheless, there were two possible dangers: (1) the attenuated virus might produce disease in the children who received it; and (2) the virus, though attenuated when administered, might undergo a mutation as it propagated in the vaccinated individual and then might be passed on to others in a more virulent form. From 1957 to 1959, Sabin's vaccine received extensive field testing in the Soviet Union, Czechoslovakia, Mexico, and Singapore (Paul, 1971; Benison, 1972). In view of the success of these large-scale trials, the United States Public Health Service, in 1961, licensed the Sabin vaccine. By that time the live-virus vaccine had already been given to 5 million persons; it appeared safe and was effective in 80 to 95 per cent of the individuals receiving it. A major attraction of live-virus vaccine was the low cost and ease of administration. The Salk vaccine had to be given by injection; the attenuated virus could be administered by mouth. It was estimated that live-virus vaccine would produce immunization against poliomyelitis at one-tenth the cost of Salk vaccine, and single doses would induce longer lasting immunity to the disease (Benison, 1972; Paul, 1971).

NEW CONCEPTS IN SUPPORT OF RESEARCH The National Foundation for Infantile Paralysis, while giving great impetus to virological research, also pioneered in the process of philanthropic giving. The Foundation was not the first voluntary health agency in the United States, but it was the first to depend on the general public rather than on the wealthy philanthropist for its funds. The March of Dimes annual collection drive made the average citizen

653

feel that he had a stake in a type of basic medical research that had a strong sentimental appeal—and the dimes and quarters and dollars poured in.

One of the most important problems faced by the Foundation during its early years was finding enough properly trained scientists to undertake the research that was required. In 1938 there were very few laboratories engaged in virus research. Of these, only a few were working on poliomyelitis. The first grants made by the Foundation went to this small group of investigators, but in order to increase the supply of qualified research workers, the Foundation, in 1940, negotiated a large, long-term grant to the Johns Hopkins University School of Hygiene and Public Health. Its aim was to create a virus research center which not only would conduct studies of poliomyelitis and other virus diseases but also would train virologists. Shortly thereafter, similar long-term grants were made to the University of Michigan School of Public Health and the Yale University School of Medicine (Benison, 1972).

These grants created a new approach to the support of medical research in the United States. Prior to this time, grants made for research by both private philanthropy and the federal government were small and were rarely made for a period of more than one year. By making large, long-term grants, the Foundation gave investigators uninterrupted time to develop their work and thus provided continuity to poliomyelitis research. Moreover, the training of virologists insured continuation of the research effort at a high level of competence.

Shortly after World War II, Foundation officials realized that many medical schools were reluctant to accept research grants because of the indirect costs which the university had to assume in administering the grants and in providing laboratory space, basic equipment, and other overhead items. Recognizing this difficulty as a threat to the development of its program, the Foundation initiated an accounting system which provided for the calculation of these indirect costs. Beginning in 1948, whenever the Foundation awarded a grant, it provided supplementary funds to the grantee institution to cover such expenses. The wisdom of this approach was recognized immediately by research administrators everywhere, and now other foundations, as well as the federal government, follow this system in allocating research grants (Benison, 1972).

COXSACKIE AND RELATED VIRUSES

Gilbert Dalldorf, pathologist at Grasslands Hospital near New York City, began some research on the poliovirus during a 1942 poliomyelitis outbreak in White Plains, New York. During these studies he first saw the "footprint" of other viruses. Dalldorf was encouraged to continue his investigations by L. T. Webster, who had explored the broad subject of neurotropic viruses (viruses with a selective affinity for nervous tissue) and who discovered the sparing effect (later called the interference phenomenon) that some other neurotropic viruses have upon poliovirus (Paul, 1971).

During the late summer of 1947, Dalldorf, who by then had become Director of Laboratories and Research in the New York State Health Depart-

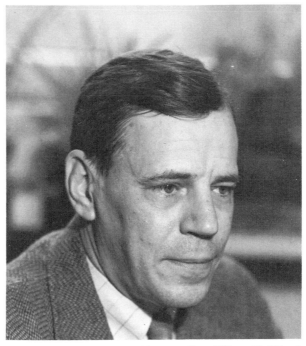

Figure 149.   Gilbert Dalldorf.

ment, and his associate, Grace M. Sickles, investigated a number of small epidemics in upstate New York with the object of finding polioviruses, or any other viruses related to cases of poliomyelitis, that would infect mice. Earlier, Dalldorf had learned the technique of infecting young mice by painting the nipples of the dams with the virus. He therefore decided to make use of suckling mice in this project. This was a decision that revolutionized research in the entire virus field, including poliomyelitis and related human infections.

Dalldorf and Sickles made several major discoveries: (1) They obtained from the feces of two patients suspected of having paralytic poliomyelitis an entirely new virus with unique properties. It caused widespread lesions in the skeletal muscles rather than in the nervous system. Animals more than one week of age were resistant to the infection. (2) They introduced a new and inexpensive animal—the suckling mouse—into the laboratory of the virologist. Other workers soon confirmed their discovery of the new virus and suggested that it be called "Coxsackie virus," since that was the name of the New York village where the first recognized human victims resided.

Within a year, other investigators had isolated related viruses from patients with different clinical syndromes, some of which resembled mild forms of poliomyelitis. By 1951 it was apparent that the growing family of Coxsackie viruses could be recovered from patients suffering from a wide variety of clinical diseases. In one major group there are central nervous system signs, typical of nonparalytic poliomyelitis or "aseptic meningitis," a term coined by Wallgren some 25 years earlier. There is also a clinical syndrome, known in Europe as Bornholm disease and in the United States

655

as devil's grippe, or pleurodynia, which Edward C. Curnen, Jr., and Joseph L. Melnick of the Yale Medical School proved to be due to a Coxsackie virus. Heubner and his colleagues at the National Institutes of Health found that a febrile illness known as "herpangina" also is caused by a Coxsackie virus (Paul, 1971).

The expanding use of cell-culture methods led to the discovery of large numbers of hitherto unknown disease-producing agents in the human intestinal tract. A new group of viruses was discovered that does not infect suckling mice or other experimental animals but that grows well in cultures of human and monkey tissues. The isolation of different strains and serotypes came so rapidly that this group became known as "viruses in search of disease." These agents finally were designated as "enteric cytopathogenic human orphans" or ECHO viruses. By 1969 this family had grown to 34 members, many of which subsequently have been associated with specific disease syndromes. The poliomyelitis, Coxsackie and ECHO viruses are similar in their predilection for the human intestinal tract, their shared physical-chemical properties, and their clinical and epidemiological behavior. These similarities eventually brought them together under the heading *enteroviruses*. There was evidence that Coxsackie and ECHO viruses interfere with the effectiveness of attenuated poliomyelitis vaccine, thus preventing satisfactory immunization. This led, in temperate climates, to the practice of administering the vaccine in winter, when infections with enteroviruses are uncommon. The task of successfully immunizing children by means of attenuated poliovirus has not been easy in semitropical or tropical areas, where enteroviruses are prevalent the year round (Paul, 1971).

VACCINES FOR MEASLES AND GERMAN MEASLES

Measles (rubeola) is a highly contagious disease. Ninety-nine per cent of persons closely exposed to a measles patient for the first time acquire the disease. As a consequence, prior to the 1960s, more than 90 per cent of the population had had measles before reaching the age of 10 years. Though the disease itself is usually relatively mild, it is often complicated by secondary bacterial infections such as otitis media and pneumonia. Since these complications usually can be controlled by antibiotics, measles became much less threatening to life after the antimicrobial drugs became available. In the 1950s an average of about 4 million cases of measles occurred in the United States each year, and in spite of antibiotics there were some 400 deaths, most of them due to pneumonia. In addition to the fatal cases, there were each year about 4000 cases of measles encephalitis, an inflammation of the brain, which though it occurs rarely, frequently leads to mental retardation. Of the 4 million cases of measles occurring annually, some 3,995,000 survived without obvious ill effects, and as a result measles too often was looked upon as an inconsequential disease. Nevertheless, it caused a vast amount of illness, and this, together with the occasional serious complications, prompted a search for preventive measures which began in the early years of the twentieth century.

Up to World War II, German measles (rubella), though highly contagious, was so mild that it attracted almost no attention. Like measles, it occurs in children at an early age; but unlike measles, serious complications almost never occur. In fact, the illness is frequently so mild that it went unnoticed, and for this reason there were no reliable statistics about the prevalence of rubella.

In 1874, J. Louis Smith, the first Professor of Pediatrics at Bellevue Hospital, New York, described an outbreak of rubella among children in an orphanage and among his private patients in the "suburbs of New York City on East 71st Street." He called this disease *German* measles because he had read about the occurrence of similar cases in Germany. Following Smith's original description, physicians frequently made a diagnosis of German measles, but no one bothered much about it until 1940 when it took on a new and gruesome aspect.

After a widespread rubella epidemic in Australia, N. McAlister Gregg, an ophthalmologist, noted a sudden rise in the incidence of congenital cataracts. By a careful study of his patients, Gregg was able to relate the occurrence of cataracts to rubella in the mother during the early months of pregnancy. This perceptive observation was the first recognition of the fact that a disease occurring during pregnancy can be teratogenic (a cause of developmental abnormalities) for the offspring. Since then many other types of congenital malformations have been traced back to the occurrence of rubella during the early months of a pregnancy. In 1960 a prospective study by Richard H. Michaels and Gilbert W. Mellin of the Columbia University College of Physicians and Surgeons reported that the fetal hazard for rubella was 47 per cent in the first month of pregnancy, 22 per cent in the second month, and 7 per cent in the third month. It was only after such facts as these became known that an all-out effort was made to develop a rubella vaccine. Before one became available, girls in their early teens were often deliberately exposed to rubella so that they would acquire immunity before becoming pregnant in later years.

THE MEASLES STORY   In 1919, when scientists at the Hospital of the Rockefeller Institute began to study measles, no causative micro-organism had been identified, and there was great uncertainty about whether the disease could be transmitted to animals. Two medical officers of the U.S. Public Health Service, J. F. Anderson and Joseph Goldberger, stated in 1911 that they had induced measles in monkeys by injecting them with blood and bacteria-free filtrates of blood from measles patients. Others attempting to repeat these experiments either failed or obtained inconclusive results. A. W. Sellards of Harvard tried again during an epidemic in a military camp in Massachusetts in 1918 and failed to infect either monkeys or human volunteers. He expressed doubt about the claim of Anderson and Goldberger that they could transmit the disease to monkeys (Paul, 1971; Corner, 1964).

Francis G. Blake, who joined the staff of the Hospital of the Rockefeller Institute in 1919, and James Trask, an assistant resident physician at the hospital, postulated that the best place to look for the causative agent of measles was in the nasal and pharyngeal secretions of the patient, during the early catarrhal stage, when the disease is highly contagious. They obtained material from the nose and throat of a measles patient and introduced it into the trachea of a monkey. Several days later the monkey developed conjunctivitis, a typical skin rash, and the telltale Koplik spots that appear in the mouth of measles patients. Obviously, the monkey had measles. After this experiment had been repeated several times, it was found that the disease could be transmitted to monkeys by nasopharyngeal drippings which had been passed through a bacteria-retaining filter. Thus it was shown that the disease is due to a filterable virus. Later it was found that measles could be passed from monkey to monkey by means of blood or ground-up skin and mucous membranes taken from measles-infected animals during the contagious stage of the disease. Finally, Blake and Trask found that monkeys which had recovered from experimentally induced measles were immune to reinfection (Paul, 1971).

The reason for the failure of previous attempts to transmit measles to monkeys was not clarified until some 25 years later. Rhesus monkeys in the wild state are highly susceptible to measles, and once they have been caught and herded together they are frequently exposed to the measles virus; they contract the disease and thereafter are immune. Blake and Trask had the good fortune to have a shipment of previously unexposed monkeys which had recently arrived from India. Otherwise they would have failed in their attempt to transmit the virus as many others had before them (Paul, 1971). It is possible that the same factors favored the earlier success of Anderson and Goldberger.

In the 1930s and early 1940s, several important peculiarities of viruses were discovered. Interference, transformation (reactivation), and hemagglutination were demonstrated, thus opening new avenues of viral research. Although the interference phenomenon was found originally with plant viruses, examples also were found among animal viruses, notably by Hoskins (1935) in strains of yellow fever virus. Studies of the mechanism of these phenomena have uncovered many important aspects of viral multiplication at the cellular level. As will be seen later, practical work with rubella virus became possible as a result of the discovery of viral interference, a process by which the virus not only fails to destroy or visibly affect the cells in a culture but also makes such cells resistant to destruction by another cytopathic virus.

In 1954 John F. Enders and Thomas C. Peebles isolated a strain of measles virus and attenuated it by passage in cell culture. They then proceeded to work toward the production of a vaccine. After nine years of development, two measles vaccines, one a live-virus preparation and the other an inactivated one, were licensed for use in the United States (1963). It was found that in order to obtain good protection with the inactivated virus, it had to be given in three injections at monthly intervals. The protection, effective at the outset, gradually diminished over a period of months. The attenuated live-vaccine, on the other hand, in a single injection evoked a rise in antibodies equal to, and as long-lasting as that of natural measles. The early batches of live-vaccine, however, produced a variety of side effects, including a fever of 103° F or higher in 30 to 40 per cent of the children receiving it. Subsequent experience demonstrated that the undesirable side effects could be lessened by administering gamma globulin along with the vaccine. Finally, a more attenuated live-vaccine was developed that made the live-vaccine suitable for general use.

With widespread use of measles vaccine, the number of cases of measles reported in 1968 had fallen to 220,000 from the pre-vaccine level of 4 million annually. In 1969 the federal government, hoping that the states would give greater support to the measles program, diverted some of its funds to the new rubella program (see later in this chapter). Unfortunately, many states did not have sufficient money for purchasing measles vaccine, and many state health departments terminated their vaccination efforts. The number of doses of vaccine administered in 1969 and 1970 was 2.3 million less than in 1967 and 1968. As a result, the incidence of measles increased to 530,000 cases in 1970 and 850,000 in 1971. Federal money for the measles vaccination programs again became available in mid-1971, and in 1971 and 1972 considerably more vaccine was administered than in any two previous years. In 1973 the case incidence was lower than it had been in 1968.

In 1975, J. J. Witte and N. W. Axnick, of the Center for Disease Control of the U.S. Public Health Service, reported on the benefits from 10 years (1963–1972) of measles immunization. They estimated that 12.700,000 cases of measles had been averted, 2400 lives saved, 7900 cases of mental retardation averted, 12,182,000 physician visits saved, and 1,352,000 hospital days saved. The economic saving during the 10-year period was placed at $1.3 billion. This was the net economic benefit after deducting the cost of preparing and administering the vaccine, which was estimated at $3 per dose. The cost of the 16.5 million doses administered in 1971 and 1972 was approximately $49.5 million. Though this was a considerable sum, it was far outweighed by the benefits achieved (Witte and Axnick, 1975).

THE RUBELLA STORY   The early attempts to cultivate a specific infectious agent from cases of rubella were unsuccessful. Some viruses can multiply in cells without killing them and, therefore, do not produce recognizable cellular disease. However, these viruses can interfere with the cellular effects of other viruses, and this *interference phenomenon* was used to discover the rubella virus. In 1960 Thomas H. Weller of the Harvard School of Public Health, who had worked with Enders on the poliomyelitis virus, had a son who contracted an unusually severe rubella-like illness. Weller decided to make some cultures to rule out the presence of a more serious disease. When the material was placed in a culture of human amniotic cells he was able to detect unique cytopathic changes. With Franklin A. Neva, he later recovered agents having similar cellular effects from patients with typical cases of rubella. At the same time Paul D. Parkman, E. L. Buescher, and Malcolm Artenstein of the Walter Reed Army Medical Center inoculated several cell types in tissue culture with throat washings taken from Army recruits with rubella. Even though there were no detectable cytopathic effects, these workers, instead of discarding the cultures, inoculated them with ECHO virus, an agent with typical cytopathic effects. They discovered that the cultures previously inoculated with the rubella specimens were resistant to a superimposed infection with ECHO virus. In addition, serum from the patients was shown to contain a specific antibody that neutralized the rubella virus. The two groups of workers at Walter Reed and Harvard concluded that they were dealing with the same virus and arranged for simultaneous publication of their findings.

Soon after this discovery, it was demonstrated by Robert H. Green, Michael R. Balsero, J. P. Giles, Saul Krugman, and George S. Mirick of the New York University School of Medicine that the virus is present in throat and serum one week before the appearance of the rubella rash. Antibody appears promptly and persists for years, being completely protective against reinfection. Green and his co-workers could not produce infection in volunteers who had even minimal levels of rubella antibody. This indicated that women exposed to rubella during pregnancy incur no risk of maternal or fetal infection if they have demonstrable antibodies at the time of exposure.

An extensive epidemic of German measles swept the United States in the late winter and early spring of 1964, producing congenital defects in some 20,000 infants. Shortly before this epidemic, Plotkin, in Philadelphia, and Weller, in Boston, had reported finding rubella antibody in infants with congenital rubella, and rubella virus itself was still present in the throat secretions and urine of several children with congenital defects. It therefore appeared that rubella contracted before birth is a chronic infection, in contrast to the acute and self-limiting disease contracted after birth. The virus in the congenital form not only is present at birth but also persists for some time after birth even though the infant's serum contains high levels of antibody. Virus was found also in fetal tissue obtained by therapeutic abortions performed months after the mother had rubella. Thus, the effect of rubella seemed to differ from that of other teratogens such as thalidomide and radiation, which do their damage with one exposure in early pregnancy. The rubella virus exerts its damaging effect on the fetus over a longer time period during gestation.

The obvious answer to the rubella problem was the development of a vaccine that would virtually eliminate the disease from the entire population. The first experimental vaccines produced a mild form of German measles followed by good antibody production. They were unacceptable, however, because the vaccinated person could transmit the disease to susceptible contacts. This feature, desirable in live poliomyelitis vaccine because it spreads the mild disease and confers widespread immunity, would be catastrophic in the case of rubella, since even the mildest infection is a dire threat to the pregnant woman. The need was to attenuate the virus so that it would not produce a transmissible disease but would still stimulate antibody production. In 1966 Paul D. Parkman and Harry M. Myer, Jr., of the Division of Biological Standards of the National Institutes of Health, reported the production of a live, attenuated rubella vaccine that met these requirements. The successful large-scale production of rubella vaccine was finally achieved in 1968, and distribution was begun by the U.S. Public Health Service.

The effectiveness of immunization against measles and rubella is shown by the experience in Alaska. During the years 1957 to 1966, the incidence of measles in Alaska was well above the average for the United States, reaching peaks of 1000 in 1959, and just under 900 in 1963, per 100,000 population. During the same years, the incidence of rubella was also usually above the national average, with peaks of about 350 in 1957 and about 450 in 1963. Measles immunization began in Alaska in 1966, and vaccination against rubella began in 1969. By 1974, 91 per cent of children under two years of age had been vaccinated against measles and 89 per cent against rubella. There was a sharp drop in the incidence of both these diseases following the institution of the immunization programs; and it was reported that in the year 1974 there had not been a verified case of either measles or rubella in Alaska (Eisenberg and Crowe, 1976).

At least 13 viruses are now known to produce intrauterine infection and fetal damage. In addition to rubella these diseases are as follows: cytomegalovirus, herpes simplex, mumps, measles, western equine encephalitis, chickenpox, herpes zoster, smallpox, cowpox, influenza, poliomyelitis, hepatitis, and Coxsackie B viruses. Blood serum from the umbilical cord and from newborn infants contains unusually high levels of IgM in cases of congenital infection, and determination of the IgM level appears to be useful for the recognition of such infections and for the diagnosis of infections in the newborn.

The Collaborative Perinatal Research Study, initiated in 1948 with 14 collaborating university-affiliated institutions at locations throughout the United States, collected data on perinatal viral infections. Chronic infection of the fetus, which may persist for months or years after birth, has been noted for rubella, cytomegalovirus, and herpes simplex. Perhaps greater susceptibility of the embryonic tissue and relative immaturity of immunological responses of the developing fetus are responsible for the chronicity of the infections.

In cytomegalic inclusion disease, many developmental abnormalities are found. During life, the diagnosis can be made by demonstrating typical inclusion-bearing cells in the urinary sediment. It is also possible to isolate the virus from the urine, throat washings, or blood, and this provides a more reliable method of diagnosis. As with rubella, the cytomegalic infection persists in the infant for months or years in spite of the presence of specific neutralizing antibody (Sever and White, 1968).

THE HEPATITIS VIRUS

Hepatitis was an ill-defined and confusing disease prior to World War II. It paraded under a variety of names: epidemic jaundice, catarrhal jaundice, Weil's disease, infective or infectious hepatitis, acute yellow atrophy of the liver, and still others. Efforts to find the causative agent of epidemic jaundice had been unsuccessful, except for the discovery in 1914 by Japanese scientists that a spirochete (leptospira) appeared to be the cause of a very severe type of epidemic disease in which jaundice and hemorrhagic phenomena were prominent. Clinically, this was the same disease that had been described in Germany in 1886 by Adolf Weil, and for a time all epidemic jaundice was called Weil's disease and was believed to be due to a spirochete. In time this was proved not to be the case.

In 1923 George Blumer at Yale was among the first in this country to point out that there is a distinct and identifiable form of infectious hepatitis which occurs in epidemics; and that catarrhal jaundice is probably a sporadic form of this disease.

Progress toward the identification of the cause of infectious hepatitis began to be made in 1937 when G. M. Findlay and F. O. MacCallum, in England, found that at least one form of hepatitis could be transmitted from one human subject to another by injection of blood serum.

During World War II hepatitis became a major health problem in all of the theatres of operation. Shortly after the United States entered the war, there was a widespread, and initially puzzling, outbreak of jaundice (hepatitis) among American troops. Epidemiological detective work disclosed that the soldiers who developed the jaundice had received immunizing doses of certain specific lots of yellow-fever vaccine. Each of these lots of vaccine contained pooled human serum as a viral neutralizing agent; and it was eventually shown that the serum was the source of the agent which caused the hepatitis—presumably the same agent that Findlay and MacCallum had identified five years earlier.

Research during the war opened an entirely new chapter in the hepatitis story. Work in the United States, particularly by John R. Paul, W. P. Havens, Jr., and others at Yale; by Joseph Stokes, Jr., John R. Neefe, and their associates at the University of Pennsylvania; and in England by Findlay, MacCallum, and their co-workers, disclosed that there are two distinct types of hepatitis and that both are due to a filterable virus. One type was designated *infectious* (type A) *hepatitis* (IH). This form of the disease has a short incubation period (two to six weeks) and occurs in epidemics, and the virus is present in the feces and blood. The other form, *serum* (type B) *hepatitis* (SH) has a long incubation period (six weeks to six months), is transmitted parenterally by injection of blood or blood constituents, and the virus is present in the blood serum. Patients who had had IH developed immunity to IH but not to SH, whereas those who had had SH developed immunity to SH but not to IH. All of these extensive studies had to be carried out on human volunteers because at that time no experimental animal was known to be susceptible to hepatitis. Subsequent studies have indicated that both types of hepatitis can be transmitted by either oral or parenteral routes; and other distinctions between the two types have become less sharp with the passage of time.

Hepatitis research was relatively unproductive during the 1950s, but it gathered momentum during the 1960s. The observation that laid the foundation for the recent advance came in 1963 when Bernard Blumberg, while studying the variation in serum constituents as a means of measuring genetic traits, discovered a previously unrecognized lipoprotein (Australia antigen) in the serum of an Australian aborigine. Four years later, Alfred M. Prince of the New York City Blood Center observed a similar substance, which is now called hepatitis B surface antigen (HB_sAg), in the blood of patients with hepatitis B. The Blumberg and the Prince substances were later shown to be identical, and to be part of the coat of the suspected B virus. As Blumberg and his associates continued their studies, additional information emerged, showing that this antigen occurred in 10 to 20 per cent of people in tropical areas. In the United States it was found to be uncommon in healthy persons but was present with significant frequency in patients with Down's syndrome, leukemia, or hepatitis. Twenty-nine per cent of individuals with hemophilia, who necessarily received many units of blood by transfusion, were found to have the antibody in their serum. The prevalence of the antigen in several of these syndromes was explained on the basis of frequent exposure to infection with hepatitis virus, either through contact or through blood transfusions. Numerous reports soon confirmed the concept that the antigen (HB$_s$Ag) is a factor specifically associated with type B hepatitis.

Discovery of HB$_s$Ag has greatly advanced our knowledge of hepatitis. Type A hepatitis (IH) was almost uniformly HB$_s$Ag-negative, and hepatitis following blood transfusions (SH) was HB$_s$Ag-positive in over 70 per cent of cases. It was found that evidence of hepatitis was demonstrable in 50 to 75 per cent of patients receiving HB$_s$Ag-positive blood, although they may not be jaundiced. The overall incidence of hepatitis following blood transfusion is 2.5 per cent. The HB$_s$Ag antigen has been demonstrated in as many as 97 per cent of cases of serum hepatitis.

Progress has also been made in identifying the virus of type A hepatitis, which as a worldwide health problem is more important than type B. In 1973 R. H. Purcell and his colleagues at the National Institutes of Health identified 27-nanometer particles in patients with type A hepatitis during the acute phase of the illness. The particles were aggregated by convalescent serum. F. Deinhardt and his group in Chicago had, since 1967, been working with the type A virus in marmoset monkeys, which had been found to be susceptible to the disease. The livers of infected marmosets contained the 27-nanometer viral particles. In human volunteers, virus particles appear in the feces five days before there is evidence of damage to the liver; they disappear when the liver damage reaches its height. Antibody to type A virus appears early in the acute attack and tends to persist in the serum. M. Hilleman has discovered the virus particles in human liver cells.

In hepatitis B, a particle in the blood, described by Dane in 1970, probably represents the complete virion. It has a core which is found in the nucleus of the liver cell and double-shelled surface particles which are formed in the cytoplasm. The surface antigen is the one routinely measured in blood as HB$_s$Ag; the corresponding antibody is HB$_s$Ab. Hoofnagle has shown that in the acutely ill patient, the core antibody level rises shortly after surface antigen is detected and that it tends to persist. Surface antibody appears later.

Immune serum globulin is of proven value in the prevention of type A hepatitis. Grady has observed that the surface antibody titer of immunogammaglobulin found in the blood of volunteer blood donors has risen in recent years; it was present in a dilution of 1 to 8 in 1947 and 1 to 256 in 1971. It must be assumed that the conventional immunoglobulin is potent enough to protect against type B as well as type A hepatitis.

Active immunization against type B hepatitis is also becoming possible. R. B. Purcell and his group at the National Institutes of Health have prepared a vaccine consisting of subunits of hepatitis B. Dane particles are removed by differential centrifugation so that only the 22-nanometer forms remain. The vaccine is effective against hepatitis B in chimpanzees. Hilleman and his group have made a potent vaccine by plasmapheresis of blood from carriers positive for surface antigen. Dane particles are removed, and this vaccine is also effective against hepatitis B in chimpanzees.

663

"SLOW" VIRUSES The term "slow infection" is not new. In the early 1950s Sigurdsson, an Icelandic pathologist, applied the name to maedi, a slowly progressive pneumonia of sheep, and to rida, a chronic encephalitis of sheep. His criteria for designating an infection as "slow" were: (1) a long latent period lasting from several months to several years; (2) a protracted course usually ending in death; and (3) strict host specificity and sometimes familial predisposition. Other characteristics of slow viral infections that have been recognized more recently are (1) persistence of the agent in the infected host for much or all of the host's life and (2) a long, continued host response which may, in itself, be part of the disease process. The concept of slow infections has influenced thinking about diseases of a progressive degenerative nature which have a protracted course and an obscure etiology. Some of the features of rabies, herpes simplex, rubella, and cytomegalovirus might place them in this category.

A number of slow virus diseases have been studied in man. Subacute sclerosing panencephalitis, known as Dawson's encephalitis, is a progressive neurological disease of children, characterized by intracytoplasmic and intranuclear inclusions in the nervous tissue. Measles virus has been grown from brain tissue of patients with this disease.

Another human neurological disease, progressive multifocal leukoencephalopathy (PML), first described in 1958, also is thought to be a slow virus disease. It is usually associated with Hodgkin's disease or chronic lymphatic leukemia. Reports indicate that PML may be a latent infection with a virus which by some unknown mechanism becomes activated and manifests itself by attacking the central nervous tissues. A viral agent has recently been isolated.

D. C. Gajdusek of the National Institute of Neurological Diseases and Blindness (NIH) and V. Zigas described a progressive, degenerative encephalopathy of natives of the Fore Tribe in New Guinea which they call *kuru*. Extensive studies have since confirmed that kuru is an infectious disease that persists for many years, during which the virus is present. The disease was reproduced by inoculation of filtered material into chimpanzees and subsequently was transmitted from one to another of these animals. The pioneering studies of Gajdusek and his colleagues have led to virtual elimination of this disease, which was formerly the commonest cause of death in the Fore tribe (Leader and Hurvitz, 1972).

THE QUEST FOR HUMAN CANCER VIRUSES Since the early period of virology there has been continuing interest in the possible relationship of viruses to cancer. In the 1950s a substantial amount of information accumulated regarding the intimate properties of oncogenic (tumor-producing) viruses and the many new tumors of rodents in which viruses have been established as the causal agents (Gross, 1952; Stewart, 1954; Friend, 1956; Maloney, 1962). Recent progress in this area of virology can be attributed to the use of newborn animals for tumor cultivation, improvements in cell-culture methodology for the propagation of viral entities, and the extensive use of the electron microscope to visualize viruses and their relation to the detailed structure of normal and malignant cells. There is still need to prove conclusively that some type of human cancer has a viral origin. Many reports have been published on the transmission of various human oncogenic agents to laboratory animals; but in view of the many pitfalls and difficulties associated with this type of work, the findings are difficult to interpret. The demonstration by Trentin and his associates in 1962 that a human virus, adenovirus type 12, possesses oncogenic properties on intrapulmonary injection of newborn hamsters, was a significant advance. Tumor induction by adenovirus was confirmed and demonstrated also, with adenovirus type 18 (Huebner et al., 1962).

THE EPSTEIN-BARR VIRUS AND INFECTIOUS MONONUCLEOSIS

When first discovered in cell lines derived from Burkitt's lymphoma, Epstein-Barr virus (EBV) seemed a breakthrough in the attempt to delineate a viral etiology in cancer. Subsequent studies revealed that EBV is an ubiquitous herpes virus of higher primates. Nevertheless, it has relationships to Burkitt's lymphoma and to nasopharyngeal carcinoma that still are unexplained. Klein and his group observed that sera from patients with Burkitt's lymphoma contained high levels of antibody to a membrane antigen (MA) on living cells, both from fresh tumor and cell lines derived from the tumor. These cell lines provided not only a means for Epstein's visualization of the herpes-like virus particle but also a source of infective virus and virus products for immunological analysis. Gertrude and Werner Henle and their colleagues, at the Children's Hospital, Philadelphia, in 1966, described a serum antibody directed toward a cytoplasmic antigen in cells of the lymphoblast cell line. This antigen is part of the virus particle itself, namely its capsid protein, VCA (virus capsid antigen). Antibody to VCA has since been found in the serum of a high proportion of American adults (Smith and Bausher, 1972).

This story is another example of a serendipitous observation, for it was only when a previously serum-negative member of the laboratory staff became VCA-positive during the course of infectious mononucleosis that the Henles obtained the first evidence, in 1968, of the probable etiological role of the Epstein-Barr virus in infectious mononucleosis. They found that patients with infectious mononucleosis regularly develop antibodies to EBV, which persist for many years (Henle et al., 1968).

In patients having classical infectious mononucleosis accompanied by increased heterophile antibody titers, anti-VCA appears in the serum within five to seven days of the onset of clinical disease. Repeated examination of sera from Yale students showed that anti-VCA was present in about 25 per cent of entering students. During the next four to six years, the number of students exhibiting the antibody increased to about 75 per cent. Those positive on entry to Yale did not develop clinically evident infectious mononucleosis during their four years in college. All cases of the disease occurred in those negative on admission (Smith and Bausher, 1972). EBV is invariably present in lymphoblastoid cell lines isolated from patients who have the active disease or have recently recovered from it. Thus, a variety of

665

evidence favors an etiological role for EBV in infectious mononucleosis, despite only fragmentary evidence for direct transmission by the virus.

CLINICAL DIAGNOSIS OF VIRAL DISEASE

One of the problems faced by the clinical virologist has been the long interval between the onset of the viral illness and the availability of laboratory confirmation of the diagnosis. Although identification of a virus or viral antigen in a specimen does not prove that it is the etiological agent, there are many diseases in which a viral agent has been shown to be the cause and where identification of virus in involved material is satisfactory presumptive evidence of the etiological diagnosis.

Some viruses, for example the smallpox virus, can be identified by electron microscopy. However, at present, this is primarily a research tool. A number of tests have been devised to identify Australia antigen (HB_sAg) by methods that will give a quick answer, including gel diffusion, complement fixation, reversed passive hemagglutination, and radioimmunoassay. Such techniques depend on high-quality immune sera which react specifically with the virus being sought and which can be applied in other diseases as well. The technique of immunofluorescence introduced by Coons in 1942 also depends on the quality of the reagents used. This method has recently been applied more extensively in the rapid diagnosis of viral disease. The presence of the virus can be identified within hours in samples taken directly from the patient. Advances in understanding and improved management of disease depend upon an early diagnosis, and the more universal use of these new techniques for rapid viral diagnosis will assist the search for better means of controlling viral diseases (Editorial, *Lancet*, 1975).

28

Cancer

Virology, immunology and chemotherapy may well stand for the first three letters that will spell victory over cancer. The day is not yet here, and we shall experience many disappointments before it dawns. But it is clearer than ever that cancer is a solvable problem, solvable by a human thought-and-action process that we call scientific research, and within the capabilities of human intelligence with which man was endowed by his creator.

(M. B. Shimkin, 1973)

Cancer may arise in any organ of the body. Its main characteristic is unrestricted growth of tissue cells. Cancer cells may be carried by the blood to distant sites of the body, where they form so-called metastases. Cancers are classified by their appearance under the microscope and by the site of the body from which they originate. The term *cancer* embraces many different entities that are dissimilar in appearance, in behavior, and perhaps in causative factors as well (Shimkin, 1973).

There has been a steady increase in cancer deaths during the past 50 years. Some of this increase, more apparent than real, has been due to more accurate diagnosis. An important factor contributing to the real increase has been the advancing age of the average citizen; the older an individual is, the more likely he is to have cancer. During the past three decades, there has been a striking increase in the incidence of cancer of the lung and of leukemia and related cancers of the blood and lymphatic system. The Third National Cancer Survey of 1969 revealed a rise of 20 per cent in the incidence of cancer among blacks, chiefly tumors of the pancreas, prostate, and esophagus. Since there are many types of cancer, there appears to be little hope of the development of a single laboratory test for diagnosis. The diagnosis in a living patient is based on the examination of a sample of the diseased tissue under the microscope — a biopsy.

If cancer can be recognized early, successful treatment may be achieved by removal of the entire cancerous area, either by surgery or by radiation. These two forms of treatment are not mutually exclusive; they may be combined.

Surgical resections of internal cancers became feasible in the nineteenth century after the introduction of anesthesia and asepsis. During the twentieth century, numerous improvements in surgical technique, and the use of blood transfusions and antibiotics, have made all portions of the human body accessible to the surgeon. Early examples of surgical triumphs were the operations for removal of intra-abdominal tumors, Harvey Cushing's operations for tumors of the brain, and the first surgical removal of a cancerous lung by Evarts Graham of Washington University, St. Louis.

The early experience with the use of X-rays and radium for the treatment of cancer was described in Chapter 14. The principles of radiation therapy have not changed, but there have been great improvements in technique and an increase in the modalities available for treatment. Radiation can now be delivered at much higher voltage over a shorter period of exposure. The electron beam of a high-voltage source can be focused more precisely, both in cross section and depth, so that it exerts its maximum effect on the target tissue without damaging surrounding parts. Descriptions of technical improvements and modern equipment are beyond the scope of this discussion. However, it should be said that modern radiation therapy is capable of completely eradicating certain types of cancer and can be employed for the palliation of symptoms in patients whose cancer cannot be eradicated either by surgery or radiation.

For many years, decisions regarding the treatment of cancer were made by the patient's physician, usually in consultation with a surgeon and a pathologist. Later, when hormones and other chemical agents became available for the treatment of certain types of cancer, decision-making became far more complicated and difficult, and as a result a new specialist—the oncologist (tumor expert)—entered the picture. At present, the treatment of cancer patients can best be guided by a team consisting of physician, surgeon, radiologist, pathologist, and oncologist. The ascendancy of the oncologist began in 1939 when Charles B. Huggins, at the University of Chicago, discovered that patients with advanced cancer of the prostate gland could, in many instances, be treated very successfully by removing their testes and giving them female sex hormones.

In the United States two organizations, one governmental and the other voluntary, have been largely responsible for providing the funds for cancer research: (1) the National Cancer Institute, established in 1937, and expanded by the National Cancer Act of 1971; (2) the American Cancer Society, a voluntary public agency, incorporated in 1945. Among the larger institutions devoted entirely to cancer research are the National Cancer Institute, a component of the National Institutes of Health; the Roswell Park Memorial Institute in Buffalo, New York; the Memorial Sloan-Kettering Cancer Center in New York City; the M. D. Anderson Hospital and Tumor Institute in Houston, Texas; and the Children's Cancer Research Foundation in Boston, Massachusetts. A number of new centers are now developing, with support being provided by grants from the NIH under a program activated by the National Cancer Act of 1971. These centers will provide coordination and leadership within their geographic regions to assure availability of up-to-date care for cancer patients (Shimkin, 1973).

CANCER: ITS NATURE AND DEVELOPMENT

Cancer now accounts for almost 20 per cent of all deaths in the United States. There are over 100 distinct varieties of malignant tumors. About half of all deaths from cancer are caused by those originating in three areas: the lung, the large intestine, and the breast. The incidence of all three rises steeply with age. The death rate from cancer of the large intestine, for example, increases about a thousandfold between the ages of 20 and 80 years, most of the increase being after the age of 60. This relationship with age suggests that each cancer is the result of successive mutational steps that occur as age advances. For example, the incidence of lung cancer is directly proportional not to the number of cigarettes being smoked today but rather to the number that were smoked 20 years ago. After exposure to a carcinogenic (cancer-producing) agent, many years may elapse before the appearance of the first cancer makes it possible to recognize the danger. It may then be too late to take the necessary preventive measures (Cairns, 1975).

Environment plays a significant role: in Japan, cancer of the stomach is far more common than in the United States, whereas cancers of the large intestine, the breast, and the prostate are less common. When Japanese move to the United States, these differences disappear within the next generation or two. The influence of environment appears to be real, but it is not easy to explain how it operates. Certainly with some types of cancer, national customs and habits play a more important role than geography. For example, cancer of the lung seems clearly to be related to the habit of cigarette smoking, which increases the risk of dying of this disease some 10 to 50 fold. Some of the commonest cancers appear to be related to diet and other habits, or to exposure to certain substances in the environment. If by appropriate public health measures, the incidence of these factors could be reduced to the lowest possible level, one might hope to effect a reduction in the incidence of cancer equal to the reduction in the incidence of infectious diseases achieved in the past half-century (Cairns, 1975).

The causation of cancer is increasingly related to the technology of our society. Each year 700 to 1000 new chemical compounds are introduced into this country; yet there is no legal requirement for chemicals other than drugs to undergo full-scale testing for safety. It seems possible that small doses of various pollutants, such as fumes in the air and chemicals in food or drinking water, may be increasing the risk of cancer (Cairns, 1975).

Out of every 100,000 Americans, 176 died of cancer in the first seven months of 1975. This was the highest death rate recorded for cancer since figures were first accumulated, some 40 years ago. The rise in the cancer death rate is a source of particular concern, since cancer treatment has improved steadily during the past decade. The rise in death rate must, therefore, be due to an increased incidence of cancer. Today the annual death rate is about 75 per cent higher than it was in 1933. This increase may be due to the growing use of, and exposure to, chemicals of various sorts.

CANCER-PRODUCING CHEMICALS IN THE ENVIRONMENT

We are exposed to innumerable chemicals in our daily lives; some estimates attribute 80 per cent of human cancer to the carcinogenic effect of these substances. In the past, the standard methods for determining carcinogenic activity of chemicals has involved the use of rodents as test animals. Such tests must be carried out under carefully controlled conditions; they are relatively costly, and a long waiting period is

669

required before a definitive answer can be obtained. Because of these and other factors, the standard rodent tests have been carried out on only a small fraction of the potential carcinogens in our environment.

Bruce N. Ames and his colleagues at the University of California (Berkeley) have recently devised a very sensitive and simple bacterial test for detecting chemical mutagens (agents that cause genetic mutations). The value of this test as an indicator of carcinogenicity is based on the fact that the active forms of a large number of proven carcinogens are known to be mutagens. In the bacterial test the bacillus *Salmonella typhimurium* is used as the test organism. The principal limitation of any bacterial system for detecting carcinogens as mutagens is that bacteria do not duplicate mammalian metabolism in activating carcinogens. Ames and his co-workers discovered that by adding a microsomal activation system from rat or human liver to the bacterial culture medium, a wide variety of carcinogens could be activated to mutagens and thus were easily detected. Ames believed that compounds that give a positive test for mutagenicity in the microbial system should be considered potentially carcinogenic for man and should be subjected to the more time-consuming standard tests in mammals (Ames et al., 1973; McCann et al., 1975).

The use of the simple bacterial test for screening potentially carcinogenic substances has wide applicability and saves both time and expense. However, there is some question about whether mutagenicity is a reliable measure of carcinogenicity. One critic views the mutagenicity test as "a bit like looking under the lamppost for the coin lost a block away because of the availability of light. . . . We must still assume the hard and expensive task of looking for carcinogens by determining a compound's carcinogenic action because that is the only way we can know what we have found" (Rubin, 1976). Nevertheless, this type of criticism does not appear to invalidate the Ames procedure as a simple screening test (Ames, 1976).

EARLY STUDIES OF EXPERIMENTAL CANCERS

THE ROUS SARCOMA

An early event in cancer research in this country was the discovery at the Rockefeller Institute by Simon Flexner and James Jobling of an epithelial tumor of the rabbit which they were able to transplant to other rabbits, a considerable feat at that time. When Jobling left the Institute, his position was offered to *Peyton Rous,* a young pathologist trained at the Johns Hopkins Medical School.

Rous was hesitant about accepting the invitation, for at that time there seemed to be little hope of any exciting new discoveries in the cancer field. Nevertheless, Flexner's offer proved irresistible, and Rous joined the staff of the Institute in 1908. Before he left Hopkins, his mentor, William H. Welch, said to him: "Whatever you do, do not commit yourself to the cancer problem." In spite of this warning Rous did commit himself, and within a few weeks he made a series of revolutionary discoveries. A dealer brought a chicken to the laboratory with a large tumor on its leg. Rous found that it was a spindle-cell sarcoma, a type of tumor highly malignant in mammals, including humans. He transplanted small portions of the tumor into other

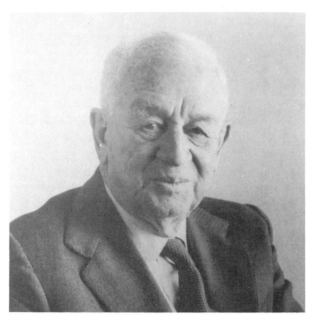

Figure 150. Peyton Rous. (National Library of Medicine, Bethesda, Maryland.)

chickens and showed that it was transmissible. Next he passed ground-up tumor through a filter that removed tumor cells and bacteria, but the filtrate was still capable of inducing sarcoma when injected into healthy chickens. This provided strong evidence that the sarcoma was due to a virus too small to be seen under the microscope. Rous succeeded in killing the sarcoma cells without destroying the virus, by freezing and drying the tumor tissue. This was the first successful application of the process of *lyophilization,* now widely used in biological research (Corner, 1964).

In order to find out whether the age of the chicken was related to the development of the tumor, Rous and James B. Murphy implanted the tumor in chick embryos, where it grew with greater rapidity than in adult fowls. This was the first use of embryos of any kind for the maintenance of grafted tumors and as a medium for the growth of viruses (Corner, 1964).

THE VIRUS OF EXPERIMENTAL LEUKEMIA

In 1940, *Ludwik Gross,* a Polish physician who had done cancer research at the Pasteur Institute in Paris, came to the United States, and five years later he was appointed Chief of Cancer Research at the Veterans' Administration Hospital in the Bronx, New York. Gross was intrigued by the role that viruses might play in the transmission of malignant tumors. He was aware of J. J. Bittner's work on the transmission of a tumor of mice. In the 1930s at the Jackson Memorial Laboratory in Bar Harbor, Maine, Bittner had demonstrated that a mammary carcinoma of mice was transmitted through the milk from mother to offspring. This was the first demonstration of natural transmission of a tumor-inducing agent

671

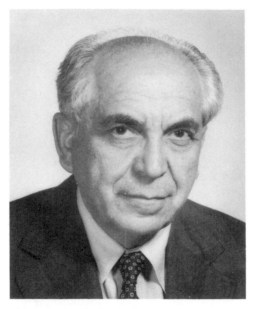

Figure 151. Ludwik Gross.

from one generation to another. Gross found other reports of a familial incidence of certain forms of cancer in successive generations of animals,
including humans. He wondered whether such a familial incidence might
mean that tumor-inducing viruses were transmitted in a latent form from
one generation to another. The virus might remain harmless in the carrier
(mother) and become activated by some triggering factor, with the production of cancer in the offspring. Gross coined the term "vertical transmission" to describe this form of transmission of oncogenic viruses, as opposed to "horizontal transmission" of contagious pathogenic agents. He
knew that at least two inbred strains of mice had a high incidence of spontaneous leukemia in each successive generation. Scientists believed that the
transmission of this leukemia was determined by genetic factors. Gross
thought that it might be due to transmission of a leukemogenic virus, and
he began attempts to transmit mouse leukemia by filtrates. At first, his
results were uniformly negative.

Then by chance, in 1951, Gross heard Gilbert Dalldorf describe the use of
suckling mice, less than 48 hours old, for the isolation of viruses. Shortly
thereafter, Gross found an elderly female mouse of the Ak strain with spontaneous leukemia and at the same time a C3H female with a litter born the
preceding day. (The C3H strain is not subject to spontaneous leukemia.) An
extract of cells from organs of the leukemic Ak mouse was inoculated into
the day-old suckling mice. All of the inoculated infant mice developed
leukemia within two weeks (Gross, 1974b). Then Ak leukemic extracts were
passed through a Berkefeld filter that held back bacteria, and the filtrate was
inoculated into newborn C3H mice. A significant number of the inoculated
animals developed leukemia after a latent period of 10 to 18 months. Later
Gross made extracts from apparently healthy normal embryos removed
from pregnant healthy Ak females and inoculated such extracts into newborn C3H mice. A significant number of the inoculated mice developed

672

leukemia, demonstrating that the mouse leukemia virus is transmitted from one generation to another through the embryos.

Gross also knew that several inbred strains of mice, such as C3H or C57-black, which are essentially free from spontaneous leukemia, would become leukemic after being exposed repeatedly to X-rays. Gross induced leukemia in C3H mice by X-ray exposure, then prepared extracts from the leukemic organs of these mice, passed the extracts through bacterial filters, and inoculated the filtrate into newborn C3H mice. A significant number of the inoculated mice developed leukemia, showing that radiation-induced leukemia is caused by a virus.

Thus the introduction, in 1951, of the newborn mouse as a basic experimental tool for the detection and bioassay of the oncogenic potential of viruses proved to be of great value in experimental cancer research (Gross, 1974b).

VIRUSES AND CANCER

A cancer occurs when a single cell undergoes permanent hereditary changes and then gives rise to billions of similarly altered cells. There are two distinguishing characteristics of cancer cells: (1) they escape the regulatory mechanisms of the body and are continuously in a cycle of multiplication; and (2) they do not remain confined to their original location but invade other tissues.

One of the important objectives of cancer research is the identification of the molecular changes that occur in the cell that becomes malignant. A change in the regulation of cell growth and multiplication must arise from distortion of the basic processes that regulate the cell, such as the synthesis of the genetic material, DNA.

In recent years, model systems for studying cancers have been developed by taking advantage of tissue culture techniques. In such systems the initial cellular changes can be observed and closely studied, using genetic, biochemical, physical, and immunological tools. Viruses have been preferable to cancer-inducing chemicals, whose action is difficult to elucidate, since chemicals have complex effects on a number of cell constituents. The number of viral genes is small, and it is easier to identify those responsible for cancer induction. Thus the problem can be reduced from one of cellular genetics to one of viral genetics. Two small DNA-containing viruses are usually used for these studies, the polyoma virus and the virus known as SV-40, both of which induce cancer when inoculated into newborn rodents. In this work, as host cells, one uses permanent lines of cellular descent, known as *clonal lines,* which are derived from a single cell.

Cell transformation can be produced by purified viral DNA, obtained by removing the protein coat from viral particles. Such experiments were first carried out by G. P. DiMayorca and his colleagues at the Sloan-Kettering Institute. Fried, at the California Institute of Technology, demonstrated directly that the function of a viral gene is required for transformation, by showing that a mutation in the viral genetic material can abolish the ability of the virus to bring about transformation. The transformed cells contain functional viral genes many cell-generations after transformation has oc-

673

curred, although they never contain or spontaneously produce infectious virus. Thus, the viral genes persisting in the transformed cells are probably instrumental in maintaining the transformed state of the cells (Dulbecco, 1967; Eckhart, 1975).

It seems probable that the viral functions responsible for cell transformation have been selected by evolutionary processes to further the multiplication of the viruses. The virus is small and contains only a limited amount of genetic information; therefore, it must exploit the synthetic mechanisms of the cell in order to survive. The cancer-producing action of viruses appears to be a by-product of viral functions that were developed to meet the requirements of viral multiplication. These viral functions can produce cancer because they are similar to cellular functions that control cell multiplication, but somehow they manage to escape the regulatory mechanisms that normally operate within the cell (Dulbecco, 1967). One of the most important investigators in this field has been *Renato Dulbecco,* who along with *Howard M. Temin* and *David Baltimore,* received the Nobel Prize for physiology and medicine in 1975. Dulbecco began his tumor-virus studies at the California Institute of Technology at Pasadena but in 1963 moved to the newly established Salk Institute at La Jolla, California.

The discovery of reverse transcriptase in 1970 by Howard M. Temin and Satoshi Mizutani of the University of Wisconsin, and independently by David Baltimore of the Massachusetts Institute of Technology (Culliton, 1972), was responsible for bringing molecular virology to the center stage of cancer research. Reverse transcriptase, or RNA-directed DNA polymerase, is an enzyme that catalyzes the flow of genetic information from RNA to DNA in a surprising reversal of the usual DNA to RNA direc-

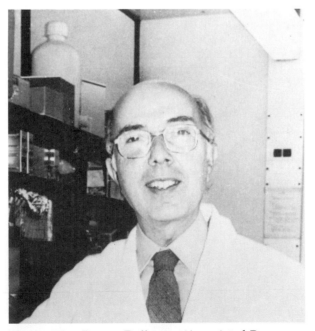

Figure 152. Renato Dulbecco. (Associated Press photo, courtesy of William Schmick, Sr.)

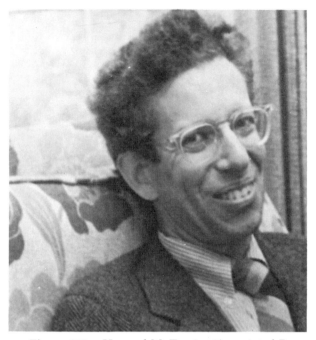

Figure 153. Howard M. Temin. (Associated Press photo, courtesy of William Schmick, Sr.)

tion of genetic expression. Because most viruses known to cause cancer in animals have an RNA core, discovery of this enzyme was of particular significance to cancer-virus studies. It explained for the first time the mechanism by which genes in the RNA of a virus can be incorporated into the DNA of a cell, where they might function like any other genes. When they are incorporated into cellular DNA and then expressed, they can transform those cells into neoplastic cells.

The search for a human tumor virus has been frustrating. Several investigators have announced the isolation of tumor viruses that were thought to be of human origin, only to discover later that they were of animal origin. However, in June, 1974, Charles McGrath, Marvin Rich, and their associates at the Michigan Cancer Foundation isolated a human virus that appears to be implicated in breast cancer. Then in January, 1975, Robert E. Gallagher and Robert C. Gallo of the National Cancer Institute reported isolation of a human virus associated with acute myelocytic leukemia. In both of these investigations, biological materials of human origin only were used. Gallagher and Gallo have shown that proteins from their new virus are closely related to proteins in two viruses that cause leukemia in subhuman primates but are more distantly related to proteins from a mouse leukemia virus. The breast cancer virus of McGrath and Rich is suspected to be a type B, AB, RNA tumor virus; a type that in animals has been associated exclusively with mammary tumors. The leukemia virus is a type C RNA tumor virus; this type is the most common class of animal tumor viruses. Type C RNA tumor viruses have been implicated in the production of leukemias, lymphomas, and sarcomas, all of which are tumors derived from

675

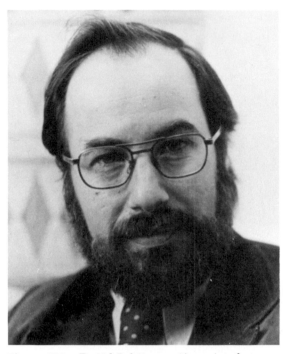

Figure 154. David Baltimore. (Associated
Press photo, courtesy of William Schmick, Sr.)

a class of tissue that includes connective tissue, cartilage, bone, muscle, and
white blood cells. The breast cancer virus is also thought to belong to another category known as endogenous viruses — viruses in which the principal
mode of transmission is from parent to progeny. It has been postulated that
endogenous viruses are produced by a gene known as a virogene, which
may be a part of the genetic complement of each member of a species. The
leukemia virus, however, may be an endogenous or an exogenous virus. Exogenous viruses are transmitted between members of a species by infection. Neither of the new viruses has been proved to be a causative agent in
human tumors.

**IMMUNOLOGY
AND ONCOLOGY** Immunological concepts are currently being explored for the early detection of cancer and for
the development of new approaches to treatment.
Immune reactions of low intensity may stimulate growth of tumor cells.
One approach to treatment utilizes various bacteria as nonspecific potentia-
tors that enhance immune responses. One of these is BCG (the attenuated
tubercle bacillus described in Chapter 12), which will retard the growth of
many cancers in experimental animals. It has been explored for its effect on
certain melanomas of human skin and its ability to enhance the effectiveness of chemotherapy in certain forms of leukemia.

W. B. Coley, as early as 1891, observed that some micro-organisms
cause the body to react more vigorously to a variety of immunological stim-

676

uli. The term "nonspecific immunopotentiators" has been used to designate micro-organisms or products of micro-organisms, as well as synthetic molecules, that have the ability to increase immunological reactivity.

In the transmission of experimental leukemia, the oncogenic virus usually must be injected into a newborn animal. Since this is the classical technique for inducing immunological tolerance, it is conceivable that leukemic animals are tolerant of their neoplastic (tumor) cells. This view is supported by the discovery that chickens infected congenitally with the Rous sarcoma virus are tolerant of that agent. In such birds there is progressive growth of the Rous sarcoma, which contains large quantities of virus. In contrast, adult chickens inoculated with the Rous sarcoma virus produce tumor-specific antibodies; as a result, the sarcoma grows poorly, if at all, and contains only a small amount of the virus.

All chemical carcinogens (cancer-producing agents) suppress antibody synthesis and retard the rejection of foreign grafts. X-rays, another type of carcinogen, also inhibit immune responses. The classical technique of inducing leukemia in mice with X-rays has immunosuppressive effects. Thymectomy in newborn animals causes impairment of immunity. The administration of polyoma virus to mice thymectomized at birth results in a high incidence of tumors in strains ordinarily refractory to this virus.

Thus, the immune system provides a defense against neoplastic cells. This function of lymphoid tissue—immunological surveillance—seems to be of central importance in resistance to lymphomas and leukemias.

The change of normal cells to neoplastic cells is associated with the appearance of new or different proteins that the body recognizes to be foreign. It has been postulated that most cancer cells are eliminated by an early immune reaction, a surveillance mechanism. Robert A. Good and others have shown that immune-deficient patients develop many more cancers of the lymphoreticular type than do normal people. Immune deficiency may be hereditary, or it may be induced by drugs such as those used in patients who receive kidney transplants, in order to keep the body from rejecting the transplant. Patients receiving these immunosuppressive drugs show an increased incidence of tumors. However, not all tumors are increased in proportion to their occurrence in the general population (75 per cent of reported tumors are either lymphoproliferative or carcinomas of the skin, lip, or cervix). This cannot be explained by impaired immunosurveillance, as pointed out by Matas and his co-workers (1975). Ninety per cent of transplant recipients develop clinical or serological evidence of herpes virus infection. Herpes viruses have been implicated in the pathogenesis of lymphoproliferative tumors and carcinoma of the skin and cervix. They may remain in latent form until reactivated by allogeneic stimulation and/or immunosuppression. These viruses localize to skin, cervix, and neural tissue; that is, exactly those sites where cancer develops following transplantations.

HORMONES AND CANCER   In 1932, the French physician A. M. B. Lacassagne first revealed the correlation between hormones and the *development* of cancer by showing that injections of estrone evoked mammary cancer in mice. The proof that

677

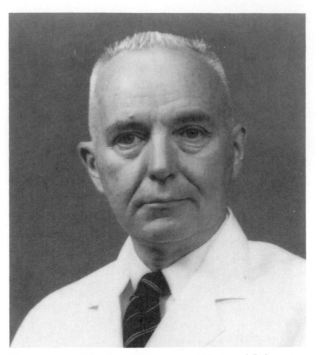

Figure 155. Charles B. Huggins. (National Library of Medicine, Bethesda, Maryland.)

hormones can influence the *growth* of cancer was derived from studies of tumors of the prostate of the dog and, later, of man.

Charles B. Huggins began his studies of the prostate at the University of Chicago because of an interest in the physiological activity of steroids and the biochemistry of organophosphorus compounds. He and his co-workers devised a simple technique for collecting prostatic secretions from dogs. They found that following castration, the prostate shrinks, the oxidative phase of carbohydrate metabolism declines, and prostatic secretion ceases. The administration of the hormone testosterone corrects these defects. The prostatic cells do not die in the absence of testosterone; they merely shrivel. Fortunately, Huggins's metabolic experiments were carried out on dogs, an animal in which tumors of the prostate occur. At first, researchers were irritated when they encountered an experimental dog with a prostatic tumor, but soon such dogs were eagerly sought. The hormone-dependent cancer cells of the prostate grow in the presence of supporting hormones but die in their absence. Huggins observed that castration or the administration of estrogenic hormones caused a rapid shrinkage of canine prostatic tumors. These experimental observations proved relevant to human prostatic cancer (Huggins, 1966).

Measurement of phosphatases in blood serum furnished proof that cancer of the human prostate is responsive to sex hormones. The measurements involved two enzymes that occur in human blood serum—acid phosphatase and alkaline phosphatase. W. Kutscher and H. W. Volbergs, in

Germany, discovered (1935) that acid phosphatase is concentrated in the prostate of adult normal males; and A. B. Gutman and E. B. Gutman (1938) found that many patients with prostatic cancer have significant increases of acid phosphatase in their blood serum. Cancer of the prostate that metastasizes to bone usually evokes a proliferation of osteoblasts, with production of new bone, which, as Kay found, gives rise to increased alkaline phosphatase levels in serum. Huggins studied human prostatic cancer that had metastasized to bone and, by periodic measurement of the two enzymes, obtained a view of the overall activity of the cancer (acid phosphatase) and the reaction of nonmalignant cells of the host to the presence of that cancer (alkaline phosphatase). This, in conjunction with the experiments with dogs, provided the proof that prostatic cancer in man is responsive to castration or the administration of estrogenic hormones (Huggins, 1966).

The control of cancer by excision of endocrine glands is known as "physiological surgery"; that is, removal of a normal structure in order to heal a disease in some other part of the body. The estrogenic hormone stilbestrol, discovered in 1938 by the English physician Edward C. Dodds, was the first synthetic substance to be employed for the control of cancer; this was the beginning of the chemotherapy of malignant disease.

Actually, excision of endocrine glands to control human cancer goes back to 1896 when G. T. Beatson, a British surgeon, removed the ovaries from two women with breast cancer. However, the modern era of endocrine surgery got its start when Huggins, R. E. Stevens, and C. V. Hodges reported the dramatic effect of castration on cancer of the prostate. The work of Huggins and his colleagues was far more impressive than any which had gone before in that it was based on a sound and experimentally based concept, namely, "hormone-dependence" (Huggins and Clark, 1940). Rous, discussing the implications of Huggins's discovery, wrote that "the significance of this discovery far transcends its practical application: for it means that thought and endeavor in cancer research had been misdirected in consequence of the belief that tumor cells are anarchic." The 1966 Nobel Prize for physiology and medicine was awarded jointly to Charles B. Huggins and Peyton Rous for their contributions to cancer research.

Huggins's work stimulated interest in the control of advanced cancers by endocrinological methods; and this has led to widespread use of endocrine-ablative procedures, particularly for cancers of the breast and prostate. That the pituitary gland plays an important role in the genesis of mammary cancer and in the maintenance of its growth has been shown in experimental animals. The first application of hypophysectomy for human malignant disease in America was reported in 1952 by several groups: W. W. Scott and A. E. Walker of Johns Hopkins Medical School, for cancer of the prostate; M. B. Shimkin of the U.S. Public Health Service and his collaborators, for malignant melanoma; and O. H. Pearson and associates of the Sloan-Kettering Institute, for breast cancer. The benefits following adrenalectomy have been similar to those from surgical hypophysectomy. Metastatic lesions at all sites regress in about 40 per cent of patients.

Tumor regression following endocrine ablation results from the removal of circulating hormones that are sustaining the growth of the neoplasm; excision of the ovaries causes estrogen deprivation; adrenalectomy removes

679

steroid hormones similar to those found in the ovaries; hypophysectomy depletes trophic-hormone activity on the adrenals, gonads, and thyroid, as well as removing growth hormone and prolactin (Dao, 1972).

TUMORS THAT PRODUCE HORMONES In Chapter 12 and elsewhere, mention has been made of endocrine tumors, some benign and some malignant, that release into the circulation excessive amounts of hormones. A number of well-known diseases result from hormonal overproduction of this type: hyperthyroidism, hyperparathyroidism, hypertension (pheochromocytoma and aldosteronoma), acromegaly and gigantism (pituitary growth hormone), Cushing's disease (pituitary basophilism), and others. In addition, some tumors that do not arise in endocrine tissue also produce hormones. For example, adenomas and carcinomas of the bronchi, thymomas, and tumors of the pancreas occasionally secrete pituitary hormones of several varieties, though usually in small amounts. The hypersecreting endocrine tumors are usually treated by surgical excision or radiation. A unique form of radiation therapy is the use of radioactive iodine for the treatment of hyperthyroidism and cancer of the thyroid.

Special types of hormone-secreting tumors, not previously mentioned, are those which secrete large amounts of chorionic gonadotropin: hydatidiform mole (a benign tumor) and choriocarcinoma (a cancer). This gonadotropic hormone is secreted by the chorionic tissue of the placenta, and it normally rises to a high level in the blood and urine in the second and third months of pregnancy. The tumors that secrete chorionic gonadotropin usually occur in relation to the pregnant uterus, but there is also a rare choriocarcinoma which occurs in the ovaries of prepubertal girls. These tumors secrete estrogen and progesterone as well as chorionic gonadotropin. The routine treatment for tumors secreting chorionic gonadotropins was surgical excision until 1956 when M. C. Li, R. Hertz, and D. B. Spencer at the National Institutes of Health found that dramatically beneficial results could be achieved in the treatment of these patients by the administration of the folic-acid antagonist, *methotrexate,* which halts the growth of choriocarcinomas and causes a sharp drop in chorionic gonadotropin secretion. It is believed that methotrexate may act on the tumor by blocking estrogen, which requires folic acid for its actions. Surgery is still the primary form of treatment for the ovarian tumors, and most of the uterine tumors require surgical evacuation of the uterus; but the use of methotrexate has reduced the need for hysterectomy and other radical forms of surgery, and it is the only form of therapy that offers any hope of success in cases of metastatic choriocarcinoma. A considerable amount of research on the chorionic-gonadotropin–secreting tumors arising in pregnancy has been carried out in the Endocrinology Branch of the National Cancer Institute, which was organized in 1947.

Studies of cancer of the adrenal cortex, also carried out at the National Cancer Institute, provided highly specific steroid indicators of tumor regression and permitted the development of a new pharmacological agent, *amphenone,* which is capable of inhibiting steroid hormone production by the normal, as well as by the cancerous, adrenal gland. Although amphenone proved capable of alleviating the metabolic burden of hyperadrenocorticism in patients with adrenal cancer, tumor growth was not arrested. However, later efforts by Bergenstal, Hertz, Lipsett, and Moy provided initial clinical data on the therapeutic value, in patients with adrenal cancer, of ortho-para-prime D.D.D., an agent that had been shown to effect a selective necrosis of normal adrenal tissue in the dog.

CARCINOGENESIS DUE TO HORMONES   Leo Loeb of St. Louis demonstrated as early as 1918 that breast cancers could be prevented in female mice if the ovaries were removed. Furthermore, breast cancer could be induced in male mice if they were castrated and ovaries were implanted under their skin. It was subsequently shown that breast cancer in mice requires the presence of three factors: genetic susceptibility, the proper hormonal status, and the milk-transmitted Bittner virus. Fortunately, the great use of estrogens and other hormones since their introduction into clinical practice over 30 years ago has not led to an increase in the incidence of breast cancer in either women or men.

However, in 1970 Arthur Herbst and his colleagues in Boston reported the occurrence of cancer of the vagina in daughters of mothers who had taken diethylstilbestrol during their pregnancy. At one time this synthetic estrogen was given in large doses to prevent abortion in women who had suffered habitual abortions. Herbst's studies indicated that diethylstilbestrol is carcinogenic for the human embryo, but the effect only becomes evident 15 years later or more. Oral contraceptives, containing estrogenic and progestational hormones, present a contemporary problem. Carefully controlled long-term observations on many women are needed in order to be sure that the risks are not increased for the development of cancers of the breast, uterus, and ovary (Shimkin, 1973).

CARCINOGENESIS DUE TO CHEMICALS   In 1775 the prominent English surgeon Percival Pott broke a leg and during his recovery wrote a book on his "Observations." In it he described cancer of the scrotum in chimney sweeps, which he attributed to long exposure to soot. This was the first clear description of an occupational cancer. Later many specific chemical compounds were found that could induce cancer in animals and, in some instances, in humans. It was noted that tars combined with a very small amount of cancer-producing chemicals are more effective in producing cancers than are the pure chemicals themselves. This discovery indicated that other substances in the mixture accelerate the reaction; Murray J. Shear called these substances *co-carcinogens.* Important contributions to the understanding of carcinogenic action were made by two husband-wife teams, the Millers of Wisconsin and the Weisburgers of the National Institutes of Health, working with cancer-producing chemicals of the azo-dye and fluorene types. One of the latter, 2-acetyl-amino-fluorene, had been recommended for use as an insecticide, but it was found to be toxic in rats and thus became a tool in cancer research. It was also found that in response to the toxic action of the chemical, an

681

enzyme was mobilized by the animal that produced carcinogenic metabolites. Participation of the host in metabolic reactions that have a carcinogenic effect was also demonstrated for polycyclic hydrocarbons. When mice were given small doses of carbon tetrachloride before receiving a carcinogenic hydrocarbon, many more tumors of the lung were produced than with the same dose of hydrocarbon alone. This results from the fact that carbon tetrachloride injures the liver, which is involved in the detoxification and elimination of hydrocarbons (Shimkin, 1973).

Carcinogens act in various ways. Some produce cancers at the site of contact, perhaps by direct injury to cells. Others produce cancer at distant sites. Some require metabolic conversion before they become carcinogenic; some do not acquire carcinogenicity unless potentiated by other chemicals. Cancer-producing chemicals are not limited to industrial products; they also occur in nature, in plants, and in molds (Shimkin, 1973).

CARCINOGENESIS DUE TO ULTRAVIOLET AND IONIZING RADIATIONS

The light of the sun is among the cancer-inducing stimuli of our environment. Paul Unna of Germany, in 1894, related cancer of the skin to exposure to sunlight; and in 1928 G. M. Findlay of England succeeded in producing skin cancer in experimental animals by exposing them to intense sunlight. Later studies by Howard F. Blum of the National Cancer Institute showed that this effect was due not to heat but to radiation from a relatively narrow band in the ultraviolet range of the wave spectrum (3000 angstrom units). Many of the carcinogenic hydrocarbons show a peak of absorption in the same wave range.

Ionizing radiation (from X-rays, radium, cobalt-60, and other sources) can cause several forms of cancer in man. The people of Hiroshima and Nagasaki who survived exposure to the two atomic bombs have been studied carefully in the past 25 years by the Atomic Bomb Casualty Commission. There is no doubt that a single exposure to ionizing radiation at high dose produces leukemia in humans and also increases the incidence of cancer of the lung, breast, and thyroid. Radiologists and others exposed to increased doses of radiation are more liable to develop leukemia than people not so exposed. Radium salts which are deposited in bone give rise to cancers there. A number of tragic deaths from bone cancer occurred in women following exposure to radium by licking brushes used in coating watch dials (Shimkin, 1973).

CARCINOGENESIS DUE TO ATMOSPHERIC POLLUTION

There are also carcinogens in the air we breathe. Lung cancer in the United States has shown the greatest increase of any type of cancer during the past 30 years. There are now over 55,000 deaths per year from this cause. Two factors have contributed to the increase: (1) cigarette smoking (Fig. 159), which accounts for over 70 per cent of the increase; and (2) pollution of the air by in-

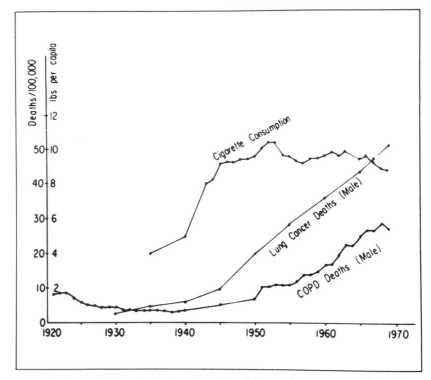

Figure 156. Deaths in the United States from cancer of the lung and chronic obstructive lung disease in relation to cigarette consumption. (From Ayres, S. M.: Cigarette smoking and lung disease: An update. Basics of Resp. Dis. 3(5):1, 1975.

dustrial waste, automobile exhaust, and pollutants in the home and place of work. The identification of cigarette smoke as a cause of lung cancer and other lung diseases ranks as one of the major scientific discoveries of this century, equivalent to the nineteenth-century discovery of water pollution as a cause of gastrointestinal diseases such as cholera and typhoid fever. Alton Ochsner and Michael DeBakey (Tulane University), in 1937, described seven patients from each of whom they had removed a cancerous lung, and they suggested that cigarette smoking was the cause of the lung disease in all seven. Cuyler Hammond and Daniel Horn of the American Cancer Society studied more than 180,000 volunteers, and Harold Dorn of the NIH followed over 200,000 holders of U.S. government life insurance policies. Among those using cigarettes there was a significantly higher incidence of lung cancer. Cigarette smoking is also closely related to conditions commonly grouped together as chronic obstructive lung disease, such as emphysema and *chronic* bronchitis. Mitchell and his co-workers introduced the term *chronic airway obstruction* to describe the condition of these patients. Most of them were cigarette smokers, and the authors were able to establish a correlation between the amount and duration of smoking and the morphological changes in the lungs (Ayres, 1975).

Gross and his co-workers demonstrated in 1965 that emphysema could be produced experimentally by instilling papain, a proteolytic enzyme, into the lungs of rats. This fact gained added significance when Eriksson, a

683

Scandinavian investigator, in the same year demonstrated that individuals with hereditary deficiencies of alpha-1-antitrypsin (a protease inhibitor) had a relatively high incidence of emphysema. Since alpha-1-antitrypsin inhibits the action of many proteolytic enzymes, an effort has been made to link proteolytic digestion of lung tissue with the development of emphysema. Mass and co-workers demonstrated that aerosolization of granulocyte contents into canine lungs produces emphysema.

Interest has been focused recently on an enzyme system, aryl hydroxylase, which is activated following exposure to an appropriate chemical stimulus. The enzyme system is under genetic control, with approximately 10 per cent of the population having a high degree of aryl hydroxylase inducibility. This substance is a microsomal oxidase that detoxifies some materials but transforms others into carcinogenic agents. Kellerman and co-workers were able to show that 30 per cent of individuals with bronchogenic carcinoma had high enzyme inducibility, compared to only 9.4 per cent of a control group. These studies raise the possibility that individuals likely to develop carcinoma may be identified by an appropriate genetic marker.

A striking example of air pollutant–cigarette interaction is the effect of asbestos inhalation. Sellicoff and others pointed out that a cigarette smoker has an 11 times greater chance of dying from lung cancer than does a nonsmoker and that a smoker who is also an asbestos worker has a 92 times greater chance. Such data suggest a synergism between cigarette smoking and certain occupational and community pollutants. A tendency to develop lung cancer has also been observed in workers handling uranium, chromium, nickel, and arsenic (Ayres, 1975).

HEREDITY AND CANCER

Around 1900 it was observed that tumors occur more frequently in certain strains of animals. It was thought that such familial predisposition might involve genetic factors, but to prove this hypothesis it was necessary to have genetically defined animals for study. This was achieved by brother-to-sister selective breeding, largely the work of geneticists, including Sewell Wright of Chicago and Clarence C. Little and Leonell C. Strong of the Jackson Memorial Laboratory in Maine. Multiple strains of mice and guinea pigs were developed which were as identical as twins and which had predictable frequencies of certain types of cancer. Studies of these inbred stains led to the conclusion that different mosaics of genetic factors are involved in susceptibility to different cancers. Studies of breast cancer in mice showed an extrachromosomal factor that resulted in the discovery of the Bittner virus. The genetic background modifies susceptibility to the virus. In humans most of the common forms of cancer do not show clear-cut familial susceptibility, though there are minor degrees of susceptibility to cancer of the breast, rectum, and lung. Such familial aggregation does not necessarily indicate a hereditary factor, since families share a common environment (Shimkin, 1973).

Until 1960 scientists believed that only germ cells were capable of fusing and forming reproducing cells. Then G. Barski and his colleagues in

Paris found that body (somatic) cells grown in tissue culture also could unite and form hybrids capable of reproduction. Such hybrids can then be produced between cells from different species such as mouse and humans. This remarkable technique of somatic cell hybridization has enhanced analysis of chromosome mapping of normal and neoplastic cells and of "the relationships of such geography" with function. It is now possible to create animals with four parents, by removing fertilized ova after a few cell-divisions, fusing them, and transplanting the tetraparental mass into the uterus of still another female. This is another technique that is contributing to our knowledge of genetics and other biochemical sciences.

Though the hybrid nature of humans makes precise genetic studies difficult, some insight into the relative roles of heredity and environment has been obtained through the study of identical and fraternal twins. If one identical twin develops leukemia, there is a one-to-six chance that the other twin will also develop leukemia, usually within one year. Some cancers and precancerous conditions in man are determined primarily by heredity. Retinoblastoma, which causes blindness and deafness in children, is inherited as a dominant trait. Familial multiple polyposis of the colon is a hereditary disease that develops into cancer during the second or third decade of life (Shimkin, 1973).

The most well-known chromosomal change in human neoplasia is the Ph^1 abnormality in marrow cells of patients with chronic myeloid leukemia. First described by P. C. Nowell and D. A. Hungerford in 1960, this involves one of the smallest acrocentric chromosomes (G 22) (Nowell and Hungerford, 1960; Sandburg and Hossfeld, 1970). It is an acquired characteristic, since in identical twins only the member with chronic myeloid leukemia has the abnormality (Sandburg and Hossfeld, 1970).

The higher incidence of acute leukemia in subjects with Down's syndrome (mongolism) with group G trisomy is of interest. The role played by the extra chromosome in the development of the leukemia is uncertain.

EXFOLIATIVE CANCER CYTOLOGY The first recorded diagnosis of cancer by the technique of exfoliative cytology (microscopic examination of cells shed by a tumor) was made in 1861; but credit for the development of this procedure as a diagnostic tool belongs principally to *George N. Papanicolaou,* who, with Herbert Traut, in 1943, published a classic monograph entitled "Diagnosis of Uterine Cancer by the Vaginal Smear."

In 1928 at the *Third Race Betterment Conference* held in Battle Creek, Michigan, Papanicolaou presented a paper entitled "New Cancer Diagnosis," describing how he had seen in vaginal smears, cells that are characteristic of uterine carcinoma. Papanicolaou had been studying the cytological variation in the sexual cycle of animals. This work was extended to humans when he realized that any cellular changes due to pathological conditions would have to be taken into account when assessing the normal situation. He made smears from patients with various lesions of the uterus and vagina and observed that characteristically abnormal cells were shed from uterine carcinoma. His contribution represents an outstanding ex-

685

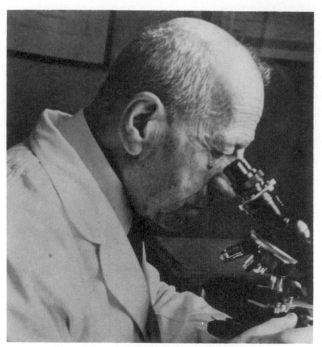

Figure 157. George Papanicolaou. (Medical Archives, New York Hospital—Cornell Medical Center.)

ample of a clinical application stemming from so-called "pure research" which had been initiated without any practical goal in mind.

Papanicolaou's early studies were received with skepticism, and the method did not gain much attention until 1943 when his earlier (1928) observations were expanded into the monograph with Traut. His discoveries then received confirmation and endorsement by J. V. Meigs, a gynecologist on the Harvard faculty, and his associates. Soon thereafter, practically every body-fluid containing well-preserved exfoliative cells was thoroughly investigated: the sputum by Wandall; the urine by Deden; and serous fluid by Louse and Reagan, among others (Naylor, 1960). Technical advances came rapidly, one outstanding improvement being fluorescence microscopy, which was first applied in this field by Friedman (Naylor, 1960). This method depends on the fact that some cancer cells emit a characteristic type of fluorescence as a result of a different content of DNA and RNA. Ultimately, mass screening programs of vaginal smears were undertaken, and this technique has brought about a significant advance in the early detection of carcinoma of the uterus.

THE CHEMOTHERAPY OF MALIGNANT DISEASE

Cancer research in the past two decades has been heavily involved with the use of chemicals as therapeutic agents. Certain outstanding successes have been achieved and palliative treatment provided in a number of instances. Choriocarcinoma has been cured in a high percentage of cases by the use of methotrexate and multiple-drug therapy has greatly lengthened the survival time of patients with acute leukemia.

The use of estrogen therapy in disseminated cancer of the prostate was the beginning of the modern era of cancer chemotherapy. Earlier work had led to the development of many of the research tools essential for experimental chemotherapy. Four of the more widely used transplantable tumors (Sarcoma 37, Sarcoma 180, Walker 256, and Ehrlich ascites tumor) were developed before 1930. The development of inbred strains of mice in the early 1920s stimulated use of mammary tumors for chemotherapy studies.

Jacob Furth initiated studies of arsenicals in experimental leukemia, but his inability to obtain financial support forced him to discontinue the work. Murray Shear of the Office of Cancer Investigations of the U.S. Public Health Service at Harvard University (later consolidated with the Pharmacology Laboratory of the Old National Institute of Health to form the National Cancer Institute in 1937) set up a screening program in the mid-1930s to test bacterial polysaccharides capable of eliciting the Shwartzman phenomenon (a necrotizing immune-type reaction) in Sarcoma 37. Toward the end of World War II, this screening program was extended to synthetic compounds and plant extracts, and it became the first project involving an interinstitutional cooperative effort. By the early 1950s, more than 3000 chemicals and several hundred plant extracts had been tested, a number of which caused necrosis of the tumors. The weak link in this program was the inability to maintain even a limited clinical activity, so that it was discontinued in 1953 (Zubrod, 1966; Shimkin, 1973).

THE NITROGEN MUSTARDS These compounds are the nitrogen analogues of the well-known vesicant war gas, sulfur mustard or "mustard gas." E. B. Khrumbaar in 1919 observed that mustard gas poisoning is characterized by leukopenia and, at autopsy, reveals aplasia of the bone marrow, dissolution of the lymphoid tissue, and ulceration of the gastrointestinal tract. This marked cytotoxic action on lymphoid tissue prompted A. Gilman, L. S. Goodman, and T. F. Dougherty to study the effects of nitrogen mustards on transplanted lymphosarcoma in mice. They demonstrated extensive regression of established tumors by doses of nitrogen mustard which were well tolerated by the host. Although the tumors returned after therapy was discontinued, these results were sufficiently encouraging to suggest a therapeutic trial in terminal cases of malignant lymphoma. A clinical trial of nitrogen mustard was conducted in 1942 at Yale University in collaboration with G. E. Lindskog. The first patient treated experienced a dramatic remission. Hematological studies revealed a severe but reversible depression of bone marrow function. The clinical remission was brief and subsequent courses of therapy proved less effective. In the following year Leon Jacobson and co-workers instituted independent clinical studies at the University of Chicago, and a third set of clinical trials carried out at the Sloan-Kettering Institute, New York, was reported by C. P. Rhoads in 1946.

At the termination of World War II these compounds, which had been on the top-secret list, were declassified, and the results of all the wartime

687

studies were published in 1946. The National Research Council Committee on Growth then established a program for the distribution of nitrogen mustards to qualified clinical investigators. Numerous other nitrogen-mustard–like compounds have been synthesized and are now among the most widely used of the "immunosuppressive" agents. These compounds are used not only for the treatment of patients with lymphoid tumors but also to suppress the immunological response in a variety of clinical diseases and in patients with renal transplants.

CHEMOTHERAPY IN THE TREATMENT OF ACUTE LEUKEMIA

The chemotherapy of acute lymphocytic leukemia in the past decade has revealed the following: (1) an occasional case can apparently be cured by a single drug or by combination therapy; (2) by using kinetic data obtained in mice with transplanted leukemias, specific dosage schedules can be devised to cure mouse leukemia with a single drug; (3) such kinetic data can be procured in human acute leukemia to serve as the basis for better drug schedules; (4) combinations of drugs can be more effective than a single agent in both mouse and human leukemia; (5) when the total care of the patient includes supportive measures such as platelet and leukocyte transfusions, newer and better antibiotics, and a protective environment, more intensive therapy can be administered; (6) Burkitt's tumor, a rapidly growing solid tumor that is somewhat analogous to acute leukemia, is curable in 50 per cent of all patients and in more than 75 per cent of those whose disease is diagnosed early.

In November, 1947, *Sidney Farber* and his associates at the Children's Hospital in Boston produced the first temporary remissions in childhood acute leukemia with *aminopterin* and later with a closely related compound, *amethopterin,* now called *methotrexate.* The materials were obtained from Y. P. Subbarow, for many years a member of the Department of Biological Chemistry of the Harvard Medical School and later the first Director of Research of the Lederle laboratories (see Chapter 22). He and his colleagues synthesized and made available a large series of these folic-acid antagonists (Farber et al., 1948).

The next agents found to be useful in the treatment of acute leukemia were the adrenal steroids and ACTH. F. R. Heilman and E. C. Kendall of the Mayo Clinic, in 1944, showed that cortisone would inhibit the growth of a lymphosarcoma in mice, or cause it to regress. In 1950 Pearson and associates and Farber demonstrated the beneficial effects of ACTH in patients with either chronic or acute lymphocytic leukemia (ALL).

In 1951 G. B. Elion, G. H. Hitchings, and H. VanderWerff demonstrated the antipurine effects of 6-mercaptopurine (6-MP), and clinical studies at Memorial Sloan-Kettering Cancer Center by J. H. Burchenal and his colleagues in 1952 showed it to be beneficial in ALL, chronic myeloid leukemia, and to a lesser degree, in acute myeloid leukemia. It was active in patients whose disease had become resistant to methotrexate or steroids.

The next effective agent for the treatment of ALL was cyclophosphamide (Cytoxan). This alkylating agent, as reported by D. J. Fernbach of Baylor University and his co-workers, is effective in producing occasional

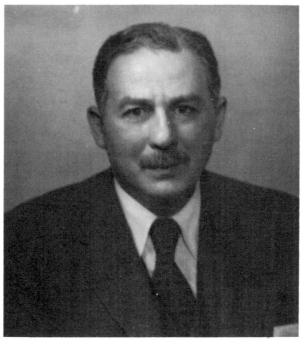

Figure 158. Sidney Farber. (National Library of Medicine, Bethesda, Maryland.)

remissions in ALL but is more beneficial in the maintenance of a remission rather than in its induction.

The *Vinca alkaloids* entered the area of cancer therapy through that familiar back door known as serendipity. The periwinkle (*Vinca rosea*), like many other plants of ancient lineage, was believed by our ancestors to have beneficial, though ill-defined, medicinal properties. In the 1940s, it was rumored that extracts of periwinkles would lower the level of the blood glucose. If this were true, such extracts might be valuable for the treatment of diabetes, and accordingly several groups of research workers began to investigate the pharmacological properties of the periwinkle. It was quickly found to have no significant effect on the blood glucose, but one of the groups of investigators (R. L. Noble and associates, 1958 and 1959) obtained from *Vinca rosea* an alkaloid which quite unexpectedly was found to depress bone-marrow activity and cause granulocytopenia in rats. Another group (I. S. Johnson and co-workers) at about the same time found that a crude extract of the periwinkle would produce some cures in mice with P1534 leukemia. Two highly active alkaloids were isolated from Vinca: *vinblastine,* of value in the treatment of Hodgkin's disease and lymphosarcoma, and *vincristine,* useful in these diseases but also in ALL.

Other agents recently found to have anticancer activity include: (1) 1-beta-D-arabinofuranosylcytosine (ara-C, cytarabine), which was shown by Evans, Farber and Brunet, and Mariano (1963) to have antileukemic activity; and (2) the antibiotics daunomycin and rubidomycin, which have both antitumor and antileukemic effects in animals and which were shown to be

689

useful clinically by Tan and her co-workers, among others. Later the two antibiotics were found to be identical compounds and were given the generic name *daunorubicin*.

L-ASPARAGINASE   Investigators have long sought to discover an exploitable metabolic difference between the normal cell and the neoplastic cell. The therapeutic effects of L-asparaginase made possible the nearest approach thus far to success in this search (Capizzi, 1970). In 1953 John G. Kidd, Professor of Pathology at Cornell Medical College, was investigating immunotherapy for lymphomas in mice and was using guinea pig serum as a source of complement. He observed unexpectedly that mice which received guinea pig serum alone experienced complete tumor regression. Broome, who started his work with Kidd, found that L-asparaginase is the active factor in guinea pig serum. In 1956 Newman and McCoy reported that L-asparagine, generally considered a nonessential amino acid, was required to support the *in vitro* growth of the Walker carcinosarcoma 256. Then in 1964 L. T. Mashburn and J. C. Wriston, Jr., of the University of Delaware, showed that L-asparaginase isolated from *E. coli* is as effective an antitumor agent as is guinea pig serum. The work of Hill and associates and Oettgen and co-workers demonstrated conclusively that remissions of short duration in acute leukemia could be achieved with large doses of L-asparaginase, but resistance to the effect of this enzyme developed rapidly.

DOSAGE SCHEDULES FOR   Initial studies with methotrexate in 1956 by
ANTILEUKEMIC AGENTS   Golden and co-workers showed that the drug was more effective when given every second or third day than when given daily, and the first curative use of methotrexate in choriocarcinoma, by Li, Hertz, and Spencer (see p. 680) in that same year, employed the drug in short four- to five-day courses of massive daily doses, followed by an interval of two to four weeks to permit recovery of the uninvolved tissues. The greater success of ara-C in mouse leukemia when given every three hours over a 24-hour period, as shown by Skipper, Schabel, and others, was due to the fact that adequate concentrations were available during the whole period of two cell-cycles. To accomplish this in human leukemia, where the cell-cycle is longer (24 to 96 hours) and where a much smaller percentage of cells are in the proliferative phase, adequate dosage over a period of at least five to nine days and repetition every three weeks for a protracted period of time are necessary. Compounds such as Cytoxan are not limited to the DNA synthesis phase for their activity and, therefore, are effective in nonproliferating cells as well as in those in an active state of proliferation. Thus, the use of short intensive courses of antimetabolites followed by intervals to allow for recovery of normal cells, interspersed with single doses or short courses of less cycle-dependent drugs, such as cyclophosphamide, vincristine, and prednisone, should help eliminate leukemic cells regardless of whether they are in the proliferative state or at rest. With the application of these techniques, improvement in long-term survival ensued, particularly with the use of intensive combination therapy.

Most of the naturally occurring viral-induced leukemias in animals are caused by RNA viruses. Temin, Baltimore, and others demonstrated that all of some 30 oncogenic viruses contain a bizarre enzyme known as RNA-dependent DNA polymerase (RDDP) or reverse transcriptase (see p. 674). Studies have shown that the RDDP from certain animal leukemia viruses is inhibited by derivatives of rifampicin in which the N-methyl of the amino-piperazine moiety is removed or substituted by a benzyl but is not inhibited by the parent compound. Gallo, using this enzyme from human ALL cells, has reported similar results, and various streptovaricin derivatives have also been shown by Brockman and associates to inhibit the RDDP from avian and murine oncogenic viruses. These findings suggest as a future possibility the use of such antiviral agents after total leukemic-cell kill has been achieved by conventional chemotherapy (Burchenal, 1972).

The approach to intensive combination drug therapy is designed to reduce the leukemic cell population from its original approximately one trillion cells down to zero cells and to do this with the least possible interference with the patient's normal life. With 99 per cent of the leukemic cells destroyed and none recognizable in either the peripheral blood or the bone marrow, there may still remain a ten-billion leukemic cell population in the patient, and any one cell among those surviving can reactivate the leukemia and give rise to a fatal outcome. Thus, the most strenuous measures are necessary if one is to achieve what now appears in many patients to be an attainable goal; the cure of the leukemia (Burchenal, 1972).

MULTIPLE-DRUG
TREATMENT PROGRAMS
Leukemia is a prevalent form of cancer, and it has been on the increase. The annual death rate from leukemia in the United States, which was less than 2 per 100,000 in the early 1920s, rose to approximately 7 per 100,000 in the late 1950s.

Since Farber's discovery shortly after World War II that folic-acid antagonists have a temporarily beneficial effect upon acute leukemia in children it has been found that many other chemical agents can effect remissions of variable duration in this disease. Included among the chemical agents most frequently used are the following: corticosteroids, 6-mercaptopurine (6-MP), and methotrexate, which interfere with nucleic acid metabolism; cyclophosphamide and other alkylating agents; vincristine and other toxic alkaloids. No one of these substances can be trusted to work in all cases; moreover, all of them lose their effectiveness if given repeatedly. However, when one agent fails, another may succeed in inducing a remission. In the early studies, evaluation of the antileukemic potency of a chemical agent was based almost entirely on its ability to induce a remission. However, the agents that induce remissions are not necessarily the most effective in maintaining them.

E. J. Freireich of the National Cancer Institute and others at various research institutions (Acute Leukemia Group B) undertook a cooperative study to evaluate antileukemic drugs on the basis of their ability to prolong rather than to induce remissions. In their model study (Freireich et al., 1963), they demonstrated how it was possible to measure in children with acute leukemia the effectiveness of 6-MP to sustain a remission that had

691

been induced by corticosteroids. This study emphasized the significantly different requirements for drugs useful in maintaining remissions as opposed to those most useful for induction of remissions. It was pointed out that this model could be employed for the evaluation of other antileukemic drugs. Subsequently, Freireich and his associates described the activity of vincristine for induction of remissions, and soon thereafter they devised the multiple-drug combination chemotherapy regime (VAMP) that proved to be highly effective for the induction of remissions in acute lymphoblastic leukemia in childhood.

J. F. Holland of Roswell Park Memorial Institute, Buffalo, New York, and the Acute Leukemia Group B worked on a combination of drugs for the treatment of acute lymphocytic leukemia of children. In 1956 no child among 39 studied lived two years. By 1966, 27 per cent survived five years, and in programs of combined chemotherapy begun in later years, the number surviving and the length of survival improved still further.

Donald Pinkel and the group at St. Jude Children's Research Hospital, Memphis, Tennessee, began their "total therapy" approach to the management of acute lymphocytic leukemia in 1962 (Simone et al., 1972). This program consists of rapid induction of complete remission with prednisone and vincristine in order to minimize early attrition; irradiation of the brain and spinal cord during the first months of complete remission in order to prevent meningeal relapse; then multiple-drug chemotherapy for two to three years to eradicate residual systemic leukemia. The data indicate that by following this program, one can expect a 50 to 55 per cent five-year leukemia-free survival rate.

The development of effective combination chemotherapy for patients with malignant lymphoma was based on clinical experience in patients with acute lymphocytic leukemia at the National Cancer Institute and specific baseline knowledge of the effects of single agents in patients with malignant lymphoma. In 1965, Paul P. Carbone of the National Cancer Institute and others reported a controlled clinical trial on the effect of a *Vinca* alkaloid or cyclophosphamide on the induction and maintenance of remissions of malignant lymphoma. They also reported the usefulness of a new agent, *procarbazine,* that appeared to be effective in patients who had become resistant to alkylating agents. The results indicated that a combination treatment program with mechlorethamine, vincristine, procarbazine, and prednisone (MOPP) was effective. Treatment was given intermittently, and the therapeutic agents were varied as seemed appropriate. The early results and subsequent long-term follow-up reports on patients with Hodgkin's disease (DeVita, Serpick, and Carbone, 1970) indicated that the complete response rate was increased from 15 to 80 per cent, and the average duration of remissions was lengthened from 3 months to 3½ years.

CHEMOTHERAPY IN THE TREATMENT OF WILMS' TUMOR

Wilms' tumors and neuroblastomas are the two most common solid tumors in infants and children. Wilms' tumor develops in kidney tissue in children usually under the age of 5 years. When treated by surgical removal alone, the cure rate was 32 per cent. Improvements in surgical technique, including the adoption of a thoracico-abdominal approach by R. E. Gross of the Children's Hospital, Boston, raised the cure rate, between 1948 and 1956, to 47 per cent. In 1946 Sidney Farber and his group at the Children's Hospital began to add chemotherapy to surgery and radiotherapy for the treatment of this condition. Between 1946 and 1954 every anticancer agent that could be given with safety to children was tried, without significantly improving the results obtained by surgery and radiation. Then in 1954, Farber received *dactinomycin,* one of the series of actinomycins first discovered by Waksman and his colleagues in 1940 (see Chapter 22). Farber demonstrated in 1954–55 that dactinomycin is a powerful anticancer agent in a number of transplanted tumors of mice. In the latter part of 1954 he used this agent in the treatment of advanced Wilms' tumor in a child with numerous metastases in both lungs. Although only a short period of treatment was possible before the child died, post-mortem examination revealed that the metastases which had been seen in X-ray films of the lungs during life had necrosed and in many instances had been replaced by noncancerous material. Additional observations of children with Wilms' tumors had demonstrated by 1960 that when treatment with dactinomycin was added to surgery and local radiation, seven of eight children not only survived but also had no detectable evidence of tumor more than two years later.

ADJUVANT CHEMOTHERAPY

The use of chemotherapy as an adjuvant (accessory) to surgery appears to be proving its worth in the treatment of cancer of the breast. Wilms' tumors, rhabdomyosarcomas, and some of the other forms of cancer in which adjuvant chemotherapy has been most successful are rare types of malignant disease; but carcinoma of the breast is one of the commonest and most serious with which we have to deal. Its lethal effect is greatest among women in the prime of life, before the menopause. A radical mastectomy, the operation perfected by Halsted in the early years of the twentieth century, is successful only when the diagnosis has been made very early, before metastases are in evidence. Even when metastases are not found at the time of operation, the cancer recurs within 10 years in 24 per cent of cases. If one, two, or three axillary lymph nodes are found to contain cancer when the operation is performed, the rate of recurrence is 65 per cent; and if four or more lymph nodes are involved, the recurrence rate is 85 per cent. The overall death rate following radical mastectomy averages about 8 per cent per year, being highest in the first three years after operation.

Studies of experimental tumors have indicated that small metastatic cancers are more susceptible than the original tumor to the killing effect of chemotherapeutic agents, presumably because they are more accessible to the circulating chemical and are in a stage of rapid growth, which makes them particularly vulnerable. It has been apparent for many years that the recurrence of breast cancer is due to minute metastases not only in the neighboring lymph nodes but also in distant parts of the body, which may not become evident until years after the operation. These were some of the factors that encouraged the development of adjuvant chemotherapy. The early work, employing single chemotherapeutic agents, was not very successful, partly because of the ineffectiveness of the agent and partly because

693

chemotherapy was not started until metastases had become evident and it was then too late to do more than a palliative job. Further research indicated that a greater degree of success could be achieved by starting treatment sooner and by using several different chemical agents in series. The current concept is that adjuvant chemotherapy should start soon after operation regardless of whether recognizable metastases are present, that it should be intensive, and that it should be continued, with intermittent rest periods, for many months. The rather spectacular results of two recent studies, one using a single chemical agent, the other using a combination of chemicals, will now be cited to indicate how far the treatment of breast cancer has advanced in the past several years.

B. Fisher, P. P. Carbone, and other American research workers engaged in a large cooperative study reported in 1975 on the use of phenylalanine mustard (L-PAM) following the surgical removal of a cancerous breast. In 103 patients treated with L-PAM, the failure rate was 9.7 per cent, as compared with 22 per cent in 108 patients who received a placebo instead of L-PAM. In premenopausal women the effect was even greater: 3 per cent failure in those receiving L-PAM and 30 per cent in those who received only a placebo. (Evaluation of these results must await a longer follow-up period.)

Early in 1976 even more spectacular results were reported by a group at the Instituto Nazionale Tumori, Milan, Italy, headed by Gianni Bonadonna, from the use of combined chemotherapy for the treatment of breast cancer. The Italian workers employed prolonged cyclic combination chemotherapy with three different agents given in series: cyclophosphamide, methotrexate, and fluorouracil (CMF). The adjuvant chemotherapy was started about one month after a radical mastectomy and in most cases was continued for one year. In all of the treated cases there were metastases in the axillary lymph nodes; hence the prognosis was unfavorable. After a maximum follow-up period of 27 months (average 14 months), the failure rate in 207 treated patients was 5.3 per cent, whereas the failure rate in 179 controls was 24 per cent. The authors reported that the toxicity produced by their long-term intensive chemotherapy was "acceptable." In not a single patient completing the full course of chemotherapy had the cancer relapsed after discontinuance of treatment. The authors state that "these results should be interpreted with caution, since, at present, the effect of this therapy on survival and possible long-term side effects remain unknown." Nevertheless, their results, when added to those reported for L-PAM, raised hope that real progress was at last being made in the chemotherapy of cancer of the breast (Bonadonna et al., 1976; Holland, 1976; Culliton, 1976).

THE EXTENT OF PROGRESS In the July 17, 1975, issue of *The New England Journal of Medicine,* there were two articles that addressed themselves to a sweeping indictment of the National Cancer Program which had appeared in the same Journal four months previously. The author of the indictment was D. S. Greenberg, who contended that although improvements in cancer therapy had occurred in the 1940s and early 1950s, there had been virtually no change during the

20 years from 1955 to 1975, in spite of the expenditure of vast sums of money.

The first of the July commentaries was by Cutler and others of the End Results Section of the National Cancer Institute, who presented a statistical study of one-year and five-year survival rates in more than 20,000 cancer patients treated in more than 100 hospitals in the United States between 1940 and 1969. The authors stated that the hard statistical data indicated that "the picture is neither as dull nor as bright as some have claimed"; and that although the improvement in survival rates was greater between 1940 and 1955 than during the next two decades, there had, nevertheless, been a substantial improvement in the survival rate of many forms of cancer after 1955.

The second commentary was in the form of an editorial by Emil Frei, III, of the Sidney Farber Cancer Center in Boston, who enumerated some of the significant advances in cancer therapy:

In *osteogenic sarcoma* the disease-free survival rate of clinically localized tumors, 12 months after the control of the primary lesion, has increased from 10–15 per cent to 60–100 per cent as a result of the use of adjuvant single-agent or combination chemotherapy.

Breast cancer is the most common neoplasm in women, and over 70 per cent of patients who die of breast cancer have axillary-node involvement when first examined. Combined modality treatment programs have been used that include surgery for the primary disease and chemotherapy for disseminated disease. Recurrence rates during the first 18 months after surgery have been reduced tenfold for premenopausal women and significantly for all patients.

It is established that chemotherapy combined with surgical management and radiotherapy is curative in 80 to 90 per cent of patients with *Wilms' tumor*. Similar progress with combined modality therapy is hoped for in Ewing's sarcoma and embryonal rhabdomyosarcoma.

It has been demonstrated that chemotherapy is far more effective against microscopic disease than against overt disease. Thus, the use of surgical and radiation therapy (or both) for the removal of primary overt disease and concurrent adjuvant chemotherapy for the control of systemic microscopic metastases is being studied in a number of types of cancer. Many investigators are convinced that useful results will be achieved in the near future in *ovarian, testicular,* and *soft-tissue tumors* and, with improved chemotherapy and immunotherapy, in *gastrointestinal cancer.*

Progress in the treatment of *acute leukemia* and *lymphomas* has been great and continues to improve. Of particular interest is the recent evidence that 40 per cent of patients with histiocytic lymphoma are cured by combination chemotherapy.

Although Frei's summary includes the more dramatic successes in many types of cancer therapy, it does not include the most recent progress in the treatment of advanced breast cancer (described earlier), soft-tissue sarcoma, and gonadal tumors. Neither does he discuss the major progress achieved in the basic and bridging sciences related to therapeutics. Increasingly, progress in the treatment of cancer has resulted from hypotheses and extrapolations developed in the basic experimental programs and from the interaction between clinical oncology investigators and their counterparts in the basic sciences.

ORGANIZED EFFORT IN THE FIGHT AGAINST CANCER

Prior to 1900, cancer research had not attracted the interest of the American public, and it had almost no financial backing. In 1897, for example, a request was made for state funds to establish a small laboratory for the investigation of cancer at the University of Buffalo, New York. The amount requested was $10,000 but the appropriation of this relatively small sum was vetoed by Governor Frank S. Black. Though the Buffalo Cancer Laboratory did succeed in obtaining some state funds the following year, such backing was exceptional for that period.

When the American Association for Cancer Research was founded in 1907, the gathering of cancer statistics was given high priority in its early proceedings. In 1913 Frederick Hoffman, statistician for the Prudential Life Insurance Company of America, warned of the increasing death rate from cancer. As a result of his study Hoffman recommended a 10-point program to deal with the cancer problem, as follows: (1) establishment of a Society for the Study and Prevention of Cancer; (2) investigations to determine the geographic distribution of cancer; (3) a study of the hospital records of cancer patients; (4) improvements in official cancer mortality statistics; (5) reapportionment of vital statistics and data analysis distributed through governmental agencies so as to provide more precise information regarding the local incidence of cancer; (6) a more exact determination of the occupational hazards with respect to cancer; (7) analysis of nutritional influences as a cause of cancer; (8) provision for better public information about cancer; (9) intensive investigation of the occurrence of cancer in domestic animals; and (10) a program to emphasize the danger signals of cancer and the necessity for early treatment.

With a view toward arousing greater public awareness of the need for cancer research, a small group of physicians (James Ewing, Howard C. Taylor, Thomas C. Cullen, Frank F. Simpson, and Joseph C. Bloodgood) met in New York City in May, 1914, and drew up plans for a new Society "to disseminate knowledge concerning the symptoms, treatment and prevention of cancer, to investigate conditions under which cancer is found, and to compile statistics in regard thereto." This new organization adopted the name *American Society for the Control of Cancer* (ASCC). Its primary objective was to put information about cancer into a language understandable by the lay public.

In 1922, the Division of Scientific Research of the U.S. Public Health Service (USPHS) was authorized to organize an Office of Cancer Investigations. Part of the assignment of the new Office involved a detailed analysis of the statistical and epidemiological evidences of cancer, a mission successfully completed in 1925 with the issuance of the now classic *Public Health Bulletin No. 155*. The data in the Bulletin disclosed an appreciable annual increase in deaths from cancer over a 20-year period. After 1925 the USPHS assumed the primary responsibility for periodic announcements of trends in cancer mortality, thus satisfying one of the fundamental aims of the ASCC.

696

The gradual increase in radiation therapy for cancer during the first quarter of the twentieth century brought to light the biological injury that could be caused by exposure to X-rays and radium. The ASCC acted vigorously to allay public fears of "radium poisoning" and to renew confidence in the beneficial effects of this form of treatment.

From the earliest time there have been nostrums for the treatment of malignant disease, usually applications of ointments, pastes, poultices, and plasters. The cancer quack has arisen in every generation to promote his "infallible" cure, whether animal, vegetable, or mineral. The magnitude of this fraudulent business was pointed out by the AMA exposé in 1914 of eight "cancer cures." In 1921 the ASCC formally endorsed the AMA's exposures of quack remedies and gave its support to legal action to prevent the distribution of unproven and secret cancer cures. By 1938, the promoters of 40 such cures were under federal indictment for unlawful flight to avoid prosecution after exposure by the AMA.

The original objectives of the ASCC did not include the support of a research campaign. However, the Association remained attuned to the latest laboratory developments. In 1918, J. Collins Warren, Chairman of the Harvard University Cancer Commission and an ASCC Director, announced the commencement of fundamental studies on the biological effects of ionizing radiation. In 1923 the value of animal experimentation received ASCC review in an editorial by William H. Woglom (Institute for Cancer Research, Columbia University), who stressed the need for laboratory projects to settle problems inherent in X-ray and radium therapy (Triolo and Shimkin, 1969).

A stimulus toward the research approach came in July, 1925, when news releases stated that the cause of cancer had been established by two scientists, William E. Gye and J. E. Bernard of the British Medical Research Council. Their investigations confirmed studies begun in 1909 by Peyton Rous of the Rockefeller Institute on the transmissible agent (virus) of chicken sarcoma. The ASCC labeled these reports as a "subject of first-class scientific and practical importance." Joseph C. Bloodgood, the Johns Hopkins surgeon who was an ASCC Director, called for a large-scale discussion of clinical and experimental oncology, and arrangements were made by the Association for a meeting of international cancer experts. This Cancer Congress assembled at Lake Mohonk, New York, in September, 1926. The discussions at the Congress left no doubt of the value of cancer research. The ASCC concluded that progress in cancer education and the advancement of cancer research must follow independent lines. The following year the ASCC impaneled a Committee to examine the status of medical service available to cancer patients in the United States. Out of this project came the idea that strategically located and financially secure Cancer Institutes should provide the basis for subsequent planning. The Committee report cited the necessity for close collaboration between each Cancer Institute and the agencies for cancer control within its geographic territory. Moreover, each Institute would form an integral part of a coordinated national network of institutes and cancer hospitals.

Thus the early activities of the American Society for the Control of Cancer paralleled a series of important developments in the public health aspects of cancer. From 1913 to 1923, an effort was made to obtain meaning-

697

ful cancer statistics and epidemiological information. From 1923 to 1933, under encouragement from the ASCC, X-ray and radium therapies were established on a firm footing, and their dangers were recognized. Research on the biological effects of ionizing radiation was also promoted. By 1933 it had become clear that fundamental research into the causes and prevention of cancer was a prime necessity (Triolo and Shimkin, 1969).

At the end of World War II, American medical science was ready for major expansion. To give financial support to the cancer effort, Mary Lasker, in 1945, began her special fund-raising effort for the American Society for the Control of Cancer (see Chapter 16). The Society had assured her that at least one quarter of the funds thus raised would be spent on research. In 1945, $4 million was raised for the ASCC, in contrast to the $780,000 that had been raised the previous year. In 1946 the Lasker group raised $10 million, and the new Board of Directors, of which Mary Lasker was a member, changed the name of the organization to the *American Cancer Society*.

The success of the American Cancer Society in raising funds demonstrated that expansion of governmental activity in cancer research (at the National Cancer Institute) stimulated rather than suppressed private interest in this field. As the budget of the National Cancer Institute increased on a yearly basis, so did the public contributions to the American Cancer Society, which in 1970 raised $70 million.

In 1945, when the American Cancer Society agreed to devote a portion of its funds to cancer research, the National Research Council agreed to provide advice on the expenditure of funds for fundamental cancer research and for training fellowships. The Council established in that year its Committee on Growth, which by the end of its sixth year was composed of 18 investigators representing clinical medicine and the basic sciences. The investigators were assisted by 16 subcommittees or panels, with a total membership of 108. Expenditures between 1946 and 1952 totaled $9 million for 1226 research grants and $1,781,000 for 381 fellowships. In addition, $5,600,000 was awarded between 1947 and 1951, in the form of institutional research grants to universities, medical schools, research institutes, and other agencies for the development of integrated programs of cancer research. The Committee on Growth exercised wide discretion in the type of grant awarded; they included all phases of the study of the cell, its growth and development, and its function. Research of this type was considered basic to the investigation of cancer.

ORGANIZATION FOR CHEMOTHERAPY RESEARCH

After World War II, a number of institutions became identified as clinical chemotherapy centers; these included the Sloan-Kettering Institute, the Columbia University College of Physicians and Surgeons, the Children's Cancer Research Foundation in Boston, and the Lankenau Hospital—National Cancer Institute Collaborative Program. A wide variety of agents were soon under study, including alkylating agents, urethane, antimetabolites, antibiotics, and hormones. The early studies in this field provided the basis for the development of major advances in cancer chemotherapy.

698

A special meeting was convened by the National Advisory Cancer Council in December, 1952, to discuss problems relating to the clinical chemotherapy of cancer. This was a key event in the development of a programmed effort in this field. Congressional appropriations committees, impressed by the successes in the wartime antibiotics and antimalaria programs, encouraged the National Cancer Institute to develop a similarly directed program for the treatment of leukemia. With the beginning of fiscal 1955, the Chemotherapy Committee of the National Advisory Cancer Council began to develop a cooperative chemotherapy program. To broaden its scope the Chemotherapy Committee extended liaison membership not only to the American Cancer Society but also to the Damon Runyon Fund, the National Research Council Committee on Growth, the Department of Defense, and the Veterans' Administration. A major objective of this program was to organize a drug development activity supported by contracts for procuring drugs, evaluating their anticancer activity in animals, performing necessary preclinical studies, and, with the support of special grants, clinical evaluation of promising drugs. The name of the new organizational unit was the Cancer Chemotherapy National Service Center (CCNSC). The American Cancer Society provided the staff for clinical programs and liaison with industry; Kenneth Endicott was appointed Chief of the new Service Center. Beginning in July, 1955, there was expanded support in research grants and authorization of funds for contracts, a virtually new activity for the NIH.

In 1965 the NCI instituted a program for drug development. This national program was operated by a large scientific team, with participants from the NIH Research Institute, industry, and universities. The program screened 15,000 new chemicals and natural products each year. The most promising compounds were studied clinically by a national network of physicians working in cooperative groups funded by National Cancer Institute grants. Important clinical gains have been possible because of the intensive use of cancer chemotherapy by such highly trained teams (Zubrod, 1966).

THE CANCER ACT OF 1971

In 1970 Senator Ralph Yarborough, Chairman of the Senate Labor and Public Welfare Committee, appointed a committee of 26 consultants on cancer to recommend what should be done to achieve cures for the major forms of cancer by 1976, the 200th anniversary of the founding of the nation. In December, 1970, the Committee recommended an all-out attack on the "implacable foe requiring the expenditure of hundreds of millions of dollars" and urged the creation of a new National Cancer Authority. President Nixon reopened the budget of the NIH in early January, 1971, and added to the figure $100 million for "an intensive campaign to find the cure for cancer." On January 21, the President launched his own cancer initiative in the course of his State of the Union Address. On January 29, Senator Edward Kennedy introduced for himself and Senator Jacob Javits the Conquest of Cancer Act, to implement the recommendation of the cancer panel. The National Cancer Institute would be absorbed by a new National Cancer Authority. The administration's plan was to raise the Cancer Insti-

699

tute to bureau level within NIH, with authority over funds for cancer research throughout the NIH. The cancer research lobby felt that it was the organizational arrangement that had to be changed if real progress were to be made.

James Shannon, the Director of NIH, was strongly opposed to the proposed Cancer Authority. Opposition began to mount, organized by the Association of American Medical Colleges. Mrs. Lasker enlisted Ann Landers, the popular guidance counselor, whose syndicated column appears in 750 newspapers, to emphasize the importance of the Conquest of Cancer Act. Congress was flooded with mail in favor of the cancer lobby's aims.

A compromise between the Nixon and Kennedy proposals was effected. The "Kennedy-Nixon" Bill was a remarkable measure because of the paradoxical alliance it seemed to symbolize. Even though the language said that the new program was to be part of the NIH, it was given special privileges that amounted to independence. The Bill passed the Senate by a vote of 79 to 1.

When the Senate passed the Kennedy-Nixon Bill, there was widespread alarm. Congressman Paul Rogers, Chairman of the Subcommittee on Public Health and Environment, expressed serious doubts about the plan, and announced that his committee would hold extensive hearings on the measure passed by the Senate. The testimony of the biomedical science community was very effective. Rogers then introduced a Bill which permitted the Cancer Institute to have an independent budget to be changed only at the presidential level but requiring that the Director of the NIH and the Secretary of HEW comment on it. Thus, no new bureau or agency would be created. In the end, this Bill passed the House by a vote of 350 to 5. Rogers had mobilized most of the significant scientific organizations in support of his Bill. For the first time in several decades of lobbying for federal support of medical research, the scientists joined issue with the would-be benefactors of medical research and opposed them. The 1971 Cancer Act was finally enacted in November and authorized the government to spend $1.59 billion in cancer research over a three-year period. It elevated the National Advisory Cancer Council to a National Cancer Board comprising five federal government officials, including the Secretary of HEW and the Director of NIH, and 19 members appointed by the President (Strickland, 1972).

THE STRUCTURE AND ACTIVITY OF CELLS

Basically, cancer is an abnormal growth of cells. Cells manufacture the chemicals that sustain life. When they do their job well, the organism is healthy; when they do it poorly, or when their function is disturbed by deleterious influences, health is impaired. The whole area of cell biology has undergone intensive study in the past three decades, and the knowledge gained has been of great importance to the disciplines discussed in this and the immediately preceding chapters: genetics, enzymology, endocrinology, immunology, virology, and oncology. It therefore seems appropriate, at the end of this chapter on cancer, to present some recent important advances in our understanding of cell biology, realizing that they are of significance not only to cancer but also to the subjects that were discussed earlier.

Our knowledge of the basic components of cells began less than a century and a half ago. The Scottish botanist Robert Brown (who, in 1828 described the dancing movement of minute particles suspended in a liquid—"Brownian movement") discovered the cell nucleus in 1831 but failed to recognize its importance. Another botanist, this time a German, M. J. Schleiden, in an extensive study of the microscopical structure of plants, carried out between 1838 and 1843, attached great importance to the nucleus. The cell theory that Schleiden developed for plants was applied to animal tissues in 1839 by the physiologist Theodor Schwann. It is difficult for the present-day student, thoroughly familiar with the details of cell structure, to realize that such an essential and conspicuous feature of the animal cell was wholly unknown 150 years ago and that it was a botanist who first pointed it out to a physiologist. Since those early years many other structural components of cells have been identified.

Today there is great interest in the minute details of the structure and function of cells, since they constitute the basic units of living tissues. Much has been learned about the myriad components that have been identified in the cellular nucleus and cytoplasm, and about the important role played by the wall (capsule) of the cell.

Three biomedical scientists, Albert Claude, George E. Palade, and Christian R. deDuve, who have been to a major degree responsible for mapping the fine structure of the cell and determining the functions of important organelles (the minute organs of cells concerned with metabolism and other functions), were awarded the 1974 Nobel Prize for physiology and medicine.

Albert Claude was born in Luxembourg; he came to the United States in the 1930s and joined the staff of James B. Murphy's oncology laboratory at the Rockefeller Institute. Claude is sometimes called the "father of the new field of cell biology." In his work at the Rockefeller Institute, he catalyzed the activities of a number of young pioneers in this field, including Palade, Keith R. Porter, W. C. Schneider, George Hogeboom, and others, who developed the techniques by which biologists could begin to use the new-found power of the electron microscope in the investigation of both intact and disrupted animal cells.

Claude recognized that morphological descriptions were insufficient for characterization of the intimate structural components of the cell. He concluded that each of the particles identified by electron microscopy must be isolated in pure form. He and his co-workers ruptured the cell in isotonic solutions, making it possible to isolate such organelles as nuclei, mitochondria, microsomes, and other small particles in a relatively pure state so that their properties could be studied in the test tube. Thus, his two major contributions, the study of cells by electron microscopy and the isolation of cellular organelles by high-speed centrifugation, depended upon two available technological advances: the coupling of high-resolution electron microscopy with special sectioning techniques and the development of high-speed centrifuges capable of providing the appropriate gravitational forces for separating the discrete organelles. He and Porter, using the electron microscope, were the first to demonstrate cancer virus particles in

701

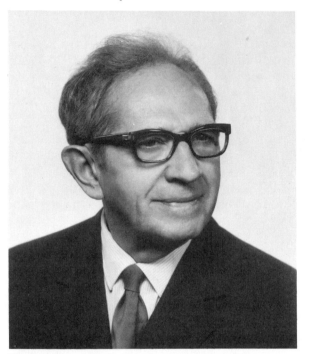

Figure 159. Albert Claude. (Courtesy of Dr. Maclyn McCarty.)

tumor cells. While working at the Rockefeller Institute and University, Claude became a United States citizen, but before the Nobel Prize was awarded he had returned to Europe to become Head of the Jules Bordet Institute in Brussels.

George Palade was born in Rumania and received his M.D. degree from the University of Bucharest in 1940. He came to the United States in 1946 and went to work in Murphy's laboratory at the Rockefeller Institute, in close association with Claude. Palade and his collaborators localized the position within mammalian cells at which proteins are synthesized. The organelles called *microsomes* were shown to be composed of a series of particles, known as *ribosomes,* structures rich in RNA, upon which proteins are synthesized. The ribosomes were shown to hang together on a lipid network—the endoplasmic reticulum. Palade later discovered the series of events that enable cells such as those of the pancreas to store proteins that have been synthesized upon the ribosomes, transporting them through the endoplasmic reticulum, sequestering them in storage granules, and finally secreting them into the bloodstream when the need for them has been signaled to the cell.

Palade used for these studies the Claude methodology (electron microscopy and fractionation by high-speed centrifuge), with additional refinements. He and his associates also isolated mitochondria, demonstrated that these minute "powerhouses" release ATP, and identified the components of the endocrine cells involved in the secretory cycle of the pancreas. In studies of the capillaries, Palade clarified the mechanisms of transport of materials through vessel walls by showing that particles are carried from the bloodstream to tissues in minute vesicles (bladderlike containers). Palade

702

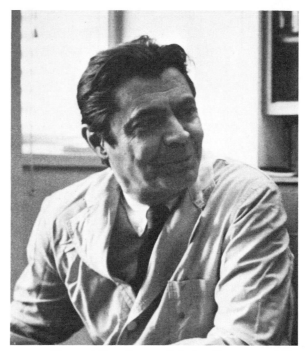

Figure 160. George Palade. (Courtesy of Dr. Maclyn McCarty.)

became an American citizen and remained at the Rockefeller Institute until 1972, when he joined the faculty at Yale.

Christian deDuve, though born in England, received his M.D. degree from the Catholic University of Louvain, Belgium, and remained there as a

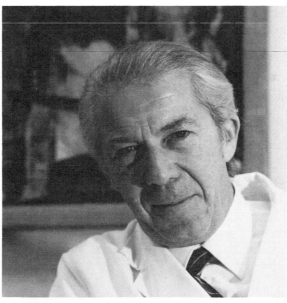

Figure 161. Christian R. deDuve. (Courtesy of Dr. Maclyn McCarty.)

member of the faculty, attaining the rank of Professor of Biochemistry in 1951. In 1962 he was appointed Professor of Biochemistry at Rockefeller University and since then has occupied simultaneously two professorial chairs; one in Belgium, the other in the United States. deDuve and his associates, utilizing the techniques developed by Claude, discovered those tiny particles known as *lysosomes,* which represent the intracellular digestive tract for various body functions. Lysosomes are capable of consuming and lysing bacteria and other foreign materials that enter cells. deDuve found that the lysosome particles contain within their sacs potent enzymes which do not escape into the surrounding medium until various procedures are used to disrupt the lipid membrane that contains them. It was demonstrated that these "contained enzymes," sequestered within lipid membranes, have the potentiality to injure tissues. This discovery opened up a new area for the investigation of tissue injury and the reactions involved in inflammatory disease.

The discovery of lysosomes has also "added an important chapter to the long developing epic begun by Metchnikoff" and has led to better insight into the functions of phagocytes. Cohn and Hirsch at the Rockefeller Institute have shown recently that the granules of white blood cells are true lysosomes. Understanding of the mechanisms that control phagocyte-invader interactions has proved to be helpful in providing an insight into the action of such anti-inflammatory drugs as cortisone, which affect the function of lysosomes in living cells. The rheumatologist, studying the release of lysosomal enzymes from synovial cells, and the gastroenterologist, studying the antibodies to mitochondria that are prevalent in some forms of liver disease, are the beneficiaries of approaches made possible by the studies that have just been described (Weissmann, 1974).

The foregoing accomplishments in cell biology can be "compared to the cracking of the atom accomplished by physicists." Just as the atom was dissected into its component particles, the mammalian cell was shown to contain within its plasma membrane a variety of discrete organelles. These organelles include not only the nucleus and its nucleoli but also the mitochondria, the lysosomes, the endoplasmic reticulum studded with ribosomes, the peroxidase-rich granules, the microtubules, and the digestive vacuoles (Weissmann, 1974).

Without the techniques for studying ultrastructure developed by these three great scientists and their co-workers, we would still be unaware of the means by which viruses are recognized and taken up by cells, how their coats are removed and how viral infections produce disease, and how they also produce animal tumors. One of Claude's first studies in cell biology was the isolation of Rous sarcoma virus and the determination of its intracellular localization. Many of the important discoveries in the past decade in immunology and pathology would not have been possible without the basic research of Claude and Palade. deDuve's study of lysosomes provided an understanding of the pathogenesis of the genetic storage diseases. Genetic abnormalities such as Tay-Sachs disease, Niemann-Pick disease, Pompe's disease, and most of the other storage diseases of childhood are due to the accumulation within lysosomes of materials ordinarily hydrolyzed by discrete lysosomal enzymes, the lack of which leads to the accumulation of the waste product (Weissmann, 1974).

29

The Neurosciences

We are a part of nature, and our mind is the only instrument we have, or can conceive of, for learning about nature or about ourselves.

(C. H. Waddington, *The Nature of Life*)

The human brain is the most highly organized structure known. It gives man his uniqueness; and in attempting to understand how it functions, science faces one of its greatest challenges. "But for man's brain, no cosmological or environmental problems would exist. 'The whole drama would be played out before empty stalls. . .'. A better understanding of the brain is certain to lead man to a richer comprehension of himself, of his fellow man, of society, and, in fact, of the whole world with its problems." Study of the brain and its functions is now being pursued vigorously by many of the leading scientists in this country and elsewhere. They are reexamining its various complex components; investigating the pathways by which it transports its functional messages; and studying how the elemental components, the nerve cells or neurons, operate. They are applying all of the knowledge of fundamental biology to the study of the chemical mechanisms involved in brain function in order to understand how drugs affect cerebral activity and how complex functions such as memory operate (Eccles, 1974).

In building the brain, the primitive cells of the embryo multiply in the neural plate, which gives rise to the central nervous system. As the process advances, these nerve cells grow fibers that connect with other nerve cells, ultimately leading to a system of connections that make even the most complex wiring in a central telephone exchange seem simple. The details of construction are coordinated primarily by the genetic instructions that come down from the embryo's parents, encoded in deoxyribonucleic acid (DNA). The DNA code determines each cell's synthesis of its many different enzyme systems. The structure and the growth characteristics of the various

705

types of cells are determined by each cell's own huge array of enzymes. As described by Eccles (1974):

> ... the enzymes and other structural components, whose synthesis is determined by the DNA, represent a source of secondary instructions, which, at all stages of development, guide the growth of neurons by sensing specific chemical signals that are believed to derive from the special protein structures in their surface membranes. Thus, for example, nerve cells in the cortex of the brain develop axonal processes, which, as they pass through a maze of other cells and their complex intermingling extensions, enter well-defined tracts in the brain stem and continue down the spinal cord for several feet, finally terminating on specific spinal nerve cells. These, in turn, also have axonal processes that grow out from the spinal cord to reach specific muscles. Sensory nerve impulses from the retina of the eye, the cochlear organ in the ear, or receptors in the skin traverse specific nerve-fiber pathways that often are interrupted by several relay stations, through which the impulse is passed on to other nerve cells before arriving at precisely localized portions of the brain. In addition, cells from different portions of the nervous system are connected in highly diffuse networks. This permits complex integrations among many separate sensory and motor functions. All of this detailed connectivity is established before any organized activity begins in the embryonic brain.

A variety of approaches are being used to determine how all of this comes about. It will be recalled that Ross Harrison developed the technique of tissue culture in order to see how nerve cells grow (p. 257). The growth of isolated fragments from embryos is still being carefully studied. The electron microscope provides a technique for visualizing the stages in the development of nerve cells. A variety of chemicals, viruses, and X-rays are employed to damage or destroy specific components of the nervous system, and the reactions of the cells remaining after such damage are then determined. Radioisotopes can be incorporated into the nuclei of nerve cells before cell division begins; hence, the behavior of the growing cells can be followed for long periods of time—a technique which is throwing light on how defects in brain development arise. This in turn may lead to more rational treatment for congenital defects in the brain that result from enzymatic or genetic disorders. Disorders due to lack of specific enzymes have already provided new information about the normal biochemistry of the brain.

Though studies of the functional performance of the nervous system have been carried out for many years, the more sophisticated microelectrode techniques have been widely utilized only in the last two decades. This approach has revealed the intimate operation of the neuronal apparatus, both in localized regions of interaction and in the long, complex pathways which are such a vital part of the machinery. The different types of communication between nerve cells in their region of close contact—the *synapse*—are now better understood. In the cerebellum, all of the neuronal constituents are known, and their synaptic connections have been rather well established. More has to be learned about the organization of these neuronal systems—how they operate over longer distances and how the more complex activities are integrated.

An area of major importance is the analysis of the "firing frequencies" of individual nerve cells. These basic elements number in the tens of thousands of millions, but in any one zone of the brain there are multitudes of similar nerve cells, so that observations of single cells should be representative of a large group of apparently identical units. At present the nervous system is regarded as being designed essentially for conveying the integrating information that is coded in the patterns of impulse discharge (Eccles, 1974).

Research into the basic aspects of cerebral function has yielded a number of practical dividends. For example, electrical recordings from the brain produce the electroencephalogram, which provides information about such brain disorders as epilepsy. This information is utilized in diagnosing abnormalities and localizing them in specific areas, where they may be treated by surgery, radiation, or other means. Another important dividend from research has been the use of electrical recordings from peripheral nerves and muscles, which help in the diagnosis, understanding, and treatment of many disorders of neuromuscular function.

The patterns of impulse frequency that have been described form the basic physiological material for the development of neurocommunications theory, which is concerned essentially with the transfer and integration of information as it passes through the nervous system. The nervous system does not operate along simple lines of communication such as we employ when we call a friend on the telephone. In nervous communications, many of the links run in parallel, and superimposed on this pattern is a complexity of "dynamic loop" operations, with a large variety of feedback controls and cross-linkages. Attempts are now being made to find out how neuronal systems operate by using the product of a human brain. Computer models have been designed to simulate the performance of portions of the brain, embodying simultaneously the principles of design that have been discovered in the neuronal system (Eccles, 1974).

IMPORTANT DEVELOPMENTS IN KNOWLEDGE OF NERVOUS SYSTEM FUNCTION

No important basic research was carried out on the nervous system in America during the first century of our nation. In the second century, thanks to the development of a variety of new tools and techniques, the American contribution has been considerable. Before describing what has occurred, it must be put in perspective.

In the latter part of the nineteenth century, it was known that the spinal cord has 31 pairs of nerve roots, representing the pathways for the entrance and exit of nerves which serve all parts of the body and communicate via the spinal cord with the brain. Microscopic studies had shown that nerve fibers are enormously long extensions of nerve cells.

Toward the close of the nineteenth century, histological controversy centered on the *neuron theory,* the doctrine of the physiological autonomy of the nerve cell and its branches. The unanswered question was: Where do the nerve fibers originate? Most people believed that they arose independently of the nerve cell. In 1850 A. V. Waller discovered that when a nerve was severed, the segment attached to the cell survived, but the portion separated from the cell underwent degeneration. This "law of wallerian degen-

707

eration" indicated that the nerve fibers are prolongations of the cells from which they receive their nourishment.

Several decades later, two European scientists made important contributions to neurology. The first one, Camillo Golgi, an Italian, in 1883 developed a method of staining nerve tissue. By this method he showed that nerve cells have two kinds of extensions from the body of the cell. One he labeled the *axon*, an elongated fiber reaching some distance from the cell and ending in a muscle, a gland, or a sense organ. The other, a thick tuft of short extensions resembling the branches of a tree, he named the *dendrite*. He also found that nerve cells are of two types: type I, those with long axons that extend outside the central nervous system; type II, those with short axons, which do not leave the central nervous system but become linked with other nerves in the brain and spinal cord. Later work demonstrated that there are so many different types of cells that the simple separation into type I and type II was no longer useful. Golgi also studied the tiny sense organs that are embedded in muscles and tendons. When a muscle is in motion, these sensory elements are stimulated, and a message is carried through the spinal cord to the brain, thus keeping the individual aware of the state of his muscles and joints. Golgi enunciated the *neuron theory*, which encompasses the operation of the nerve cell with all its processes. The cell and processes together constitute the neuron.

The other European scientist, Santiago Ramón y Cajal, a Spaniard, established the neurotropic theory of the growth of nervous tissue. He believed that the nerve cells release special chemicals, which he called "neurotropic" because he believed they had an attraction for nerve tissue. They are catalysts, formed in the embryonic connective tissue surrounding the nerve sheaths; and they spread in the direction of growth, guiding the growth bud along its special pathway. Moreover, when a nerve is severed after birth, the stump attached to the nerve cell continues to grow in the direction laid down by its original path; this is why the nerve fiber regenerates always in the direction of its end-organ.

During this early period, there were opposing views about how the neurons were formed. An important advance came when Ross Harrison (see p. 257) demonstrated (in 1907) the outgrowth of nerve fibers from a nerve cell in tissue culture.

Golgi and Cajal were to an important degree instrumental in establishing the neuron concept, and Harrison contributed important evidence to support this concept. In substance, the neuron theory asserts three principles:

(1) The neuron is the unit of which the nervous system is composed. Each neuron stems from a single embryonic cell. Each is a functional unit, and nothing less than the complete neuron can carry nerve impulses. (Though it was long believed that neurons are the only elements that can conduct nerve impulses, it is now known that *parts* of neurons under certain conditions can serve as conductors. For example, in many neurons, an impulse initiated at the base of the axon is conducted down the neuron and never invades the dendrites nor even the cell body. This new discovery is the basis of the concept of integrative action of single cells. If the all-or-nothing impulse invaded the entire cell on each occasion, it would wipe out all subsequent events, and cellular integrative action would not eventuate.

This is one of the most important concepts to be advanced in the past 20 years—how a single neuron integrates its inputs, both excitatory and inhibitory, into a running integral, which it expresses in terms of frequency of output.) Each nerve cell is responsible for its own nutrition and integrity. Hence, when an axon is severed from its cell body, it dies.

(2) Neurons carry impulses from one to the other across spatial gaps, the neurons being related to each other by contiguity and not by continuity. (It was later shown by Otto Loewi and Henry Dale [in the 1930s] that chemical transmitter-substances are released by the axonal endings and stimulate the cell beyond them, providing the chemical mechanism for the transmission of the impulse from one neuron to another.)

(3) Neurons conduct in one direction only. Each nerve pathway will permit only one-way traffic, and the direction of the traffic is never reversed. In the dendrites, the nerve impulses travel toward the cell body, whereas in the axons it is away from the cell body.

Neurons display many different patterns of action: some obey the classic laws outlined above, others do not. Moreover, the neuron theory itself must be modified in the light of recent discoveries of close junctions and locales of decreased impedance to ionic flow between cells. So-called electrical synapses have now been shown to exist in many nuclei of the mammalian brain. The links between cells connected in this manner are so close that impulse conduction between them is unconditional, immediate, and invariant: hence, the two cells act as if they were one. The structural individuality of cells is not brought into question by these findings; it is the special contact between them that accounts for the physiological unity of the two.

S. WEIR MITCHELL   One of the most interesting personalities in American medicine was S. Weir Mitchell (1829–1914). For over 50 years he was a busy practitioner, yet he was known internationally as an experimental physiologist, a neurologist, and a man of letters.

Most of his ideas for research arose from his clinical experience. He was one of the first American examples of the class of investigators who have the ability to weld together their laboratory observations and their clinical experience in such a way as to benefit their patients while they are advancing science. Mitchell never wrote endless speculations, as was the custom of the times; rather, he resorted to experiment and analysis for the solution of his clinical problems.

As a result of his Civil War experience, he was able to write a treatise on "Injuries to Nerves and Their Consequences." His knowledge of the peripheral nervous system and sense organs was profound. He showed that cutting a cutaneous nerve does not destroy all sensibility and that sensory areas in the skin overlap. In all of these observations he was far ahead of his contemporaries. In a series of papers presented in the *American Journal of the Medical Sciences,* he described his well-known investigations on the knee jerk and its reinforcement.

The studies by Mitchell of the functions of the cerebellum demonstrate his skill as an experimental physiologist. Over 350 experiments were per-

709

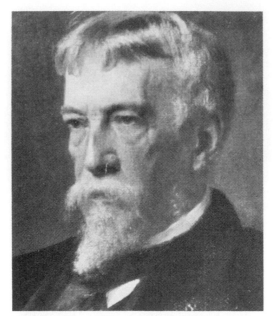

Figure 162. S. Weir Mitchell. (From
Riesman, D.: History of the Interurban
Clinical Club, 1905–1937. Philadelphia,
The John C. Winston Co., 1937.)

formed on pigeons, rabbits, and guinea pigs, mainly along three lines: ablation, freezing, and irritation of the cerebellum. He pointed out the vicarious
functioning of other parts of the central nervous system after cerebellar
removal. As a result of these studies, he proposed his well-known augmen-
tor theory for the function of this important part of the brain.

When Weir Mitchell was still a young man, he hesitated between medicine and literature as a career. He went to Oliver Wendell Holmes for advice. Holmes urged him to devote himself to science, remarking that after
he had succeeded in medicine, he might devote himself to literature. The
"Old Autocrat" no doubt thought he had spared the world one more bit of
mediocrity. Mitchell took his advice. In later life, after world fame had come
to him as a physician, physiologist, and neurologist, he began a series of
historical novels which marked him as a literary figure of considerable talent.

NEUROMUSCULAR PHYSIOLOGY   Major advances in understanding of how muscles
and nerves work together were made by two
brilliant English neurophysiologists, Charles
Scott Sherrington and Edgar Douglas Adrian, who received the Nobel Prize
for medicine and physiology in 1932 for their studies of the function of the
neuron. Every neurologist depends on the work of Sherrington when he attempts to diagnose and treat patients with abnormalities of muscular function. Sherrington became interested in the knee jerk, the involuntary kick of
the leg when the tendon just below the kneecap is tapped lightly. Because it
is an involuntary movement, it is called a reflex. Sherrington found that the
spinal cord coordinates such reflex responses. He further concluded that the

710

location of reflex centers for various muscles at different levels in the spinal cord indicated that the cord had a segmental pattern. He developed his researches on the "spinal animal" experimentally deprived of its brain. Its reactions are controlled entirely by centers in the spinal cord. The same is true of humans paralyzed as a result of injury to the cord; they still retain some of these automatic responses to stimulation. By his deep insight and ingenious experiments, Sherrington explained how the complicated workings of the body are integrated by the billions of nerve cells in the central nervous system (Riedman and Gustafson, 1963).

Adrian was interested in finding out more about our sensory perceptions: how we know how heavily an object is pressing on our skin, how loud a sound is, how bright a light, how heavy the weight we are holding in our hands, how cold an object we are touching — simple questions but very difficult to answer. How do we perceive stronger and weaker sensations from our sensory organs, as we obviously do? Adrian began his neurological research with Keith Lucas. Together they discovered the "all or none" law of nerve conduction: when a nerve is stimulated, an impulse either does or does not develop, depending on the strength of the stimulus; there is no such thing as a partial impulse.

Adrian found that sense organs and nerve cells discharge whole series of impulses. In each individual fiber, the nerve impulse is of constant size; but the stronger the stimulus, the greater the frequency of the impulses traveling along the nerve. Nerve cells communicate with each other by a system of repetitive impulses similar to the firing of a machine gun (Riedman and Gustafson, 1963).

JOSEPH ERLANGER AND HERBERT GASSER In 1907 the Swedish physiologist Gustaf Gothlin made the assumption that conduction velocity in thick nerve fibers is greater than in thin ones. The basis for his view was Thompson's formula for conduction in electrical cables. Joseph Erlanger and Herbert Gasser furnished the scientific proof for this hypothesis. A new and highly important technical development was responsible for the success of their experimental approach. At a meeting of the American Physical Society held in Chicago in 1920, J. B. Johnson of Western Electric Company described a cathode-ray oscillograph possessing a greatly increased sensitivity. This instrument allowed Erlanger and Gasser to record the brief electrical phenomena associated with nervous impulses.

Joseph Erlanger, after graduating from the Johns Hopkins School of Medicine in 1899, served his internship at the Johns Hopkins Hospital. He then became an assistant in the Department of Physiology under William H. Howell. When the University of Wisconsin organized a medical school in 1907, Erlanger became its first Professor of Physiology. It was here that he met his celebrated pupil, *Herbert S. Gasser.* While Gasser was still a student, in 1910, Erlanger moved to Washington University in St. Louis, as head of its newly organized Department of Physiology. Gasser received his M.D. degree from Johns Hopkins in 1915. The following year he taught pharmacology at the University of Wisconsin and then joined Erlanger in St. Louis. In 1921 he was made head of the Department of Pharmacology. He then studied in Europe for two years and on his return resumed his work

711

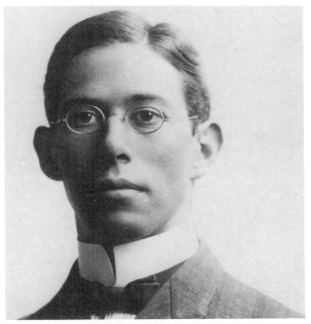

Figure 163. Joseph Erlanger. (From The Archives Office, The Johns Hopkins Medical Institutions.)

on muscle-nerve physiology, which he had begun earlier with Erlanger. It was then that he first hooked up the cathode-ray tube to a precision amplifier in order to measure accurately the weak currents generated by activity in the nerve fibers. He and Erlanger recorded the action potential as it passed down the conducting nerve fiber and found that the resulting electric wave had three distinct peaks. The peaks are due to the different rates at which the nerve impulse is conducted by the different types of fibers in the nerve. The perception of pain is mediated largely by slowly conducting fibers, the sensation of touch by rapidly conducting fibers. The muscles of the body were shown to be activated by very fast conducting fibers.

In 1931 Gasser went to Cornell Medical College as Professor of Physiology. Four years later, when Simon Flexner retired as Director of the Rockefeller Institute, Gasser succeeded him. In 1937, Erlanger and Gasser collaborated on a book entitled *Electrical Signs of Nervous Activity,* which summarized their earlier work. In 1944 they received the Nobel Prize for physiology and medicine "for their discoveries regarding the highly differentiated functions of single nerve fibers." A *New York Times* editorial, commenting on the award, said: "Such work is less spectacular than that which gave us the sulfa drugs and penicillin, but hardly less important" (Riedman and Gustafson, 1963).

As we have seen from the work of Adrian, understanding of the way that sense organs work is vital to our knowledge of how the brain works. The 1967 Nobel Prize for physiology and medicine was shared by H. K. Hartline and George Wald of the United States and Ragnar Granit of Sweden for their discoveries concerning the primary chemical and physio-

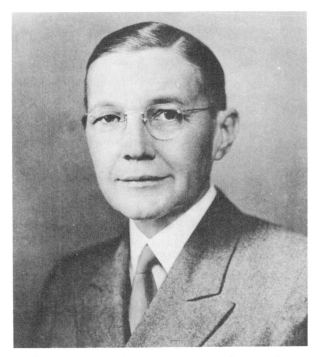

Figure 164. Herbert Gasser. (From Corner, G. W.: A History of the Rockefeller Institute. New York, The Rockefeller Institute Press, 1964.)

logical visual processes. Wald was a biologist who had received his Ph.D. degree from Columbia University in 1932 and had been a member of the Harvard University faculty since 1934. He had been concerned with the chemical events in the retina that underlie vision. Hartline and Granit were concerned with the nerve impulses that are induced as a consequence of the chemical events in the retina. A graduate of Johns Hopkins University Medical School and, at the time of his award, a faculty member of Rockefeller University, Hartline devised methods for recording the nerve impulses from single cells of the eye of the horseshoe crab and cold-blooded vertebrates. He and his associates were the first to demonstrate that "individual nerve cells in the retina never act independently; it is the integrated action of all units of the visual system that gives rise to vision."

THE GROWTH OF NERVE CIRCUITS Severe damage to the principal motor nerve of the face may leave a person afflicted with a condition which results in the production of "crocodile tears." As the injured nerve regenerates, fibers that should have gone to a salivary gland may go astray and connect themselves to the tear gland of one eye. Thereafter, every situation calling for the production of saliva causes, instead, weeping from the eye with the misplaced nerve.

713

The concern of the patient in such cases is whether or not normal function can be restored. Physicians were once agreed that the central nervous system is plastic enough so that any motor nerve might be reconnected to any gland or muscle with an appropriate result. It was believed that learning determined not only the function but also the structure of the nervous system.

The doctrine of the functional plasticity of the nervous system was sharply challenged in 1938 by Frank R. Ford and Barnes Woodhall of the Johns Hopkins School of Medicine. In an account of their clinical experience with functional disorders following the regeneration of nerves, they declared that these disorders persisted in many patients for years without improvement. Their report cast serious doubt not only upon the accepted methods of therapy but also upon the theory of functional plasticity.

That same year Roger Sperry of the University of Chicago and later of the California Institute of Technology began a series of experiments, the initial aim of which was to find out whether functional plasticity is a property of the higher brain centers only or whether it extends to the lowest levels of the spinal cord.

Sperry switched the nerve connections between opposing muscles in the hindlimb of rats in such a way as to reverse the movement at the ankle joint. The rats never adjusted to this change: when they tried to lift the affected foot, it pulled downward; when they tried to rise on the ball of the foot, their toes swung up and they fell back on their heels. In spite of a program of special training, the rats' feet continued to work backward.

Then Sperry turned to the sensory system. He transposed the nerves of the skin from the left to the right hindfoot, and vice versa. As the crossed hindlimb nerves regenerated, the rats began to exhibit false reference of sensations. In response to a mild electric shock to the sole of the right foot, the animals withdrew their left foot.

In similar experiments on monkeys, Sperry believed at first that the monkeys were making a better adjustment than the rats. But after three years of testing and observation, they too failed to achieve any functionally beneficial correction in the action of the cross-innervated muscles (Sperry, 1959).

In most cases, human subjects can learn to control transplanted muscles only in simple, slow, voluntary movements. They seem to have a greater capacity for adjustment than do the subhuman primates. Such re-education as does occur would appear to be due to the greater development of higher learning centers in the human brain. Contrary to earlier thought, it does not reflect an intrinsic plasticity of nerve networks in general.

NEUROCHEMISTRY AND NEURO-PHARMACOLOGY

Neurochemistry, having evolved from the crude experiments of the past century, is now a sophisticated science utilizing many microchemical procedures and radio-tracer techniques. By use of histochemical fluorescence methods, the nervous system has been "mapped" by tracing the predominant transmitter substance along fiber pathways. In this manner unique neuronal pathways have been identified that contain mainly dopamine, noradrenalin (called also levarterenol or norepine-phrine), or serotonin—three transmitter substances that are known to be involved in neuronal function. Knowledge of such pathways, together with other pharmacological, physiological, and pathological data, has led to advances in our understanding of nervous-system functions and their alteration in disease.

An outstanding example of the achievements of research in the neurosciences is the present-day therapy of Parkinson's disease with L-dopa. Another key area of research has been concerned with the molecular structure of cell membranes, with synaptic receptor sites, and with the associated transport of sodium, potassium, and chloride ions. These ions bring about the changes in membrane potentials that are a vital part of neuronal function. Equally important are the neurotransmitters released at the synapses, which activate the specific receptor sites to permit the passage of an impulse from one nerve to the next. These transmitters are a vital part of the molecular machinery that carries out the specialized communications between nerves in the brain. Acetylcholine has been known for years to be one of these transmitters, but only recently have investigators succeeded in extracting from the specialized receptor membrane of nerve cells the specific molecular component that combines with acetylcholine. This is an important step toward explaining the actual mechanism by which communication among neuronal structures is achieved and regulated. It has practical application in the study and treatment of myasthenia gravis, a disease of neuromuscular synapses (Eccles, 1974).

Other research areas being explored by neurochemists include enzyme systems and metabolic cycles. The brain has "pumps" that help to maintain the correct ionic composition within nerve cells and the associated electrical potentials across the surface membranes of the cells. Also under study is the energy needed to push the trophic substances along the nerve fibers in order to maintain the lines of communication both within the central nervous system and in the peripheral nerves.

Closely allied to neurochemistry is neuropharmacology, which is concerned with the action of the various synaptic transmitters and how they work. The technique of micropharmacology is now well developed. It has clarified the role of such substances as acetylcholine, glycine, gamma-aminobutyric acid, and noradrenalin as synaptic transmitters in the central nervous system. An important problem for the neuropharmacologists is that of determining how the brain manufactures, releases, and removes the synaptic transmitters. These substances appear to operate by acting at receptor sites on the surface membranes of nerve cells, and their action can be enhanced or blocked by pharmacological agents. Once the specific action of such agents has been identified, they can be used to exert control over particular aspects of brain function. Already there have been improvements in anesthetics, in drugs for the control of epileptic seizures, and in agents used for the treatment of the peripheral neuromuscular paralysis of myasthenia gravis. Pharmacological advances sometimes create problems, as evidenced by the widespread use of drugs that affect the brain and nervous system. Specific hallucinogens such as LSD (lysergic acid diethylamide) may cause serious psychotic disorders and even permanent destruction of the personality (Eccles, 1974).

715

NEURO-TRANSMITTERS

In 1901 the noted English physiologist J. N. Langley observed that the injection of an extract of the adrenal gland into an animal stimulated tissues innervated by the sympathetic nerves—the nerves of the autonomic nervous system that increase the heart rate, raise the blood pressure, and cause smooth muscle to contract. Langley's observation prompted T. R. Eliott, his student at Cambridge University, to inject Adrenalin (which had just become available) into experimental animals. Eliott saw that the hormone, like the crude extract, produced a response similar to that evoked by electrical stimulation of sympathetic nerves. He then made the brilliant suggestion that Adrenalin (epinephrine) might be released from sympathetic nerves and thus stimulate muscle cells with which the nerves form junctions. Eliott was the first to enunciate the concept of neural communication by means of chemical transmitters.

W. H. Howell, at Johns Hopkins, observed in 1906 that when an experimental animal's heart was perfused with a solution containing no potassium salts, stimulation of the *vagus nerve* (a nerve of the parasympathetic system that reduces the heart rate) was less effective in slowing the heart rate. On the other hand, if potassium ions were increased in the perfusion fluid, the effect of vagal stimulation was enhanced. Two years later Howell and W. W. Duke discovered that during vagal stimulation of the mammalian heart, potassium is liberated and appears in the perfusion fluid. Howell interpreted these results as evidence of the indirect action of the vagus nerve: stimulation of the nerve first liberates potassium in the heart tissue, and the increase in free potassium ions then retards the heart's action.

Though Howell was the first to produce evidence that chemicals may be liberated at nerve terminals, the first *conclusive* evidence for neurochemical transmission was obtained in 1921 by Otto Loewi in Austria. Loewi put the heart of a frog in a bath in which the heart could be kept beating. The fluid bathing the heart was allowed to perfuse a second heart. When Loewi stimulated the first heart's vagus nerve, the beat of the second heart was slowed, showing that some substance liberated by the stimulated vagus nerve was transported by the fluid and influenced the perfused heart. This substance was later identified by Sir Henry Dale as acetylcholine.

Very important contributions to our knowledge of neurotransmission in the sympathetic nervous system were made by Walter B. Cannon of Harvard, whose early experiments with X-rays were described in Chapter 14. In 1946 Ulf von Euler, a Swedish physiologist, isolated the neurotransmitter of the sympathetic nervous system and identified it as noradrenalin. Noradrenalin, which differs from epinephrine only by lacking the methyl attached to the amino group, is present in peripheral nerves, brain, and spinal cord and in the medulla of the adrenal gland. In peripheral tissues and in the brain, noradrenalin acts as a neurotransmitter. In the adrenal medulla it functions as a hormone; that is, it is released into the bloodstream and acts on distant target organs. Dopamine, once thought to be simply an intermediate in the synthesis of noradrenalin and epinephrine, is also a neurotransmitter, in its own right, in the brain, where it functions in nerves that influence movement and behavior. The third catecholamine, epinephrine, is concentrated largely in the adrenal medulla. It is discharged into the bloodstream during fear, anger, or other stress reactions, as described

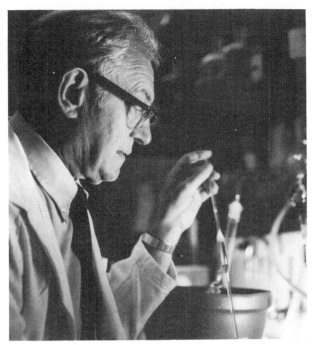

Figure 165. Julius Axelrod. (National Library of Medicine, Bethesda, Maryland.)

by Cannon, and acts as a hormone on a number of organs, including the heart, liver, and intestines.

In 1960 Georg Hertting, Gordon Whitby, and *Julius Axelrod,* at the National Institutes of Health, showed that radioactive noradrenalin is taken up selectively and retained in sympathetic nerves. Electron micrographs of sympathetic neurons from rats injected with labeled noradrenalin show that noradrenalin is stored within the nerve.

The discharge of neurotransmitter from the nerve ending is the final episode in a complex chain of events that follow one another with extraordinary rapidity. When a nerve is stimulated, its membrane is depolarized, with sodium moving into the nerve as potassium moves out; the wave of depolarization moves along the nerve axon to its end, where it causes a tiny spurt of the transmitter to be discharged from the nerve ending into the synaptic cleft. Once the transmitter is liberated, it diffuses across the cleft from the nerve terminal to the effector cells. The capacity of a neighboring effector cell to respond to the transmitter depends on whether a receptor on the cell's surface recognizes and combines with the neurotransmitter. When the receptor and transmitter interact, a series of events is triggered that causes the effector cell to carry out its special function. There are two receptors that recognize noradrenalin, alpha- and beta-adrenergic receptors, and one that recognizes dopamine. These receptors can be distinguished from one another by the specific response that each elicits and by the ability of specific drugs to block those responses.

Once the neurotransmitter has interacted with the effector cell, its action must be terminated quickly; otherwise its effect would be continued so long that precise control of the effector mechanism would be lost. One of

717

the neurotransmitters, acetylcholine, is inactivated rapidly by the enzyme acetylcholinesterase. In the past 10 years it has become clear that the inactivation of neurotransmitters through enzymatic transformation is the exception rather than the rule. Julius Axelrod and his associates at the National Institutes of Health devised experiments that clearly demonstrated that noradrenalin is taken up into as well as released from sympathetic nerves. Leslie L. Iversen of Cambridge University has since shown that this neuronal recapture by sympathetic nerves is highly selective for noradrenalin and compounds resembling it in chemical structure.

In view of the long chain of chemical events that is involved in neuromuscular actions, one wonders how a fencer or boxer ever succeeds in striking his adversary or defending himself, or how a finger can be so quickly withdrawn when it has inadvertently made contact with a hot iron.

L-DOPA AND PARKINSONISM

The physiologically important catecholamines are dopa, dopamine, noradrenalin, and epinephrine. There are precise methods of measuring catecholamines in body fluids and tissues, and drugs are available that alter their formation, storage, release, and metabolism. As a result, more is known about catecholamines than about other neurotransmitters. Fluorescence photomicrography and drugs that selectively destroy catecholamine-containing nerves have made it possible to locate the noradrenalin and dopamine cell bodies and to trace the pathways of their axons and nerve endings. The cell bodies of the dopamine-containing nerves are in the area of the brain stem called the substantia nigra; from here the dopaminergic axons course through the brain stem, many of them terminating in the caudate nucleus. The dopamine-containing tracts in the caudate nucleus play an important role in the integration of movement.

The Swedish pharmacologist Arvid Carlsson noted in 1959 that when reserpine was given to rats, it sharply reduced the dopamine content of the caudate nucleus in the brain and also caused a tremor resembling that of patients with Parkinson's disease. The administration of dopa, a dopamine precursor that can get from the blood into the brain more easily than dopamine, abolished the tremors. These findings prompted Oleh Hoanykie-wicz, who was then working at the University of Vienna, to measure the content of dopamine in the brain of patients who had died of Parkinson's disease. He found that there was virtually no dopamine in the caudate nucleus. This basic observation led to a major therapeutic advance. George C. Cotzias of the Brookhaven National Laboratory found that when L-dopa, the dopamine precursor that can enter the brain, is administered, it corrects the dopamine deficiency and effectively relieves the symptoms of Parkinson's disease. This is a good example of how basic research can lead to a new form of treatment.

OTHER DRUGS ACTING ON THE NERVOUS SYSTEM

In the late 1940s the group at the Cleveland Clinic interested in the study of hypertension isolated from blood serum a pressor substance which they named *serotonin*. M. M. Rapport of the Clinic staff determined that serotonin is 5-hydroxytryptamine (5-HT), pharmacologi-

718

cally a highly active substance. In the early 1950s pharmacologists recognized that the hallucinogenic agent lysergic acid diethylamide (LSD) not only resembles serotonin in chemical structure but also counteracts some of its pharmacological actions (by occupying sites intended for serotonin). It was suggested that serotonin must have something to do with insanity. Other hallucinogenic agents, such as mescaline and amphetamine, are related in structure to noradrenalin. In the mid-1950s clinical investigators were learning that chemicals such as chlorpromazine could mitigate psychotic behavior and that monamine oxidase inhibitors and imipramine could relieve depression. At about the same time it was discovered that reserpine, which was proving valuable for the treatment not only of hypertension but also of schizophrenia, reduces the levels of noradrenalin and serotonin in the brain. These observations suggested that these drugs exert their actions on the brain by interfering with neurotransmitters.

After Axelrod and his colleagues found that radioactive noradrenalin can be taken up and released from nerves, they investigated the ways in which various drugs influenced the disposition of injected, radioactively labeled transmitters. Cocaine, a potent stimulant that can produce psychosis, intensifies the action of noradrenalin by preventing its capture and inactivation, thus leaving large amounts of the catecholamine to react with the effector cell. Antidepressant drugs such as imipramine have the same effect. Amphetamine, which is both a stimulant and a mind-altering drug, affects noradrenergic nerves in two ways: it blocks the uptake of noradrenalin and also promotes the release of the neurotransmitter from nerves.

Many drugs used in the treatment of hypertension affect the storage and release of noradrenergic transmitters. Reserpine and guanethidine prevent the storage of noradrenalin in the nerves that raise the blood pressure. Drugs such as alpha-methyldopa are transformed by enzymes in the nerve into substances that resemble noradrenalin chemically. These "false transmitters" are stored and released along with natural neurotransmitters, thus diluting them and reducing their effect.

Drugs that relieve mental depression produce their results by mechanisms which increase the amount of catecholamine that is available to stimulate the receptor. Conversely, reserpine, a compound that decreases the amount of the chemical transmitters, may produce depression. These considerations led to the hypothesis that mental depression is associated with a decreased availability to the brain of catecholamine and is relieved by drugs that increase the amount of these transmitters at the adrenergic receptor. Although not fully substantiated, this hypothesis has stimulated new approaches to the study of mental depression.

The introduction in the 1950s of antipsychotic drugs such as chlorpromazine and haloperidol revolutionized the treatment of schizophrenia, dramatically reducing the stay of schizophrenics in mental hospitals. Such antipsychotic drugs also exert an effect on the catecholamine neurotransmitters. Carlsson observed that antischizophrenic drugs cause an increase in the formation of catecholamines in the rat brain by blocking dopamine receptors.

Amphetamine produces a psychosis indistinguishable from that exhibited by paranoid schizophrenics. Solomon H. Snyder of the Johns Hopkins Medical School has proposed that the psychosis induced by this drug is due

719

to excessive release of dopamine. The ability of antischizophrenia drugs, which block dopamine receptors, to relieve symptoms of amphetamine-psychosis is consistent with this hypothesis.

The Nobel Prize for medicine and physiology in 1970 was awarded to Julius Axelrod of the National Institutes of Health along with Sir Bernard Katz of London and Ulf von Euler of Stockholm for their discoveries concerning the humoral transmitters in the nerve terminals and the mechanisms for their storage, release, and activation.

CYCLIC AMP IN BRAIN: ROLE IN SYNAPTIC TRANSMISSION

The formation and degradation of cyclic AMP (see Chapter 24) have been shown to be regulated, at least partially, by the same factors that affect the conduction of impulses by neurons. In addition, some central neurons appear to transmit their messages to other nerve cells by releasing chemicals called neurohormones that diffuse across the synapses and stimulate the production of cyclic AMP by the target cells. Rall and Sutherland discovered that brain is an unusually rich source of adenyl cyclase, the enzyme that catalyzes the synthesis of cAMP from adenosine triphosphate, and also of phosphodiesterase, the enzyme that inactivates cAMP.

Rall and his colleagues found that stimuli known to cause depolarization of neurons produced increases in the cyclic AMP concentration. For stimulation they employed neurohormones (norepinephrine, serotonin, and histamine) and electrical stimuli. It has been postulated by Greengard at Yale that stimulation of protein kinases by cAMP may result in both transient and persistent alterations (including the establishment of short- and long-term memory) in the properties of neurons. They identified in human brain a member of a family of enzymes called protein kinases, which catalyze the transfer of the terminal phosphate group of ATP to an acceptor protein. Cyclic AMP causes a marked stimulation of the activity of protein kinases, and it has been suggested that this is the factor that enables cyclic AMP to produce its many different effects. Histones, basic proteins associated with chromosomal DNA and thought to be involved in the regulation of gene expression, are good substrates for the cyclic AMP–dependent protein kinases. A similar kinase has been found in the caudate nucleus of rat brain. This type of preparation may be useful in the search for new drugs with a biochemical action similar to that of dopamine and which might be effective in the treatment of Parkinsonism (Axelrod, 1972).

NEURO-REGULATORS AND SLEEP MECHANISMS

In the past 15 years several important advances have been made in our understanding of sleep. First, the introduction of the electroencephalogram (EEG) by the German psychiatrist Hans Berger meant that sleep could be correlated with electrical changes occurring in the brain. G. Moruzzi and H. W. Magoun of Northwestern University Medical School reported in 1949 that in the cat,

720

lesions or stimulation within the reticular system of the midbrain would cause sleep or waking, respectively. This suggested that mechanisms within the midbrain are capable of altering brain function, producing sleep or arousal. E. Aserinsky and N. Kleitman (1953) of the University of Chicago described two states of sleep based mainly on electrophysiological components: slow wave sleep (SWS) and rapid eye movement (REM) sleep. In attempts to determine the specific areas of the brain that are involved in regulating these different features of sleep, investigators have found that lesions, particularly in the brain stem, can selectively suppress either waking, or SWS or REM sleep (Holman et al., 1975).

Fluorescence histochemistry has also influenced the study of sleep. This technique, originally developed by Erenko and associates, has enabled investigators to isolate, visualize, and map specific neurotransmitter cells, their axons and their terminal endings. It has been possible to develop anatomical maps of the catechol-indolamine systems in the central nervous system. As a result, stimulation and specific lesions that alter sleep and waking have taken on neurochemical significance.

Finally, the work of von Euler, Vogt, Brodie, Axelrod, Carlsson, Udenfriend, and their colleagues has permitted the design of drugs which have aided the examination of the relationship of various processes to sleep. Drugs have been developed that permit pharmacological dissection of the mechanisms involved. From this background the present-day theories of sleep have arisen. The data point to the presence of many neuroregulators at numerous integrative levels of the process. What triggers and maintains the process, what stops sleep, and what happens to the body and brain during sleep are questions still to be answered (Holman et al., 1975).

MEMORY   Studies of memory have proceeded along two lines. One is concerned with the way in which use and disuse affect the ability of the synapses to transmit information and to correlate the changes with synaptic growth and breakdown. As Eccles (1974) has stated:

> ... in the incredibly complex communication system of the brain, each memory must involve some stabilization of specific channels. A sensory input — something seen or heard, for example — would thus be able to trigger a whole series of patterned activities that are much the same as those produced by an earlier input of the same kind. One can say that this replaying in the brain results in remembrance in the mind.

The other type of study concerns itself with postulated chemical mechanisms of memory. Postulated specific chemical molecules that have a unique relationship, each with a specific "memory," cannot be effectively correlated with neuroanatomy and neurophysiology, and they provide no basis for recall, which is, of course, the essence of memory. However, chemical investigations are important in that memory must in the end be the result of a neuronal change that has a chemical and metabolic basis. It has been shown, for example, that long-term memories cannot be established if the enzymes responsible for protein synthesis in the brain are inactivated.

721

Moreover, the RNA responsible for the production of these enzymes is essentially concerned in the laying down of long-term memory traces.

SPEECH AND CONSCIOUSNESS Of the greatest importance both neurologically and philosophically have been the unique investigations of Roger Sperry and his associates at the California Institute of Technology. They have studied patients in whom epilepsy was so uncontrollable that in order to relieve the seizures it was necessary to cut the commissure (the *corpus callosum*) connecting the two cerebral hemispheres.

The two halves of the mammalian brain each have a full set of centers for the sensory and motor activities of the body. When an area in one hemisphere is damaged, the corresponding area in the other hemisphere often takes over its work and controls the function for both sides of the body.

Anatomically the two halves of the brain are united not only by the common stem that descends from the brain into the spinal cord but also by cross-bridges between the hemispheres. The cerebral hemispheres are linked by discrete bundles of nerve fibers called *commissures,* the most prominent of which is the great cerebral commissure, the corpus callosum. This structure contains most of the nerve fibers that connect the two halves of the cerebral cortex, the highest integrating portion of the brain.

Brain surgeons discovered that cutting the corpus callosum produced no noticeable change in the patient's capacities. Experiments in severing the corpus callosum in monkeys tended to confirm this observation. The purpose of the corpus callosum remained a mystery.

Starting in the early 1950s Sperry and his colleagues began to delve into the mystery of the corpus callosum. From their studies a new technique for analyzing the organization and operation of the brain emerged. This technique consists in the study of the brain divided surgically so that the performance of each half can be tested separately. These experiments began with cats and continued with monkeys and chimpanzees. There was also an opportunity to study human patients in whom the corpus callosum had been divided for treatment of severe epilepsy and who, freed of convulsive attacks, still were in possession of most of their faculties, in spite of having a "split brain." These split-brain studies have confirmed the fact that cutting the entire corpus callosum results in little disturbance of ordinary behavior.

The first convincing demonstration that the split brain is not, after all, entirely normal was provided by Ronald E. Myers, in research started in 1951 in Sperry's laboratory. Testing the performance of the two hemispheres separately, he found that what was learned by one side of the brain was not transferred to the other half. The two sides could learn opposite solutions to the same experimental problem, so that the animal's response in a test situation depended on which side of the brain was receiving the triggering stimulus. The split-brain animal behaved as if it had two entirely separate brains (Sperry, 1964).

722

The initial experiment involved animals that had had a special operation which left each eye feeding its visual messages solely to the hemisphere on the same side of the head. The animal was then trained to discriminate between a square and a circle presented to one eye only, the other eye being covered with a patch. After the animal had demonstrated that it could distinguish the square from the circle using one eye and one half of its brain, the problem was then presented to the other eye and hemisphere, the first eye now being blindfolded. When the subject used the second eye, it reacted as if it had never been faced with the problem before. The number of trials required to relearn the problem with the second eye showed that no benefit carried over from the earlier learning with the first eye. The transfer of learning and memory from one hemisphere to the other occurred readily in animals with the corpus callosum intact but failed completely in those with the corpus callosum cut. Subsequent studies dealing with other forms of learning supported the same conclusion (Sperry, 1964).

Thus, the corpus callosum has the important function of allowing the two hemispheres to share learning and memory. There were two possible mechanisms: transmission of the information at the time the learning takes place, or supplying it on demand later. In the first, the memory traces of what is learned are laid down both in the directly trained hemisphere and, by way of the corpus callosum, in the other hemisphere as well. In other words, intercommunication via the corpus callosum at the time of learning results in the formation of a double set of memory traces, one in each half of the brain. In the second process, a set of memory traces is established only in the directly trained half, but this information is available to the other hemisphere, when it is required, by way of the corpus callosum.

Sperry's studies showed that the cat tends to form memory traces in both hemispheres. In humans, where one hemisphere is nearly always dominant, only a single memory trace results, particularly in memory relating to language.

In one such man, Philip J. Vogel and Joseph E. Bogen, surgeons at the Institute of Nervous Diseases of Loma Linda University in Los Angeles, cut through the corpus callosum and other commissures, with successful relief of epileptic attacks. In the months after the operation, the patient appeared to be normal when engaged in casual conversation. Michael S. Gassaniga of Sperry's laboratory carefully studied the man's performances with one or both sides of the brain and body. The patient was right-handed, and his dominant cerebral hemisphere was the left one. He was able to perform most activities involving only the left half of the brain and the right side of the body. For example, he could easily read material in the right half of his visual field, name and locate objects in that half, execute commands with his right hand or foot, and so on.

He appeared to see clearly in the left half of his visual field and had normal sensitivity to touch and good motor function on his left side. However, in any task that required judgment or interpretation based on language, which was stored in his left cerebral hemisphere only, he clearly showed the effects of the cerebral disconnection. He could not read any material that fell in the left half of his visual field. He could not write anything meaningful with his left hand and could not carry out verbal commands with his left hand or left leg. When an object was presented solely in the left

723

half of his visual field, he might react to it appropriately, but he could not name or describe it. When his dominant left hemisphere was questioned about nonverbal activities that had just been carried out successfully by the left hand via the right hemisphere, it could not recall them. The dominant hemisphere of the brain did not know or remember anything about the experiences of the other hemisphere.

Once it was established that the commissure does serve important communication functions, Sperry's interest shifted to more general questions. Such a brain offered an opportunity to examine the many functions and interrelations of parts of the brain, structure by structure and control center by control center. Each half was intact with its internal organization; the inflow of sensory messages and the outflow of motor commands were normal. Each retained its cerebral control centers and the potentiality for performing essentially all the functions of a whole brain.

Even the human brain, in spite of the normal dominance of one side, could adapt itself to carry on reasonably well when one hemisphere was eliminated early in life because of a tumor or an injury. A monkey with one cerebral hemisphere removed got along better than a human in a comparable condition, and a cat did much better than a monkey. These results seem to reflect the evolution of the brain. As the accumulation of memories, or the storage of information, becomes more important in the higher animals, the duplication of memory files in the two brain hemispheres is given up for a more efficient system; the division of labor by the assignment of specialized files and functions to each hemisphere. This evolution has culminated in the human brain. Here a distinct separation of functions prevails: language is the task of the dominant hemisphere, and lesser tasks are largely taken over by the other hemisphere. The question of dominance is crucial for the effective functioning of the brain as the master control system. What happens, then, if the two halves of an animal's split brain are taught to give completely conflicting responses to a given situation? The split-brain monkey learns, remembers, and performs as if it were two different individuals, its identity depending on which hemisphere it happens to be using at the moment (Sperry, 1964).

When the split brain is confronted with a situation in which it must make a choice between two "correct" answers, one hemisphere or the other takes command and governs the monkey's behavior. This dominance may shift from time to time, each hemisphere taking its turn at control, but it would appear that no serious conflict disrupts any given movement.

Evidence of conflict between the separated hemispheres may be seen in tests given to human patients. Incorrect responses by the left hand may so exasperate the more sophisticated dominant hemisphere that the subject reaches across with the right hand to grab the left and force it to make the correct choice. As in the split-brain cats and monkeys, however, one hemisphere or the other generally prevails at any given time. Any incompatible messages coming down from the other hemisphere are inhibited or disregarded.

Work with these split-brain subjects has enabled investigators to pinpoint various centers of specific brain activity, has suggested new concepts and new lines of thought, and thus has opened up a fruitful approach to unraveling the mysteries of the mind (Sperry, 1964).

"PATHWAYS TO PERCEPTION" One of the most important foci of neurophysiological work was that carried out over several decades in the laboratories of Walter B. Cannon, Professor of Physiology at Harvard. In addition to Cannon himself, there were other outstanding men: Alexander Forbes (the founder of American electrophysiology), Alfred Redfield, Cecil Drinker, Hallowell Davis, and William B. Castle. The central theme of Cannon's own investigations was the autonomic nervous system. Almost every aspect of the subject was studied: its anatomical origin, distribution, and peripheral effector actions; its neurohumoral mediators; the holistic action of the sympathetic nerves under conditions of stress; its central nervous system regulation; the control systems regulating bodily states — the concept of homeostasis; the interrelation of endocrine and autonomic systems in those regulations; and the central nervous mechanisms in emotional expression. One of Cannon's most famous pupils, Philip Bard, became interested in the last of these subjects. In a long series of experiments he showed that the integration of sympathetic and somatic efferent discharge that characterizes the expression of rage in carnivores depends upon the integrity of the posterior hypothalamus. The excessive and readily evoked "quasi-emotional" behavior displayed by decorticated animals was conceived to be an example of the release of function, in the tradition of Jackson and Head. These studies provided for the first time an experimental definition of a neural center, a concept that has guided the later work of many investigators.

The integrating and regulating function of the hypothalamus was pursued by Bard in a long series of investigations, with many collaborators, which included: studies of hypothalamic function in regulating sexual behavior and the reproductive cycle; in governing the pituitary gland and its target organs; and in regulation of body temperature, including the production of fever. Bard in 1933 became Professor of Physiology at the Johns Hopkins School of Medicine and initiated there a continually productive program of research in the physiology of the nervous system. A central feature of this program was the general problem of the localization of function in the cerebral cortex. His particular interest was in the motor and the sensory cortices, and he used as a measure of function the integrity of the placing and hopping reactions. With Clinton Woolsey and Chandler Brooks he carried out an extensive comparative study of the cortical control of these postural reactions, showing their increasing corticalization in phylogeny, their loss following discrete local lesions of the somatotopically related portions of the sensory and motor cortices. Bard, with Wade Marshall, then introduced the evoked potential method to the Hopkins laboratory, using it to map the sensory somatic area of the monkey.

The present operational point of view taken by sensory neurophysiologists has been presented by one of Bard's pupils, Vernon Mountcastle (1975b):

> ... we can define in precise terms the central neural events evoked by sensory stimuli, and discover the neural transforms of the qualitative, static and dynamic parameters of those stimuli. The goal is based upon the idea of Psychoneural Identity; that is, that the total ensemble of neural events set in motion by a sensory input and leading after successive central transformations to storage, to discrimination, to an output of any kind, is in and of itself the essence of sensation and perception. For

725

the physiologist functioning as an experimentalist, there are no ghosts in the neural machinery. In this endeavor we build upon descriptions of the topology of the brain in general, and of sensory and motor systems in particular. The external world is represented in detail in the neural space of the brain, a representation distorted by differential peripheral innervation, but topologically intact. This we owe to the study of human beings by neurosurgeons using methods of electrical stimulation and recording, and to the careful and persistent application of the evoked potential method in animals. These central representations depend upon a precise linkage between the peripheral sensory sheet and the cerebral cortex. That linkage is present at birth in full detail, but depends for its persistence upon continued, patterned stimulation of the peripheral sensory sheet, especially during the early weeks and months of life. In the nervous system the position of active elements in a neural field signals the spatial position of peripheral stimuli; the spatial distribution of activity is a description of the spatial contour of stimuli. Within the active population of central neurons excited by a peripheral stimulus, labeled lines and cellular identity signal stimulus quality, though how the position of a neuron within a neural field is used as a code for the transmission of information is still unknown.

Beyond topography and quality, the mainstream of current work is aimed at understanding the dynamic and quantitative aspects of evoked neural activity, ranging from first-order fibers to the cerebral cortex, and the method of single neuron analysis is the favorite weapon. We seek to determine which of the dynamic aspects of peripheral stimuli are transduced or abstracted; which codes are used for frequency and temporal pattern; which for periodic movement and spatial translation; and which for even more specific and behaviorally meaningful events. An important question is how the code in peripheral nerve fibers is transformed at central neural stations and how those transformations may reveal or be the result of central integrative action.

An important conceptual advance of recent years is the understanding that the study of sensory performance by quantitative methods, called Psychophysics, and the study of the neural events that follow sensory stimuli by the method of electrical recording, called Sensory Neurophysiology, represent only different approaches to what are generically the same set of problems. The methods and the concepts of the two can be combined to yield greater insight into those problems than is possible with either alone.

Mountcastle (1975b) has made many important contributions using this type of combined experiment. Scientists employing these approaches are endeavoring to learn how humans live in and cope with their environment:

Each of us lives within the universe — the prison — of his own brain. Projecting from it are millions of fragile sensory nerve fibers, in groups uniquely adapted to sample the energetic states of the world around us; heat, light, force and chemical composition. That is all we ever know of it directly: all else is logical inference. *Sensory stimuli reaching us are transduced at peripheral nerve endings, and neural replicas of them dispatched brainward, to the gray mantle of the cerebral cortex. We use them to form dynamic and continually updated neural maps of our place and orientation in the external world, and of events within it. At the level of sensation, your images and my images are virtually the same, and readily identified one to another by verbal descriptions, or common reactions. Beyond that, each image is conjoined with genetic and stored experiential information that makes each of us uniquely private. From that complex integral each constructs at a higher level of perceptual experience, on my view in brain regions like those of the parietal lobe, his own, very personal,* view from within.

30

Psychiatry

A bodily disease, which we look upon as whole and entire within itself, may after all, be but a symptom of some ailment in the spiritual part.

(Nathaniel Hawthorne)

THE FIRST CENTURY   The early history of the United States reflected its cultural heritage from the European peoples. The Salem witchcraft trials may have been a shameful example of intolerance and delusional nonsense, but the people of Massachusetts were never as completely victimized by this hysteria as were the French and Germans. Likewise the establishment of "asylums" for mental patients in the United States was no more than a reflection of similar developments abroad. The early settlers had not knowingly brought with them many who were thought to be mentally abnormal, but as time passed, the colonial villages were populated with the same type of mentally ill as were seen in European communities. To the degree that mental disease is either hereditary or the result of cultural factors, this was to be expected. In the petition drawn up by Benjamin Franklin for the founding of the Pennsylvania Hospital in 1751 he noted that "the number of persons distempered in mind . . . has greatly increased in this province." He attributed the increase to the growth in total population.

The witchcraft hysteria became widespread during the post-reformation era, when the American colonies were being settled. In Europe the hysteria caused thousands of the mentally ill to be tortured and executed. In North America, the one significant outbreak of this delusion (at Salem, Massachusetts, in 1691–1692) occurred in New England, the only section of the British colonies in which a single church (Congregational or "Puritan") dominated community life. The clergy of this church were active leaders in the persecutions of witches, just as certain Roman Catholic clergy had led the persecutions on the European continent.

In 1691–92, 250 persons were tried for witchcraft in Salem, a town with

727

no more than 4000 inhabitants. Fifty of the "witches" were condemned, 19 were executed, 2 expired in prison, and 1 died of torture. The hysteria subsided promptly when several prominent citizens were accused of witchcraft, and it was never revived in Salem or elsewhere in America, although the execution of witches continued in Europe through the first quarter of the eighteenth century (Shryock, 1944).

The treatment of the mentally ill in the colonies reflected that in the mother country. American villages were usually too small to provide almshouses or even jails, but local authorities were held responsible for relief for the poor, including the "insane." The violent were confined at home both for their own protection and because mental illness was considered to be a family disgrace.

When the population of a colonial town rose to several thousand, an almshouse was built. The insane were then placed in these institutions, which served as both workhouses and penal institutions. In addition, the almshouse usually had a small infirmary or primitive hospital. Such an almshouse was established in Philadelphia in 1732 and in New York City in 1736. When the Pennsylvania Hospital was established in 1752, it was the first institution in the British colonies to care exclusively for the sick; and the sick included mental patients (see Chapter 5).

Benjamin Rush was a pioneer among American physicians in giving attention to mental disease. As usual, he prescribed bleeding and purging; and he observed that if the bleeding were continued long enough, "excessive action" in the patient declined. Rush also recommended rapidly alternating hot and cold baths, an early form of "shock therapy." In the psychological realm, he advocated a sort of moral suasion—patients should have pleasant companions—and even occupational therapy. Most important was his practice of having the patient report his own recollections and experiences; in this he anticipated what was to come a century later in the era of psychoanalysis.

The period of Enlightenment began in the late eighteenth century with the work of Philippe Pinel in France and William Tuke in England (see Chapter 5). It was Pinel who first "struck off the chains" in the mental institutions of Paris. American psychiatrists insisted on a degree of physical restraint long after it had been renounced by British leaders. Rush devised the "tranquilizer chair" which, to the modern psychiatrist, has a rather brutal aspect. To quiet the morbid excitement in the brain, Rush also advocated the use of a "whirling gyrator," or forcing patients to stand erect for 24 hours at a time. However, he denounced the cold cells, the whips, and the chains of the old regime. This was important, since Rush's *Medical Inquiries and Observations upon the Diseases of the Mind* was the only American guide when the first institutions devoted exclusively to the care of the mentally ill were established in this country.

Some 15 years after the founding of the Pennsylvania Hospital, the Virginia Assembly was requested to provide a state institution for "idiots, lunatics and other persons of unsound mind." When a hospital was established at Williamsburg, Virginia, in 1768, reliance on chains prevailed. The principle of state aid was involved in the establishment of this hospital, and the major "insane asylums" built in this country after 1845 were to be state institutions. By 1840 most general hospitals in the United States were

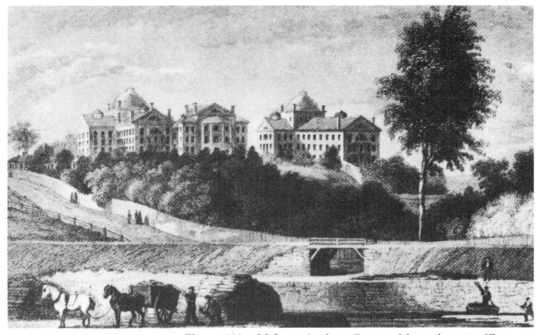

Figure 166. McLean Asylum, Boston, Massachusetts. [From Zilboorg, G. (ed.): One Hundred Years of American Psychiatry. New York, Columbia University Press, 1944.]

private institutions, but insane asylums and municipal hospitals grew out of the almshouse tradition and were supported and controlled by government. However, in the first quarter of the twentieth century, a few mental hospitals were founded by private philanthropy: the New York Lunatic Asylum (1808), the *McLean Asylum of Boston* (1818), the Friends Asylum at Frankford near Philadelphia (1817), and the Hartford Retreat (1824).

The establishment of numerous state asylums after 1825 was due to the rising tide of humanitarianism and a growing belief among physicians as to the curability of mental illness. In 1830, there were only some 24 hospitals for the mentally ill, with a total bed capacity of about 2500, for a national population of over 12 million. The Prison Discipline Society of Massachusetts estimated in 1833 that there were about 12,000 "lunatics" in the United States, a ratio of 1 to 1000. The census of 1840 included estimates of the number of insane and idiotic persons, which was reported to be 17,500 for that year, giving a ratio to the total population of 1 to 977.

The best run mental hospitals were those that had physicians as superintendents. A number of able physicians served in this capacity; for example, physicians of the Galt family, who long presided over the first Virginia hospital, had enviable records as superintendents. In these hospitals, little was done to foster research. Education in psychiatry also suffered. It would have been desirable to have psychiatric chairs in the medical schools, but the medical teachers of that period were not interested in psychiatry (Shryock, 1944).

The legal implications of mental illness gained little attention until the mid-nineteenth century. Psychiatrists themselves were the first to become concerned about this problem, and in 1838 Isaac Ray published his "Trea-

729

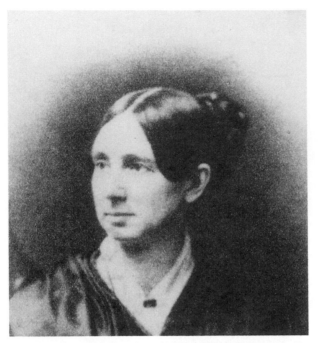

Figure 167. Dorothea Lynde Dix. [From Zilboorg, G. (ed.): One Hundred Years of American Psychiatry. New York, Columbia University Press, 1944.]

tise on the Medical Jurisprudence of Insanity." This was the beginning of an effort to persuade jurists to reconcile their procedures with medical findings. Before progress began in this direction, many of the mentally ill were imprisoned for crime.

In 1841 *Dorothea Lynde Dix,* an ex-schoolteacher reared in the social idealism of the Unitarians, first observed the sufferings of lunatics in the jail of East Cambridge, Massachusetts. She became a vigorous advocate of humane care of the mentally ill. Legislatures responded with enthusiasm, and asylums began to be built throughout the Union. Dorothea Dix was probably this country's greatest social reformer. Not only did she succeed in getting the insane out of the jails but also she fought successfully to keep orphans out of the almshouses. During the Civil War she made still another contribution to medicine when she served as Superintendent of Women Nurses, with headquarters in Washington, D.C. She was not a professional nurse, but neither was any other American woman at that time.

THE AMERICAN PSYCHIATRIC ASSOCIATION   On October 16, 1844, there was founded in Philadelphia the *Association of Medical Superintendents of American Institutions for the Insane,* later to be called the *American Medico-Psychological Association* and later still the *American Psychiatric Association* (Overholser, 1944).

Overholser (1944) has given the background against which this important event took place. In 1844 it was estimated that the number of mentally ill in the United States was 17,457, but only 2561 of these were in institutions. Most of the population of the 26 states was concentrated in the northeastern corner of the nation. There were approximately 20 mental hospitals in the entire country, only three of these being west of the Alleghenies. These institutions, since it was the custom for the superintendent to care for each patient personally, were quite small; the largest, at Worcester, Massachusetts, had a total of 255 patients. Dorothea Dix was just starting on her campaign to upgrade mental hospitals which was to last for the next 40 years and which would result in the establishment or expansion of 30 institutions. Bleeding, blistering, and purging were not yet obsolete forms of treatment. Phrenology was generally accepted as scientific dogma, and mental disease was regarded as a disorder of the brain, which was considered to be "the organ of the mind."

All of the men assembled at Philadelphia on that day in 1844 had had experience in the general practice of medicine. Four were surgeons of repute who looked upon mental disorders as something closely related to general medicine—a viewpoint which was soon abandoned and was considered obsolete for many years. The emphasis of the first Association was on the administration and organization of hospitals and the day-to-day care of the patients. The promotion of scientific psychiatry was not one of its objectives. It should be recalled that the denigration of science in that period of American medicine was not peculiar to psychiatry.

Included among the 13 superintendents who founded the Association in 1844 were two who deserve an important place in the history of psychiatry. One was Thomas S. Kirkbride, who had an enormous influence on the architecture of mental hospitals. He was the superintendent of the Psychiatric Division of the Pennsylvania Hospital and planned the new structure when that division moved its patients to West Philadelphia in 1841. He also played a large role in designing the famous Trenton State Hospital. There his trail crossed that of Dorothea Dix, who had a significant part in the establishment in 1845 of the first state hospital at Trenton. She was very proud of this institution, and when she became an old lady, worn out from her long years of devotion to the cause of better treatment of the mentally ill, she was given a room in the Administration Building in which to spend her remaining years (Hamilton, 1944).

Kirkbride's chief interest was the rational planning of hospital buildings. He developed a practical set of floor plans for mental hospitals, which was first adopted at Trenton in 1845. This type of building consisted essentially of a series of blocks with a characteristic arrangement. The center block held offices, quarters for staff and employees, and an amusement hall. Other blocks housed patients. These blocks were attached to each other either directly or by an offset passage, but each was set back far enough from its more central neighbor to let light and air travel from end to end of the central corridor of every section. When an institution outgrew its original plan, the number of blocks could be increased, thus lengthening the frontage. A picture of one such hospital showed no less than ten blocks arranged in this traditional way. When the Buffalo (New York) Institution was opened in 1880, the distance a physician had to walk in making rounds, to get from one end of the structure to the other, was a half-mile. Since there were few physicians in these institutions, such distances made medical supervision difficult.

731

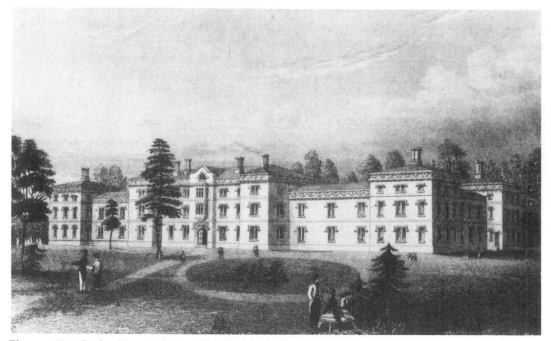

Figure 168. Butler Hospital, Providence, Rhode Island. [From
Zilboorg, G. (ed.): One Hundred Years of American Psychiatry.
New York, Columbia University Press, 1944.]

The other important member of the founding group, *Pliny Earle,* was
appointed Professor of Psychological Medicine at the Berkshire Medical Institution in Cooksfield, Massachusetts, in 1853. This was probably the first
time in the United States that a chair of this sort had been established and
that the study of mental disorders was recognized as an appropriate part of
medical education. In 1877 Earle published a volume entitled *The Curability
of Insanity.* He had a mathematical mind and indicated clearly the errors in
the claims of cures made by some of his colleagues. Earle lived in the early
days of what Deutsch has called the "cult of curability." In his book, Earle
traced the history of the "curability delusion," showing that the hopes of
his colleagues had influenced their interpretation of statistics. Earle's articles often bore titles which sound quite modern. In 1867, for example, he
published his inaugural lecture at the Berkshire Medical Institution, which
was entitled "Psychological Medicine—Its Importance as a Part of the Medical Curriculum." He advocated small hospitals aimed at cure, separate
asylums for the incurable, and family care. He felt that the state should care
for the mentally ill. In addition to being one of the organizers of the Association of Hospital Superintendents, he was also an organizer of the American Medical Association and the New York Academy of Medicine.

**THE SECOND
CENTURY**

When St. Elizabeth's Hospital was opened in
Washington in 1855, it made provisions for the
mentally ill from the District of Columbia and
also for those in the permanent services of the government. The next federal

732

venture into the field of institutional psychiatry was the Asylum for Insane Indians at Canton, South Dakota, which functioned from 1903 to 1934. The federal government assumed responsibility for the mentally ill along with other casualties of the First World War. In a related field, the U.S. Public Health Service (USPHS) was called on to give institutional treatment to drug addicts in hospitals organized for this specific purpose at Lexington, Kentucky, in 1935, and at Fort Worth, Texas, in 1938.

The Association of Medical Superintendents played an important role in establishing good care in mental hospitals. They maintained a united front and adopted principles of organization, management, and construction that were carefully formulated. Their unified platform gave them a strong position before governors, legislators, and other public authorities. They formulated a plan that would limit each hospital to 250 beds, the intent being to limit the patients to the number for whom the superintendent could provide close personal supervision. The limit originally proposed was raised to 600 in the year 1866. The Association had a continuing interest in many causes, including schools of nursing, occupational therapy, after-care, and the treatment of general paresis. The whole mental hygiene movement in the United States was a development of the work carried on over many years by the founders of this Association.

The National Committee for Mental Hygiene was founded in 1909 under the leadership of Clifford W. Beers, a young businessman who had recovered from a severe mental upset. He stands second only to Dorothea Dix in influencing improvements in the care of psychiatric patients. When the National Committee was still young, it was awarded money by the

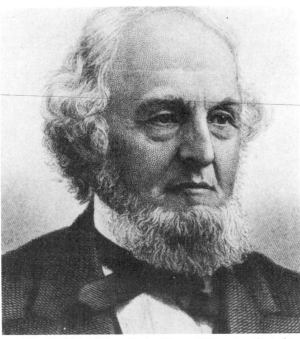

Figure 169. Pliny Earle. [From Zilboorg, G. (ed.): One Hundred Years of American Psychiatry. New York, Columbia University Press, 1944.]

Rockefeller Foundation to finance surveys of mental hospitals. The leaders of the Committee were prominent members of the Association of Medical Superintendents, and its first Medical Director, W. Salmon, had a sound understanding of hospital administration.

At the end of World War I, the federal government became responsible for the care of many mental patients who had been in the military services. Contracts were placed for much of this care. To speed this work, a Committee of members of the Association was called together by the National Committee for Mental Hygiene. They helped to set standards for the treatment of the mentally ill veterans.

During the nineteenth century, the mental hospital was the place where a family, concerned about the mental state of one of its members, sought advice. The needs of those who required office treatment only but could not afford a private physician led to the establishment of outpatient services for psychiatric care. In 1885 John B. Chapin inaugurated an outpatient service that was open twice a week in the downtown Pennsylvania Hospital. In 1891 Walter E. Fernald assigned one day each week for consultations at the Massachusetts State School, and by 1913 there were clinics for mental defectives in several states. In New York City, Cornell Medical College developed a mental clinic in 1904, which was carried on under the guidance of Adolf Meyer.

PSYCHIATRIC
RESEARCH
IN AMERICA

On May 16, 1894, S. Weir Mitchell gave an address before the American Medico-Psychological Association that was a strong denunciation of the organized psychiatry of that day in the United States. He said: "Once we spoke of asylums with respect; it is not so now. We, neurologists, think you have fallen behind us, and this opinion is gaining ground outside of our own ranks, and is, in part at least, your own fault. . . . Where [are] your careful scientific reports? . . . You live alone uncriticized, unquestioned out of the healthy conflicts and honest rivalries which keep us (neurologists) up to the mark of the fullest possible competence." Mitchell then went on to sketch his ideal hospital, designed and organized primarily to stimulate and encourage scientific investigation and progress. This scolding served as a stimulus. The next year Edward Cowles replied to Mitchell's criticism by describing the "new" McLean Hospital in Boston, where provision was made for intensive laboratory research in pathology, physiology, and biochemistry as related to psychiatry.

The scientific framework of medical investigation was then undergoing change, and Cowles was in the front rank of medical thought when he decided to support biochemical research. Around 1900, he obtained the services of a young biochemist, Otto Folin, and his assistant, Philip A. Shaffer, who developed new methods for the study of metabolism in the mentally ill. Folin's publications served to discredit rash speculations about the metabolic etiology of the psychoses. (Folin's brilliant career in metabolic research began at the McLean Hospital.)

Another important event for psychiatric research came in 1895 with the founding of the Association of Assistant Hospital Physicians, organized for

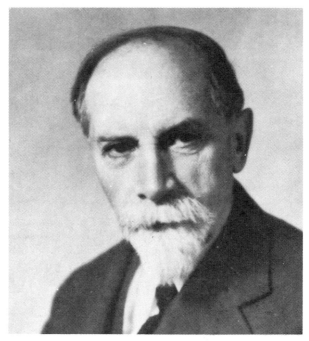

Figure 170. Adolf Meyer. (From The Archives Office, the Johns Hopkins Medical Institutions.)

the discussion of scientific rather than administrative problems. The secretary was *Adolf Meyer* of the Kankakee State Hospital in Illinois. Meyer had begun his career as a pathologist, but he had developed an intense interest in studying the personalities of patients with dementia and was a strong supporter of psychiatric research.

From 1894 to about 1919, research became a definite aim of the leaders in psychiatry. Institutions were built, laboratories were equipped, and men who had been trained in scientific methods were recruited to investigate the causes of insanity. This quarter of a century was important because it set certain patterns for the institutional organization of psychiatric research. Weak points in this style of research organization lay in its relative isolation; its lack of correlation with the basic sciences; and its loss of contact with significant clinical investigations in other branches of medicine (Whitehorn, 1944).

The financial resources of state governments were tapped to provide research funds for the *New York Psychiatric Institute* (established as the Pathological Institute in 1895) and for the Psychopathic Hospital at Ann Arbor (1906) and at Boston (1912). Private philanthropies helped to establish and endow the Henry Phipps Psychiatric Clinic (1913) of the Johns Hopkins Hospital. At a later period Yale University and its Institute for Human Relations sought to coordinate a very broad research program that included psychiatry. The influence of Adolf Meyer and the clinical interest of August Hoch were responsible for the growth of the New York Psychiatric Institute and Hospital, which later found a home in the Columbia-Presbyterian Medical Center. These were teaching hospitals as well as research centers. The University of Michigan, with its Psychopathic Hospital in Ann Arbor, Har-

735

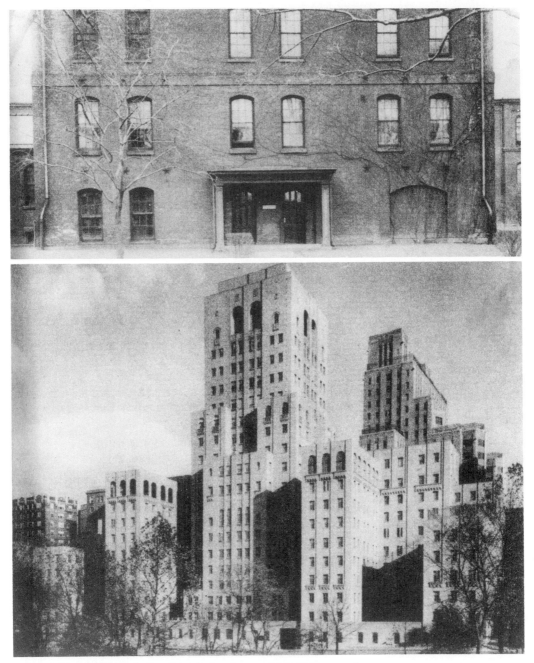

Figure 171. New York Psychiatric Institute, old building and present building. [From Zilboorg, G. (ed.): One Hundred Years of American Psychiatry. New York, Columbia University Press, 1944.]

vard with its Psychopathic Hospital in Boston, and the Johns Hopkins University with its Phipps Institute launched more graduates into careers in psychiatry than any other medical schools. At the Phipps Clinic and the Boston Psychopathic Hospital, Adolf Meyer and Elmer Southard, respectively, stimulated and inspired numerous young psychiatrists who came to them for advanced study.

At the Phipps Clinic, Meyer, who was its first Director, attempted to gain scientific recognition of the functioning human being as the central feature in psychiatry and in general medicine as well. He wanted to insure a practical acknowledgement and a realistic handling of the psychological modes of human functioning. To this end he developed and taught a type of orientation to psychiatry which came to be known as "psychobiology." The voluminous case records gathered by him and his staff became the main research material of the Phipps Clinic. There was a behavior chart for the day-by-day notation of each patient's conduct. Meyer, moreover, objected to the deceptive implications of a mere categorical diagnosis in psychiatry, and sought instead to develop formulations of "reaction patterns" which would give appropriate consideration to the plasticity, spontaneity, and individuality of the patient. He had a special terminology of the "ergasias," by which the reaction-pattern concepts were given verbal expression. During the first half of the twentieth century, Meyer exerted a profound influence on psychiatric research in America. This was strengthened by his great capacity for recognizing and encouraging younger workers who exhibited an interest in psychiatry (Whitehorn, 1944).

The Boston Psychopathic Hospital had two successive directors who were brilliant psychiatrists, E. E. Southard and C. Macfie Campbell. The long-term study of neurosyphilis, started under Southard and continued under Harry Solomon, was a notable research contribution. Bowman, while at the Boston Psychopathic Hospital, made significant studies of prepsychotic personalities in both schizophrenic and affective disorders.

Research became an accepted responsibility in most state and private psychiatric hospitals in the first quarter of the twentieth century. The Binet-Simon test to determine mental age stimulated the development of scientific methodology. Public attention was called to the relation between social problems and mental deficiencies by Henry H. Goddard's study of the Kallikak family. William Healy brought a psychiatric perspective to bear on the problems of the juvenile delinquent. Southard and Mary C. Jarrett established a significant working liaison between psychiatry and the professionally trained social worker. World War I introduced a new term, *shellshock*; curiosity about the emotional dynamics of war neuroses led to increased interest in psychiatric problems. "Dynamic consideration" (a term meaning the psychology of motivation) received a great stimulus in America as a result of Sigmund Freud's visit to Clark University (1909) and the subsequent organization of a psychoanalytic society. Psychoanalytic doctrines found able exponents in A. A. Brill, S. E. Jelliffe, and W. A. White. This approach did not markedly influence the course of research until after World War I. At that time an increasing number of American psychiatrists with psychoanalytic training and a number of Europeans who had immigrated to this country carried out an increasing amount of research utilizing psychoanalytic methods.

From about 1894 to 1945 the field of psychiatry was predominantly organicist and impersonal in its scientific philosophy. By 1945, there was a growing measure of practical interest in the personal; "disorders of personality" became recognized as a practical synonym for psychiatry. Adolf Meyer was among the leaders in this new direction of psychiatric study. Of the various papers in which he dealt with this matter, probably the most constructive was one with a characteristically involved title, "Objective psychiatry or psychobiology with subordination of the medically useless contrast of mental and physical," in which he said: "As soon as mental attitude and mental activity are accepted as definite functions of a living organism, mentation and behavior is treated as a real chapter of the natural history of man and animal and psychology ceases to be a puzzle supposedly resisting the objective methods of science."

In the organicist tradition, the outstanding psychiatric achievement in the early twentieth century was the demonstration of the etiological role of syphilis in general paresis. This was accomplished by Noguchi and Moore at the Rockefeller Institute in 1913, when they demonstrated the spirochete in the brain of patients suffering from this type of organic brain disease.

During the first quarter of the twentieth century, the major centers for psychiatric research were located principally on the Atlantic seaboard: at St. Elizabeth's Hospital in Washington, D.C., under W. A. White, who continued his active interest in the dynamic forces of the personality; at the Henry Phipps Psychiatric Clinic, under Meyer's guidance, where many excellent people were trained, including Oskar Diethelm, Frederick Wertham, Solomon Katzenelbogen, Wendell Muncie, Curt Richter, and Horsley Gantt; at the Pennsylvania Hospital, where Douglas Bond and Edward Strecker maintained active research teamwork with younger staff members; at the Boston Psychopathic Hospital; at Bloomingdale Hospital, where Henry and Zilboorg contributed to physiological and psychoanalytic investigations; at McLean Hospital, where Whitehorn began his combination of biochemical, physiological, and clinical investigations of emotional reactions and attitudes; at the Psychiatric Institute in New York, where Flanders Dunbar and Daniels made pioneer studies in psychosomatic medicine; at the Worcester State Hospital in Massachusetts, where Roy Hoskins assembled a group especially qualified for endocrine and statistical studies under the Memorial Foundation for Neuroendocrine Research. One of their particular interests was schizophrenia. In the psychoanalytic field, the Institute of Psychoanalysis in Chicago, under Alexander, French, Saul and Benedek, provided teaching in this area, with a research interest in psychosomatic medicine.

Activities at Harvard in the 1940 to 1945 period illustrate the great diversity of scientific interest in psychiatric research. Murray's group concerned itself with the experimental validation of the Freudian concepts. Lashley was studying the cerebral cortex and behavioral capacity of rats. Allport developed a personalistic social psychology. Sheldon systematized new formulations regarding the physical and mental constitution. Zipfa, a philologist, studied schizophrenic language with John Whitehorn, who was originally a biochemist. Epilepsies were the special field of study for Stanley Cobb, Lennox, the Gibbses, and Houston Merritt and Tracy Putnam, resulting in a new formulation of this problem as a paroxysmal cerebral dysrhythmia and the development of a new and effective remedy, diphenylhydantoin. Cobb and Finesinger investigated physiological psychology. John Romano, at the Peter Bent Brigham Hospital, studied patients on the medical and surgical wards from the psychiatric point of view, while Myerson explored the potentialities of adrenergic and cholinergic drugs and electroshock. The Davises studied the electroencephalogram in psychoses. Stolz, in the biochemical laboratory at McLean, studied the enzyme systems and vitamins important in cerebral metabolism. Campbell and Solomon, carrying the mass of the clinical teaching, continued their studies on schizophrenia and general paresis.

All in all, the Harvard studies form an impressive array of work in the field of psychiatry. A comparable complexity of psychiatric research was also in progress at Johns Hopkins and at Columbia. Shortly after World War II, Leo Kanner contributed a much-needed textbook that provided better organization for the neglected field of child psychiatry.

The psychoneuroses gradually became an accepted responsibility of psychiatry, as part of the general reorientation toward personality and its disorders. To some degree this was stimulated by the interest that internists developed in the problem of the psychoneuroses as a result of their World War II experience; they saw the need for more emphasis on these aspects in the teaching and practice of internal medicine.

PSYCHOSOMATIC MEDICINE

Psychosomatic medicine has been an area of controversy. There have been expansive claims and great therapeutic expectations for it. In its broadest sense it refers to the study and treatment of those conditions which are related to the interaction of psychic and somatic phenomena. It includes psychological reactions to physical illness; psychological disturbance resulting from disorders affecting brain function; medical complications of maladaptive behavior; emotional disorders manifested by somatic symptoms with no organic basis; physiological concomitants of emotional states; and psychosomatic diseases (organic disorders in which there is structural change or tissue damage and in which it is postulated that psychological factors contribute importantly to etiology) (Imboden, 1976).

After World War II, psychosomatic medicine became a very active research field. Flanders Dunbar's monumental compilation of emotions and bodily changes was a significant landmark in this field of study, and the journal *Psychosomatic Medicine* provided an avenue for publications on this subject. Among the early investigators were Franz Alexander (peptic ulcer and asthma), Stanley Cobb (mucous colitis and arthritis), Harold Wolff (gastric disorders), and Felix Deutsch.

SHOCK THERAPY, FRONTAL LOBOTOMY, AND THE RORSCHACH TEST

During the 1930s, psychiatry in America received a great stimulus from the discovery by Manfred Sakel in Vienna of the improvement seen in schizophrenic patients subjected to insulin hypoglycemia. From 1935 on, many American workers contributed to the extensive literature on insulin-shock treatment. A short while later, Metrazol shock was devised by L. von Meduna of

739

Budapest; and then electroshock by Cerletti of Rome. These several types of shock therapy were used extensively in this country, chiefly because of their apparent effectiveness in shortening the course of affective disorders, as first reported by Bennett.

Another radical innovation in this same period was the surgical attack upon the frontal lobes, introduced in the United States by Freeman and Watts. Frontal lobotomy was found useful for relieving the anxiety of chronically agitated patients, with less diminution of intellectual capacity than earlier theories of brain localization would have led one to expect.

During the 1930s also the Rorschach experiment prompted much psychological study in psychiatry. This movement in the United States was accelerated by the European physician immigrants who were adept and experienced in the interpretation of Rorschach findings. In the Rorschach test, the subject reports what he sees when he examines a series of ink blots. What he sees, when interpreted by an experienced person, reveals in an extraordinary way the style of the subject's approach to life situations. The employment of unorganized stimuli, to which there is no "correct" response, permits and even solicits the spontaneous organizational reactivity of the subject, giving more abundant opportunity than do question-and-answer tests for the exhibition of personal characteristics. Such methods for studying personality have been called "projective"; they have close similarities to the type of clinical attitude-study described by Whitehorn for investigating personality functions.

ANIMAL EXPERIMENTATION

In psychiatric research the methods of animal experimentation have been employed far less frequently than in other fields of medicine. However, in one area, productive animal research has been in progress for over 75 years. In 1904 the Russian physiologist Ivan P. Pavlov received a Nobel prize for his work on the physiology of digestion. In the course of a long series of experiments, both before and after 1904, Pavlov demonstrated that experimental animals (chiefly dogs) could be conditioned to respond to "psychic stimuli" and that the experimental events could be so arranged that a "neurosis" would be induced in the dogs. Pavlov's research stimulated many studies of experimental neurosis. The outstanding American experimentalists in the early period were Liddell, Gantt, Dworkin, Maier, and Masserman. More recently, new techniques have been devised by B. F. Skinner at Harvard, and it has become possible to study animals over a long period and in a variety of behavioral situations. Extensive experimental facilities are available for utilizing these animal techniques for the production of conditions simulating human abnormalities, and potential drug therapy for these conditions is under study.

PSYCHIATRY AFTER WORLD WAR II

A great change in American psychiatry took place after World War II with the passage of the National Mental Health Act of 1946, which provided generous financial support for education and research in this special field (Brandt, 1965).

In a retrospective review of the National Mental Health Act of 1946, Jeanne L. Brandt (1965) points out that the passage of the Act represents a significant facet of some major social developments that have taken place in the United States in the past 25 years—developments which have extended society's and the government's responsibility for the health and welfare of the nation's citizens.

During the war it became obvious that there were many mentally ill persons in the United States. Vannevar Bush's report at the end of the war stated that "despite great strides in the war against disease, approximately 7 million persons in the United States were mentally ill and that their care cost the public over $175,000,000 a year" (Brandt, 1965).

The role of the federal government in mental illness developed late in the U.S. Public Health Service (USPHS) program. The medical inspection of aliens which the USPHS carried out for the Immigration and Naturalization Service was one of its first activities in the mental health field. From 1900 to 1920 the high incidence of first admissions of foreign-born persons into New York state mental hospitals helped to develop public awareness of mental illness as a national health problem. By 1914 the PHS had assigned Dr. Walter Treadway to carry out a series of sampling studies on the physical and mental health of schoolchildren, including an evaluation of state and local policies relating to dependency, delinquency, crime, and other problems associated with mental illness and mental deficiency.

In 1840 the incidence of mental illness in America was estimated at one per 1000 population. Bush's estimate of 7 million in 1940 would be 50 per 1000, an increase of some 50 times, which seems scarcely credible even if one takes into account the fact that clinicians were better trained in the recognition of mental disease. It would seem that a marked broadening of the definition of mental illness contributed substantially to the increase: (1) all neuroses, character disorders, mental deficiency, and even illiteracy were included as mental illnesses; (2) psychoanalysis and Meyerian psychobiology had tended to blur the distinction between mental health and illness; and (3) the American type of humanitarianism supported the view that deviant behavior of all kinds, including criminal behavior, is the product of mental illness. This broadening of the definition made it so inclusive that some people began to question the validity of the concept of mental illness. This view was expressed in the movement initiated by the publication of the book, *The Myth of Mental Illness,* by Dr. Thomas Szasz.

Required to provide psychiatric care in federal penal and correctional institutions (Public Law 203, Seventy-first Congress), the USPHS in 1930 renamed the Narcotics Division the Division of Mental Hygiene, with Treadway as its first Director. In 1938 Treadway was succeeded by Lawrence Kolb, and when he retired in 1944, Robert Felix was appointed to the post and later became the first Director of the National Institute of Mental Health. It was under Dr. Lawrence Kolb in the immediate prewar years that the concept of a National Neuropsychiatric Institute was born. The Kolb plan called for extensive laboratories and animal facilities (Brandt, 1965).

During World War II, some 1,100,000 men were rejected for military duty because of mental or neurological disorders. When these were added to the rejectees for mental and educational deficiencies, the total came to

1,767,000 out of 4,800,000. Of those inducted into the Army and sub-sequently given medical discharges, 40 per cent were dismissed for psychiatric reasons. By 1946, 60 per cent of all hospitalization under the Veterans' Administration was for psychiatric disorders. The severe shortage of trained psychiatric personnel, absence of knowledge of the etiology of mental illness, lack of adequate methods for dealing with large numbers of psychiatric cases, and lack of understanding of the role of psychiatry in the prevention and treatment of mental illness were emphasized by the Navy's Captain Braceland, by the Army's Brigadier General William C. Menninger, and by the Public Health Service's Robert H. Felix. Many conscientious objectors were assigned to duty in hospitals during the war, and for the first time intelligent attendants witnessed the neglect, overcrowding, and often barbarism in public mental hospitals throughout the country.

At the end of the war a favorable atmosphere for action existed, and Dr. Felix outlined a program to Dr. Thomas Parrin, the Surgeon-General of the USPHS. By February, 1945, a draft Bill for a National Neuropsychiatric Institute was ready. The House Bill set forth four general purposes: (1) fostering and aiding research relating to the cause, diagnosis, and treatment of neuropsychiatric disorders; (2) provision for the training of professional personnel through the award of fellowships to individuals and grants to public and nonprofit institutions; (3) aid to the states to enable them to establish clinics and treatment centers; and (4) the provision of pilot and demonstration studies in the prevention, diagnosis, and treatment of neuropsychiatric disorders. To implement these provisions, the Bill also called for the creation of a new National Advisory Council and the establishment of a National Neuropsychiatric Institute. The testimony in favor of this Bill was overwhelming, and the National Mental Health Act was signed into law in July, 1946. The National Institute of Mental Health (NIMH) was not established until April, 1949, at which time the Division of Mental Hygiene was abolished, the two federal drug addiction hospitals were transferred to the Bureau of Medical Services, and the NIMH joined the administrative structure of the NIH.

With the federal assistance authorized by this Act, thousands of psychiatrists, psychologists, psychiatric social workers, and nurses have obtained their education. Hundreds of research workers in a wide range of social, medical, and biological disciplines have also been trained. When the Act was passed, it was estimated that only $2.5 million from all sources was being spent annually in the United States on research in psychiatry and related fields. In 1947 the total federal expenditure for all medical and health-related research was only $27 million. By 1963 the National Institute of Mental Health alone was investing some $69 million in its intramural and extramural research programs. The Institute's research interests crossed through psychiatry, psychology, anthropology, and all of the social sciences, in addition to such biological disciplines as neuro-anatomy, neurophysiology, biochemistry, neurochemistry, and genetics. From the beginning, support was provided for research in all fields related to mental illness, whether clinical or nonclinical, basic or applied, empirical, methodological, or theoretical in the medical, biological, social, or behavioral sciences. The result has been an unparalleled growth of the behavioral sciences in this country.

742   In December, 1963, the federal mental health program entered a new

era through the passage of the Community Mental Health Centers Act (Public Law 88-164), authorizing the appropriation of $150 million to finance up to two thirds of the cost of constructing community mental health centers throughout the country. An additional $126 million was made available to construct research and treatment facilities for the mentally retarded. In the years since the passage of the National Mental Health Act of 1946, there has been increasing acceptance of mental health concepts in promoting individual and community well-being.

PSYCHIATRIC
INTERVENTION

The problems associated with the major mental disorders have been altered significantly as a result of the availability of new and effective drugs and changes in the methods of delivering care. These advances have been made even though our knowledge of the basic causes and mechanisms of mental disorders has increased very little. However, the striking effects of chemotherapy have stimulated a major effort in basic research of the biochemical and genetic mechanisms underlying psychiatric illness.

In spite of the widespread use of psychotherapy (the psychological treatment of mental disorders, psychoanalysis, behavior therapy, and family therapy), the value of these approaches is still doubtful; and whether the psychological treatment of neurotic patients should be looked upon as an exclusive medical specialty remains uncertain. The available studies suggest that in the treatment of neurotic disorders, psychiatrists are little more effective than psychologists, social workers, and counselors. On the other hand, the psychiatrist can deal more effectively with the psychoses, notably, schizophrenia and manic-depressive states.

An objective measure of the change in psychiatric practice resulting from the availability of drugs for treatment of psychotic illness is the number of patients in mental hospitals. The patient census of mental hospitals reached a peak of 560,000 in 1955. Over the preceding decade the number of hospitalized patients had increased at the rate of 3 per cent per year, or twice the growth rate of the population. After 1955 this trend was sharply reversed. From 1962 to 1969 *first* admission rates rose from 130,000 to 164,000 and *readmission* rates from 150,000 to 216,000, while the average daily census of resident patients fell from 516,000 to 370,000; showing a dramatic decline in the average length of hospital stay. The number of hospital-resident mental patients fell to 276,000 by 1972, in spite of the increase in the general population (Eisenberg, 1973).

In contrast, the total number of patient-care episodes (inpatient plus outpatient) in the United States increased from 1,675,000 in 1955 to 4,038,000 in 1971. In that period the number of inpatient episodes rose from 1,296,000 to 1,721,000 and the number of outpatient episodes from 379,000 to 2,317,000. Considered from another point of view, the inpatient episodes per 100,000 population rose only from 799 to 847, whereas outpatient episodes increased from 234 to 1,134. Thus, the site of care had shifted from the wards of state hospitals to newly created yet not always adequate facilities in the community itself. Eisenberg points out that there is no wholly satisfactory explanation for these changes but that two important transformations in psychiatric care were largely responsible: the rediscovery of the

743

principle of "moral" (humane) treatment and the development of effective psychotropic drugs. In the late 1940s and early 1950s, sociologists began to examine the way in which care was provided in mental institutions and the interactions between patients and staff. It became clear that the behavior of patients with chronic mental disease was the result not only of a mental disorder but also of the dehumanization produced by the mental hospital environment. Innovative hospital superintendents opened locked doors, introduced a measure of patient self-government, and reestablished contact with the surrounding community. With these changes many of the chronic inpatients were able to return to the community. With the advent of effective chemotherapy for acute psychotic disorders, the patient census in mental hospitals fell still further (Eisenberg, 1973).

The discovery of the first effective psychotropic agent, *chlorpromazine* (Thorazine), another example of serendipity, resulted from efforts to synthesize a more effective antihistamine. In 1949, a French surgeon, H. Laborit, used chlorpromazine to reinforce ordinary anesthesia and produce a hibernation syndrome in patients undergoing prolonged surgery. He noticed that the patients exhibited a striking indifference to environmental stimuli. In 1952 J. Delay and P. Deniker discovered the drug's effect in aborting acute psychotic episodes both in schizophrenia and in manic-depressive disorders. These observations were confirmed by controlled clinical trials, and Francis Boyer of the Smith Kline and French Company was responsible for bringing this drug to the United States (see Chapter 22).

Ayurvedic medicine in India had for thousands of years made excellent use of the snakeroot plant, *Rauwolfia serpentina*, for its sedative properties. A noticeable side effect was the production of severe depression in some patients. It was introduced into psychiatry to cut short the acute psychotic episodes seen in schizophrenia. Although it has been supplanted to a large degree by the phenothiazines (chlorpromazine), reserpine still has an important role in the experimental pharmacology of the psychoses.

About the same time that chlorpromazine was introduced, physicians using iproniazid in patients with tuberculosis discovered that many developed euphoria prior to any improvement in the pulmonary disease. This led to the trial of this drug in depressed patients, and it proved to have a definite effect in relieving depression. It was soon discovered that iproniazid is an inhibitor of the enzyme monamine oxidase (monamines, such as serotonin, norepinephrine, and dopamine, are thought to act as chemical transmitters in the brain). Following this discovery, organic chemists soon synthesized the drug imipramine, which has a beneficial effect on the depressed schizophrenic.

In Australia, J. F. J. Code discovered that when lithium was given to laboratory animals, it acted as a sedative. Clinical trials suggested that this element could control mania. This lead was ignored for a decade because toxicity had been observed when lithium salts were used in high doses as a substitute for sodium in the treatment of hypertension. After 10 years it was reintroduced with careful monitoring of blood levels, and it has been shown to be a safe agent for the treatment of mania.

These various clinical observations have served as a stimulus for much study of the biochemical mechanisms in the brain. It appears (as mentioned earlier) that the biogenic amines (including serotonin, norepinephrine, and dopamine) function in specific regions of the central nervous system as chemical transmitters between nerve cells or as modulators of transmission by other substances such as acetylcholine. There seems to be a relatively close relation between the effects of the psychoactive drugs on monamine level and on affective and behavioral states. Drugs that result in an inactivation and depletion of norepinephrine in the brain (such as reserpine and lithium) produce sedation and depression. Drugs such as imipramine, together with monamine oxidase inhibitors that increase or potentiate norepinephrine, are associated with behavioral stimulation and usually have an antidepressant effect. The evidence appears to be increasing that cyclic AMP mediates some of the effects of norepinephrine and dopamine in the brain. Cyclic AMP is present in large concentrations in the central nervous system and is known to be important in the induction of enzymes and the synthesis of other proteins. Recent experiments have indicated that protein synthesis may play an important role in long-term memory. When chemicals that inhibit protein synthesis are used in the experimental animal, the formation of long-term memories is impeded. Drugs that release or enhance norepinephrine in the brain counteract this suppression. These findings of Seymour S. Kety of the Harvard Medical School support a tentative model of memory in which protein synthesis, stimulated by the release of norepinephrine, serves as the biochemical basis for the consolidation of learning.

Evidence has been accumulating that points toward a genetic basis for schizophrenia and for manic-depressive disorders. Research on twins has shown that schizophrenia in both twins is much commoner in monozygotic (identical) pairs than in dizygotic (fraternal) pairs. The emergence of these mental disorders probably requires a predisposition involving more than one gene and still unspecified environmental precipitants (Eisenberg, 1973).

As Eisenberg points out, the fundamental task of psychiatry is to understand behavior that results from interaction of stimulus (environmental) conditions and the response (psychobiological) capacities of the organism, capacities that reflect the organism's genetic endowment as well as its history. Psychiatry, he emphasizes, has two faces; one represented by treatment at the psychosocial level and the other by treatment at the pharmacological level. These two forms of treatment often act to reinforce one another.

Although psychiatry is still a complex area of medical practice, disorders once crudely lumped together as insanity have now been differentiated and categorized. One type, a dementia accompanied by variable degrees of general paralysis, is now known to be the result of syphilis of the central nervous system and can be prevented by the effective treatment of the disease in its early stages. The complex of mental disturbances that one sees in pellagra is now known to result from a dietary deficiency of B-complex vitamins (tryptophan, nicotinic acid, and pyridoxine). Similar disturbances, in the absence of dietary inadequacy, have been shown to be the result of an inherited metabolic defect (Hartnup's disease) that leads to an inability to absorb tryptophan from the gut. These disturbances of nature or of disease, which produce clearly recognizable psychiatric illnesses, and the accumulating experience with drugs that influence cerebral function have encouraged the belief that we can look forward to important advances in

745

our understanding of and ability to manage mental disease (Eisenberg, 1973).

PSYCHOCHEMICAL
RESEARCH STUDIES
IN HUMANS

Research in psychology and psychiatry is drawing heavily on the area opened by the basic neurophysiologists who studied (in the 1940s and 1950s) electrical potentials produced by cells and brain systems in animals. During this period, the electroencephalogram was a popular instrument of research. In the early and middle 1950s, behavior-oriented neurochemists and neuropharmacologists began to discover new things about the brains of animals. Various animal models came into existence for comparison with human psychological states. Changes in excitability of peripheral autonomic synapses as a result of chemical manipulation with natural substrates or drugs were used as models for generalization to the central synapses of animals and man. These research areas were many, but four have been outstanding: (1) the neuropharmacological and neurochemical manipulation of animal brain with agents having established behavioral effects in humans; (2) the administration to humans, by the "load" technique, of precursors of metabolic substances hypothesized to be active in the central nervous system, with resulting behavioral effects; (3) the use of sleep-stage as an electrophysiological state that is relatively stereotyped across species so that various chemically induced changes in this parameter can be studied in both animals and humans; (4) the search for metabolic errors reflected in changes in both body chemistry and behavior so that either absences of normal metabolites or the excess of usually insignificant substances may be correlated with behavioral phenomena and suggest underlying chemical mechanisms (Mandell and Spooner, 1968).

It has been far more difficult to determine in the brain the type of basic data obtained in peripheral neurotransmitter situations where acetylcholine plays a prominent role. The central nervous system has little in the way of focal synaptic regions. In spite of these difficulties, a great deal has been accomplished. New methods have been developed, but the kinds of assumptions, operations, and conclusions that prevail in this field are still relatively crude. Nevertheless, when one compares work from earlier decades in this area with current activity, it is clear that the psychochemist is benefiting from the basic advances that have been made in chemistry and biology (Mandell and Spooner, 1968).

PROVISION OF
PSYCHIATRIC CARE

Romano has drawn attention to the fact that many persons other than psychiatrists will be increasingly involved in both individual and group psychotherapeutic procedures in the future. The general physician, including the internist, will continue to be active in the identification and treatment of most of the neurotic patients whom he encounters in his practice.

The Community Health Program, which in a sense is the vanguard of health care delivery in all fields of medicine, reflects an awareness of current deficiencies in the continuity of medical care and encourages a search for better measures to serve the patient's need. Many now insist that the major objective of psychiatry (whether in the field of education, research, or service) should be that of primary prevention. The need is emphasized by the fact that in the Veterans' Administration system alone there are 5000 schizophrenic male patients who have been hospitalized for 10 years or more. No matter what the number of practicing physicians may be, they will never be able to deal effectively with this disease when it is in an advanced stage. Prevention seems the only logical answer to this problem.

Another development in the past few decades has been family psychotherapy. The pioneers in this field were Lidz at Yale, Ackerman in New York, Minuchin at Pennsylvania, and Bowen at Georgetown, as well as Jackson and his associates at Stanford. This development has had a major impact on child psychiatry, since it emphasizes that emotional disturbances in a child are frequently symptomatic of family problems and that therefore the family as a whole needs treatment and not just the individual child. The applications of family therapy, however, are by no means limited to disturbed children. Some feel that the development of theories of family systems and therapeutic approaches to them represent a more substantial and lasting contribution than far-out offshoots of group therapy, although the latter has perhaps received more attention.

PSYCHIATRIC TEACHING   American psychiatric teaching had its origin in the work of Benjamin Rush, who in 1821 published his *Medical Inquiries and Observations upon the Diseases of the Mind,* which was the first American general treatise on the subject of mental diseases. It was the only American text of its kind until 1883, when William Hammond and E. C. Spitzka published textbooks on insanity. However, the subject continued to be neglected by all but a few medical schools in this country.

Pliny Earle was appointed visiting physician to the New York Asylum in 1853, during which year he delivered his first course of lectures on mental diseases at the College of Physicians and Surgeons. Until the 1870s, even occasional lectures on mental and nervous diseases were rarities in our medical colleges. This lack of psychiatric instruction was recognized in 1871 when the Association of Medical Superintendents of American Institutions for the Insane adopted a resolution recommending the need for lectures and clinical experience as well. Later, Adolf Meyer pointed out the need to develop a systematic curriculum of psychiatry in medical schools.

In 1909 the Council on Medical Education of the AMA published a model medical curriculum that included a total of 30 hours of psychiatry, all in the fourth year. In 1912 the Association of American Medical Colleges set a minimum standard of 20 hours of psychiatric teaching in medical schools. Through Adolf Meyer's influence, a number of surveys were undertaken in the intervening years. These surveys were followed by conferences supported by the National Committee for Mental Hygiene. The first, in 1933, considered the formation of the American Board of Psychiatry and Neurology; the second (1934) discussed the curriculum for psychiatric teaching; the third (1935), psychiatry in pediatrics; and the fourth (1936), methods of psychiatric teaching. Two famous conferences were held at Ithaca, New York, in the summers of 1951 and 1952, and the recommendations that issued

747

from them were generously implemented by federal funds which had been made available for the development of new types of undergraduate and graduate teaching programs.

The most important changes in departments of psychiatry in the United States since the end of World War II have resulted from the National Mental Health Act, which provided funds for education and research. More than 80 per cent of psychiatric units in general hospitals have opened since 1947. Much of this came about as a result of the expansion and liberalization of health insurance programs and the Hill-Burton Act, which provided federal matching funds for construction of psychiatric facilities in general hospitals.

An important contribution was that of John Romano and his colleagues, which began in 1939 at the Peter Bent Brigham Hospital in Boston. Romano's experiment in medical education was motivated by the belief that an awareness of the psychological components of illness could not be imparted to students when there were artificial lines of cleavage in teaching. He set up a closely knit liaison service. The psychiatric problems in the setting of the general hospital, while differing from those in a psychiatric hospital, enabled the teacher to make all students aware of the emotional factors in all sick people. Soon liaison services were set up in other institutions; notably successful was that of Dr. Theodore Lidz in Baltimore. In 1946 George L. Engel and his co-workers developed at the University of Rochester a graduate and undergraduate teaching program in the psychological aspects of medicine, jointly sponsored by the Departments of Medicine and Psychiatry. It was unique in a number of respects, not the least of which was that the staff were trained first as internists and then received psychological training. Teaching and research in this unit were, accordingly, carried on by physicians sophisticated in both disciplines, thus creating a broader perspective than that of either the internist or the psychiatrist separately and providing for the student and physician-in-training models for identification.

Romano (1973a) has attempted to list the important accomplishments in psychiatry of the last few decades:

(1) The establishment of psychiatric units in general hospitals and community hospitals. (2) The teaching of psychiatry to all undergraduate medical students. (3) The considerable increase in the manpower pool of career psychiatrists through resident teaching programs in university and affiliated clinics and hospitals, providing psychiatrists for private and group community practices. (4) The furtherance of research through research educational opportunities at the National Institute for Mental Health and the university departments. (5) The introduction of psychology and the social sciences into the matrix of the medical school teaching hospital. (6) Multiple ventures in psychotherapeutic procedures, from psychoanalytic origins into diverse group and family techniques; from learning theory to behavior modification and to several combinations of these. (7) The extensive use of the major psychoactive drugs in treatment of psychotic patients, and the use of minor tranquilizers by the general practitioner in the treatment of neurotic conditions. (8) The growth of the general practice of psychiatry as well as the more restrictive therapeutic special practices, and the role of such practices in returning the care of the chronically ill patients from the state to the local community. (9) The expansion of educational programs for psychiatric nurses and psychiatric social workers and

748

their assumption of new roles in therapy and care. (10) The creation of new types of paraprofessional persons in child and adult care-nursing assistants, mental health workers, etc., who participate at many points in the health service network. (11) The beginning of systematic studies in the nature of health delivery systems, emergency, triage, neighborhood centers, home visit, outpatient, inpatient, chronic hospitals, the remarkable changes in distribution of patients from inpatients to outpatient services, etc. (12) Attention to areas of neglect, the chronically sick, the poor, the black, the addict, the alcoholic, and the criminal. (13) Expansion of child psychiatry beyond its traditional engagement with the middle class neurotic child, with concern for children with brain damage, psychosis, retardation, and delinquent behavior. (14) Increased interest and attention to human genetics, biological studies of mind and brain and mind and body. (15) Greater precision in clinical diagnosis, with greater attention to physical examination of the patient.

Romano believes that the major contribution psychiatry has made to medicine has been in the education of the medical student. It has become possible for the medical student today to study and care for mentally sick patients in the same hospital setting in which he studies medical, surgical, and obstetrical patients. This was accomplished in the past 25 years in part by federal subsidies for the establishment of psychiatric units in general teaching hospitals. The founding of the National Institute of Mental Health and the support by the provision of federal funds for training programs and research studies have resulted in the creation of models which include the clinician, investigator, and a new mutation — the behavioral scientist (Romano, 1970).

31

Medical Practice

The perpetual enemies of the human race, apart from man's own nature, are ig-norance and disease.

(Alan Gregg, 1941)

In contrast with the almost imperceptible change in the skills of the medical practitioner during the nation's first century, today's physician has made great strides forward in many areas of medical practice. His professional mission is the same, but there is a profound difference in his ability to make accurate diagnoses and to take the necessary steps to cure disease and to prevent its spread. This enhanced power has come about through an extraordinary advance in our understanding of how the human organism grows and functions and how it defends itself or may be defended against disease. To gain this type of understanding the physician has had to become an educated person. In 1876, with a sub–high-school education and eight months of medical lectures, practitioners embarked on their professional careers confident that they could deal, at least as well as their competitor down the road, with any and every problem "whether in medicine, surgery, or midwifery" (p. 40). They may have been weak in their ability to prevent or cure, but they were strong in compassionate management—an aspect of medical practice that many patients value almost as highly as a cure.

The man or woman who enters the practice of medicine today must be a better than average college student; and before receiving a medical degree he or she must have acquired the underpinnings of a scientist, grounded in chemistry, physics, and biology, and thoroughly acquainted with the concepts and much of the substance of anatomy, physiology, psychology, pharmacology, bacteriology, virology, genetics, immunology, radiology, oncology, enzymology, endocrinology, and nutrition. With this scientific foundation the student enters upon a long period of training to acquire the special knowledge and specialized techniques that will enable him or her to practice, usually in some narrow branch of medicine or surgery.

751

The individual who has gone through this long period of preparation, not surprisingly, frequently enters the practice of medicine more as a scientist than as a humanist and often is more responsive to the challenge of a complex problem in diagnosis or treatment than to the seemingly trivial complaints—the common colds, the constipation, the anxieties, and other minor disturbances—that bring most patients to the doctor.

Though medical students are now selected almost exclusively from those with high intellectual ability, they are often overwhelmed by the intricacies of medical science—the sheer enormity of the subject—and are happy to devote their energies to a manageable segment of that vast, proliferating, complex domain; hence the trend away from general practice and toward the specialties in which one can become a recognized expert in a circumscribed area. Moreover, in a specialty, unless one chooses obstetrics or traumatic surgery, one has a greater degree of control over one's work, less night work, relatively undisturbed weekends, more time for recreation and study, and greater freedom to attend medical meetings and to take refresher courses. The solo general practitioner not only lacks these advantages but also must dwell with the consciousness of being second best to the specialist in many of his technical undertakings. With present-day transportation, there are very few communities that are out of reach of well-trained surgeons, obstetricians, and other specialists. Today no general practitioner should, and few do, pretend to be a jack-of-all-medical-trades.

It took time for medical educators and others to realize that an important gap was being created in medical service by the rise of specialism and the fade-out of general practice. Only when those who were trained during the early decades of the twentieth century were dying off rapidly after World War II did the gap become apparent. Then the question arose as to who was going to take care of the day-to-day health problems of the family and who was going to steer the family members to the proper specialist when one was needed. As the significance of this widening gap was realized, there began to be talk about the need for *primary* physicians, and medical schools began to offer courses in "family medicine." Soon family practice became recognized as a specialty in its own right, and hospitals began to offer residency training in this specialty. The family practitioner, as presently conceived, is the primary physician, the one to be called in to give advice about any health problem. He or she takes care of the common illnesses from infancy to old age, arranges and supervises preventive measures, educates the family in health matters, sets fractures and performs the surgery needed to care for minor trauma, and may or may not engage in obstetrical care, depending on whether a qualified obstetrician is available in the community.

In addition to the family physician, two new types of primary health personnel have come into existence during the past decade: (1) the *nurse practitioner,* a registered nurse who has received special postgraduate training in either general medicine or a specialty such as obstetrics or pediatrics; (2) the *physician's assistant,* an individual who usually has had some college education and frequently some experience in the medical corps of one of the armed services and who is given a year of concentrated medical education followed by a year of on-the-job training, usually in a hospital setting. Both the nurse practitioner and the physician's assistant work under the general supervision of a physician. They may become involved in a highly specialized practice, such as midwifery, but for the most part they work as "physician extenders," practicing the type of primary family medicine that made up most of the work of a practicing physician a century ago. It would appear that we may be moving in the direction of training two classes of medical practitioners, as has been done in some other countries, to meet the health needs of the people without having to put all practitioners through the long and expensive period of education and training required of today's physicians and surgeons.

A program designed to meet the needs of communities with insufficient medical service came into being in 1970 when Congress adopted the National Health Service Corps Act. This Act provides scholarships for medical students who agree to serve for two years in a rural or metropolitan area that lacks doctors. Applications from needy communities are reviewed, and the scholarship students, after graduation and additional hospital training, are assigned to approved communities in teams of two. It was hoped that at least some of these doctors would decide to remain in the communities after their two-year obligatory service. By 1974 there were more applicants for NHSC scholarships than there were openings. It is too early to tell how successful this program will be in filling the gaps in the distribution of medical practitioners. In 1974 the Secretary of Health, Education and Welfare identified 524 geographic areas needing and requesting physicians under the NHSC Act. Swanson (1975) has calculated that if 6 to 15 per cent of each year's 14,000 medical graduates were to serve in the NHSC for two years, the identified needs would be met. Congress gave serious consideration to going even further than this: prior to the adoption of the Health Professions Educational Assistance Act of 1974, there was debate as to whether all students in schools funded by the Act should be *required* to enter the NHSC after graduation. A mandatory requirement of this type may come up for reconsideration at a later date (Swanson, 1975).

In addition to those mentioned above, there are several types of non-M.D. practitioners who play an important role in the provision of health services. Included among these are: (1) Optometrists, who perform a large share of the refractions for eyeglasses. Some optometrists are associated with ophthalmologists as members of a team, but most of them have their own independent offices or shops. (2) Podiatrists, who confine their practice to the study and treatment of disorders of the feet. This group of specialists have a long period of education and training before they enter practice. They are examined by special state examining boards, and although their license restricts them to work on the feet, within this narrow field they function largely as a licensed physician would function.

CHANGES IN THE PREVALENCE OF DISEASES	Along with the change in the practitioner, there has been an equally drastic change in the type of medicine that he is called upon to practice. A century ago, the infectious diseases presented the

most formidable problems: intestinal infections killed countless infants and children; puerperal infections brought death to many young women; tuberculosis was a leading cause of illness among young adults of both sexes. Then, at intervals, came the great epidemics of cholera, typhoid fever, yellow fever, diphtheria, typhus, and smallpox. In addition, there were endemic parasitic diseases such as malaria and hookworm disease. Nutrition-deficiency diseases (pellagra, rickets, endemic goiter, and others) also were prevalent in some areas. The causes of all of the diseases just mentioned and of many others are now well known, and the diseases can be prevented by appropriate measures; indeed, many of them have been virtually eliminated and are never seen by the present-day physician. In addition to the diseases that can be prevented, many of those which were once debilitating or lethal can now be cured by modern drugs. There are far too many of these to mention here; they include pneumonia and other pneumococcal infections, a wide variety of acute streptococcal infections, epidemic meningitis, tuberculosis, syphilis, gonorrhea, typhoid fever, and diseases due to nutritional deficiencies. Many diseases, such as diabetes, hypertension, and pernicious anemia, which cannot be cured, can be kept under control so that the patients can lead productive, near-normal lives.

In addition to the diseases that can be treated by chemicals, hormones, diet, and other therapies, there are a large number of once fatal or debilitating diseases that can now be treated by surgery. Today one of the commonest surgical operations is appendectomy, and we are inclined to look upon appendicitis as a rather benign illness. We forget that in 1876 appendicitis was frequently a fatal disease; the studies by Reginald Fitz that brought appendicitis to the attention of the medical profession in 1886 were based largely on over 250 *autopsies* carried out at the Massachusetts General Hospital. In addition to the operations that are lifesaving, there are many that are designed to restore function; these include the repair of hernias; replacement of worn-out, painful joints such as the hip or knee by new metal joints; the operations on congenitally malformed hearts; restoration of vision with a new cornea, or restoration of hearing by microsurgery of the middle ear.

One of the effects of the prevention and successful treatment of so many different diseases has been a considerable lengthening in the life span of the average individual. As a result, the practitioner's most difficult and discouraging problems are no longer among infants and children but among the steadily increasing number of the aged. The major disease problems at present are cancer, heart disease, arteriosclerosis, stroke, senile mental deterioration, and chronic arthritis. One hears it said that almost nothing has been done to cope with these diseases, but this is far from the truth.

There are many different types of cancer, and although the majority of them still run a fatal course, some can now be completely cured and others can be controlled so that the affected individual can lead a useful, pain-free life for a period of years. When the diagnosis can be made early, a complete cure often can be effected by surgical excision or radiation. When a cure cannot be effected, palliation can be achieved sometimes for a period of years by the use of surgery, radiation, and chemotherapy, singly or in various combinations.

In recent years there have been some curious and not well understood changes in the death rate from various types of cancer. For example, in 1930, among 100,000 male members of the population, 28 died of cancer of the stomach while 2 died of cancer of the lung, but by 1968 the deaths from cancer of the stomach had fallen from 28 to 9 while the deaths from cancer of the lung had risen from 2 to 45. The deaths from cancer of the lung were more than double those of any other single form of cancer in men. The next highest in 1968 was carcinoma of the large intestine (colon and rectum), with a death rate of 18. In 1930 among 100,000 females, the death rate from cancer of the uterus was 28 while that from cancer of the stomach was 22, and from cancer of the lung it was only 2. In 1968 the death rate for cancer of the uterus had fallen from 28 to 11, and that for cancer of the stomach had fallen from 22 to 5, while that for cancer of the lung had risen from 2 to 8. Though carcinoma of the uterus was the commonest fatal cancer among women in 1930, carcinoma of the breast had replaced it in 1968, with a death rate of 25.

The striking decline in the death rate from cancer of the stomach in both men and women has no satisfactory explanation. The deaths from this cause have diminished at a rate of about 5 per 100,000 population per decade since 1930. A peculiar feature of the decline is that it has been limited largely to the United States; in most other countries the death rate from gastric cancer is at least as high as it was in 1930. It is of interest that the decline occurred during a period when there was a great increase, in the American diet, of those additives which are now suspected of being carcinogenic. The only form of treatment that, at present, offers any hope of curing gastric carcinoma is surgical excision of all or part of the stomach. However, very few lives are saved by surgery, and the lower death rate is due almost entirely to a reduction in the incidence of this form of cancer.

Though the reduced death rate from cancer of the stomach cannot be attributed to improvements in medical practice, the decline in the rate for carcinoma of the uterus definitely *can* be attributed to such improvements. More frequent and more thorough pelvic examinations and the routine use of the Papanicolaou smear have made possible earlier diagnoses, and improved methods of surgery and radiotherapy have increased the cure rate.

Great progress has also been made in the prevention and management of heart disease. The correction of congenital defects in childhood prevents cardiac failure later in life. Effective treatment of syphilis at an early stage in the disease has virtually eliminated syphilitic aortitis with resulting incompetence of the aortic valve and heart failure. Likewise the use of antibiotics to prevent or treat streptococcal infections has reduced the incidence of rheumatic fever, with its damaging effect upon the heart muscle and valves. Moreover, when the heart has been crippled by disease of one or more of its valves, the defective valve can now be replaced by an artificial one. One of the most important causes of congestive heart failure has been high blood pressure. The effective large-scale treatment of hypertension goes back less than 10 years and is still not being utilized to the extent that it should be. We do not yet know what effect the modern treatment of hypertension will have in reducing the incidence of cardiac enlargement and failure; the present indications are that the effect may be very great. While the incidence of cardiac failure resulting from congenital defects, syphilis, rheumatic heart disease, and hypertension has been reduced, there has been an increase in the incidence of myocardial infarction and heart failure resulting from disease of the coronary arteries. The recently devised coronary artery bypass has a definitely favorable effect upon angina pectoris, but it is still too early to predict what the effect will be on congestive heart failure and long-term survival.

Owing to the great progress that has been made in the prevention and treatment of disease during the past century, no single practitioner and, in fact, no small group of practitioners can absorb all the information and master all the techniques required to provide the best type of medical care that modern methods will afford. This is perhaps the most important reason for the growing popularity of group practice and for the development of "health maintenance organizations," in which a number of physicians, surgeons, and other personnel can work together for the prevention and treatment of disease.

EARLY AMBULATION

Many physicians who have entered the practice of medicine in the past 30 years are unaware of the radical change in the management of patients that occurred during and after World War II. Prior to the war, prolonged bed-rest had been an important feature of therapy. Patients undergoing the common types of surgical operations were kept at complete bed-rest for long periods: appendectomy, 10 days; hernia repair, 14 days; gall bladder surgery, 14 to 18 days; hysterectomy, 14 to 18 days. The long stay in bed necessitated a long period of hospitalization: about two weeks for appendectomies and three to four weeks for cholecystectomies and hysterectomies. After returning home, the patient had to devote another three to six weeks to getting into shape before resuming his usual activities. The routine of the obstetrician was similar to that of the surgeon: after delivery, the mother remained at strict bed-rest for two to three weeks and in the hospital for three to four weeks; and after returning home, activities were very slowly resumed over a period of six to eight weeks. Bed-rest also was prescribed generously for medical patients after febrile illnesses and for those with tuberculosis, myocardial infarction, and many other conditions. In addition, there were prolonged "rest cures" for patients with "nervous breakdowns."

Bed-rest had not always been accorded such a high therapeutic rating. It is well known that women in primitive societies, for example among the American Indians, resume their usual activities two or three days after the birth of a baby. In the latter part of the eighteenth century, Charles White of Manchester, England, one of that country's leading obstetricians, said that the sooner "the patient gets out of bed, the better, and this should not be deferred beyond the second or third day at the furtherest." However, several decades later, a different expert opinion was put forth. Robert Gooch, also a leading British obstetrician, warned in 1820 that women should be kept in bed for three weeks after delivery because of the danger of prolapse of the uterus (a miserable condition in which the uterus descends and inverts the vagina). Three weeks in bed following delivery seems to have become the rule in the United States in the nineteenth century, at least for city dwellers, though it would hardly have applied to the rugged women of the frontier areas.

The early surgeons, like the early obstetricians, were not so insistent on bed-rest. It will be recalled that Ephraim McDowell, in 1809, was the first surgeon deliberately to open the abdominal cavity to remove an ovarian tumor. No anesthesia was used. The tumor was very large (22 pounds), and during the operation the intestines "ran out upon the table, remained out about 20 minutes and, being upon Christmas Day, they became so cold that I thought proper to bathe them in tepid water previous to my replacing them." The patient recovered from this ordeal without incident, and McDowell was pleased to find her on her feet making up her bed five days after the operation.

In surgery, the therapeutic value of bed-rest was promoted by those who developed modern operative procedures. In the late nineteenth century, surgeons were always fearful that the wound which they had stitched together so carefully would break down. W. S. Halsted was one of the most cautious of the innovators. When he developed the modern operation for the repair of inguinal hernias, he is said to have placed the first patients in plaster casts to assure complete immobility and rest. In his original description of this operation (1889), Halsted does not mention plaster casts, but he says that the patients were not permitted to get out of bed until the twenty-first day after the operation. In 1893, after Sir William MacEwen, the famous Glasgow surgeon, had said that a patient need not be kept in bed more than eight days following the repair of a hernia, Halsted (1893) made the following statement:

> *The time to be spent in bed depends upon the judgement of the surgeon and not. . . upon the particular method. Our patients are kept upon their backs for twenty-one days. Wounds thoroughly healed throughout per primam are not strong in eight days. One can easily tear open a typically healed wound which is not more than six or seven days old. . . . A wound is certainly stronger on the fourteenth day than on the seventh, and stronger on the twenty-first than on the fourteenth. . . . I sometimes question the propriety of allowing, as I do, my patients to walk about on the twenty-first day.*

This statement regarding the time required for a wound to heal, expressed by such a prominent surgeon, had a long-lasting influence. Nevertheless, an occasional surgeon refused to be a worshiper of bed-rest. Emil Ries, Professor of Gynecology at the Post-Graduate Medical School, Chicago, while visiting a clinic in Naples, Italy, in 1893, was shown a patient who got out of bed and walked across the ward during the evening of the day on which a pelvic operation had been performed. There was no evidence that this early postoperative activity damaged the wound in any way. When Ries returned to Chicago, he started a program of getting his patients up and walking about within hours of recovery from anesthesia. In 1899 Ries reported what he considered to be the very gratifying results of this program: "The changes which I have reported here have not to my knowledge been carried out anywhere else to this extent. I can assure you that . . . they can be introduced anywhere, not only without detriment to our patients, but to their positive gain and advantage. It means a great deal for a businessman or a laborer, or their wives, to be put on their own feet in a short time and to be able to return to their work two or three weeks after an abdominal operation." H. J. Boldt of New York City, a gynecologist and friend of Ries, also adopted this early activity program: "Occasionally I have done abdominal hysterectomies . . . in the morning and have had my patients out of bed in a rocking chair late in the afternoon of the same day." In 1907 Ries and Boldt had a combined series of nearly 900 patients who had been allowed up on the first or second day after laparotomy with "not a single instance of untoward result which could in any way be attributed to the early rising from bed." The advantages noted by these two surgeons were: less nausea and vomiting, less abdominal bloating, earlier return to normal bowel action, fewer bronchial and pulmonary complications, less circulatory disturbance, better appetite and assimilation of food, less general weakness, and a more rapid recovery to normal working ability (Ries, 1899; Boldt, 1907).

In spite of this seemingly convincing report of the advantages of early activity after operations, surgeons in general refused to abandon their time honored routine of prolonged bed-rest. The change did not come until the 1940s.

In 1941 John H. Powers, a surgeon at the Mary Imogene Bassett Hospital in Cooperstown, New York, had several unhappy experiences with young adults following operation. At that time he knew nothing about the work of Ries and Boldt. He had been brought up in the surgical tradition of Halsted, as one of Harvey Cushing's surgical residents at the Peter Bent Brigham Hospital. The postoperative events that disturbed him in 1941 were occasioned by thrombosis in the veins of the legs, followed by pulmonary infarcts. Powers suspected that these events were related to the prolonged period of enforced inactivity following operation. He knew that children who could not be kept quiet in bed and became active almost immediately after operation did not develop such complications; and that the incidence of complications was lessened in elderly men following prostate operations if they were gotten out of bed the day after the operation. Powers wondered why young and middle-aged adults should be treated differently from children and old men; he therefore decided to carry out some carefully controlled experiments to determine whether patients who were gotten out of bed and forced to exercise within the first day or two after operation did better or worse than those who were kept flat in bed for periods of ten days to three weeks. These experiments were going forward in 1942, 1943, and 1944.

After the United States entered the war, several factors combined to arouse interest in a more rapid turnover of patients in hospitals. Very few new hospitals had been constructed during the period of the Great Depression, and there was a serious shortage of beds in many areas, particularly those areas where there had been a marked increase in the population, around munitions factories, airplane factories, and shipyards. There was also the need to get soldiers and sailors back to duty as rapidly as possible following illness or operations. Late in the winter of 1943–44, the Division of Medical Sciences of the National Research Council heard about the experiments on early activity of postoperative patients that were being carried out in Cooperstown, and Powers was invited to come to Washington to tell the Council about what he had learned in the course of his studies. On March 17, 1944, Powers presented a paper describing the results of his experiments at a meeting of the Committee on Convalescence and Rehabilitation of the

National Research Council. This paper was given wide circulation in mimeographed form by the National Research Council as *Convalescence and Rehabilitation Report No. 2,* dated April 15, 1944, and entitled "Early activity of postoperative patients."

On June 15, 1944, at the Annual Session of the American Medical Association, the Section on Experimental Medicine and Therapeutics held a symposium on "The Abuse of Rest in the Treatment of Disease." The six papers presented in the symposium were published in the August 19, 1944, issue of the *Journal* of the AMA, and they attracted a great deal of attention not only because of the timeliness of the subject but also because the speakers were all such distinguished men within their special fields. In addition to Powers, who presented his work on postoperative convalescence, Tinsley R. Harrison of Dallas, Texas, spoke on cardiovascular disease, Nicholson J. Eastman of Baltimore spoke on obstetrics, William Dock of Los Angeles spoke on general medicine, Ralph K. Ghormley of the Mayo Clinic spoke on orthopedic surgery, and Karl Menninger of Topeka, Kansas, spoke on psychiatry. It is worthy of note that all of these individuals, with the exception of one, spoke in rather general anecdotal terms. Eastman's paper seemed particularly wide of the mark: never once mentioning early ambulation after delivery, he concentrated his attention on the time that should be allowed between pregnancies and the amount of work that pregnant women should be permitted to do in industry.

The one person who presented a convincing, controlled clinical study was Powers. He confined his attention to four types of operations: appendectomy, hernia repair, gall bladder operations, and abdominopelvic operations. For each operation he had two groups of equal numbers of patients, one group who were kept in bed for the usual 10 to 15 days, and the other group who were gotten out of bed usually on the day of operation or the following day. Powers's studies were carried out in a small rural hospital, and he reported results on only 200 patients, 100 in the early and 100 in the late activity group. However, his work obviously was carried out with meticulous care. He was dealing with matched pairs for each type of operation, and the follow-up information on the patients was unusually complete. The results of this study are summarized in Table 8. It may be seen that every factor favors early postoperative activity: fewer days in the hospital, less loss of weight, much shorter convalescence, and fewer complications, when all complications from minor to major were considered.

Powers's final report on early postoperative ambulation appeared in 1958. This was a report on hernia repair only, in 847 patients. The result bore out the conclusions of the 1944 report. In the meantime, many other studies had contributed to the wealth of information on this subject. Today, appendectomy patients are kept in hospital for only two or three days instead of two or three weeks; and hernia wounds do not break down when the patient walks around a few hours after operation and goes home a week later.

In obstetrics it took longer for early ambulation to gain general acceptance than it did in surgery. In 1943 a brief note by W. F. Guerriero appeared in the *American Journal of Obstetrics and Gynecology,* stating that in New Orleans the maternity services of the hospitals had been faced with a critical shortage of beds, and "in order to prevent crowding . . . after deliv-

759

TABLE 8.   EARLY VS. LATE POSTOPERATIVE ACTIVITY*

Type of Operation	P.O. Activity	
	Early	*Late*
Hernia repair	39	39
Appendectomy	22	22
Gall bladder surgery	14	14
Abdominopelvic surgery	25	25
TOTAL	100	100
Additional Data		
Average age of patient (years)	43.4	38.7
Average loss of weight per patient (lb.)	2.9	4.4
Days in bed	1.0	12.7
Days in hospital	10.3	16.1
Weeks of convalescence	5.7	10.3
Complications (all types)	17.0	46.0

*Adapted from Powers (1944).

ery, it was decided to institute a policy of early discharge of patients who had normal deliveries. . . . In the past twelve months, 2926 patients have been sent home between the second and fifth post-partal days." Of these patients, only three had to be readmitted to hospital, two with pyelitis, which seemed unrelated to early discharge. In 1946, Guerriero followed up his earlier report by giving a few more particulars about the 2926 patients mentioned above, and a detailed report of 323 who experienced early controlled ambulation. Guerriero concludes from his studies that early ambulation offers "advantages to the obstetric patient without imposing any disadvantages."

In 1962 L. M. Hellman and co-workers reviewed the subject of "early hospital discharge in obstetrics" and in a controlled study of over 2000 patients concluded that no harm resulted to either mother or baby when they were released from the hospital within 72 hours postpartum. Hellman's comment on the general attitude of obstetricians toward this subject was of interest: "Such early discharge is not mentioned in the British literature except for the Bradford experiment described by Theobald in 1959. Even in America, early hospital discharge is not generally accepted, and investigations are limited to the publications of Guerriero (1946) and Herndon (1956)." Though obstetricians may have been slow to accept early ambulation, it has certainly been widely accepted during the past decade, and recent statistics indicate that many patients are being discharged two or three days after delivery.

Powers (1976) says that one of his most difficult problems back in the 1940s and 1950s was to convince patients that early ambulation was to their advantage. All their lives they had been conditioned to the traditional doctrine that prolonged bed-rest is necessary after surgery, and they were hesitant about accepting any other point of view. Obstetrical patients exhibited an even stronger resistance to change; this was particularly true of those who had already enjoyed, in an earlier pregnancy, the luxury of the long rest and personal attentions that were part of the prewar maternity routine.

The change in attitude toward the therapeutic value of prolonged bed-rest has resulted in a tremendous saving in the cost of medical care. The amount of the saving has been obscured by the rapid and extensive rise in the cost of hospital operation. If patients were kept in hospital in the 1970s for as long as they were in the 1930s, the cost per hospital-stay might be some 50 per cent greater than it is. Moreover, we would need many additional hospital beds, with the heavy construction and operating costs that this would entail.

HOSPITALS

Many factors have combined to make institutional care of the sick and disabled an increasingly prominent feature of health services. Only in hospitals can one receive the full benefit of the massive technical facilities that are required for the application of the advances in medical science and technology. In the first two decades of the twentieth century, many babies were still being born at home, but today, except in case of accident or miscalculation, almost all births take place in hospitals. The care of the elderly, the crippled, and the chronically ill, which formerly was provided in the home, now has shifted largely to the "long-term care" institution—the nursing home or the "health-related facility." This important shift has come about not because of changes or improvements in medical care but as a result of social factors: smaller homes, husband and wife both working, no servants, no one to take care of grandfather or old aunt Suzie, generous provision of governmental funds for institutional care of the poor and the aged, but inadequate funds for their care at home.

Along with the increased use of institutional care, there has been a fantastic increase in the cost per patient-day of such care. Before World War II, good hospital care could be provided at an average cost of $4 per patient-day. In 1974, depending upon the location of the hospital and the type of services provided, the average cost was rarely less than $80, was usually more than $100, and was occasionally more than $150 per patient-day. In a survey of hospital costs reported in *American Medical News* (Breo, 1976), it was found that when the entire period of hospitalization was taken into account, the lowest average *charge* (in 1974) was for hospitals in the state of Wyoming, $652 for 8.2 days ($79.50 per patient-day), while the highest average charge was for hospitals in New York City, $2486 for 13.3 days ($187 per patient-day). The average charge rarely exceeds the average cost; in fact, in New York State, the average charge for Blue Cross and Medicaid patients, who made up the majority of those hospitalized, may not, under the law, exceed the cost. Even in nursing homes the cost per patient-day frequently lies between $20 and $30.

What explanation can one offer to a bewildered public for this extraordinary increase in costs? Many factors are involved:

(1) Inflation has been an important factor, but it can account for only a fraction of the increase.

(2) The payroll is the largest factor. Seventy to eighty per cent of a hospital's cost is in the payroll. A hospital has a 168-hour week rather than the 40-hour week that is the standard for industrial plants. Many of a hospital's most important services operate at night and during weekends. Prior to

761

1940, the average pay of hospital workers was pitifully low, and they often worked a 48- to 60-hour shift. Since then their work-week has been reduced to 40 hours, and they have gone a long way toward catching up with the wages and fringe benefits of industrial workers. Highly trained nurses, technicians, dietitians, psychologists, social workers, physical therapists, inhalation therapists, maintenance workers, professional secretaries, and business office personnel all now command good pay. Moreover, the number of hospital workers per patient has in some cases more than doubled, not only because of the shorter work-week, more holidays, and longer vacations, but also because of the many new skills required to keep up with the advances in science and technology, and the large clerical force required to do the paperwork (medical records, insurance forms, government forms, etc.). The result has been a tremendous increase in payroll expense.

(3) Equipment costs have increased greatly. For example, improvements in diagnostic and therapeutic radiology apparatus have made this equipment much safer and more effective, but at a high cost. The latest addition to diagnostic X-ray equipment is the computerized axial tomograth (CAT), which sells for just under $400,000. This is a high price to pay, but the benefits are very great. The CAT procedure is benign, no more discomforting to a patient than an ordinary X-ray picture. It can be used in the outpatient department to obtain important diagnostic information that ordinarily is obtained by admitting the patient to a hospital and employing methods which cause great discomfort and involve definite risks of permanent injury. Many hospital boards are now trying to decide whether to purchase this expensive piece of equipment, which will provide great benefits at less risk for a relatively small number of patients but at the same time will contribute significantly to the cost of hospital care. This is the type of dilemma that hospital trustees and administrators have had to face over and over again during the past 30 years. When the decision is affirmative, as it has had to be in many instances, hospital costs rise. The equipment costs for postoperative recovery rooms, intensive care units, and coronary care units are considerable, and when one adds to these the cost of the nursing and technical skills required to operate such units, the contribution to over-all costs is very great. Then there are artificial kidneys, cardiac catheterization laboratories, heart-lung machines, and a host of other items.

(4) There has been a great increase in the number of effective drugs, and as noted in Chapter 22, the research, development, and production costs that have been involved before many of these products are made available for clinical use make a high price tag inevitable.

(5) Great efforts have been made to shorten the number of days that each patient remains in the hospital. Few people realize that this results in an increase in the cost per patient-day. The major cost occurs almost always during the patient's first day or two in the hospital, when there are many laboratory tests, X-ray examinations, anesthesia and operating room or delivery room costs, and possibly the high costs of intensive care or coronary care. Before early ambulation for surgical and maternity cases was introduced in the late 1940s, patients remained in the hospital for long periods of convalescence. The daily hospital cost during the convalescent phase was much less than during the first few hospital days, and this served to bring down the *average* cost per day while the patient was in the hospital.

(6) There has been a great increase in the cost of the malpractice insurance which all hospitals must carry. This may add several dollars to the cost per patient-day.

(7) The cost of caring for the hopelessly ill, who formerly were allowed to die quietly at home, is now a very significant one. The attitude of most hospital authorities is that when patients are admitted to the hospital for care, every effort must be made to prolong their lives. As a result much equipment, many supplies, and a large segment of professional time are devoted to keeping alive the hopelessly ill, those with irreversible coma, and the elderly who wish to be allowed to die. In such cases it is hard to draw the line between social, religious, and medical responsibilities. Until the moral, ethical, and legal aspects of this problem are solved, it is likely to continue to add more and more to the cost of hospital care.

(8) About 90 per cent of the hospital bills are now paid not by the patient but by a third party: Blue Cross, commercial insurance, Medicare, Medicaid, and other organizations. Prior to World War II the patient usually was responsible for paying the hospital bill, and this had a restraining effect on hospital costs. The patient then wanted to get out of the hospital as soon as possible to save expense. Now, with a third party paying the bill, the patient does not object to being hospitalized, and when admitted, he is in no hurry to be discharged.

(9) Construction costs have risen to very high levels, and almost all hospitals, when the time comes for them to modernize their buildings, must borrow large sums of money. The amortization of these loans or the depreciation on buildings and equipment adds greatly to the cost per patient-day. It might be added that some hospitals are more elaborate than necessary. Local pride sometimes leads to extensive grounds, gardens, and fountains, all of which may be fine for the convalescent patient; however, few patients today remain in the hospital to convalesce. Other luxuries that help to increase the cost are air-conditioning in northern areas where it is not necessary, a telephone and a television set for every bed, extensive lobbies and sitting rooms for visitors, and individual bathing and toilet facilities for every room. Such luxuries, now often viewed as necessities, add significantly to the cost of construction and operation.

KEEPING UP WITH MEDICAL PROGRESS One of the great problems for the practitioner of the twentieth century has been that of keeping up with the rapid advances in medical science. The need for some mechanism to keep abreast of new developments began to be felt in the first decade of the century. It will be recalled that when Joseph McCormack, in 1909 to 1911, was organizing the state and local medical societies for the grassroots movement of the AMA, he emphasized the role that they could and should play in the continuing education of practicing physicians by sponsoring publications, lectureships, and university extension courses (see p. 365). Among the other organizations involved in the continuing education of practitioners, the American College of Surgeons and the American College of Physicians have played leading roles.

THE AMERICAN
COLLEGE OF
SURGEONS

Soon after 1900 Franklin Martin, a forward-look-ing Chicago surgeon, saw that surgery had be-come a specialized branch of medical practice, that it required special training, and that it should have its own journals and other methods of keeping abreast of de-velopments. In 1905 Martin founded the journal *Surgery, Gynecology and Obstetrics*. This publication filled a need for a practical, well-illustrated surgical journal, and it soon had an extensive list of subscribers. In 1910 an editorial appeared in *SG&O* inviting its readers "to a clinical meeting, *not* a limited number to see the work of a few surgeons, but, as far as practicable, every man in the United States and Canada who is particularly interested in surgery, to observe the principal clinics in one of the large medical centers. The initial test of this experiment will be inaugurated in Chicago, No-vember 7th to 19th [1910] — the program will consist of operative clinics ex-tending from 8:00 A.M. to 5:00 P.M. each day during the two weeks."

In arranging for this meeting, which was called "The Clinical Congress of Surgeons of North America," Martin evidently was expressing agreement with his Chicago colleague, J. B. Murphy, one of the surgical giants of that period, who had said, "Hearing papers and reading papers is one thing. Seeing men do things is another. We all know that no such benefit can be derived from hearing papers read as one can obtain from seeing the work done right before you."

Martin's experiment was a great success, and similar congresses were held in Philadelphia in 1911 and in New York in 1912. The enrollment for the 1912 meeting was 2600. The Congress had a very loose organizational structure, and its annual meetings were dependent upon an invitation from the surgeons of one or another city. In 1913 Franklin Martin decided that there should be a national organization of surgeons similar to the Royal College of Surgeons of England. Such an organization could sponsor and manage an annual Congress and could perform other activities designed for the improvement of surgery and surgeons. Hawley (1955) has pointed out that in the founding of most professional societies, organization comes first and a program is arranged later. "The American College of Surgeons is a notable exception to this general rule. The program came first, and the College was founded to ensure the continuation of the program." The pro-gram to which Hawley referred was, of course, the two-week Congress for the continuing education of surgeons. The purposes of the American College of Surgeons (ACS) were stated in the original by-laws as follows (Hawley, 1954):

The object of the College shall be to elevate the standard of surgery, to establish a standard of competency and of character for practitioners of surgery, to provide a method of granting fellowships in the organization, and to educate the public and the profession to understand that the practice of surgery calls for special training, and that the surgeon elected to fellowship in this college has had such training and is properly qualified to practice surgery.

In 1916 the ACS took the initiative in a movement to upgrade hospitals by establishing *Minimum Standards for Hospitals*. This was undertaken in co-operation with the American Hospital Association, the Catholic Hospital Association, the Protestant Hospital Association, the Board of Hospitals and

764

Homes of the Methodist Episcopal Church, and the Baptist Hospitals. A plan was drawn up for surveying hospitals to see whether they met the Minimum Standards. The hospitals accepted this plan, cooperated with the surveying teams, and invited criticism and advice regarding their shortcomings. Of the 692 hospitals surveyed in 1918, only 83 merited full approval. The number of approved hospitals gradually increased, and by 1952, of 4100 hospitals surveyed, 2834 were fully approved and 431 provisionally approved. Until 1952 the ACS assumed the responsibility and bore the expense for inspecting, rating, and accrediting hospitals. In January, 1952, this work was turned over to a new organization, *The Joint Commission on Accreditation of Hospitals,* composed of representatives of the American Medical Association, Canadian Medical Association, American Hospital Association, American College of Surgeons, and American College of Physicians. The Commission has revised and modernized the standards and has maintained and expanded the program of hospital surveys started by the College.

The ACS Committee on Graduate Training in Surgery began in 1937 to evaluate postgraduate (residency) training programs for surgeons. In 1940 the ACS published a list of 200 hospitals that met its Minimum Standards for Graduate Training in Surgery. In 1950 the ACS joined with the AMA and the American Board of Surgery to form the Conference Committee on Graduate Training in Surgery. Subsequently, similar conference committees were established for graduate training programs in various surgical specialties. By 1953 there were 1430 approved training courses in general surgery and the surgical specialties. Since then there has been a steady and marked increase in the number of approved programs.

Apart from its interest in upgrading hospitals and assuring good training programs in surgery, the ACS still devotes much of its work to the continuing education of surgical practitioners. The College takes the point of view that the postgraduate education of a surgeon is never-ending. There is an annual Clinical Congress, with forums, panel discussions, symposia, postgraduate courses, demonstration of operations (now usually by moving pictures or television), and demonstrations of new instruments, equipment, and methods, all designed to bring the surgeon up to date. In addition to the National Congress, there are Sectional Meetings in various regions of the United States and Canada and local Chapter Meetings for smaller groups, at which papers are read and new methods are demonstrated and discussed.

THE AMERICAN COLLEGE OF PHYSICIANS

The American College of Physicians (ACP) did not get off to such a quick and impressive start as did the ACS. Dr. Heinrich Stern of New York, during a visit to London in 1913, attended a meeting of the Royal College of Physicians of London and was so deeply stirred by what he saw that he resolved to try to establish a similar organization in the United States. He could not arouse much enthusiasm for his project, but by 1915 he had gathered together a large enough group of interested practitioners to have the American College of Physicians incorporated. The first meeting was held in New York City in June of that year.

765

During its first three years, the ACP grew only slightly and remained largely a New York City organization. It signed up a few scattered members from other cities, but when Dr. Stern died in 1918 there was serious question as to whether the still very small organization could be held together. In the early years, in order to increase the size of the College, the qualifications for membership were kept at a minimal level, and in order to be nearer the nation's center of population, the headquarters were moved to Chicago in 1921. As a further attraction to members, the College undertook the publication of a new clinical journal, the *Annals of Medicine*, but this venture failed after only three numbers had been published. Publication was started again in 1922 with a new name, *Annals of Clinical Medicine*, but without attracting many subscribers. Finally in 1927, after another change of name and with a new editor (Maurice C. Pincoffs), the *Annals of Internal Medicine* became a successful and much respected journal.

By 1925 the ACP had about 1000 members, but the names of most of the leaders of the profession and the heads of university departments of medicine were conspicuously lacking from its roster. One of the few leaders of academic medicine who took an interest in the College was the Professor of Medicine at the University of Pennsylvania, Alfred Stengel. Stengel was elected President of the ACP in 1925 and remained in office for two years, during which he put the organization on a much more businesslike footing. The headquarters were moved from Chicago to Philadelphia, and a layman with administrative experience was hired as full-time Executive Secretary. In 1928, when Charles F. Martin, Professor of Medicine at McGill University, was elected President he startled the College by refusing to accept the position unless certain fundamental changes were made in its policies. Martin had interviewed leaders in internal medicine from all parts of the country and had secured from many of them signed applications for membership in the College, but Dr. Martin stated that he was authorized to submit these applications "only on the promise of certain radical modifications in your policy and organization." The modifications that Martin said would have to be accepted by the Board of Regents of the College before he would submit the applications or accept the Presidency were as follows (Martin, 1940):

1. A new Board of Regents with adequate representation from the academic leaders, and I must ask the privilege of designating at least four.

2. This new Board must be given full power to raise the standards of admission; the present generous policy of expansion must be restricted so that the membership will be in keeping with our ideals.

3. There must be an entirely new and appropriate application form.

4. The headquarters of the Association must be established in Philadelphia.

5. There must be a readjustment of fees, on a lower scale.

To Martin's surprise his conditions were accepted unanimously by both the Board of Regents and the Board of Governors of the College. The prominent physicians whose applications Martin held in escrow became Fellows of the College and were soon numbered among its leaders. Since that time the ACP has risen steadily in importance and influence. Like the

766

ACS, the ACP has concentrated much of its effort on programs for the continuing education of physicians. There is an Annual Session of national scope (usually attended by several thousand physicians) and regional and state meetings, lectures, and demonstrations.

OTHER SPONSORS OF CONTINUING EDUCATION   In addition to the educational activities sponsored by the ACS and ACP, many medical schools now offer programs and courses (sometimes lasting for several weeks) to bring practicing physicians and surgeons up to date in both general and specialized fields. Two-way radio programs, with question-and-answer periods, for physicians, nurses, medical and X-ray technicians, and other categories of health personnel have also been organized under the auspices of the Regional Medical Program (RMP) and other agencies. One of the original objectives of the RMP was to acquaint practicing doctors with the most advanced methods for treating those suffering from heart disease, cancer, or stroke. The National Library of Medicine is also playing an increasingly important role in keeping the practitioner abreast of new developments.

NATIONAL LIBRARY OF MEDICINE— INFORMATION AND COMMUNICATION   The ghost of John Shaw Billings would never recognize the giant tree which has grown from the seedling that he tended so hopefully as the nation entered its second century. In 1864, the year before Billings became its Director, the Library of the Surgeon-General's Office contained 1365 volumes. The rate of growth before then had been slow (there were 200 volumes in 1840). Under the vigorous leadership of its new Director, the Library grew rapidly and in 1880 contained 50,000 volumes and 60,000 pamphlets. Since then the annual rate of growth has increased almost every year, and in 1975, after having undergone several changes in its name, the National Library of Medicine (NLM) contained more than 1.5 million items. By then the Library had moved to Bethesda, Maryland, where it is now housed in an imposing structure on the grounds of the National Institutes of Health.

The NLM places at the disposal of American physicians an information resource unsurpassed by that available for any other scientific discipline. At the core of its service to the profession are the two media that Billings conceived and initiated (p. 382): (1) the *Index-Catalogue of the Library of the Surgeon-General's Office,* now known as the *NLM Current Catalog;* and (2) the *Index Medicus,* which after going through several permutations and temporary lapses, is now published annually as originally planned. However, instead of the single volume that Billings produced annually, eight fat, heavy volumes are produced each year: two for items listed under the authors' names and six for listing by subject. The *Index Medicus* today carries indexed journal article entries from 2500 periodicals, selected from the more than 20,000 titles received by the NLM.

In the early days, the indexing and cataloging were the personal chores of Billings and his friend and colleague, Robert Fletcher. A government van delivered clothes baskets full of journals to Billings's house in Georgetown

767

each evening so he could review them for indexing. "He acknowledged that much of it was rubbish, 'for the proportion of what is both new and true is not much greater in medicine than in theology'" (Cummings, 1975).

Later, when data processing was coming to the fore, the items for indexing were placed on punch cards. In the 1950s, as the size of the task mounted, efforts were made to introduce a greater degree of automation into the process of indexing, assembling, and publishing the material. In 1959 a semiautomatic process was devised, using *Flexowriter* composing machines, *IBM* key-punches and sorters, and a *Listomatic* camera for composing column-width film. The final production of what was then called the *Cumulated Index Medicus* was shared by the NLM and the American Medical Association. The Library cumulated and filed the cards in proper sequence and photographed the cumulation in December. The photographic film was then delivered to the AMA, which printed, bound, and distributed each annual publication.

Because of the enormous number of items that were being cumulated and indexed each year, it became highly desirable to develop some means to search out items bearing upon a particular subject, such as a disease or a drug or an operation. This could have been done by utilizing the punch cards to conduct a search. But in the early 1960s, the fastest card sorter then available would handle only about 1000 cards per minute. To search a five-year file of 750,000 subject cards would have taken 12½ hours—obviously not a feasible way to cope with an anticipated large number of searches. Some better means had to be found. The means came into view in the years 1961 to 1964 with the development of MEDLARS (Medical Literature Analysis and Retrieval System). MEDLARS, which is a computer-based system, achieved automation of the publication of the *Index Medicus* and at the same time made possible searches of the literature on a wide range of medical subjects. In 1971 a refinement of the system became operational: MEDLINE (MEDLARS On-Line). MEDLINE is a system for making accessible a data base of recent journal article references—some 600,000 of them—indexed from 3000 biomedical journals, including all those indexed for the *Index Medicus*. The references are stored in the Library's computer and are accessible from terminals in some 300 hospitals, medical schools, and medical research institutions throughout the country (Cummings, 1975).

MEDLINE services are coordinated in each geographical area by a regional medical library, of which there are 10, located in established libraries in Boston, New York, Philadelphia, Detroit, Atlanta, Chicago, Omaha, Dallas, Seattle, and Los Angeles. In addition, the NLM in Bethesda serves as a regional library for the mid-Atlantic region.

At the regional libraries and the 300 institutions tied into the network, there are computer terminals resembling an ordinary electric typewriter. Each terminal is connected with the NLM computers through a telephone circuit. The individual who wishes to have a search made for articles on a particular subject utilizes the terminal (often with the assistance of a librarian) to carry on a dialogue with the computer to identify which of the 9000 medical subject headings recognized by the computer will best satisfy the searcher's needs. It may be a combination of several elements. Once the identification has been made, the computer locates the references, and the terminal typewriter prints out the requested bibliography in a series of individual citations, each of which lists author, title, and journal source. The entire search usually takes less than 15 minutes. If more than 25 references are involved, they are printed out at the NLM and mailed to the requester. The charge for a search depends upon length and complexity, but for an ordinary search in 1975 the charge did not exceed $8.50 (Cummings, 1975).

In addition to MEDLINE, there are other on-line data bases in the NLM computer system. These include TOXLINE, which provides access to about 350,000 references and abstracts in the field of toxicology and pharmacology, and CANCERLINE, sponsored in collaboration with the National Cancer Institute, which has some 40,000 *abstracts* of articles related to cancer research. The system also includes other specialized data bases.

Of special importance to the practicing physician is the National Medical Audiovisual Center in Atlanta, which has been part of the NLM system since 1967. The Center attempts to identify, collect, and evaluate audiovisual materials used in medical and dental education. The collected items judged to be accurate, sound in content, of good educational design, and high in technical quality become part of an on-line retrieval system known as AVLINE. This system went into operation on an experimental basis in May, 1975, when a test data base containing 250 references to material about the nervous system was released to 31 United States medical institutions. After the on-line retrieval system has been tested, it will be released nationwide, starting with a data base of about 900 citations to audiovisual materials. Through AVLINE, teachers, students, and practitioners will be able to search for the instructional audiovisuals that they desire. In order to supply these materials to requesters, the NLM in 1973 began a sales program for self-instructional audiovisuals, which are packaged at the Atlanta Center. These packages should be of great value for the continuing education of practitioners.

Before leaving this subject, mention should be made of the Lister Hill National Center for Biomedical Communications, which was established by act of Congress in 1968 and is now an organizational component of the NLM. This Center is concerned with coordinating interagency efforts within the federal government toward improving biomedical communications; and promoting research, development, and evaluation of advanced communications and computer technology, so as to improve networks and information systems for the betterment of health education, medical research, and the delivery of health services.

THE MEDICAL SECTS

In the nation's first century, practicing physicians had competition from homeopaths, eclectics, osteopaths, and several other sects (p. 41). When Abraham Flexner made his survey of the medical schools in 1910, he noted that most of the sectarian schools were unable to provide the type of education required for modern medical practice and that the sects were rapidly losing ground (p. 163). By the 1920s the eclectics had ceased to exist, and the once flourishing educational institutions of the homeopaths were rapidly going out of business. In 1921 the Regents of the University of Michigan voted to merge the homeopathic school (see p. 45) with the orthodox medical school and to provide only a single medical course leading to the M.D. degree. In 1922, Boston University, which had been an important homeopathic educational center, did not graduate a single homeopath, the Hahnemann College in Philadelphia graduated only 17, and throughout the nation there were only 62 homeopathic graduates. By 1923 only two homeopathic colleges were left—New York Homeopathic and Hahnemann of Philadelphia (Kaufman, 1971).

In spite of the small number of recent graduates, there were still many practicing homeopaths in the 1920s, and for the next three decades the leaders of the sect made a variety of efforts to preserve their identity as medical practitioners and to strengthen their educational institutions. A serious blow fell upon them in 1935 when the AMA Council on Medical Education and Hospitals resolved that after 1938 it would not include in its list of approved hospitals and medical schools any institution of "sectarian medicine." As a result, in 1936, the New York Homeopathic Medical College decided to change its name to the New York Medical College and to strive to maintain a *Class A* rating under the AMA criteria. Hahnemann of Philadelphia did not change its name, but it made some changes in its curriculum and also strove to be a *Class A* school. In 1960 the International Hahnemann Association voted itself out of existence, and at about this same time the American Board of Homeotherapeutics was established, with the hope that it would be accepted as a subspecialty of internal medicine within the structure of the AMA. This suggestion was refused by the AMA, and homeopathy continued to move toward extinction.

Osteopathy had done better than homeopathy in preserving its independence. In the early years of the twentieth century, the osteopathic colleges raised their educational standards and moved far enough in the direction of orthodox medicine to gain a degree of respectability in the eyes of the AMA. In the 1950s osteopaths began to gain greater recognition as physicians. In 1967 the House of Delegates of the AMA voted to authorize negotiations for the conversion of schools of osteopathy to orthodox schools. Although the leaders of osteopathy were striving to preserve their schools and maintain their identity, it seemed probable that they were following the same course that had led to the amalgamation of the homeopaths into the orthodox profession.

In discussing homeopathy (p. 163) Abraham Flexner said, "One cannot simultaneously assert science and dogma. . . . Homeopathy has two options: one to withdraw into the isolation in which alone any peculiar tenet can maintain itself; the other to put that tenet into the melting-pot." Flexner believed that "science, once embraced, will conquer the whole." This, it would seem, is what happened to both homeopathy and osteopathy. However, one healing-cult—chiropractic—escaped this fate by refusing to put its tenet into the melting-pot and by rejecting all rational science. For 80 years the chiropractors have clung doggedly to their tenet that disease is due to a misalignment of the vertebrae and may be cured by manipulating the vertebrae back into proper alignment. This doctrine was expounded by D. D. Palmer, a storekeeper and self-styled healer in Davenport, Iowa, who founded chiropractic medicine in 1895; and while orthodox medicine was learning how to prevent many diseases and how to cure many others with drugs or surgery, the chiropractors refused to deviate from their irrational tenet and continued to insist that the best treatment for any disease is manipulation of the spine. By 1910 chiropractic had not attained great enough prominence among the cults to warrant any comments by Flexner. But it evidently gave serious thought to what Flexner had said about the other cults. Carefully avoiding the melting-pot, it refused to permit its tenet to be tainted by science and not only survived but prospered. In 1971 there were 19,151 practitioners of chiropractic in the United States. In four states they cannot obtain a license to practice, and in most states they have only a limited license, which does not allow them to prescribe drugs, attend maternity patients, or perform surgery. As Firman and Goldstein have recently remarked: "The chiropractor functions to fulfill a need by 'legitimizing' the sick status of patients with whom physicians can find nothing wrong" (Firman and Goldstein, 1975).

Epilogue

There are perhaps few things upon which all men are so agreed as that the problems which beset them today surpass in difficulty those which confronted any previous generation. It is maintained that never has knowledge been so complex nor the pace of life so insistent; that never has it been so difficult to take thought on those larger considerations which allow men to appreciate the trend of events and the measures by which they might be controlled.

(Harold Himsworth, 1953)

As one contemplates the developments in American medicine during the past 200 years, one is impressed by the sharp contrast between the first and second centuries. During the first century, evidence of progress was barely detectable: medical education worsened; medical research was minimal; medical practice crept ahead a pace or two owing to the introduction of anesthesia and the abandonment of the fanciful system and harsh therapy of Benjamin Rush. The second century, on the other hand, presented an almost overwhelming crescendo of progress in all aspects of medicine: medical science, preventive medicine, medical education, and medical therapy. Along with these great advances, two other phenomena assumed major importance — the ascendency of government in medical affairs and the fantastic increase in medical costs.

The new knowledge that began to accumulate early in the second century had its initial impact upon preventive medicine. The discovery of bacteria and other parasitic causes of disease, the detection of the vectors (insects, etc.) that spread disease, and the disclosure that illness may result from the lack of certain substances in the diet all made possible effective prevention by the use of hygienic measures, insect and rodent control, antitoxins, vaccines, and surgical asepsis and by the addition of vitamins and other essential substances to the diet. The gains in the treatment of disease were at first less spectacular than the gains in prevention, but with improvements in medical education and clinical training, clinicians began to understand and apply the discoveries of their colleagues in the basic sciences and soon started to undertake investigations and make their own discoveries. Thus the physician came into possession of new diagnostic tools and effective therapeutic agents and techniques: antitoxic and antibacterial sera; antimicrobial chemicals such as salvarsan and the sulfa drugs; manipulation of dietary factors and electrolytes; diuretic agents; and hormones. With improved instruments and techniques and with the use of asepsis, intravenous fluids, and blood transfusions, surgeons found that they could operate on any area and enter any body cavity — abdomen, skull, thorax — to remove tumors and to correct defective or malfunctioning organs.

773

After World War II, explosive advances occurred almost simultaneously in many areas of medical science. The micro-organisms of the soil gave the chemists a series of lessons in how to synthesize powerful antimicrobial agents, and as a result penicillin, streptomycin, and a host of related antibiotics followed one another in rapid succession. The new immunology, working in partnership with the new virology, made it possible to prevent yellow fever, poliomyelitis, and rubella and thus head off premature death, crippling disability, and congenital defects. Stunning achievements in genetics disclosed how abnormal genes and chromosomes lead to physical and mental defects and made it possible to prevent certain abnormalities by (1) better selection of marital partners; (2) amniocentesis followed by selective interruption of pregnancies; and (3) supplying genetically deficient chemicals. New hormonal substances became available for the treatment of endocrine deficiencies and cancer and for the prevention of pregnancy. New drugs for the treatment of psychiatric disorders allowed many patients to leave mental institutions for a more normal life in the home environment. Improved methods for the prevention and/or treatment of syphilis, rheumatic fever, and hypertension brought about a reduction in the incidence of secondary heart disease, and it was expected that the prevention of rubella and improved genetic surveillance would result in a reduction in congenital heart disease. Of the many advances in operative surgery, none gave better evidence of the enhanced skills of the surgeon than the new operations on the heart, the transplantation of organs, and the operations on the hands for arthritic deformities and on the ears for the relief of certain types of deafness. There were also many new mechanical, electrical, and electronic devices for extending the useful life of those who had defective or malfunctioning organs: artificial kidneys, cardiac pacemakers, prosthetic joints, and hearing aids.

American scientists were at the forefront of these advances, making many of the fundamental discoveries, and American public health workers and medical practitioners successfully applied the discoveries for the prevention and treatment of disease. Between the basic scientists and the practicing physicians were the clinical investigators, who occupied a position of major importance in education and training for both practice and research and whose contributions to new knowledge raised clinical science to a level equal to that of other biological sciences.

Many of the great advances, particularly those of the last three decades of the nation's second century, would not have been possible without the vast financial and physical resources made available by the federal government. Philanthropic giving, which had played such a vital role in the progress during the early years of the twentieth century, continued to be important (Blendon, 1975), but its contributions were dwarfed by the magnitude of the expenditures by the federal government. The extent and rapidity of the rise in federal expenditures for research is indicated by the following figures. The appropriations for research by the National Institutes of Health (NIH) amounted to only $85,000 in 1945; by 1950, total federal support for medical research reached $74 million, of which $25 million went to the NIH; by 1955, the total federal contribution had reached $139 million and by 1974, $2.75 billion, of which 71 per cent was expended through the NIH (including the National Institute for Mental Health). The total national expenditure for medical research in 1974 was $4.25 billion; of this sum, $2.75 billion was expended by the federal government, $1.18 billion by industry (research on drugs, medical equipment, supplies, and other areas), and the remaining $320 million came largely from private, nonprofit organizations, whose contributions made up less than 6 per cent of the total (Burger, 1975).

Lewis Thomas (1971) has pointed out that it is assumed that medical technology simply exists and that our only problem today is to determine how best to deliver this technology with equity to all people. Thomas holds that such a simplistic view does not represent the true situation. In order to provide a better understanding of the current status of the delivery of medical care, he divides the technology of medicine into three categories: (1) nontechnology, (2) halfway technology, and (3) decisive technology.

(1) *Nontechnology* cannot be measured in terms of its capacity to alter either the force of disease or its eventual outcome. It is supportive or standby therapy, not directed at the underlying causes of disease, but nevertheless is indispensable; and it consumes a large portion of any good doctor's time. The diseases that require this type of nontechnological management are exemplified by intractable cancer, severe arthritis, multiple sclerosis, stroke, and advanced cirrhosis of the liver. Long periods of institutional care are required, and many professional and nonprofessional personnel are involved both in and out of the hospital. The cost is very high and getting higher as time passes; it represents a substantial segment of today's expenditures for health.

(2) *Halfway technology* involves efforts to compensate for the incapacitating effects of diseases whose course one is unable to do very much about. The spectacular quality of these halfway techniques has attracted the attention of the news media, who tend to present each new device as a triumphant breakthrough in therapy instead of the makeshift that it really is. Much of what is done in the treatment of cancer by surgery, irradiation, and chemotherapy, though sometimes impressive, is no more than halfway technology; it is treatment after-the-fact and would be unnecessary if we knew how to prevent cancer. The new bypass operations for occlusion of the coronary arteries fall into this same class and would not be needed if we knew how to prevent arteriosclerosis. Similarly, artificial kidneys and kidney transplants would not be required if we knew how to prevent the glomerular destruction associated with certain diseases. It is characteristic of halfway technology that it costs an enormous amount of money and requires continuing expansion of hospital facilities and equipment. There is no end to the need for new highly trained people to run such an elaborate medical empire, and there is every prospect that the empire will continue to expand in the present state of our knowledge. Medicine can move away from this level of technology only if new information is brought forth by research.

(3) Examples of *decisive technology* are immunization against bacterial and viral diseases, the treatment of infectious diseases with antibiotics and chemicals, the use of hormones to treat endocrinological disorders, the prevention of hemolytic disease of the newborn, and the prevention and treatment of nutritional disorders. Though the benefits of these decisive measures have not yet been fully realized, the shortcomings are due to social rather than medical factors. The important consideration is that this type of technology comes as the result of research that has provided a genuine under-

standing of the mechanisms of disease; and when the mechanisms are known, effective prevention or treatment is relatively inexpensive, relatively simple, and relatively easy to deliver. The cost is never as great as that of managing the same disease by nontechnology or halfway technology. For example, if typhoid fever had to be managed today by the approved methods of 1935, the expense would be staggering: 50 days in hospital; the most demanding type of nursing care around the clock; obsessive concern for the details of diet; daily monitoring of various laboratory procedures; and, on occasion, surgical intervention for intestinal hemorrhage or perforation. The bill for all this would probably be of the order of $20,000. This stands in sharp contrast with today's cost of treatment: a bottle of chloramphenicol and two or three days in bed at home. Another illustration of contrasting costs is the huge expense of caring for a case of paralytic poliomyelitis versus the cost of vaccination.

Thomas concludes his note with the following paragraph:

> It is when physicians are bogged down by their incomplete technologies, by the innumerable things they are obliged to do in medicine when they lack a clear understanding of disease mechanisms, that the deficiencies of the health-care system are most conspicuous. If I were a policy-maker, interested in saving money for health care over the long haul, I would regard it as an act of high prudence to give high priority to a lot more basic research in biologic science. This is the only way to get the full mileage that biology owes to the science of medicine, even though it seems, as used to be said in the days when the phrase still had some meaning, like asking for the moon.

Thomas sees the problems of medicine through the eyes of an experienced and thoughtful physician, and he is convinced that the best solution will come through greater emphasis on basic research. In his view, only when we have the information that will enable us to prevent more diseases or to treat them more decisively will we be able to dispel the image of the costly incubus that medicine has assumed in the eyes of many people.

Several years ago the news media were full of disturbing information about the "national health-care crisis" and the "non-system of American medicine," and a frantic search was on for those who were responsible for the crisis and for ways quickly to put the medical profession back on a proper course (Schwartz, 1975a). Fortunately, precipitate action was avoided, and a more careful analysis of the defects in the American system and of alternative means to overcome those defects is now in progress. The major concerns of the public, as voiced by politicians, social workers, and others closely in touch with human problems, are as follows: (1) the already high and continually rising cost of medical care; (2) the declining number and the maldistribution of family (primary) physicians; (3) the inequitable distribution of the fruits of medical progress. These concerns will be considered in order:

(1) Medical expenditures have, indeed, risen at an alarming rate. A report released on April 25, 1976, by the President's Council on Wage and Price Stabilization stated that health costs in 1975 had reached $118.5 billion, 40 per cent of it paid by federal, state, and local governments and that an average American family had to spend 10 per cent of its income to meet health costs (Hicks, 1976). The Consumer Price Index for 1975 indicated that health costs, compared with the preceding year, had risen 10.3 per cent while the cost of services other than health had risen 7.7 per cent.

Fein (1975) has pointed out that in considering the rising cost of medical care, one must make a distinction between prices and expenditures. He cites estimates made by the Social Security Administration, which indicated that of the $38.4 billion increase in the national health expenditures during the fiscal years 1965 to 1972, about 52 per cent reflected a rise in prices, while 10 per cent was the result of population growth, and the remaining 38 per cent was attributable to greater utilization of services and the introduction of new techniques. It may be added that the rise in prices was due in part to the general inflation. In brief, about half the rise in expenditures was due to increased charges for services and half to population growth and the utilization of additional services. Fein also points out that in the almost two years of federal price controls (in the early 1970s), medical care prices rose by less than 4 per cent per annum and yet medical care expenditures rose at about 12 per cent per annum. Similarly, in the fiscal years 1960 to 1966, while medical expenditures rose 11 per cent per annum, the rise in medical prices was only 3 per cent per annum.

It is necessary, therefore, when one reads the frightening reports of increased national medical expenditures, that one should have in mind the distinction between increased prices and increased expenditures. Nevertheless, regardless of economic niceties, the total effect is brought home to the individual by the increase in the cost of his or her Blue Cross and other health insurance premiums; and it is impressed on local, state, and federal governments by what they must pay on behalf of Medicaid and Medicare patients. The increased expenditures are due in part to an increase in the price of specific services and in part to an increase in the number and variety of services provided, and, in the case of Medicaid and Medicare, an additional factor is the increase in the number of eligible individuals.

Apart from increased prices and utilization, a major component of higher health expenditures is the rise in hospital costs. The factors responsible for these increased costs have been discussed in Chapter 31. As Thomas has pointed out, the treatment of patients by nontechnology and halfway technology accounts for a large share of the expenditures for hospital care. Included among the patients who receive such treatment is the increasing number of those who are hopelessly ill, sometimes in an irreversible coma, sometimes demented, sometimes old and wanting to die (Netsky, 1976). Until we can solve the moral and legal problems posed by this type of care, the cost will inevitably mount. The PSRO mechanism and the efforts of state and federal authorities may succeed in slowing the rise in hospital costs, but it is difficult to see how the effect can be very great upon the hopelessly ill, who "require" hospitalization, unless there is a radical change in the attitude toward the treatment of such patients.

(2) With regard to primary-care physicians, efforts that are being made to deal with this problem are meeting with some success. More physicians are being trained for family practice. The National Health Service Corps is providing doctors for some areas that lacked them. "Physician extenders" such as nurse practitioners and physician's assistants are helping to fill some of the gaps. The final answer to this problem is not yet in sight, but it may come from training two types of practitioners, one to serve as primary physicians, the other to serve as specialists. This has been done in other countries.

(3) The equitable distribution of the fruits of medical progress presents many problems, of which the most formidable is the price that has to be paid. As a result of the advances in medical science and technology, there is now almost no limit to the cost of the best in medical care. With modern drugs, respirators, cardiac pacemakers, intravenous feedings, artificial kidneys, expert nursing care, and other developments, death can be postponed for weeks, months, even years for those who are beyond any hope of recovery. There is general agreement that the full benefit of decisive technology should be available to everyone. There is less agreement about whether it is economically feasible to give equitable distribution to the many "halfway" technological advances.

A recent report from the Massachusetts General Hospital (Cullen et al., 1976) describes a study of 226 consecutive critically ill patients entering the Recovery Room–Acute Care Unit (RR–ACU) of that hospital between July 1, 1972, and June 30, 1973. The average age of these patients was 59 years, and the average period of hospitalization was 35 days. All of them were admitted to the RR–ACU in critical condition, and all were treated by the best methods that a fine modern hospital can offer. At the end of one month, 54 per cent of the patients were dead, 31 per cent were still in the hospital, and only 1 of the 103 survivors had fully recovered. By 12 months, 73 per cent had died, and 12 per cent had made a satisfactory recovery. The hospitalization charges for the 226 patients came to $3,232,647 (exclusive of physicians' fees), or an average of $14,304 per patient. The greatest expenditures were for the one-to-one expert nursing care required in such cases and for the transfusions of blood and blood fractions, which alone accounted for 21 per cent of the total cost. In speaking of the high mortality rate in these elaborately treated, critically ill patients, the authors point out that:

> Although these costly deaths do not occur nationwide, they become commonplace as more rather than fewer patients receive intensive care until their death. Medical science continues to improve the physicians' ability to maintain and prolong life. Quite properly, those responsible for advancing medical frontiers do not consider the financial impact of providing increasingly costly, high quality medical care on a large scale. Yet economically these costs are becoming intolerable and will be self-limiting in yet undetermined ways. We believe that once accepted for intensive care, cost restraints should not compromise efforts or be factors in providing less than the best care available.

Cullen and his colleagues suggest that cost control in such cases might be achieved in two ways: by refusing to accept patients for whom intensive care is inappropriate, and by discontinuing intensive care for patients whose survival to a successful outcome is highly unlikely. These decisions must be guided by adequate diagnostic evaluation and must be based on "a consideration of ethics, logic, sound information, and prospective data." The authors note that three hospitals have already developed guidelines to aid in these matters.

The dilemma presented by Cullen's cases is one that has to be faced with increasing frequency: whether to utilize every resource of modern medicine to prolong the life of the individual, or whether, in the best interest of society (i.e., keeping down the overall cost of medical care), to utilize the high-powered resources only when there is a reasonable prospect of a successful outcome. Many physicians would feel that in choosing the second of these alternatives they would be forsaking their traditional position, which since the days of Hippocrates has been to favor the individual rather than society (Bunker, 1976). Moreover, the second alternative would be more attractive if prognosis could be determined with greater precision, if, for example, Cullen had been able to select for intensive care only the 12 per cent who were destined to make a satisfactory recovery, thus avoiding the tremendous expense of treating the other 88 per cent. Unfortunately, prognosis cannot be made with such a high degree of accuracy, though, doubtless, it would have been possible to predict inevitable failure in many of the 88 per cent.

To place a lid on the steadily escalating medical costs and to achieve better distribution of both family physicians and top-quality medical care, some of our most eminent political leaders have been advocating, for close to half a century, that we adopt a compulsory system of national health insurance (NHI). Whatever merits such a system may have, a saving in overall costs without impairment in quality is not likely to be among them. Previous efforts by the federal government to improve the delivery of health services — the Hill-Burton program, Medicare, Medicaid, and the mental health program — have invariably cost far more than their legislative proponents estimated. The blame for the overruns has been placed on unconscionable doctors' fees, unrestrained hospital administrators, and the lack of adequate controls over the American "nonsystem" of medical service, but certainly part of the blame should be attributed to the open-ended character of any system that undertakes to deliver all of the fruits of medical progress. When financial restraints are removed, there is almost no limit to the tests and examinations and the medical and surgical therapy that can be justified in the interest of preventive medicine and prolongation of life. When face to face with the problems of a sick individual, doctors are not inclined to give first consideration to the cost effectiveness of the treatment they recommend.

In Britain, where tax-supported medical care is said to be "free" for everyone, rationing of services has been necessary. Dr. David Owen, who is in charge of the British National Health Service, in answer to complaints about inadequacies in the Service, recently stated: "The health service is a rationed service. There will never be a government or a country that has enough resources to meet all of the demands any nation will make on a national health service" (Schwartz, 1975b).

The nominal leadership of the medical profession has been in the hands of the American Medical Association. In 1975 this organization had 173,000 dues-paying members, up from 70,000 in 1910. Over the years the AMA has exhibited impressive political strength, much of it directed toward defeating legislative measures to which it was opposed. It has consistently taken a strong stand against compulsory national health insurance (see p. 368). Some of the arguments in support of its position have seemed sound and reasonable; they have, at least, served to postpone the adoption of a national insurance scheme until its pros and cons can be aired and debated more thoroughly.

In the first decade of the twentieth century, when the affairs of the AMA were guided by such progressive and innovative leaders as W. H. Welch, W. J. Mayo, W. C. Gorgas, and Frank Billings, there was no inclination to doubt that its leadership represented all classes of physicians. But after World War II, increased specialization, the advent of full-time medical teachers, and the growing emphasis on research tended to attract many of the

779

best medical minds to interests and associations other than the AMA. As a result, the voice of the AMA became increasingly the voice of medical practitioners rather than the voice of all segments of the profession. In recent years much of the lay press has assumed an antagonistic attitude toward the AMA. These journalists have nurtured the impression that the Association's chief interest is in preserving the favorable financial status of practicing physicians and surgeons and that its opposition to NHI and certain other national programs has been motivated by this overriding concern for the doctors' pocketbook. This unfortunate public image has served to obscure the outstanding achievements, in the public interest, that should be credited to the AMA, its Councils, Bureaus, and Committees. Nevertheless, the leaders of the Association are not the leaders of medical education and medical research, and although its membership includes outstanding specialists in various fields of medicine, most of them consider that their primary allegiance is to their specialty society.

The leadership of the AMA has also been weakened by its failure to obtain solid backing from the medical profession; in spite of its large membership, there are areas where the majority of physicians are not AMA members. It was recently reported, for example, that less than half of the doctors in the State of Massachusetts were members (American Medical News, April 26, 1976). From time to time various groups of the medical profession, chiefly among educators and research workers, have been outspoken in their opposition to AMA policies.

It has, therefore, not been possible for the AMA as presently constituted, or for any other medical organization, to exert the type of leadership that is required to guide the health affairs of the nation. This is not as it should be, for as Edwards (1975) has said, the health professions should not "assign to others a role that we alone can fully discharge, the role of health leadership for the nation." It is not difficult to see that a wise, well-informed, unselfish type of medical leadership is badly needed, but no one seems to know just how it can be generated. Perhaps the reincarnation of William Henry Welch would suffice.

In addition to the need for a more effective leadership, there is also a need for the provision of better public information on health matters. Many people seem totally unaware of the great forward strides that have been made during the past hundred years.

One of the purposes of this book has been to show how medical science has advanced during the past two centuries and how the advance in science has been translated into the prevention and cure of disease. The practitioner of medicine is today far more effective than he was in 1776 or 1876 because of the resources that have been made available to him by medical research. Many of the basic discoveries that have been responsible for the most far-reaching improvements in prevention and therapy have been made not by those engaged in the practice of medicine but by those, often not possessors of the M.D. degree, who have worked in laboratories. For example, the sensational advances in surgery, though attributable in part to the new technical skills of surgeons, would not have been possible without basic discoveries in other fields: the development of anesthesia by Morton, a dentist; the discovery of the relation of bacteria to infections by Pasteur, a chemist turned bacteriologist; the discovery of blood groups by Landsteiner, an immunologist; and the discovery by Fleming, a bacteriologist, that a mold can produce a powerful antibacterial substance. Without anesthesia, asepsis, blood transfusions, and antibiotics, surgery would be little better today than it was in 1825.

This book should have made it clear that our incomplete technologies (in Thomas's sense) are extraordinarily costly methods of administering medical care. Though one can sympathize with the public demand for a wider distribution of these technologies, the public should be made aware that their demands can be met only at greater cost and that there is no evidence that the cost can be reduced under a national health insurance program without resort to some sort of rationing of services.

This book should also have made it clear that basic medical research in the past century has led to the development of simple, effective, and inexpensive methods for preventing and curing many diseases. And, again, the public should know that the promotion of research of this basic, noncategorical type offers the best hope of achieving a wider distribution of effective medical care at an affordable cost.

Shortly before the Rockefeller Institute celebrated its tenth anniversary, two laymen who had played important roles in altering the course of American medical history, President Eliot of Harvard and Frederick T. Gates, John D. Rockefeller's principal advisor, were strolling down Broadway together. Mr. Gates remarked that the Rockefeller Institute was to him "the most interesting thing in the world." President Eliot said that he felt precisely the same way and asked, "Why is this so?" To which Gates replied (Morison, 1975):

> "It is so for one thing: if one stops to think about it for a moment, because the values of research are universal values. The nations have their racial antagonisms and their peculiar ideals and their distinctive literatures. Authors, the greatest of them, can speak in a single language only and are little heard in the other tongues. Statesmen, in general, are confined in their influence to single nations; the empires of kings are limited. But here is an institution or in this medical research is a work, the value of which touches the life of every man that lives. Think of that!"

Appendix A

POPULATION OF THE UNITED STATES, URBAN AND RURAL

	Total	Urban		Rural	
Year	Population	Number	Per Cent	Number	Per Cent
1800	5,300,000*	200,000	3.8	5,100,000	96.2
1850	23,200,000	3,500,000	15.3	19,600,000	84.7
1870	38,600,000	9,900,000	25.7	28,700,000	74.3
1880	50,200,000	14,100,000	28.2	36,000,000	71.8
1890	62,900,000	22,100,000	35.1	40,800,000	64.9
1900	76,000,000	30,200,000	39.7	45,800,000	60.3
1910	92,000,000	42,000,000	45.7	50,000,000	54.3
1920	105,700,000	54,200,000	51.2	51,600,000	48.8
1930	122,800,000	69,000,000	56.2	53,800,000	43.8
1940	131,700,000	74,400,000	56.5	57,300,000	43.5
1950	151,300,000	96,800,000	64.0	54,500,000	36.0
1960	179,300,000	125,300,000	69.9	54,000,000	30.1
1970	203,200,000	149,400,000	73.5	53,800,000	26.5
1975	213,100,000**				

*The population figures have been rounded off to the nearest 100,000.
**Mid-decade estimate of Census Bureau.

Appendix B
Chronological Summary of Major Events in American Medical History

1776 Declaration of Independence.

1777 William Shippen chosen Director General of Army Medical Department.
Scheele's experiments with silver chloride lay groundwork for photography.

1778 William Brown publishes first American *Pharmacopoeia* in Philadelphia.
Rush describes dengue fever in Philadelphia.

1779 Mesmer's memoir on animal magnetism published.

1780 Benjamin Franklin invents bifocal lenses.
American Academy of Arts and Sciences founded in Boston.

1781 Massachusetts Medical Society founded.

1782 Medical Department of Harvard University founded.

1783 Royal Society of Edinburgh founded.

1784 King's College (New York) rechartered as Columbia College.
James Watt constructs steam radiator for his workroom.

1785 Watt patents device for smoke abatement.

1786 Parry describes exophthalmic goiter.

1787 College of Physicians of Philadelphia founded.
Adoption of the U.S. Constitution.

1789 Edward Wigglesworth constructs first American life-table.
Medical and Chirurgical Faculty of Maryland incorporated.

1790 First United States Census.

1791 Medical Department of Columbia College (New York) reorganized.
William Baynham of Virginia operates for extrauterine pregnancy.
Opening of the New York Hospital.

1792 Cotton gin invented by Eli Whitney.

1793 Matthew Cary describes yellow fever epidemic in Philadelphia.
Bell differentiates between syphilis and gonorrhea.

1794 Dalton describes colorblindness.
Board of Health started in Philadelphia.

1796 Jenner vaccinates William Phipps.
Board of Health established in New York City.
Yellow fever epidemic in Boston.

1797 Medical Department of Dartmouth College founded.
First publication of the *Medical Repository*.

1798 United States Marine Hospital Service established.
Jenner's *Inquiry* published.
Paul Revere heads Board of Health in Boston.

1799 Death of George Washington.
Medical School of Transylvania University founded (opened 1817).
Davy discovers anesthetic properties of "laughing gas" (nitrous oxide).

1800 Benjamin Waterhouse introduces jennerian vaccination in New England.

1801 Pinel publishes his treatise on psychiatry.
Ritter experiments with ultraviolet rays.

1802 United States Marine Hospitals established at Norfolk and Boston.

1803 Otto describes family with hemophilia in New England.

1804 Dalton states atomic theory.

1805 First Boston Medical Library founded.
Sertürner isolates morphine.
Philip Syng Physick appointed to Chair of Surgery at University of
 Pennsylvania.

1806 Fulton invents the steamboat.

1807 University of Maryland Medical School founded.
College of Physicians and Surgeons (New York) founded.
John Stearns of Saratoga County (New York) publishes first account of the
 physiological effects of ergot.

1809 McDowell performs first ovariotomy.
Yale Medical School founded.

1810 Daniel Drake publishes first clinical description of "milk sickness."

1811 Elisha North describes cerebrospinal meningitis and is among first to emphasize importance of the clinical thermometer.
Massachusetts General Hospital founded.

1812 First independent village medical school founded at Herkimer, N.Y.
(College of Physicians and Surgeons of the Western District).
Bellevue Hospital (New York) established.
Rush publishes his famous *Diseases of the Mind.*
New England Journal of Medicine and Surgery first published.

1815 Laennec discovers mediate auscultation.

1816 Laennec perfects stethoscope.

1818 Vermont Medical Academy established.
Valentine Mott successfully ligates innominate artery.

1819 Medical College of Ohio founded.

1820 First official U.S. *Pharmacopoeia* published.

1821 Opening of the Massachusetts General Hospital.
Philadelphia College of Pharmacy founded.
McGill University founded.

1822 Widespread epidemic of yellow fever along East Coast.
James Jackson describes alcoholic neuritis.

1823 James Fenimore Cooper publishes *The Pioneers.*

1824 Purkinje establishes a laboratory of physiology in Breslau.

1825 Liebig establishes first chemistry laboratory open to students and investigators (Giessen).
American Journal of Pharmacy published (first in English).
Beaumont begins his studies on Alexis St. Martin.

1829 Daguerre introduces photography.

1831 Chloroform discovered by Samuel Guthrie.

1832 Bobiquet isolates codeine.
British Medical Association founded.
Year of the great cholera epidemic on the Atlantic coast.
Boston Lying-in Hospital established.
Faraday describes galvanic and magnetic induction.

1833 William Beaumont publishes studies on gastric digestion.

1834 Runge isolates carbolic acid and discovers analine.
Dumas obtains and names pure chloroform.

1835 *Discourse on Self-Limited Diseases* published by Jacob Bigelow.
Louis first uses statistics in clinical analysis.
Berzelius coins the term "catalysis."

1836 First dermatological clinic in U.S. (Broome St. Infirmary, New York City).
Rush Medical College (Chicago) chartered (opened 1843).

1838 Tremont Street School founded (Boston).
Medical College of Richmond (Virginia) founded.
Isaac Ray's treatise *On the Medical Jurisprudence of Insanity* published.

1839 American Statistical Association founded (Boston).
Pennock invents first flexible-tube stethoscope.
Schwann publishes treatise on the cell theory.

1840 Basedow describes exophthalmic goiter.
Samuel Gross conducts experimental study of wounds of the intestine.
Henle publishes statement of germ theory of communicable diseases.

1841 Dorothea Lynde Dix becomes interested in the plight of lunatics.

1843 Publication of Oliver Wendell Holmes's classic paper, *The contagiousness of puerperal fever.*

1844 Wells begins to use "laughing gas" for anesthesia.
Founding of the forerunner of the American Psychiatric Association.

1846 J.C. Warren performs first operation using anesthesia after ether introduced by Morton.
Marion Sims invents vaginal speculum.

1847 Founding of the American Medical Association.
Boylston Medical School founded (Boston).
New York Academy of Medicine founded.
Simpson introduces chloroform anesthesia.
Semmelweis discovers pathogenesis of puerperal fever.

1848 American Association for the Advancement of Science founded.
Fehling introduces test for sugar in the urine.
Claude Bernard demonstrates that glycogen is synthesized in the liver.

1849 Marion Sims operates for vesicovaginal fistula.
John Snow publishes views on waterborne cholera.

1850 Women's Medical College of Philadelphia founded.
Daniel Drake publishes his classic, *The Diseases of the Interior Valley of North America.*
Founding of the University of Michigan Medical School.
First thoracentesis by Henry Bowditch.
William Detwold (New York) opens an abscess of the brain.
Claude Bernard publishes his studies on arrow poisons (curare).

1851 Reid devises reduction of dislocations by simple manipulation.
Medical faculty of Georgetown University founded.
Helmholtz invents the ophthalmoscope.

1852 American Pharmaceutical Association founded.

1853 Pliny Earle appointed visiting physician to New York Asylum and gives first lectures on mental disease at College of Physicians and Surgeons.

1854 California Academy of Sciences founded.

1855 Marion Sims founds Hospital for Women's Diseases (New York City).
Louisiana establishes first State Board of Health.
St. Elizabeth's Hospital opened in Washington, D.C.
Goedcke extracts cocaine from coca leaves.

1856 Perkin obtains analine dyes.
Virchow establishes first laboratory of pathology in Berlin.

1857 Pathological Society of Philadelphia founded.

1859 Chicago Medical College (later Northwestern) founded by Nathan Smith Davis.
Publication of Florence Nightingale's *Notes on Hospitals.*
Darwin's *Origin of Species* published.

786

1860 Pasteur demonstrates presence of bacteria in the air.

1861 Massachusetts Institute of Technology founded.

1862 Florence Nightingale establishes training school for nurses at St. Thomas'
     Hospital (London).
     Péan devises first hemostat.

1863 American Veterinary Medical Association organized.
     National Academy of Sciences founded.

1864 Weir Mitchell describes causalgia.
     Use of milk from diseased cows prohibited (Boston).

1865 Lister introduces antiseptic treatment of wounds.
     Woodward first to use analine dyes for histopathological studies in the U.S.
     Gregor Mendel publishes his notes on plant hybridity.
     Billings becomes Surgeon-General's librarian.
     Cornell University founded.

1866 Metropolitan Health Board founded (New York City).
     Marion Sims publishes *Clinical Notes on Uterine Surgery.*

1867 Lister introduces antiseptic surgery.
     Bobbs performs cholecystectomy.
     First International Medical Congress (Paris).
     Canadian Medical Association established.

1868 James Lenox founds Presbyterian Hospital (New York).
     American Otological Society founded (Boston).

1869 Brown-Séquard introduces doctrine of internal secretions.
     Wunderlich publishes treatise on clinical thermometry.
     American Journal of Obstetrics founded.
     Liebreich demonstrates hypnotic effect of chloral hydrate.
     Ludwig establishes Physiological Institute at Leipzig.

1870 Fritsch and Hitzig study localization of brain function.

1871 First American physiological laboratory established at Harvard (Bowditch).
     Darwin's *Descent of Man* published.
     Hoppe-Seyler discovers nuclein (DNA) in white blood corpuscles.
     First American filter for water supply (Poughkeepsie, N.Y.).
     Hammarsten discovers role of fibrinogen in coagulation of the blood.

1872 Wyman describes "autumnal catarrh" (hay fever).
     American Public Health Association holds first meeting.
     Spencer Wells improves hemostat.
     Hoppe-Seyler establishes laboratory of physiological chemistry (Strassburg).

1873 Budd's treatise on *Typhoid Fever: Its Nature, Mode of Spreading and Pre-
     vention* published.
     Gull describes myxedema.

1874 First laboratory of physiological chemistry in U.S. founded at Yale
     (Chittenden).
     Miescher investigates nucleoproteids (DNA).
     Illinois law regulating food supply.

1875 Pepper describes bone marrow changes in pernicious anemia.
     Weir Mitchell introduces "rest cure."
     Chesebrough obtains vaseline.
     Landois discovers hemolysis from transfusion of alien blood.
     Hardy and Gerard introduce pilocarpine.

1876 The Johns Hopkins University founded.

Billings publishes *Specimen Fasciculus* (forerunner of *Index Catalogue of the Surgeon-General's Library*).

American Dermatological Association founded.

American Chemical Society founded.

Horner describes X-linked recessive pattern of colorblindness.

Construction of new Cook County Hospital (Chicago) begins.

Kohle isolates salicylic acid.

Pictet invents artificial manufacture of ice.

Nitze introduces the cystoscope.

1877 Sayre introduces plaster-of-Paris jacket for treatment of Pott's disease.

Bollinger and Israel describe actinomycosis.

Opening of the Hospital of the University of Michigan Medical School.

Esmarch introduces aseptic bandage.

Pasteur discovers bacillus of malignant edema.

1878 Edison invents platinum-wire electric lamp.

Marine Hospital Service takes over national quarantine duties.

Welch, Prudden, Sternberg, and Salmon introduce bacteriology into the U.S.

Halsted invents new hemostat (the Halsted clamp).

Pettenkofer opens first experimental laboratory for hygiene.

1879 Billings and Fletcher start *Index Medicus.*

First chemically standardized pharmaceutical preparation, *Liquor Ergotae Purificatus,* introduced by Parke-Davis.

Congress creates National Board of Health.

Neisser discovers the gonococcus.

Manson discovers transmission of filariasis by the mosquito.

1880 Pasteur discovers streptococcus, staphylococcus, and pneumococcus (latter described independently by Sternberg).

American Surgical Association founded.

J. S. Billings constructs life-tables from data of U.S. Census.

Eberth discovers the typhoid bacillus.

Laveran discovers the parasite of malarial fever.

1881 Pasteur produces vaccine against anthrax.

Food and Drug Law passed in New York State.

Carlos Finlay surmises transmission of yellow fever by mosquito.

American Federation of Labor founded.

Koch introduces gelatin bacteriological media and steam sterilization.

1882 Michael Reese Hospital (Chicago) opened.

Atwater and Rosa construct first calorimeter in U.S.

Koch discovers the tubercle bacillus.

1883 Conner (Cincinnati) performs a gastrectomy.

Pennsylvania Anatomical Law passed.

Publication of the *Journal of the American Medical Association* begins.

Martin, Howell, and Donaldson give early statement of the *law of the heart* (later known as Starling's law).

Klebs discovers the diphtheria bacillus.

Kjeldahl introduces method of estimating nitrogen.

Golgi introduces silver stain for nervous tissue.

Koch discovers cholera bacillus.

Metchnikoff states phagocytic theory of immunity.

1884 Nicolaier discovers tetanus bacillus.

Emmerich isolates colon bacillus, subsequently described in more detail by Escherich in 1886.

1885 Halsted introduces conduction anesthesia.

Reilly (U.S. Army) constructs first incinerator.

First Visiting Nurse Association organized in Buffalo, N.Y.
Pasteur first uses his anti-rabies vaccine.
Corning of New York discovers spinal anesthesia.
von Ziemssen establishes first clinical laboratory.

1886 Nuttall notes bactericidal power of the blood serum, leading to humoral
    theory of immunity.
Fitz describes pathology and clinical features of appendicitis.
Weir Mitchell and Reichert investigate serpent venoms.
Association of American Physicians organized.
Salmon and Smith show that killed bacterial cultures can be used as vaccines.
von Bergman introduces steam sterilization in surgery.
Marie establishes relationship of acromegaly to the pituitary gland.

1887 Sewall immunizes pigeons against rattlesnake venom.
American Orthopedic Association founded.
Mall and Halsted develop technique of bowel suture—essential for bowel
    surgery.

1888 Marine Biology Laboratory at Woods Hole, Mass., founded.
American Association of Anatomists founded.
Artificial drinking straws introduced.
Vaughan establishes Michigan State Hygiene Laboratory.
Sternberg opens first private bacteriology laboratory (Brooklyn).
Roux and Yersin discover diphtheria toxin.
Osler describes hereditary form of angioedema.

1889 The Johns Hopkins Hospital opens.
Vaughan and Novy teach formal course in bacteriology at University of
    Michigan.
The Mayo Clinic opens.
Halsted introduces rubber gloves into surgery.
McBurney describes "McBurney's point" and advises early operation for
    appendicitis.
Halsted devises new operations for inguinal hernia and cancer of the breast.

1890 Bowditch demonstrates nonfatigability of nerves.
Babcock develops method of estimating fats in milk.
Henry Newell Martin reports use of isolated blood-perfused mammalian
    heart for the first time.
Behring and Kitasato develop antitoxin treatment of diphtheria.
Koch announces discovery of tuberculin and describes tuberculin reaction.

1891 First child treated with diphtheria antitoxin.
Association of American Medical Colleges founded.
Welch describes the bacillus of gas gangrene.
Dalton first to repair stab wound of the heart.

1892 Sternberg first describes viral neutralizing antibodies (vaccinia).
Opening of New York City Bacteriological Laboratory.
Smith and Kilbourne demonstrate tick transmission of bovine piroplasmosis
    (Texas fever).
Halsted successfully ligates first portion of subclavian artery.
Frank Hartley resects gasserian ganglion for trigeminal neuralgia.
Sedgwick emphasizes necessity of fly-control in prevention of typhoid fever.
Wistar Institute of Anatomy and Biology (Philadelphia) founded.

1893 Gilbert discovers paracolon bacilli and paratyphoid bacilli.
Hermann M. Biggs establishes diagnostic laboratory in New York City.
First class admitted to the new Johns Hopkins School of Medicine.
First School of Public Health organized at the Army Medical School.
Ewing describes what is now known as complement.
Halsted removes infected kidney in the male.
Müller describes increased oxygen utilization in hyperthyroidism.

789

1894 Walcott organizes a laboratory to produce diphtheria antitoxin.
First large epidemic of poliomyelitis in the United States.
Wellcome physiological research laboratories founded (London).

1895 Robb's book on *Aseptic Surgical Technique* published, first such work in English.
First pharmaceutical research laboratory started by Parke-Davis.
James Brown first to catheterize the male ureter.
Roentgen announces discovery of X-rays.
John Cox first in U.S. to use X-rays as an adjunct to surgery.
Association of Assistant Hospital Physicians organized, with Adolf Meyer as secretary—to promote research in psychiatry.
Calmette introduces antitoxin against snake venoms.

1896 Murphy performs successful circular anastomosis of blood vessels.
Welch founds *Journal of Experimental Medicine.*
Schenck describes sporotrichosis.
F. H. Williams does pioneer work in radiology (Boston).
Walter Cannon achieves X-ray visualization of the gastrointestinal tract.

1897 Nuttall demonstrates fly-transmission of plague bacilli.
Horton Smith shows danger of chronic (urinary) typhoid carriers.
New York State adopts law for compulsory notification of tuberculosis.
MacCallum demonstrates sexual conjugation of parasites of avian and human malaria.
Cancer research facility (Roswell Park) opens at University of Buffalo.
George Stewart formulates indicator-dilution principle for measuring cardiac output.

1898 Theobald Smith isolates and cultivates bovine tubercle bacillus.
Vincent describes spirillobacillary angina.
Davis and Varnier employ X-rays in obstetric diagnosis.
Cornell University Medical College founded.
W. T. Porter demonstrates that ventricular fibrillation is not irreversible and helps to found *American Journal of Physiology.*

1899 Society of American Bacteriologists founded.
Reed, Carroll, Lazear, and Agramonte demonstrate mosquito transmission of yellow fever.
Medical Library Association founded.
Epinephrine isolated by John J. Abel.
Dreser introduces aspirin.
Beijerinck isolates filterable virus of tobacco mosaic.
Stenbeck treats cancer with X-rays.

1900 American Association of Pathologists and Bacteriologists founded.
American Roentgen Ray Society founded.
Landsteiner describes ABO blood groups.
Compilation of official mortality statistics begins.
Theobald Smith describes hypersensitivity reaction to foreign protein.
Solis-Cohn introduces epinephrine in the treatment of asthma.
Park recommends control of milk by bacteriological tests (New York).

1901 Rockefeller Institute for Medical Research opened.
Nuttall founds *Journal of Hygiene.*
Frazier introduces section of posterior (sensory) root of trigeminal nerve for neuralgia.

1902 First perineal prostatectomy performed by Hugh Young.
Hygienic Laboratory of Public Health and Marine Hospital Service (later to become U.S. Public Health Service) opens.

1903 Luther L. Hill, father of Senator Lister Hill, is first U.S. surgeon to suture a wound of the heart.

Carrel introduces new methods of vascular anastomosis and transplantation of organs.

McClung isolates sex chromosome.

Finney performs gastroduodenostomy.

General Education Board (Rockefeller Foundation) organized.

Lina Rogers becomes first full-time school nurse (New York City).

von Pirquet outlines concept of allergy.

American Society of Clinical Surgeons organized.

Pauli uses potassium sulfocyanate in treatment of hypertension.

American Genetic Association founded.

Henry Phipps Institute for Study of Tuberculosis opened.

Jensen propagates cancer through several generations of mice.

License No. 1 "for the manufacture of viruses, toxins, serums, and other analogous products" issued by U.S. Treasury Department to Parke-Davis.

Einthoven uses string galvanometer for electrocardiography.

Arrhenius first to use the term "immunochemistry."

Riva Rocci devises a practical sphygmomanometer for blood pressure measurements.

1904 Atwater constructs a respiration calorimeter.

National Tuberculosis Association founded.

First radical operation for cancer of prostate performed by Hugh Young.

Construction of Panama Canal begins, with Gorgas heading disease control division.

1905 Osler founds Interurban Clinical Club.

Barker replaces Osler as Professor at Johns Hopkins and organizes first full-time clinical research divisions.

American Social Hygiene Association organized.

American Child Health Association founded.

Schaudinn discovers *Treponema pallidum* (causative agent of syphilis).

Folin's classic paper, *Laws governing composition of normal urine,* published.

Wilson first uses frozen sections for surgical diagnosis in the U.S.

Winter resuscitates heart by injection of epinephrine.

Novacaine introduced by Einhorn.

1906 Federal Food and Drug Act passed.

American Society of Biological Chemistry founded.

Howell demonstrates amino acids in the blood.

Flexner and Joblin transplant a rat epithelioma.

Wasserman introduces serum diagnosis of syphilis.

Ehrlich develops arsenical (606) treatment of syphilis.

1907 Theobald Smith suggests use of toxin-antitoxin in diphtheria.

Ricketts demonstrates tick transmission of Rocky Mountain spotted fever.

Ross Harrison introduces tissue culture.

S. Flexner develops an antiserum for cerebrospinal meningitis.

von Pirquet introduces the tuberculin skin test.

Miles introduces operation for cancer of the rectum.

1908 Maude Abbott's studies on *Congenital Malformations of the Heart* published.

Buerger describes thromboangiitis obliterans.

Cushing operates on the pituitary gland.

Garrod interprets pattern of inheritance of alkaptonuria in mendelian terms.

Rous discovers first viral-induced experimental cancer.

Landsteiner transmits poliomyelitis to monkeys.

Peking Union Medical College founded by the Rockefeller Foundation.

S. Flexner transmits poliomyelitis from humans to monkeys.

1909 National Committee for Mental Hygiene organized.

Meltzer organizes Society of Biology and Medicine.

F. F. Russell vaccinates U.S. Army against typhoid fever.

791

American Society for Clinical Investigation founded.

Marine and Lenhart standardize iodine treatment of endemic goiter.

MacCallum and Voegtlin clarify relation of parathyroid glands to calcium metabolism.

Blum notes importance of sodium in water retention.

1910 W. D. Coolidge announces new and improved X-ray tube.

Adelaide Nutting establishes course of public health nursing at Columbia University in New York City.

Rockefeller Sanitary Commission for hookworm prevention organized.

Libman publishes his classical description of bacterial endocarditis.

A. Flexner publishes his study, *Medical Education in the United States and Canada.*

Cushing, Crowe, and Horsley develop experimental hypophysectomy.

Opening of the Hospital of the Rockefeller Institute.

Rowntree and Geraghty introduce PSP test of renal function.

Auer and Lewis demonstrate bronchial spasm in acute anaphylaxis, and Meltzer suggests that this reaction characterizes bronchial asthma.

Vedder demonstrates amebicidal effect of emetine.

1911 Morgan and Wilson associate pattern of inheritance of hemophilia and color-blindness with X chromosome.

Funk coins term "vitamine."

Walter Cannon publishes *The Mechanical Factors of Digestion.*

Peyton Rous publishes study of viral cancer in chickens.

Goldberger and Anderson transmit measles from man to monkey.

Van Slyke begins development of method for estimating amino nitrogen.

1912 Nobel Prize awarded to Alexis Carrel for work on vascular suturing and organ transplantation.

Cannon begins work on effect of adrenal secretions on the emotions.

Discovery of vitamin A (Osborne and Mendel; McCollum).

Cushing's treatise on *The Pituitary Body and Its Disorders* is published.

Act of 1912 creates the United States Public Health Service.

Schloss introduces "scratch test" for human hypersensitivity.

Herrick publishes his classic description of coronary thrombosis.

Edsall organizes research ward and emphasizes clinical investigation at the Massachusetts General Hospital.

1913 Rockefeller Foundation chartered (New York).

Incorporation of the American College of Surgeons.

Dochez, Gillespie, and Avery type pneumococci (1913–1916).

Maude Slye performs experiments regarding hereditary susceptibility to and immunity from cancer (1913–1927).

Full-time clinical professorships begin at Johns Hopkins.

Abel isolates amino acids from blood by vividiffusion.

Association of Experimental Pathology founded.

1914 Pasteurization of milk begins in large cities.

Dandy and Blackfan demonstrate pathogenesis of hydrocephalus.

Passage of the Harrison Anti-Narcotic Act.

Association of Immunologists founded.

1915 Incorporation of the American College of Physicians.

Carrel-Dakin treatment of infected gunshot wounds introduced.

Cannon publishes *Bodily Changes in Pain, Hunger, Fear and Rage.*

Goldberger demonstrates that pellagra results from nutritional deficiency.

Death certificates come into general use.

Rous develops trypsin digestion method for isolation of individual cells from tissues for study.

Cooke introduces intracutaneous diagnostic test for hypersensitivity.

Jackson devises apparatus for closed-system anesthesia.

Kendall isolates and identifies thyroxin.

1916 Bull introduces antitoxin for treatment of gas gangrene.
The Johns Hopkins School of Hygiene and Public Health founded.
Heparin discovered by McLean and Howell.

1917 Dandy introduces ventriculography with air.
Avery and Dochez describe specific soluble substance of pneumococcus.
Stockard and Papanicolaou demonstrate vaginal epithelial changes during
estrous cycle.

1918 Ellerman establishes transmission of leukemia in chickens by virus.
Benedict devises basal metabolism test.
Fahraeus introduces erythrocyte sedimentation test.
Johns Hopkins School of Hygiene and Public Health opens in Baltimore.

1919 Krumbhaar describes leukopenia and dissolution of lymphoid tissue by
"mustard gas."
Loeb induces mammary cancer by ovariectomy in mice.
Blake and Trask demonstrate viral origin of measles.
Herrick publishes first electrocardiogram in myocardial infarction.
Huldschinsky demonstrates curative effect of sunlight on rickets.

1920 Cutler performs surgery on the mitral valve.
Marine describes endemic goiter due to iodine deficiency.
Allen rediscovers use of the salt-free diet for treatment of edema.
Saxl introduces mercurial diuretics for treatment of cardiac edema.

1921 Evans and Long identify growth-stimulating and gonadotropic properties
of anterior pituitary lobe extracts.
Osborne and Rowntree use sodium iodide as contrast medium for kidney
X-rays.
Banting and Best first isolate insulin.

1922 McCollum and Steenbock discover vitamin D.
Insulin first administered to a patient with diabetes mellitus.
U.S. Public Health Service opens Office of Cancer Investigation, with
laboratory for cancer research at Harvard.
Whipple shows regenerative effect of liver on experimental anemia in the
dog.
Association of Clinical Pathologists founded.

1923 George and Gladys Dick discover hemolytic streptococcus of scarlatina and
devise a susceptibility test.
Graham and Cole introduce cholecystography by use of an opaque dye.
Nobel Prize for discovery of insulin to Banting and McLeod.
Avery and Heidelberger demonstrate that the specific soluble substance of
the pneumococcus is a polysaccharide.
Murlin and Kimball discover glucagon.
Plummer introduces iodine therapy before surgery for Graves' disease.

1924 Chen and Schmidt introduce ephedrine.
Association of Parasitologists founded.

1925 Parker and Nye grow vaccinia virus in tissue culture.
Rowntree and Adson report first sympathectomy for hypertension.

1926 Minot and Murphy report liver treatment for pernicious anemia.
Cushing receives Pulitzer Prize for his *Life of William Osler.*
Vitamins B_1 and B_2 described.
Goldberger isolates pellagra-preventive factor.
Abel isolates insulin in crystalline form.
Kennaway extracts first known cancer-causing chemical, 3,4-benzpyrene.

1927 Wilder reports first pancreatic islet cell tumor producing hyperinsulinism.
Charles Mayo first successfully removes a pheochromocytoma.

793

1928 Alexander Fleming discovers penicillin.
Castle describes role of stomach in pathogenesis of pernicious anemia.
Forssmann performs first heart catheterization (on himself).

1929 Institute of the History of Medicine established at Johns Hopkins.
Smith demonstrates failure of growth and atrophy of sex glands, thyroid, and adrenal after hypophysectomy.
Corner and Allen describe corpus luteum hormone.
Master and Oppenheimer introduce exercise test for angina pectoris.
Berger constructs electroencephalograph.
Churchill performs first American pericardiectomy for constrictive pericarditis.
Best and Murray use heparin to prevent venous thrombosis experimentally.

1930 Nobel Prize to Landsteiner for discovery of the blood groups.
Theiler develops immunization against yellow fever in animals.
Duke University Hospital and Medical School open.
Wilson, MacLeod, and Barker introduce the precordial lead.

1931 *American Standard Nomenclature* first published.
Webster and Fite transmit St. Louis encephalitis by intracerebral inoculation of mice.
Goodpasture adopts technique of inoculation on chorioallantoic membrane of chick for use in virology.
Wolferth and Wood introduce chest lead for routine use in suspected myocardial infarction.
Development of the electron microscope.

1932 Riboflavin discovered.
Urey describes heavy hydrogen.
Lawrence develops the cyclotron.
Cushing describes the syndrome that bears his name.
Goldblatt produces experimental hypertension by renal artery stenosis.
Domagk discovers Prontosil (first sulfa drug).

1933 Nobel Prize to T. H. Morgan for his studies of genetics.
Hamilton designs manometer for measurement of intravascular pressure.

1934 Nobel Prize for physiology and medicine to Whipple, Minot, and Murphy.
Dam discovers vitamin K.

1935 Kendall and Reichstein isolate cortisone.
Stanley crystallizes tobacco mosaic virus.
Nucleic acids found to be principal components of viruses and genes.
Beck does first operation to vascularize heart muscle in patients with angina pectoris.
Gibbon successfully uses extracorporeal pump in the dog.
First hospital for drug addicts founded at Lexington, Kentucky.
Trefouël, Nitti, and Bovet show that Prontosil's action is due to sulfanilamide.
Murray uses heparin clinically to prevent venous thrombosis.

1936 Bittner describes transmission of mammary cancer through virus in milk (mice).
Long and Bliss introduce sulfa drugs in the United States.

1937 American Foundation Studies in Government: Report published on *American medicine: Expert testimony out of court.*
Fantus establishes first blood bank.
National Cancer Institute established.
Ochsner and DeBakey describe lung cancer in cigarette smokers.
Chargoff and Olsen discover protamine antagonism to heparin.
Introduction of angiocardiography.

1938 Pickering and Prinzmetal and Landis rediscover renin.

1939 Doisy isolates vitamin K from alfalfa and determines structure.
   Dubos introduces tyrothricin (gramicidin), which led Florey to the revival
      of penicillin.

1940 Landsteiner and Wiener describe Rh factor.
   Huggins describes effects of hormones on prostatic secretion.
   Gregg describes congenital malformations following German measles.
   Hinshaw and Feldman show beneficial effect of Promin on experimental
      tuberculosis.
   Link discovers dicumarol.

1941 First clinical use of oral anticoagulants.
   Office of Scientific Research and Development organized under Vannevar
      Bush. Committee on Medical Research chaired by A. N. Richards.
   Huggins describes estrogen therapy and orchiectomy for prostatic cancer.
   Hirst demonstrates influenza virus by agglutination of red blood cells.
   Coons fluorescent labeling of antibody introduced.
   First clinical trials of penicillin by Florey et al.

1942 Collection of blood by Red Cross for treating battle casualties.
   Atomic energy released and controlled in first nuclear chain reaction.
   Gilman and co-workers describe effect of nitrogen mustard on lymphomas.

1943 Earle demonstrates conversion of normal cells to cancer cells in tissue culture.
   Papanicolaou and Trout publish *Methods of Exfoliative Cytology.*
   Selman Waksman announces discovery of streptomycin.
   ACTH isolated from anterior pituitary gland.
   Dam and Doisy receive Nobel Prize for work on vitamin K.
   Birthyear of bacterial genetics (work of Delbruck and Luria).

1944 Nobel Prize to Erlanger and Gasser for research on nerve fibers.
   Avery, McLeod, and McCarty identify transforming factor in pneumococci
      as DNA.
   Heilman and Kendall describe beneficial effect of cortisone in experimental
      lymphosarcoma.
   Hinshaw and Feldman show effectiveness of streptomycin in experimental
      tuberculosis.
   Synthesis of quinine accomplished.
   Negarski performs first resuscitation after clinical death.
   First "blue baby" operation by Blalock and Taussig.
   Introduction of early ambulation after surgery and childbirth.

1945 Promin therapy proven effective against leprosy.
   American Cancer Society incorporated.
   Williams and Wycoff develop shading technique to demonstrate viruses by
      electron microscopy.
   Hinshaw and Feldman report successful use of streptomycin in treatment of
      human tuberculosis.

1946 Nobel Prize to H. J. Muller for research on X-ray mutations.
   Penicillin produced synthetically.
   Passage of Hospital Survey and Construction (Hill-Burton) Act.
   Passage of the National Mental Health Act.
   Communicable Disease Center established at Atlanta.

1947 Parke-Davis announces discovery of Chloromycetin.
   Nobel Prize to the Coris and Houssay for studies on the metabolism of
      glycogen and sugar.
   Farber induces remissions in acute leukemia with the anti-folates.
   Work on the artificial kidney begins at Peter Bent Brigham Hospital.
   Dalldorf uses suckling mice for virus inoculation.
   Lederle announces discovery of Aureomycin.
   Bing catheterizes the coronary sinus.
   Kempner advocates rice-fruit diet for treatment of hypertension.

795

1948 Bailey performs first mitral commissurotomy.
Rickes and Smith describe vitamin B_{12}.
Kinesy report on sex behavior of the male published.
Kendall and Hench describe therapeutic properties of cortisone.
Dalldorf and Sickles isolate first Coxsackie virus.

1949 Pauling and co-workers describe first molecular disease—sickle cell anemia.
Enders, Robbins, and Weller cultivate poliovirus in human cells from tissues other than the nervous system.
Vaskil reports antihypertensive effect of *Rauwolfia*.
National Institute of Mental Health established.
Lithium first used in the treatment of psychiatric disease.
Zaimis and Paton introduce ganglionic blocking agents.

1950 Pfizer announces discovery of Terramycin.
Nobel prize to Hench, Kendall, and Reichstein for studies on treatment of rheumatoid arthritis with cortisone and ACTH.
Isolation in crystalline form of vitamin B_{12}.
Pearson et al. describe effect of ACTH in leukemia.

1951 Ludwik Gross shows virus transmission of leukemia in mice.
Nobel Prize to Max Theiler for yellow fever vaccine.
Hitchins et al. describe effect of 6-mercaptopurine in leukemia.
Hammon conducts field trial with gamma globulin as prophylaxis against poliomyelitis.
Effect of fluoride in prevention of dental caries discovered.

1952 Zoll introduces first practical cardiac pacemaker.
Hufnagel inserts first artificial heart valve.
First open-heart operation by Bailey.
Nobel Prize to Waksman for discovery of streptomycin.
The Coris demonstrate first enzyme-deficiency disease (hepatic G-6-phosphatase deficiency in a glycogen storage disease).
The Hershey-Chase experiment identifies DNA as the genetic material.
Bodian and Horstman demonstrate viremia in poliomyelitis.
Discovery of isoniazid announced.
External cardiac stimulation used in cardiac arrest by Zoll.
Bahnson removes an aneurysm of the arch of the aorta.

1953 Nobel Prize to Lipmann and Krebs for studies on carbohydrate metabolism and coenzyme A.
Announcement by Watson, Crick, and Wilkins of the "double helix" configuration of DNA.
ACTH isolated in pure form by White et al.
Gross discovers polyoma virus inducing multiple experimental neoplasms.
Kidd discovers dissolution of experimental lymphoma by guinea pig serum (asparaginase).
First open-heart operation using extracorporeal pump (Gibbon).

1954 Enders, Robbins, and Weller receive Nobel Prize for work on tissue culture of poliomyelitis virus.
Farber describes effect of daunomycin in experimental tumors.
Sourkes reports antihypertensive effect of alpha-methyldopa.
Successful preoperative diagnosis of unilateral renal disease as a cause of hypertension (Howard et al.).

1955 Introduction of the Salk polio vaccine.
Nobel Prize in chemistry to du Vigneaud and Theorell for studies of chemical synthesis of oxytocin and oxygen transport system in living tissues.
Lawrence describes transfer factor.
Conn describes syndrome of primary aldosteronism due to adrenal adenoma.
DeBakey, Creech, and Harris remove aortic aneurysm and replace with a homograft.

1956 Nobel Prize to Forssmann, Cournand, and Richards for cardiac catheterization.

Tigo and Levan describe true diploid chromosome number in man (48).

Kalchar and co-workers report first inborn error of metabolism to be studied in cell culture.

Zoll introduces external defibrillator.

Passage of Health Research Facilities Construction Act.

James Shannon appointed Director of the National Institutes of Health.

1957 Ingraham discovers specific amino acid change in sickle-cell hemoglobin.

Li, Hertz, and Spencer describe effect of methotrexate on choriocarcinoma.

Sabin's oral polio vaccine tested in Russia.

Witebsky offers postulates for diagnosis of autoimmunization.

Freis and Hollander note antihypertensive effect of thiazide derivatives.

1958 Nobel Prize to Beadle, Tatum, and Lederberg for genetic research.

First use of closed chest cardiac massage combined with mouth-to-mouth respiration for cardiac resuscitation.

1959 Ochoa and Kornberg share Nobel Prize for work on synthesis of RNA and DNA by enzymes.

Ford and Jacobs discover role of Y chromosome in sex determination in humans.

Nowell and Hungerford describe Ph' chromosome in chronic myeloid leukemia.

Fernbach et al. describe effect of Cytoxan in acute leukemia.

Guanethidine introduced by Ciba for treatment of hypertension.

Avery and Mead discover surfactant deficiency in lungs of premature infants.

1960 Farber describes effect of daunomycin on Wilms' tumor.

Barski describes technique of cell hybridization.

P. C. Nowell discovers that the lymphocyte is not an end-stage cell.

Li synthesizes ACTH.

Berson and Yalow describe technique of radioimmunoassay of hormones.

Laragh discovers that angiotensin stimulates secretion of aldosterone.

Introduction of the laser.

1961 Gamma globulin used for prevention of hemolytic disease of the newborn by Gorman, Frida, and Pollack.

Lyon hypothesis advanced (genetics).

U.S. Public Health Service licenses Sabin's oral polio vaccine.

Good and Miller show that thymectomy in the newborn prevents normal development of the immune system.

1962 Trentin et al. demonstrate that a human virus (adenovirus type 12) has oncogenic potential in animals.

Lown introduces electrical conversion for treatment of cardiac arrhythmias.

Nobel Prize to Watson, Crick, and Wilkins for the "double helix."

Passage of the National Vaccination Assistance Act.

1963 Johnson et al. describe effect of vincristine in leukemia.

Blumberg describes Australia antigen and relates it to hepatitis B.

Donaldson and Evans demonstrate absence of C'-1 esterase in hereditary angioedema (described by Osler).

Community Mental Health Center Act passed by Congress.

Passage of the Health Professions Educational Assistance Act.

1964 Nobel Prize to Bloch and Lynen for work on the mechanism and regulation of cholesterol and fatty acid metabolism.

Establishment of Commission on Heart Disease, Cancer and Stroke.

National Library of Medicine introduces a computer-based system (MEDLARS) for analysis and retrieval of medical literature.

1965 Proinsulin discovered by Steiner and Oyer.
Passage of Regional Medical Program (RMP) Act.
Introduction of immunization against measles.
Passage of Medicare, Medicaid, and Higher Education acts.

1966 Nobel Prize to Huggins and Rous for their contributions to cancer research.
Passage of Comprehensive Health Planning (CHP) Act.
Parkman and Myer develop rubella vaccine.
Ishizaka describes IgE and its association with allergic states.

1967 Favaloro performs first coronary artery bypass utilizing a vein.
Hartline and Wald receive Nobel Prize for work on the visual process.
NIH budget passes the billion dollar mark.

1968 Nirenberg, Khorana, and Holley receive Nobel Prize for work on the genetic code.
Henles relate Epstein-Barr virus to infectious mononucleosis.
Cotzias introduces L-dopa treatment for Parkinson's disease.
Passage of Health Manpower Act.

1969 Man first walks on the moon.
Nobel Prize to Delbruck, Luria, and Hershey for work on bacteriophage and viral genetics.
Good et al. describe homograft treatment of thymic agenesis.
Guillemain synthesizes the thyrotropic-releasing hormone of the hypothalamus.
Introduction of immunization against rubella (German measles).

1970 Khorana synthesizes the first artificial gene.
Discovery of "reverse transcriptase" by Temin and Mizutani.
Herbst describes cancer of the vagina in daughters of mothers who used diethylstilbestrol.
Implantation of the first cardiac pacemaker.
Nobel Prize to Axelrod, Katz, and von Euler for work on humoral transmission in nerves.

1971 National Cancer Act of 1971—the "crusade against cancer."
Structure of gonadotropin-releasing factor determined.
Sutherland receives Nobel Prize for discovery of cyclic AMP.

1972 Nobel Prize for chemistry to Anfinsen, Moore, and Stein for studies on ribonuclease.
Cost of medical education reaches $9700 per student per year.

1973 Construction of molecules that combine genetic information from two somas (Chang and Cohen; Bayer and Heiling).
Guillemain isolates somatostatin.

1974 Nobel Prize to Claude, deDuve, and Palade for their pioneer work in cell biology.
Passage of National Health Planning and Resources Development Act.

1975 Nobel Prize to Dulbecco, Baltimore, and Temin for studies relating to cancer.

References

Chapter 1

Blanton, W. B.: Washington's medical knowledge and its sources. Ann. Med. Hist. (N.S.) 5:52, 1933.

Lewis, F. O.: Washington's last illness. Ann. Med. Hist. (N.S.) 4:245, 1932.

Trousseau, A.: Lectures on Clinical Medicine, Delivered at the Hôtel-Dieu, Paris. 5 vols. Translated from the edition of 1868. London, The New Sydenham Society, 1870.

Chapter 2

Bard, S.: Two Discourses Dealing with Medical Education in Early New York. New York, Columbia University Press, 1921. (The first Discourse was delivered in 1769, the second in 1819.)

Bell, W. J., Jr.: The medical institution of Yale college. Yale J. Biol. Med. 33:169, 1960.

Bell, W. J., Jr.: Nathan Smith Davis—an autobiographical letter, previously unpublished. JAMA 224:1014, 1973.

Butterfield, L. H. (ed.): Letters of Benjamin Rush. 2 vols. Princeton, N.J., Princeton University Press, 1951.

Cooper, J. F.: The Pioneers. (The 1st edition appeared in 1823. The description of Elnathan Todd is found in Chapter VI.)

Cunningham, E. R.: A short review of the development of medical education and schools of medicine. Ann. Med. Hist. (N.S.) 7:228, 1935.

Davis, N. S.: Address on the progress of medical education in the United States. In Transactions of the International Medical Congress of Philadelphia, 1876. Philadelphia, printed for the Congress, 1877, pp. 265–285.

Drake, D.: Practical Essays on Medical Education and the Medical Profession in the United States. Cincinnati, Roff and Young, 1832. (Reprint: Baltimore, Johns Hopkins University Press, 1952.)

Drake, D.: A Systematic Treatise, Historical, Etiological, and Practical, on the Principal Diseases of the Interior Valley of North America, as they Appear in the Caucasian, African, Indian, and Esquimaux Varieties of its Population. Cincinnati, Philadelphia, and New York, W. B. Smith and Co., 1850. (Reprint: New York, Plenum Publishing Corp., 1969.)

Flexner, A.: Medical Education in the United States and Canada. New York, Bulletin of the Carnegie Foundation for the Advancement of Teaching, No. 4, 1910.

Garrett, W. D.: Thomas Jefferson Redivivus. Barre, Mass., Barre Publishers, 1971.

Harrington, T. F.: The Harvard Medical School: A History, Narrative and Documentary. 3 vols. New York, Lewis, 1905.

Hudson, R. P.: Patterns of Medical Education in Nineteenth-Century America. Thesis for M.A. degree, Institute of the History of Medicine, Johns Hopkins University, 1966.

James, H.: Charles W. Eliot, President of Harvard University, 1869–1909. 2 vols. Boston and New York, Houghton Mifflin Co., 1930.

Morgan, J.: A Discourse upon the Institution of Medical Schools in America. Philadelphia, 1765. (Reprint: Baltimore, Johns Hopkins University Press, 1937.)

Morison, S. E.: Three Centuries of Harvard. Cambridge, Mass., Harvard University Press, 1965.

Packard, F. R.: History of Medicine in the United States. 2 vols. New York, Paul B. Hoeber, 1931.

Pepper, W.: Higher Medical Education, The True Interest of the Public and of the Profession. (Address Introductory to the 112th course of lectures of the Medical Department of the University of Pennsylvania.) Philadelphia, Collins, Printer, 1877.

Putnam, J. J.: A Memoir of Dr. James Jackson. Boston, Houghton Mifflin Co., 1906.

Sabin, F. R.: Franklin Paine Mall—The Story of a Mind. Baltimore, Johns Hopkins University Press, 1934.

Vaughan, V. C.: A Doctor's Memories. Indianapolis, Bobbs-Merrill Co., 1926.

Waite, F. C.: Birth of the first independent proprietary medical school in New England, at Castleton, Vermont, in 1818. Ann. Med. Hist. (N.S.) 7:242, 1935.

Warren, E.: The Life of John Warren, M.D. Boston, Noyes, Holmes and Co., 1874.

White, A. D.: Selected Chapters from the Autobiography of Andrew D. White. Ithaca, N.Y., Cornell University Press, 1939.

Wood, G. B.: Early History of the University of Pennsylvania from Its Origin to the Year 1827, 3rd ed. (With supplementary chapters by F. D. Stone.) Philadelphia, J. B. Lippincott Co., 1896.

Chapter 3

Ball, J. M.: Samuel Thomson (1769–1843) and his patented "system" of medicine. Ann. Med. Hist. 7:144, 1925.
Bragman, L. J.: The medical wisdom of Mark Twain. Ann. Med. Hist. 7:425, 1925.
Bryan, L. S., Jr.: Blood Letting in American Medicine. Bull. Hist. Med. *38*:516, 1964.
Butterfield, L. H. (ed.): Letters of Benjamin Rush. 2 vols. Princeton, N.J., Princeton University Press, 1951. (An account of the Cobbett-Rush feud is given in Vol. II, Appendix III.)
DeJong, R. N.: The first American textbook on psychiatry. A review and discussion of Benjamin Rush's "Medical inquiries and observations upon diseases of the mind." Ann. Med. Hist. (3rd S.) 2:195, 1940.
Gardner, F. T.: King Cole of California. (Presented in three parts). Ann. Med. Hist. (3rd S.) 2:245, 319, 432, 1940.
Garrison, F. H.: History of Medicine, 4th ed. Philadelphia, W. B. Saunders Co., 1966.
Gross, S. D.: Surgery. *In* Clarke, E. H., et al.: A Century of American Medicine, 1776–1876. Philadelphia, H. C. Lea, 1876. (Reprint: New York, Burt Franklin, 1968.)
Hertzler, A. E.: The Horse and Buggy Doctor. New York, Harper and Brothers, 1938.
Holmes, O. W.: Medical Essays, 1842–1882. Boston, Houghton Mifflin Co., 1891.
Kaufman, M.: Homeopathy in America. The Rise and Fall of a Medical Heresy. Baltimore, Johns Hopkins University Press, 1971.
Lloyd, J. H.: Benjamin Rush and his critics. Ann. Med. Hist. (N.S.) 2:470, 1930.
Mason, J. M.: Early medical education in the far south. Ann. Med. Hist. (N.S.) 4:64, 1932.
Rosenberg, C. E.: The Cholera Years. Chicago, University of Chicago Press, 1968.
Rucker, M. P.: Benjamin Rush, obstetrician. Ann. Med. Hist. (3rd S.) 3:487, 1941.
Rush, B.: An Account of the Bilious Remitting Yellow Fever as it Appeared in the City of Philadelphia in the Year 1793, 2nd ed. Philadelphia, Thomas Dobson, 1794.
Rush, B.: Medical Inquiries and Observations. Vol. IV. Philadelphia, Thomas Dobson, 1796. (The last section, pp. 181–258, is entitled "A defense of blood-letting.")
Shryock, R. H.: The medical reputation of Benjamin Rush—contrasts over two centuries. Bull. Hist. Med. *45*:507, 1971.
Smith, G.: Plague on Us. New York, Commonwealth Fund, 1941.
Spiller, R. E., et al.: Literary History of the United States, 4th rev. ed. New York, Macmillan, 1974.
Tucker, L. L. (ed.): Our Travels, Statistical, Geographical, Mineorological, Geological, Historical, Political and Quizzical. Written by myself XYZ. (A Knickerbocker Tour of New York State, 1822). Albany, N.Y., The State Education Department, 1968.
Yandell, L. P.: Address on American medical literature. Transactions of the International Medical Congress, 1876. Philadelphia, printed for the Congress, 1877.

Chapter 4

Bowditch, H. I.: Address on Hygiene and Preventive Medicine. Transactions of the International Medical Congress of Philadelphia, 1876. Philadelphia, printed for the Congress, 1877.
Hume, E. E.: Max von Pettenkofer's theory of the etiology of cholera, typhoid fever and other intestinal diseases—a review of his arguments and evidence. Ann. Med. Hist. 7:319, 1925.
Malloch, A.: Lead poisoning (editorial). Ann. Med. Hist. (N.S.) 3:455, 1931.
Rolleston, H.: The progress and pioneers of preventive medicine. Ann. Med. Hist. (N.S.) 6:95, 1934.
Rosenberg, C. E.: The Cholera Years. Chicago, University of Chicago Press, 1971.
Shryock, R. H.: The origins and significance of the public health movement in the United States. Ann. Med. Hist. (N.S.) 1:645, 1929.

Chapter 5

Ashhurst, A. P. C.: The centenary of Lister (1827–1927): a tale of sepsis and antisepsis. Ann. Med. Hist. 9:205, 1927.
Butterfield, L. H. (ed.): Letters of Benjamin Rush. Princeton, N.J., Princeton University Press, 1951. (The letter cited is found on p. 1063.)
Cohen, I. B. (ed.): "Some Account of the Pennsylvania Hospital from Its First Rise to the Begin-

ning of the Fifth Month, Called May, 1754." By Benjamin Franklin. Baltimore, Johns Hopkins University Press, 1954.

Deutsch, Albert: The Mentally Ill in America. New York, Doubleday, Doran & Co., 1937.

Freidson, E. (ed.): The Hospital in Modern Society. London, Collier-MacMillan, Ltd., 1963.

Greenblatt, M.: Psychiatry: the battered child of medicine. N. Engl. J. Med. *292*:246, 1975.

Lane, J. E.: Jean Devèze, 1753–1826?; notes on the yellow fever epidemic at Philadelphia in 1793. Ann. Med. Hist. (N.S.) *8*:202, 1936. (Contains an excellent account of the Bush Hill Hospital.)

Morton, T. G.: The History of the Pennsylvania Hospital—1751–1895, revised ed. Philadelphia, Times Printing House, 1897.

Myers, G. W.: History of the Massachusetts General Hospital—June, 1872 to December, 1900. Boston, Griffith-Stillings Press. (Undated but Preface is dated 1929.)

Packard, F. R.: Some Account of the Pennsylvania Hospital from Its First Rise to the Beginning of the Year 1938. Philadelphia, Eagle Press, 1938.

Putnam, James J.: A Memoir of Dr. James Jackson. Boston, Houghton Mifflin Co., 1906.

Roberts, K., and Roberts, A. M. (translators and eds.): Moreau de St. Méry's American Journey—1793–1798. Garden City, N.Y., Doubleday and Co., 1947.

Waring, J. I.: St. Philip's Hospital in Charleston in Carolina—medical care of the poor in colonial times. Ann. Med. Hist. (N.S.) *4*:283, 1932.

Washburn, F. A.: The Massachusetts General Hospital—Its Development. Boston, Houghton Mifflin Co., 1939.

Wylie, W. Gill: Hospitals: Their History, Organization and Construction. New York, D. Appleton and Co., 1877.

Chapter 6

Billings, J. S.: Literature and institutions. *In* Clarke, E. H., et al.: A Century of American Medicine, 1776–1876. Philadelphia, H. C. Lea, 1876. (Reprint: New York, Burt Franklin, 1968.)

Billings, J. S.: Our medical literature. Transactions of International Medical Congress, London, 1881.

Derbyshire, R. C.: Medical Licensure and Discipline in the United States. Baltimore, Johns Hopkins University Press, 1969.

Morton, T. G.: The History of the Pennsylvania Hospital—1751–1895, revised ed. Philadelphia, Times Printing House, 1897.

Shafer, H. B.: Early medical magazines in America. Ann. Med. Hist. (N.S.) *7*:480, 1935.

Shryock, R. H.: Medical Licensing in America, 1650–1965. Baltimore, Johns Hopkins University Press, 1967.

Yandell, L. P.: Address on American Medical Literature. Transactions of the International Medical Congress, Philadelphia, 1876. Philadelphia, printed for the Congress, 1877.

Chapter 7

Bishop, W. J.: Thomas Dimsdale, M.D., F.R.S. (1712–1800) and the inoculation of Catherine the Great of Russia. Ann. Med. Hist. (N.S.) *4*:321, 1932.

Blanton, W. B.: Washington's medical knowledge and its sources. Ann. Med. Hist. (N.S.) *5*:52, 1933.

Butterfield, L. H. (ed.): Letters of Benjamin Rush. 2 vols. Princeton, N.J., Princeton University Press, 1951. (Letter of December 29, 1798, to R. Bushe, Jr.)

Deutsch, A.: The Mentally Ill in America. New York, Doubleday, Doran & Co., 1937.

Freidson, E. (ed.): The Hospital in Modern Society. London, Collier-MacMillan, Ltd., 1963.

Gross, S. D.: Autobiography of Samuel D. Gross, M.D. with Sketches of His Contemporaries, 2 vols. Philadelphia, George Barrie, Publisher, 1887. (Reprint: New York, Arno Press, 1972.)

Rosen, George: Fees and Fee Bills—Some Economic Aspects of Medical Practice in Nineteenth Century America. Bull. Hist. Med. (Supplement No. 6). Baltimore, Johns Hopkins University Press, 1946.

Shryock, R. H.: Public relations of the medical profession in Great Britain and the United States—1600–1870. A chapter in the social history of medicine. Ann. Med. Hist. (N.S.) *2*:308, 1930.

Walsh, J. J.: Physicians' fees down the ages. International Clinics *4*:259, 1910.

Chapter 8

Atwater, E. C.: Morrill Wyman and the aspiration of acute pleural effusions, 1850. A letter from New England. Bull. Hist. Med. *46*:235, 1972.

Ball, J. M.: The ether tragedies. Ann. Med. Hist. 7:264, 1925.

Benjamin Waterhouse, American Pioneer. (Editorial.) Ann. Med. Hist. 9:195, 1927.

Bigelow, H. J.: A History of the Discovery of Modern Anesthesia. *In* Clarke, E. H., et al.: A Century of American Medicine, 1776–1876. Philadelphia, H. C. Lea, 1876. (Reprint: New York, Burt Franklin, 1968.)

Christian, H. A., and others: Sesquicentenary of the professorship of the theory and practice of physic. Harvard Med. Alumni Bull. 7:17, 1933.

Clarke, E. H.: Practical Medicine. *In* Clarke, E. H., et al.: A Century of American Medicine, 1776–1876. Philadelphia, H. C. Lea, 1876. (Reprint: New York, Burt Franklin, 1968.)

Gerhard, W. W.: On the typhus fever, which occurred at Philadelphia in the spring and summer of 1836; showing the distinction between this form of disease and dothinenteritis or typhoid fever with alteration of the follicles of the small intestine. Am. J. Med. Sci. 19:289, 1837.

Gibbon, J. H.: Samuel D. Gross. Ann. Med. Hist. 8:136, 1926.

Gray, Laman A.: Ephraim McDowell—Father of Abdominal Surgery. Reprint of paper read before the Filson Club, Louisville, Ky., January 8, 1968.

Gross, S. D.: Surgery. *In* Clarke, E. H., et al.: A Century of American Medicine, 1776–1876. Philadelphia, H. C. Lea, 1876. (Reprint: New York, Burt Franklin, 1968.)

Leikind, M. C.: The evolution of medical research in the United States. Int. Rec. Med. 171:455, 1958.

Miller, W. S.: William Beaumont and his book; Elisha North and his copy of Beaumont's book. Ann. Med. Hist. (N.S.) 1:155, 1929.

Miller, W. S.: William Beaumont, M.D. (1785–1853). Ann. Med. Hist. (N.S.) 5:28, 1933.

Osler, W.: The first printed documents relating to modern surgical anesthesia. Ann. Med. Hist. 1:329, 1917.

Otto, J. C.: An account of an hemorrhagic disposition existing in certain families. Med. Repository 6:1, 1803.

Pleadwell, F. L.: A new view of Elisha North and his treatise on spotted fever (based on a recently discovered manuscript). Ann. Med. Hist. 6:245, 1924.

Roth, G. B.: The "original Morton inhaler" for ether. Ann. Med. Hist. (N.S.) 4:390, 1932.

Shryock, R. H.: American Medical Research Past and Present. New York, The Commonwealth Fund, 1947.

Thomas, T. G.: Obstetrics and Gynaecology. *In* Clarke, E. H., et al.: A Century of American Medicine, 1776–1876. Philadelphia, H. C. Lea, 1876. (Reprint: New York, Burt Franklin, 1968.)

Wells, Horace, Dentist, Father of Surgical Anesthesia. Published by the Horace Wells Centenary Committee of the American Dental Association, 1948.

Woglom, W. H.: Discoverers for Medicine. New Haven, Yale University Press, 1949.

Chapter 9

In collecting the general information for this section we have made use of the following:

Boorstin, D. J.: The Americans—The Democratic Experience. New York, Random House, 1973.

Bradley, H. W.: The United States from 1865. New York, Charles Scribner's Sons, 1973.

Morison, S. E.: The Oxford History of the American People. New York, Oxford University Press, 1965.

Morison, S. E., Commager, H. S., and Leuchtenburg, W. E.: The Growth of the American Republic, 6th ed. 2 vols. New York; Oxford University Press, 1969.

The following references, with a few exceptions, were taken from medical sources. In relating medical progress to other historical developments the two articles by Shryock and the slender treatise by Stern have been helpful. Brieger's book contains a wealth of skillfully edited gleanings from nineteenth-century medical literature, nicely placed in context. We learned about Erichsen's visit to the United States from Brieger.

Billings, J. S.: A review of higher medical education. Am. J. Med. Sci. 76:174, 1878.

Brieger, Gert H.: Medical America in the Nineteenth Century—Readings from the Literature. Baltimore, Johns Hopkins University Press, 1972.

Erichsen, J. E.: Impressions of American surgery. (Address delivered at University College Hospital.) Lancet 2:717, 1874.

Flexner, A.: Medical Education in the United States and Canada. New York, Bulletin of the Carnegie Foundation for the Advancement of Teaching, No. 4, 1910.

Hertzler, A. E.: The Horse and Buggy Doctor. New York, Harper and Brothers, 1938.

Huxley, Thomas H.: American Addresses. London, MacMillan and Co., 1886.

Jaffe, Bernard: Crucibles—The Lives and Achievements of the Great Chemists. London, Jarrolds Publishers, Ltd., 1931.

Keuchel, E. F.: Master of the art of canning: Baltimore, 1860–1900. Maryland Historical Magazine, 67:351, 1972.

Pepper, W.: Higher Medical Education, the True Interest of the Public and the Profession. An Address Introductory to the 112th Course of Lectures of the Medical Department of the University of Pennsylvania. Philadelphia, Collins, Printer, 1877.

Shryock, R. H.: Public relations of the medical profession in Great Britain and the United States, 1600–1870. A chapter in the social history of medicine. Ann. Med. Hist. (N.S.) 2:308, 1930.

Shryock, R. H.: The interplay of social and internal factors in the history of modern medicine. Scientific Monthly 56:221, 1953.

Stern, Bernhard J.: American Medical Practice in the Perspectives of a Century. New York, Commonwealth Fund, 1945.

Welch, W. H.: Some of the conditions which have influenced the development of American medicine, especially during the last century. Bull. Johns Hopkins Hosp. 19:33, 1908.

Chapter 10

Boorstin, D. J.: The Americans—The Democratic Experience. New York, Random House, 1973.

Bradley, H. W.: The United States from 1865. New York, Charles Scribner's Sons, 1973.

Keefer, C. S.: Dr. Richards as Chairman of the Committee on Medical Research. Ann. Intern. Med. (Supplement 8) 71:64, 1969.

Knowles, J. H. (ed.): Hospitals, Doctors and the Public Interest. Cambridge, Mass., Harvard University Press, 1965.

Means, J. H.: Doctors, People, and Government. Boston, Little, Brown and Co., 1953.

Morison, S. E., Commager, H. S., and Leuchtenburg, W. E.: The Growth of the American Republic. 2 vols. New York, Oxford University Press, 1969.

Turner, T. B.: Heritage of Excellence. Baltimore, Johns Hopkins University Press, 1974.

Chapter 11

Billings, J. S.: A review of higher medical education. Am. J. Med. Sci. 76:174, 1878.

Billings, J. S.: Commemoration of the one hundredth anniversary of the birth of, with various papers including two papers by Billings on medical education. Bull. Johns Hopkins Hosp. 62:283, 1938.

Burrow, J. G.: A.M.A.—Voice of American Medicine. Baltimore, Johns Hopkins University Press, 1963.

Cannon, W. B.: President Eliot's relations to medicine. N. Engl. J. Med. 210:730, 1934.

Carter, B. N.: Fruition of Halsted's concept of surgical training. Surgery 32:518, 1952.

Chesney, A. M.: The Johns Hopkins Hospital and the Johns Hopkins University School of Medicine. 3 vols. Baltimore, Johns Hopkins University Press, 1943, 1958, and 1963.

Corner, G. W.: George Hoyt Whipple and His Friends. Philadelphia, J. B. Lippincott, 1963.

Crowe, S. J.: Halsted of Johns Hopkins. Springfield, Ill., Charles C Thomas, 1957.

Cushing, H.: The Life of Sir William Osler. Oxford, The Clarendon Press, 1926.

Davis, A. W.: Dr. Kelly of Hopkins. Baltimore, Johns Hopkins University Press, 1959.

Davison, W. C.: The Duke University Medical Center (1892–1960)—Reminiscences. Privately printed, 1960.

Flexner, A.: Medical Education in the United States and Canada. New York, The Carnegie Foundation for the Advancement of Teaching, No. 4, 1910.

Flexner, S.: A half century of American medicine. Science 85:505, 1937.

Flexner, S., and Flexner, J. T.: William Henry Welch and the Heroic Age of American Medicine. New York, Dover Publications, Inc., 1966. (Originally published by the Viking Press, 1941.)

Fluhmann, C. F.: The department of obstetrics and gynecology of Stanford University School of Medicine. Am. J. Obstet. Gynecol. 51:285, 1946.

Fosdick, R. S.: The Story of the Rockefeller Foundation. New York, Harper and Bros., 1952.

French, J. C.: A History of the University Founded by Johns Hopkins. Baltimore, Johns Hopkins University Press, 1946.

Gonda, T. A.: Stanford University School of Medicine. Calif. Med. 110:74, 1969.

Hamilton, A.: Exploring the Dangerous Trades. The Autobiography of Alice Hamilton. Boston, Little, Brown and Co., 1943.

Holman, E.: Sir William Osler and William Stewart Halsted—two contrasting personalities. Pharos 34:134, 1971.

Holman, E.: William Stewart Halsted. Johns Hopkins Med. J. 135:418, 1974.

James, H.: Charles W. Eliot, President of Harvard University, 1869–1909. 2 vols. Boston and New York, Houghton Mifflin Co., 1930.

Kubie, L. S.: The half-failure of the full-time system as an instrument of medical education. Pharos 34:63, 1971.

803

Littlemeyer, M. H. (ed.): Association of American Medical Colleges Archives: Preliminary Survey—1876–1973. Pamphlet. April, 1974.

MacCallum, W. G.: William Stewart Halsted. Baltimore, Johns Hopkins University Press, 1930.

Osler, W.: The license to practice. Maryland Med. J. 21:61, 1889.

Osler, W.: The inner history of the Johns Hopkins Hospital (edited, annotated, and introduced by D. G. Bates and E. H. Bensley). Johns Hopkins Med. J. 125:184, 1969.

Penfield, W.: The Difficult Art of Giving: The Epic of Alan Gregg. Boston, Little, Brown and Co., 1967.

Robinson, G. C.: Adventures in Medical Education. Cambridge, Mass., Harvard University Press, 1957.

Rogers, F. B.: Selected Papers of John Shaw Billings, Compiled with a Life of Billings. Chicago, Medical Library Association, 1965.

Roland, G. C., and others: William Osler, 1849–1919—commemorative issue. J.A.M.A. 210: 2213–2271, 1969.

Sabin, F. R.: Franklin Paine Mall—The Story of a Mind. Baltimore, Johns Hopkins University Press, 1934.

Shryock, R. H.: The Unique Influence of the Johns Hopkins University on American Medicine. Copenhagen, E. M. Munksgaard, 1953.

Shryock, R. H.: Medical Licensing in America, 1650–1965. Baltimore, Johns Hopkins University Press, 1967.

Thom, H. H.: Johns Hopkins—Silhouette. Baltimore, Johns Hopkins University Press, 1929.

Thomas, H. M., and others: Symposium on the development of the Johns Hopkins Medical School and Osler influence. Bull. Johns Hopkins Hosp. 30:185, 1919.

Turner, T. B.: Heritage of Excellence. Baltimore, Johns Hopkins University Press, 1974.

Walsh, J.: Stanford School of Medicine (1): problems over more than money. Science 171:551, 1971.

Welch, W. H.: Higher medical education and the need of its endowment. Med. News (Philadelphia) 65:63, 1894.

Welch, W. H.: Papers and Addresses. 3 vols. Baltimore, Johns Hopkins University Press, 1920.

Zinsser, H.: As I Remember Him. Boston, Little, Brown and Co., 1940.

Chapter 12

Abel, J. J., Rowntree, L. G., and Turner, B. B.: On the removal of diffusible substances from the circulating blood by means of dialysis. Trans. Assoc. Am. Physicians 28:51, 1913.

Baldwin, E. R.: History of tuberculosis research in America. Yale J. Biol. Med. 15:301, 1943.

Banting, F. G., and Best, C. H.: The internal secretion of the pancreas. J. Lab. Clin. Med. 7:251, 1922.

Barker, L. F.: Medicine and the universities. Am. Med. 4:143, 1907a.

Barker, L. F.: The organization of the laboratories in the medical clinic of the Johns Hopkins Hospital. Johns Hopkins Hosp. Bull. 18:193, 1907b.

Bayliss, W. M.: Principles of General Physiology. London, Longmans, Green and Co., 1924.

Bean, W. B.: Walter Reed—a biographical sketch. Arch. Intern. Med. 134:877, 1974.

Best, C. H.: Reminiscences of the researches which led to the discovery of insulin. Can. Med. Assoc. J. 47:398, 1942.

Best, C. H.: Victory over the sugar sickness (as told to J. D. Ratcliff). Today's Health 42(3):56, 60, 64, 1964.

Billings, J. S.: The plans and purposes of the Johns Hopkins Hospital. Bull. Johns Hopkins Hosp. 65:7, 1939. (Reprinted: address originally delivered in 1889 at opening ceremonies of the Johns Hopkins Hospital.)

Bondy, P. K., and Brainard, E. R.: The American Society for Clinical Investigation, 1909–1959, and the Journal of Clinical Investigation, 1924–1959. J. Clin. Invest. 38:1783, 1959.

Bordley, J., III, and Richards, A. N.: Quantitative studies of the composition of glomerular urine. VIII. The concentration of uric acid in glomerular urine of snakes and frogs, determined by an ultramicroadaptation of Folin's method. J. Biol. Chem. 101:193, 1933.

Buchman, D. D.: The Sherlock Holmes of medicine: Dr. Joseph Goldberger. New York, Messner, 1969.

Cameron, V., and Long, E. R.: Tuberculosis Medical Research. National Tuberculosis Association, 1904–1955. New York, National Tuberculosis Association, 1959.

Carrel, A.: Some physiologic aspects of blood vessel surgery. JAMA 51:1658, 1908.

Carrel, A., and Guthrie, C. C.: Anastomosis of blood vessels by the patching method and transplantation of the kidney. JAMA 51:1658, 1908.

Carrel, A., and Lindbergh, C. A.: The Culture of Organs. New York, Paul B. Hoeber, 1938.

Castle, W. B.: The contributions of George Richards Minot to experimental medicine. N. Engl. J. Med. 247:585, 1952.

Castle, W. B.: A century of curiosity about pernicious anemia. Trans. Am. Clin. Climatol. Assoc. *73*:54, 1961.

Christie, A.: The disease spectrum of human histoplasmosis. Trans. Assoc. Am. Physicians *64*: 147, 1951.

Clark, P. F.: Theobald Smith, student of disease (1859–1934). J. Hist. Med. *14*:490, 1959.

Corner, G. W.: George Hoyt Whipple and His Friends. Philadelphia, J. B. Lippincott Co., 1963.

Corner, G. W.: A History of the Rockefeller Institute: 1901–1953. Origins and Growth. New York, The Rockefeller Institute Press, 1964.

Crowe, S. J., Cushing, H., and Homans, J.: Experimental hypophysectomy. Johns Hopkins Hosp. Bull. *21*:127, 1910.

Cushing, H.: Partial hypophysectomy for acromegaly with remarks on the function of the hypophysis. Ann. Surg. *50*:1002, 1909a.

Cushing, H.: The hypophysis cerebri—Clinical aspects of hyperpituitarism and of hypopituitarism. JAMA *53*:249, 1909b.

Cushing, H.: The function of the pituitary body. Am. J. Med. Sci., *139*:473, 1910.

Cushing, H.: The basophil adenomas of the pituitary body and their clinical manifestations (pituitary basophilism). Bull. Johns Hopkins Hosp. *50*:137, 1932.

Dandy, W. E.: Ventriculography following the injection of air into the cerebral ventricles. Ann. Surg. *68*:5, 1918.

de Kruif, P.: Microbe Hunters. New York, Harcourt Brace and Co., 1926.

Dolman, C. E.: Texas cattle fever: A commemorative tribute to Theobald Smith. Clio. Med. *4*:1, March, 1969a.

Dolman, C. E.: Theobald Smith (1859–1934). Life and work. N.Y. State J. Med. *69*:2801, 1969b.

Duclaux, E.: Pasteur–The History of a Mind. (Translated into English.) Philadelphia, W. B. Saunders Co., 1920.

Flexner, S., and Flexner, J.: William Henry Welch and the Heroic Age of American Medicine. New York, Viking Press, 1941.

Flint, A.: Conservative medicine. Am. Med. Monthly *18*:1, 1862. (Quoted from Brieger, G. H.: Medical America in the Nineteenth Century. Baltimore, Johns Hopkins University Press, 1972.)

Galdston, I.: Progress in Medicine: A Critical Review of the Last Hundred Years. New York, Alfred A. Knopf, 1940.

Garrison, F. H.: An Introduction to the History of Medicine. Philadelphia, W. B. Saunders Co., 1929.

Goldberger, R. F.: Dr. Joseph Goldberger. His wife's recollections. J. Am. Diet. Assoc. *32*:724, 1956.

Haagenson, C. D., and Lloyd, W. E. B.: A Hundred Years of Medicine. New York, Sheridan House, 1943.

Halsted, W. S.: Practical comments on the use and abuse of cocaine suggested by its invariably successful employment in more than a thousand minor surgical operations. N.Y. Med. J. *42*: 294, 1885.

Halsted, W. S.: The operative story of goitre. The author's operation. Johns Hopkins Hosp. Reports *19*:71, 1919.

Harris, S.: Banting's Miracle. Philadelphia, J. B. Lippincott Co., 1946.

Harrod, K. E.: Man of Courage: The Story of Edward L. Trudeau. New York, Messner, 1959.

Harvey, A. McG.: Johns Hopkins—the birthplace of tissue culture: The story of Ross G. Harrison, Warren H. Lewis, and George O. Gey. Johns Hopkins Med. J. *136*:142, 1975.

Hench, P. S.: Presentation of the Kober Medal to Edward Calvin Kendall. Trans. Assoc. Am. Physicians *65*:42, 1952.

Hume, E. E.: Victories of Army Medicine. Philadelphia, J. B. Lippincott, 1943.

Hume, E. E.: Editorial: Surgeon-General Sternberg's centenary, 1838–1938. Ann. Med. Hist. *10*: 266, 1938.

Kelly, H. A.: George Miller Sternberg, 1838–1915. Johns Hopkins Hosp. Bull. *32*:1, 1921.

Kendall, E. C.: The isolation in crystalline form of the compound containing iodine which occurs in the thyroid. JAMA *64*:2042, 1915.

Krause, A. K.: Studies on tuberculous infection. I. A note on experimental tracheo-bronchial node tuberculosis. Am. Rev. Tuberculosis *3*:1, 1919.

Lechevalier, H. A., and Solotorovsky, M.: Three Centuries of Microbiology. New York, Dover Publications, Inc., 1974.

Leikind, M. C.: The evolution of medical research in the United States. International Record of Medicine, July, 1958, p. 455.

MacCallum, W. G., and Voegtlin, C.: Influence of various salts upon tetany following parathyroidectomy. J. Pharmacol. Exp. Ther. *2*:421, 1911.

McCollum, E. V.: A History of Nutrition. Boston, Houghton Mifflin Co., 1957.

Mayo, C. H.: Paroxysmal hypertension with tumor of retroperitoneal nerve. JAMA *89*:1047, 1927.

805

Meltzer, S. J.: The science of clinical medicine: What it ought to be and the men to uphold it. JAMA 53:508, 1909.

Mendel, L. B., et al.: The Vitamins. A symposium of 11 articles which appeared in the Journal of the American Medical Association between April and August, 1932. Reprinted in a special edition by Mead Johnson and Co., Evansville, Indiana, 1932.

Minot, G. R.: Treatment of pernicious anemia by a special diet. JAMA 87:470, 1926.

Minot, G. R.: Development of liver treatment in pernicious anemia. (Nobel Lecture.) Lancet 1:361, 1935.

Mitchell, J. F.: The introduction of rubber gloves for use in surgical operations. Ann. Surg. 122: 902, 1945.

Nicholas, J. S.: Ross Granville Harrison, 1870–1959. Yale J. Biol. Med. 32:407, 1960.

Orloff, J., and Berliner, R. W. (eds.): Handbook of Physiology. Section 8: Renal Physiology. Washington, D.C., American Physiological Society, 1973.

Parsons, R. P.: The adventurous Goldberger. Ann. Med. Hist. 3:534, 1931.

Peery, T. M.: The new and old diseases—a study of mortality trends in the United States, 1800–1969. Am. J. Clin. Pathol. 63:453, 1975.

Pincoffs, M. C.: A case of paroxysmal hypertension associated with suprarenal tumor. Trans. Assoc. Am. Physicians 44:295, 1929.

Porter, J.: Louis Pasteur Sesquicentennial. (1822–1972). Science 178:1249, 1972.

Rackemann, Francis M.: The Inquisitive Physician—The Life and Times of George Richards Minot. Cambridge, Mass.: Harvard University Press, 1956.

Richards, A. N.: Methods and Results of Direct Investigations of the Function of the Kidneys. (Beaumont Foundation Lecture No. 8.) Baltimore, Williams and Wilkins Co., 1929.

Richards, A. N.: Processes of urine formation. (Croonian Lecture before the Royal Society, June 30, 1938.) Proc. R. Soc. Med., Series B, 126:398, 1938.

Richmond, P. A.: The 19th Century American physician as a research scientist. Symposium on the history of American medicine. International Record of Medicine, 171:317, June, 1958.

Ricketts, H. T.: Contributions to Medical Science by Howard T. Ricketts, 1870–1910. Published as a tribute to his memory by his colleagues under the auspices of the Chicago Pathological Society. Chicago: Chicago University Press, 1911.

Rowntree, L. G.: Amid Masters of 20th Century Medicine. Springfield, Ill.: Charles C Thomas, Publ., 1958.

Sabin, F. R.: Franklin Paine Mall, The Story of a Mind. Baltimore: The Johns Hopkins Press, 1934.

Shope, R. E.: An intermediate host for the swine influenza virus. J. Exp. Med., 54:373, 1931.

Shope, R. E.: Influenza. History, epidemiology and speculation. Pub. Health Rep., 73:165, 1958.

Shryock, R. H.: Factors affecting medical research in the United States, 1800–1900. Bull. Soc. Med. Hist. (Chicago), 5:1, 1943.

Shryock, R. H.: Trends in American medical research during the nineteenth century. Proc. Am. Philos. Soc. 91:59, 1947a.

Shryock, R. H.: American Medical Research: Past and Present. New York, The Commonwealth Fund, 1947b.

Shryock, R. H.: The Development of Modern Medicine. New York, Alfred A. Knopf, 1947c.

Shryock, R. H.: Changing outlooks in American medicine over three centuries. *In* Essays in Honor of David J. Davis. Chicago, Illinois University College of Medicine, 1965, p. 182.

Shryock, R. H.: The Historical Significance of the Tuberculosis Movement. Transactions of 38th Annual Meeting of the National Tuberculosis Association, 1942. (Reprinted in Medicine in America. Baltimore, Johns Hopkins University Press, 1966.)

Singer, C., and Underwood, E. A.: A Short History of Medicine, 2nd ed. New York and Oxford, Oxford University Press, 1962.

Smith, G.: Plague On Us. New York, The Commonwealth Fund, 1941.

Smith, Homer W.: Lectures on the Kidney. Lawrence, Kan., University Extension Division, University of Kansas, 1943.

Smith, P. E.: The disabilities caused by hypophysectomy and their repair. JAMA 88:148, 1927.

Smith, P. E.: Hypophysectomy and a replacement therapy. Am. J. Anat. 45:205, 1930.

Sternberg, M. L.: George Miller Sternberg—A Biography by His Wife. Chicago, American Medical Association, 1920.

Stevenson, L. G.: Sir Frederick Banting. Toronto, Ryerson Press, 1946.

Stevenson, L. G.: Nobel Prize Winners in Medicine and Physiology. 1901–1950. New York, Henry Schuman, 1953.

Thorn, G. W., Dorrance, S. S., and Day, E.: Addison's disease: Evaluation of synthetic desoxycorticosterone acetate therapy in 158 patients. Trans. Assoc. Am. Physicians 57:199, 1942.

Vaughan, V. C.: A Doctor's Memories. Indianapolis, Bobbs-Merrill Co., 1926.

Wilder, R. M., Allan, F. M., Power, M. H., and Robertson, H. E.: Carcinoma of the islands of the pancreas—hyperinsulinism and hypoglycemia. JAMA 89:348, 1927.

Windhager, E. E.: Micropuncture Techniques and Nephron Function. New York, Appleton-Century-Crofts, 1968.

Chapter 13

Brieger, G. H.: Medical America in the 19th Century. Baltimore, Johns Hopkins University Press, 1972.

Corwin, E. H. L.: The American Hospital. New York, The Commonwealth Fund, 1946.

Doolen, R. M.: Founding of the University of Michigan Hospital: An innovation in medical education. J. Med. Educ. *39*:50, 1964.

Eaton, L. L.: Charles Bulfinch and the Massachusetts General Hospital. Isis *41*:8, 1950.

Faxon, N. W.: The Massachusetts General Hospital, Its Development, 1935–1955. Cambridge, Mass., Harvard University Press, 1959.

Flexner, A.: Medical Education in the United States and Canada. New York, Carnegie Foundation, 1910.

Freidson, E.: The Hospital in Modern Society. Chicago, The Free Press of Glencoe, 1953.

Hertzler, A. E.: The Horse and Buggy Doctor. New York and London, Harper & Bros., 1938.

Knowles, J. H. (ed.): Hospitals, Doctors, and the Public Interest. Cambridge, Mass., Harvard University Press, 1965.

Ranson, J. E.: Beginnings of hospitals in the United States. Hospitals *15*:75, 1941.

Rappleye, W. C.: The Current Era of the Faculty of Medicine. Columbia University, 1910–1958. New York, Columbia University Press, 1958.

Rideing, W. H.: Hospital life in New York. Harper's New Monthly Magazine, *57*:171, 1878.

Robinson, G. C.: Adventures in Medical Education. Cambridge, Mass., Harvard University Press, 1957.

Thomas, D. G.: History of founding and development of the first hospitals in the United States. Am. J. Insanity *24*:131, 1867–68.

Wylie, W. C.: Hospitals: Their history, organization and construction. Boylston Prize Essay of Harvard University for 1876. New York, D. Appleton & Co., 1877.

Chapter 14

Braasch, W. F.: Early Days in the Mayo Clinic. Springfield, Ill., Charles C Thomas, 1969.

Brecher, E., and Brecher, R.: The Rays—A History of Radiology in the United States and Canada. Baltimore, Williams and Wilkins Co., 1969.

Brown, P.: American Martyrs to Science through Roentgen Rays. Springfield, Ill., Charles C Thomas, 1936.

Chesney, A. M.: The Johns Hopkins Hospital and the Johns Hopkins University School of Medicine. 3 vols. Baltimore, The Johns Hopkins University Press, 1943, 1958, 1963.

Clapesattle, H.: The Doctors Mayo. Minneapolis, University of Minnesota Press, 1941.

Crile, G.: George Crile, an Autobiography. Edited, with sidelights, by Grace Crile. 2 vols. Philadelphia, J. B. Lippincott Co., 1947.

Crowe, S. J.: Halsted of Johns Hopkins: The Man and His Men. Springfield, Ill., Charles C Thomas, 1957.

Diamond, L. K.: History of blood banking in the U.S. JAMA *193*:40, 1965.

Fitz, R. H.: Perforating inflammation of the vermiform appendix: With special reference to its early diagnosis and treatment. Trans. Assoc. Am. Physicians *1*:107, 1886.

Fulton, J. F.: Harvey Cushing, a Biography. Springfield, Ill., Charles C Thomas, 1946.

Haagensen, C. D., and Lloyd, W. E. B.: A Hundred Years of Medicine. New York, Sheridan House, 1943.

Halsted, W. S.: Refusion in the treatment of carbonic acid poisoning. Ann. Anat. Surg. *9*:7, 1884.

Halsted, W. S.: Circular suture of the intestine. Am. J. Med. Sci. *94*:436, 1887.

Halsted, W. S.: Radical cure of inguinal hernia in the male. Bull. Johns Hopkins Hosp. *4*:17, 1894a.

Halsted, W. S.: Results of operation for cure of cancer of the breast. Ann. Surg. *20*:497, 1894b.

Halsted, W. S.: Ligature and suture material. JAMA *60*:1119, 1913.

Halsted, W. S.: The operative story of goitre. The author's operation. Johns Hopkins Hosp. Reports *19*:71, 1919.

Harvey, A. McG.: Pioneers in urology: James R. Brown and Howard A. Kelly. Johns Hopkins Med. J., *134*:291, 1974a.

Harvey, A. McG.: Neurosurgical genius—Walter Edward Dandy. Johns Hopkins Med. J., *135*:358, 1974b.

Harvey, A. McG.: Early contributions to the surgery of cancer: William S. Halsted, Hugh H. Young and John G. Clark. Johns Hopkins Med. J. *135*:399, 1974c.

Hutchins, P.: History of blood transfusion. Surgery *64*:685, 1968.

Johnson, V.: Origins and development of the Mayo Foundation. Minn. Med. *47*:1161, 1964.

Kelly, H. A.: Asepsis not antisepsis. A plea for principles, not paraphernalia in laparotomy. Maryland Med. J. *15*:110, 1886.

MacCallum, W. G.: William Stewart Halsted—Surgeon. Baltimore, Johns Hopkins University Press, 1930.

807

Myers, Grace W.: History of the Massachusetts General Hospital, June, 1872, to December, 1900. Boston, Griffith-Stillings Press, ND. (Preface dated 1929.)

Nagel, G. W.: The Mayo Legacy. Springfield, Ill., Charles C Thomas, 1966.

Rosenberg, C.: The practice of medicine in New York a century ago. Bull. Hist. Med. *41*:223, 1967.

Rynearson, E. H.: The Drs. Mayo: Their influence upon young men. Minn. Med. *47*:1073, 1964.

Stern, B. J.: American Medical Practice in the Perspectives of a Century. New York, The Commonwealth Fund, 1945.

Thomson, St. Clair: A house-surgeon's memories of Joseph Lister. Ann. Med. Hist. *2*:93, 1920.

Walker, Kenneth: The Story of Medicine. New York, Oxford University Press, 1955.

Walters, W.: Forty years of surgery at the Mayo Clinic. Perspect. Biol. Med. *7*:3, 1963.

Wangensteen, O. H.: The Mayo enterprise: A study in the anatomy of success. Minn. Med. *47*: 1067, 1964.

Wilder, Lucy: The Mayo Clinic. Springfield, Ill., Charles C Thomas, 1936.

Chapter 15

Cannon, W. B.: President Eliot's relation to medicine. N. Engl. J. Med. *210*:730, 1934.

Cassedy, J. H.: The registration area and American vital statistics—development of a health research resource. Bull. Hist. Med. *39*:221, 1965.

Chapin, C. V.: History of state and municipal control of disease. *In* Ravenel, M. P. (ed.): A Half Century of Public Health. New York, The American Public Health Association, 1921.

Dock, L. L.: The history of public health nursing. *In* Ravenel, M. P. (ed.): A Half Century of Public Health. New York, The American Public Health Association, 1921.

Flexner, S., and Flexner, J. T.: William Henry Welch and the Heroic Age of American Medicine. New York, Viking Press, Inc., 1941.

Fosdick, R. B.: The Story of the Rockefeller Foundation. New York, Harper and Bros., 1952.

Gorham, F. P.: The history of bacteriology and its contribution to public health work. *In* Ravenel, M. P. (ed.): A Half Century of Public Health. New York, The American Public Health Association, 1921.

Grove, R. D., and Hetzel, A. M.: Vital Statistics Rates in the United States, 1940–1960. Washington, D.C., United States Department of Health, Education and Welfare, Public Health Service, 1968.

Morison, S. E.: The Oxford History of the American People. New York, Oxford University Press, 1965.

Peery, T. M.: The new and old diseases. A study of mortality trends in the United States, 1900–1969. Am. J. Clin. Pathol. *63*:453, 1975.

Penfield, W.: The Difficult Art of Giving: The Epic of Alan Gregg. Boston, Little, Brown & Co., 1967.

Ravenel, M. P.: The American Public Health Association: past, present, future. *In* Ravenel, M. P. (ed.): A Half Century of Public Health. New York, The American Public Health Association, 1921.

Rosen, G.: A History of Public Health. New York, MD Publications, Inc., 1958.

Singer, C.: History of Medicine. Oxford, Oxford University Press, 1928.

Smillie, W. G.: Public Health: Its Promise for the Future. New York, The Macmillan Company, 1955.

Smith, S.: The history of public health, 1871–1921. *In* Ravenel, M. P. (ed.): A Half Century of Public Health. New York, The American Public Health Association, 1921.

Turner, T. B.: Heritage of Excellence, the Johns Hopkins Medical Institutions, 1914–1947. Baltimore, Johns Hopkins University Press, 1974.

Vaughan, V. C.: A Doctor's Memories. Indianapolis, Bobbs-Merrill Co., 1926.

Vedder, E. B.: Medicine, Its Contribution to Civilization. Baltimore, The Williams and Wilkins Co., 1929.

Wattenberg, B. J.: This U.S.A. An Unexpected Family Portrait of 194,067,296 Americans Drawn from the Census. Garden City, New York, Doubleday and Co., 1965.

Welch, W. H.: Public Health in Theory and Practice: An Historical Review. New Haven, Yale University Press, 1925.

Welch, W. H., and Rose, W.: Institute of Hygiene. *In* Papers and Addresses of William H. Welch. Vol. 1. Baltimore, Johns Hopkins University Press, 1920.

Chapter 16

Keefer, C. S.: Dr. Richards as chairman of the Committee on Medical Research. Ann. Intern. Med. (Suppl. 8) *71*:64, 1969.

Leikind, M. C.: The evolution of medical research in the United States. Int. Rec. Med., July, 1958, p. 455.

Shannon, J. A.: The advancement of medical research: A 20-year view of the role of the National Institutes of Health. J. Med. Educ. *42:*97, 1967.

Shryock, R. H.: American Medical Research: Past and Present. New York, The Commonwealth Fund, 1947.

Strickland, S. P.: Politics, Science, and Dread Disease: A Short History of the United States Medical Research Policy. Cambridge, Mass., Harvard University Press, 1972.

Vaughan, V. C.: A Doctor's Memories. Indianapolis, Bobbs-Merrill Co., 1926.

Chapter 17

Barrow, J. G.: AMA—Voice of American Medicine. Baltimore, Johns Hopkins University Press, 1963.

Davis, N. S.: History of the AMA from its organization up to January, 1855. Philadelphia, Lippincott, Grambo and Co., 1855.

Fishbein, M.: A History of the AMA. Philadelphia, W. B. Saunders Co., 1947.

Young, J. H.: The Medical Messiahs: A Social History of Health Quackery in Twentieth Century America. Princeton, N.J., Princeton University Press, 1967.

Chapter 18

Derbyshire, R. C.: Medical Licensure and Discipline in the United States. Baltimore, Johns Hopkins University Press, 1969.

Flexner, A.: Medical Education in the United States and Canada. New York, Carnegie Foundation, 1910.

Flexner, S., and Flexner, J. T.: William Henry Welch and the Heroic Age of American Medicine. New York, Dover Publications, Inc., 1966. (Originally published by Viking Press, 1941.)

Osler, W.: The license to practice. Maryland Med. J. *21:*61, 1889.

Rogers, F. B.: Selected Papers of John Shaw Billings, with a Life of Billings. Chicago, Medical Library Association, 1965.

Sabin, F. R.: Franklin Paine Mall—The Story of a Mind. Baltimore, Johns Hopkins University Press, 1934.

Shindell, S.: The Law of Medical Practice. Pittsburgh, University of Pittsburgh Press, 1966.

Shryock, R. H.: Medical Licensing in America. Baltimore, Johns Hopkins University Press, 1967.

Chapter 19

Boorstin, D. J.: The Americans: The Democratic Experience. New York, Random House, 1973.

Chapter 20

Allen, E. M.: Fiscal relations between the medical schools and the federal government. J. Med. Educ. *43:*697, 1968.

Beeson, P. B.: The ways of academic clinical medicine in America since World War II. (The Cartwright Lecture.) Man and Med. *1:*65, 1975. (The lecture is followed by Commentaries by M. D. Bogdonoff, R. J. Glaser, G. T. Perkoff, and W. McDermott, and an Editorial.)

Bromberg, J.: State roles in financing medical education. J. Med. Educ. *49:*1193, 1974.

Burrow, J. G.: AMA—Voice of American Medicine. Baltimore, Johns Hopkins University Press, 1963.

Checker, A., Fribush, S., and Larson, T.: U.S. medical school faculty members who earned their M.D. degrees in foreign medical schools. J. Med. Educ. *49:*876, 1974.

Colwill, J. M.: Medical school admissions as a reflection of societal needs. Pharos *36:*91, 1973.

Crispell, K. R.: Task force report: Graduates of foreign medical schools in the United States: A challenge to medical education. J. Med. Educ. *49:*809, 1974.

Dubé, W. F.: COTRANS and the U.S. citizen studying medicine abroad. J. Med. Educ. *49:*394, 1974.

Dubé, W. F.: COTRANS after five years. J. Med. Educ. *50:*208, 1975a.

Dubé, W. F.: U.S. medical school enrollment, 1970–71 through 1974–75. J. Med. Educ. *50:*303, 1975b.

Dublin, T. D.: Foreign physicians: their impact on U.S. health care. International migration aids domestic supply but raises issues of quality. Science *185:*407, 1974.

Education cost set at $2,650 yearly—capitation figure lower. Am. Med. News, March 4, 1974.

Education for family practice. *In* Medical Education in the United States, 1972–73. JAMA *226*: 896, 1973.

Fagan, S. K.: Salaries of strict full-time faculty in U.S. medical schools. J. Med. Educ. *49*:913, 1974.

Funkenstein, D. H.: Implications of the rapid social changes in universities and medical schools for the education of future physicians. J. Med. Educ. *43*:433, 1968.

Goldhaber, S. Z.: Medical education: Harvard reverts to tradition. Science *181*:1027, 1973.

Ham, T. H.: Medical education at Western Reserve University—a progress report for the sixteen years, 1946–62. N. Engl. J. Med. *267*:868, 916, 1962.

Kerr, C.: We are building too many medical schools—and in the wrong places. Am. Med. News, March 17, 1975.

Lambson, R. O.: Medical school admissions—a glimpse at the future by looking back. J. Med. Educ. *50*:912, 1975.

Levit, E. J., Sabshin, M., and Mueller, C. B.: Trends in graduate medical education and specialty certification. A tracking study of United States medical school graduates. N. Engl. J. Med. *290*:545, 1974.

Magraw, R. M., Hahn, J. J., Autrey, H. L., and Preissig, J. L.: Perspectives from new schools—the costs and financing of medical education. N. Engl. J. Med. *289*:558, 1973.

Margulies, H., Bloch, L. S., and Cholko, F. K.: Random survey of U.S. hospitals with approved internships and residencies; a study of the professional qualities of foreign medical graduates. J. Med. Educ. *43*:706, 1968.

Marks, P. A.: Report of the Vice President for health services. P & S Quarterly, Summer, 1974.

Mason, H. R.: Foreign medical graduates—profiles for those qualifying for practice in the United States, 1957 to 1971. JAMA *229*:428, 1974.

McGuinness, A. C.: Performance of U.S. citizen candidates on the January 1974 ECFMG examination. JAMA *229*:431, 1974.

Millis, J. S.: The Shattuck Lecture: The graduate education of physicians. N. Engl. J. Med. *276*: 1101, 1967.

O'Malley, C. D. (ed.): The History of Medical Education. Berkeley, University of California Press, 1970.

Painter, D. D., and Carow, R.: House staff salaries: An analysis of interinstitutional and longitudinal variations. J. Med. Educ. *49*:1128, 1974.

Payer, L. J.: American medical students abroad: Group finds way in French system. Science *185*: 594, 1974.

Rogers, D. E.: Health care and the academic medical center. Pharos *36*:49, 1973.

Ronaghy, H. A., Cahill, K., and Baker, T. D.: Physician migration to the United States: One country's transfusion is another country's hemorrhage. JAMA *227*:538, 1974.

Senate rejects restrictive education bill. Am. Med. News, August 30, 1974.

Sprague, C. C.: National health policy: objectives and strategy. J. Med. Educ. *49*:3, 1974a.

Sprague, C. C.: The foreign medical graduate—a time for action. (Editorial.) N. Engl. J. Med. *290*:1482, 1974b.

Stetten, D.: Projected changes in medical school curriculum: Are three years really better than four? Science *174*:1303, 1971.

Stevens, R., Goodman, L. W., and Mick, S. S.: Physician migration reexamined: The magnitude of the migration of foreign physicians to the United States since 1965 has been overstated. Science *190*:439, 1975.

Stross, J. K., Hiss, R. G., Rinaldo, J. A., Dykman, C. J., and Vanselow, N. A.: A statewide approach to graduate medical education. N. Engl. J. Med. *291*:701, 1974.

Summer, S. J., and Dove, D. D.: Income analysis of university owned or operated teaching hospitals. J. Med. Educ. *50*:486, 1975.

Swanson, A. G.: Mandatory requirement versus voluntary opportunity for service in the National Health Service Corps. (Editorial.) J. Med. Educ. *50*:406, 1975.

Turner, T. B.: Accounting of a Stewardship. Privately printed, ND. (about 1970).

Visscher, M. B.: Basic scientific education for the future of medicine. Fed. Proc. *33*:1996, 1974.

Weiss, R. J., Kleinman, J. C., Brandt, U. C., Feldman, J. J., and McGuinness, A. C.: Foreign medical graduates and the medical underground. N. Engl. J. Med. *290*:1408, 1974a.

Weiss, R. J., Kleinman, J. C., Brandt, U. C., and Felsenthal, D. S.: The effect of importing physicians—return to a pre-Flexnerian standard. N. Engl. J. Med. *290*:1453, 1974b.

Chapter 21

Bush, V.: Carnegie Institute. Washington Yearbook *45*:1, 1946.

Cooper, J. A. D.: Letter to the Editor. Wall Street Journal, July 30, 1975.

DeBakey, M. D.: Report to the President—A National Program to Conquer Heart Disease, Cancer and Stroke. 2 vols. Washington, D.C., U.S. Government Printing Office, 1964.

Ebert, R. H.: Biomedical research policy. Trans. Assoc. Am. Physicians *86*:1, 1973.

Edwards, C. C.: The federal involvement in health—a personal view of current problems and future needs. N. Engl. J. Med. *292*:559, 1975.

Keefer, C. S.: Dr. Richards as chairman of the Committee on Medical Research. Ann. Intern. Med. (Suppl. 8) *71*:64, 1969.

Rogers, P. G.: Letter to the Editor. Wall Street Journal, August 11, 1975.

Strickland, S. P.: Politics, Science and Dread Disease: a Short History of the United States Medical Research Policy. Cambridge, Mass., Harvard University Press, 1972.

Chapter 22

Astwood, E. B.: Treatment of hyperthyroidism with thiourea and thiouracil. JAMA *122*:78, 1943.

Astwood, E. B.: Thyroid disorders—a half century of innovation. Ann. Intern. Med. *63*:553, 1965.

Bender, G. A.: Great Moments in Medicine. Detroit, Michigan, Northwood University Press (Parke, Davis and Co.), 1966.

Brunel, J.: Antibiosis from Pasteur to Fleming. J. Hist. Med. *6*:287, 1951.

Campbell, G. D.: Oral hypoglycemic agents, pharmacology and therapeutics. Med. Chem., Vol. 9. New York, Academic Press, 1969.

Chain, E., Florey, H. W., et al.: Penicillin as a chemotherapeutic agent. Lancet *2*:226, 1940.

Clarke, F. H.: How modern medicines are discovered. Mount Kisco, N.Y.: Futura Publishing Co., 1973. (This reference has been used extensively as source material.)

Cluff, L. E., Caranosos, G. J., and Stewart, R. B.: Clinical problems with drugs. Vol. 5, *In* Smith, L. H., Jr. (ed.): Major Problems in Internal Medicine. Philadelphia, London, Toronto, W. B. Saunders Co., 1975.

Cooley, D. G.: The Science Book of Modern Medicines. New York, Pocket Books, Inc., 1963.

Davies, W.: The Pharmaceutical Industry. A Personal Study. Oxford and New York, Pergamon Press, Ltd., 1967.

DeFelice, S. L.: An analysis of the relationship between human experimentation and drug discovery in the United States. Drug Metabolism Reviews *3*:167, 1974.

Dubos, R.: Medicine's living history. Medical World News, May 5, 1975, p. 77.

Duggar, B. M.: Aureomycin: A product of continuing search for new antibiotics. Ann. N.Y. Acad. Sci. *51*:177, 1948.

du Vigneaud, V.: Trail of sulfur research: From insulin to oxytocin. Science *123*:967, 1956.

Ehrlich, J., Bartz, X. R., et al.: Chloromycetin, a new antibiotic from a soil actinomycete. Science *106*:417, 1947.

Engel, L.: Medicine Makers of Kalamazoo. New York, McGraw-Hill, 1961.

Feldman, W. H.: Streptomycin: Some historical aspects of its development as a chemotherapeutic agent in tuberculosis. Am. Rev. Tuberc. *69*:859, 1954.

Galdston, I.: Behind the Sulfa Drugs. New York, Alfred A. Knopf, 1940.

Goodwar, L. S., and Gilman, A.: The Pharmacological Basis of Therapeutics, 2nd ed. New York, Macmillan Co., 1955.

Gray, G. W.: The antibiotics. Sci. Am. *181*:26, 1949.

Hawkins, F., and Lawrence, J. S.: The Sulfonamides. London, H. K. Lewis, 1950.

Hinshaw, H. C.: Historical notes on the earliest use of streptomycin in clinical tuberculosis. Am. Rev. Tuberc. *70*:9, 1954.

Hitchins, G. H.: A quarter century of chemotherapy. JAMA *209*:1339, 1969a.

Hitchins, G. H.: Chemotherapy and comparative biochemistry. G.H.A. Clowes Memorial Lecture. Cancer Res. *29*:1895, 1969b.

Hudson, R. P.: Action and reaction in medical research. Ann. Intern. Med. *67*:660, 1967.

Lechevalier, H. A., and Solotorovsky, M.: Three Centuries of Microbiology. New York, Dover Publications, Inc., 1974.

Loubatieres, A.: The use of certain sulfonamides in the treatment of experimental diabetes mellitus. Ann. N.Y. Acad. Sci. *67*:185, 1956.

Mackenzie, C. G.: Differentiation of the antithyroid action of thiouracil, thiourea and PABA from sulfonamides by iodine administration. Endocrinology *32*:185, 1943.

Mahony, T.: The Merchants of Life: An Account of the American Pharmaceutical Industry. Freeport, N.Y., Books for Library Press, 1949. (This reference has been used extensively as source material.)

Martin, H. N.: The study of the physiological action of drugs. *In* Physiological Papers of H. Newell Martin. Baltimore, Johns Hopkins University Press, 1895.

Owen, C. A., Jr.: The discoveries of vitamin K and dicumarol and their impact on our concepts of blood coagulation. Mayo Clinic Proc. *49*:912, 1974.

Richter, C. P., and Clisby, K. H.: Toxic effects of bitter tasting phenylthiocarbamide. Arch. Path. *33*:46, 1942.

Starr, I., et al.: Alfred Newton Richards, scientist and man. Ann. Intern. Med. *71* (Suppl. 8): 7, 1969.

811

Waksman, S. A.: My Life with the Microbes. New York, Simon and Schuster, 1954a.

Waksman, S. A.: Tenth anniversary of the discovery of streptomycin. The first chemotherapeutic agent found to be effective against tuberculosis in humans. Am. Rev. Tuberc. *70*:1, 1954b.

Weatherall, M.: Chance and choice in the discovery of drugs. Proc. R. Soc. Med. *65*:329, 1972.

Webster, B., and Chesney, A. M.: Studies in the etiology of simple goiter. Am. J. Path. *6*:275, 1930.

Welch, H., and Lewis, C. N.: Antibiotic Therapy. Washington, D.C., Arundel Press, 1951.

Woods, D. D.: Relation of p-aminobenzoic acid to mechanism of action of sulphanilamide. Br. J. Exp. Pathol. *21*:74, 1940.

Woodward, T. E., Smodel, J. E., et al.: Preliminary report on the beneficial effect of Chloromycetin in the treatment of typhoid fever. Ann. Intern. Med. *29*:131, 1948.

Chapter 23

Abbott, M. D.: Atlas of Congenital Cardiac Disease. New York, American Heart Association, 1936.

Ball, J. M.: Dr. Adam Hammer, surgeon and apostle of higher medical education. J. Miss. State Med. Assoc. *6*:155, 1909.

Beyer, K. H., et al.: Electrolyte excretion as influenced by chlorothiazide. Science *127*:146, 1958.

Bing, R. J.: Heart metabolism. Sci. Am. *196*:51, 1957.

Bing, R. J., Vandam, L. D., and Gray, F. D.: Physiological studies in congenital heart disease. Bull. Johns Hopkins Hosp. *80*:107, 1947.

Bing, R. J., et al.: The measurement of coronary blood flow, oxygen consumption, and efficiency of the left ventricle in man. Am. Heart J. *38*:1, 1949.

Boucher, R., Veyrat, R., De Champlain, J., and Genest, J.: New procedure for determination of renin activity in human plasma and measurement of renin activity in some physiological and pathological states. Can. Med. Assoc. J. *90*:194, 1964.

Brannon, E. S., Weens, H. S., and Warren, J. V.: Atrial septal defect: Study of hemodynamics by the technique of right heart catheterization. Am. J. Med. Sci. *210*:480, 1945.

Braun-Menendez, E., Fasciolo, J. C., Leloir, L. F., Munoz, J. M., and Taquini, A. C.: Renal Hypertension. (Translated by Lewis Dexter, M. D.) Springfield, Ill., Charles C Thomas, 1946.

Buckler, H.: Doctor Dan: Pioneer in American Surgery. Boston, Little, Brown and Co., 1954.

Burch, G. E., and De Pasquale, N. P.: A History of Electrocardiography. Chicago Year Book Medical Publishers, 1964.

Calder, R.: Profile of Science. London, George Allen and Unwin, 1951.

Chamberlain, W. E.: Fluoroscopes and fluoroscopy. Radiology *38*:383, 1942.

Coltman, J. W.: Fluoroscopic image brightening by electronic means. Radiology *51*:359, 1948.

Comroe, Jr., J. H.: What's locked up? Am. Rev. Resp. Dis. *110*:111, 1974.

Conn, J. W.: Presidential Address. Part II. Primary aldosteronism, a new clinical syndrome. J. Lab. Clin. Med. *45*:6, 1955.

Conn, J. W., Cohen, E. L., Rovner, D. R., and Nesbit, R. M.: Normokalemic primary aldosteronism. JAMA *193*:200, 1965.

Corday, E.: Status of coronary bypass surgery. JAMA *231*:1245, 1975.

Cournand, A., and Ranges, H. A.: Catheterization of the right auricle in man. Proc. Soc. Exp. Biol. Med. *46*:462, 1941.

Day, H. W.: An intensive coronary care area. Dis. Chest *44*:423, 1963.

Davis, J. O., Hartroft, P. M., Titus, E. O., Carpenter, C. C. J., Ayers, C. R., and Spiegel, H. E.: The role of the renin-angiotensin system in the control of aldosterone secretion. J. Clin. Invest. *41*:378, 1962.

Deane, H. W., Shaw, J. H., and Gelep, R. O.: The effect of altered sodium or potassium intake on the width and cytochemistry of the zona glomerulosa of the rat's adrenal cortex. Endocrinology *43*:133, 1948.

Deming, Q. B., and Luetscher, J. A.: Bioassay of desoxycorticosterone-like material in urine. Proc. Soc. Exp. Biol. Med. *73*:171, 1950.

Dexter, L., et al.: Studies of congenital heart disease. I. Technique of venous catheterization as a diagnostic procedure. J. Clin. Invest. *26*:547, 1947.

Dock, G.: Some notes on the coronary arteries. Med. Surg. Reporter *75*:1, 1896.

Dole, V. P.: Transport of non-esterified fatty acids in plasma. *In* Page, I. H. (ed.): Chemistry of Lipids as Related to Atherosclerosis. Springfield, Ill., Charles C Thomas, 1958, pp. 189–204.

Dotter, C. T., and Frische, L. H.: Visualization of the coronary circulation by occlusion. Aortography: A practical method. Radiology *71*:502, 1958.

Dotter, C. T., and Steinberg, I.: Angiocardiography: clinical progress. Circulation *4*:123, 1951.

Driscol, T. E., Ratnoff, O. D., and Nygaard, O. F.: The remarkable Dr. Abildgard and counter shock. Ann. Intern. Med. *83*:878, 1975.

Effler, D. B.: Surgery for coronary disease. Sci. Am. *219*:36, 1968.

Ehrlich, E. N.: Aldosterone, the adrenal cortex and hypertension. Ann. Rev. Med. *19*:373, 1968.

Elam, J. O., Brown, E. S., and Elder, J. D.: Artificial respiration by mouth to mask method. N. Engl. J. Med. *250*:749, 1954.

Erlanger, J.: A new instrument for determining systolic and diastolic blood pressure in man. J. Am. Physiol. Soc. *6*:22, 1901.

Erlanger, J.: Sinus stimulation as a factor in the resuscitation of the heart. J. Exp. Med. *16*:452, 1912.

Erlanger, J., and Hooker, D. R.: An experimental study of the blood pressure and pulse pressure in man. Johns Hopkins Hosp. Rep. *12*:145, 1904.

Farmer, H.: Daniel Hale Williams, M.D., L.L.D., F.A.C.S. Ann. Med. Hist. *1*:252 (Ser. 3), 1939.

Fishman, A. P., and Richards, D. W. (eds.): Circulation of the Blood: Men and Ideas. New York, Oxford University Press, 1964.

Freis, E. D.: The chemotherapy of hypertension. JAMA *218*:1009, 1971.

Gibbon, J. H., Jr.: Development of the artificial heart and lung extracorporeal blood circuit. JAMA *206*:1983, 1968.

Gibbon, J. H., Jr.: The development of the artificial heart-lung apparatus. Rev. Surg. *27*:231, 1970.

Gofman, J. W., et al.: The role of lipids and lipoproteins in atherosclerosis. Science *111*:166, 1950.

Goldblatt, H.: Hypertension due to renal ischemia. Bull. N.Y. Acad. Med. *40*:745, 1964.

Goldblatt, H., et al.: Studies on experimental hypertension. I. The production of persistent elevation of systolic blood pressure by means of renal ischemia. J. Exp. Med. *59*:347, 1934.

Gunnels, J. L., Jr., and McGuffin, W. L., Jr.: Low renin hypertension. Ann. Rev. Med. *26*:259, 1975.

Harvey, A. McG., Grob, D., and Holaday, D. A.: Some preliminary observations on the neuromuscular and ganglionic blocking action in man of bis-trimethylammonium decane and pentane diiodide. Trans. Am. Clin. Climatol. Assoc. *60*:133, 1948.

Heart Pacemaker. Interactions of Science and Technology in the Innovative Process: Some case studies prepared for the NSF by Battelle Laboratories under contract NSF-C677, March 19, 1973.

Helmer, O. M., and Judson, W. E.: The quantitative determination of renin in the plasma of patients with arterial hypertension. Circulation *27*:1050, 1963.

Herrick, J. B.: Clinical factors of sudden obstruction of the coronary arteries. JAMA *58*:1971, 1912.

Hill, L. L.: A report of a case of successful suturing of the heart, and table of thirty-seven other cases of suturing by different operators with various terminations, and the conclusions drawn. Med. Rec. *62*:846, 1902.

Hollander, W., and Wilkins, R. W.: Chlorothiazide: A new type of drug for the treatment of arterial hypertension. Boston Med. Quart. *8*:69, 1957.

Hosler, R. M.: Historical notes on cardiopulmonary resuscitation. Am. J. Cardiol. *3*:416, 1959.

Howell, W. H.: Vagus inhibition of the heart and its relation to the inorganic salts of the blood. Am. J. Physiol. *15*:280, 1905.

Howell, W. H., and Brush, C. E.: A critical note upon clinical methods of measuring the blood pressure. Boston Med. Surg. J. *145*:146, 1901.

Howell, W. H., and Duke, W. W.: Experiments on the isolated mammalian heart to show the relation of the inorganic salts on the action of its nerves. Am. J. Physiol. *35*:131, 1906.

Howell, W. H., and Duke, W. W.: The effect of vagus stimulation on the output of potassium from the heart. Am. J. Physiol. *211*:51, 1908.

Humphries, J. O., Kuller, L., Ross, R. S., Friesinger, G. C., and Page, E. E.: Natural history of ischemic heart disease in relation to arteriographic findings: A 12-year study of 224 patients. Circulation *49*:489, 1974.

Hyman, A. S.: Resuscitation of the stopped heart by intracardial therapy. Arch. Intern. Med. *50*:283, 1932.

Janeway, T. C.: A clinical study of hypertensive cardiovascular disease. Arch. Intern. Med. *12*:755, 1913.

Janeway, T. C.: Important contributions to clinical medicine during the past thirty years from the study of human blood-pressure. Trans. Assoc. Am. Physicians *30*:27, 1915.

Johnson, S. L.: The History of Cardiac Surgery (1896–1955). Baltimore, The Johns Hopkins University Press, 1970. (This reference has been used extensively as source material.)

Kannel, W. B., et al.: Risk factors in coronary heart disease: An evaluation of several serum lipids as predictors of coronary heart disease. The Framingham Study. Ann. Intern. Med. *61*:888, 1964.

Karmen, A., Wroblewski, F., and LaDue, J. S.: Transaminase activity in human blood. J. Clin. Invest. *34*:126, 1955.

Keith, N. M., Wagener, H. P., and Barker, N. W.: Some different types of essential hypertension: Their course and prognosis. Am. J. Med. Sci. *197*:332, 1939.

Keith, N. M., Wagener, H. P., and Kernohan, J. W.: The syndrome of malignant hypertension. Arch. Intern. Med. *41*:141, 1928.

813

Kempner, W.: Treatment of kidney disease and hypertensive vascular disease with rice diet. N. C. Med. J. *5*:125, 1944.

Kountz, W. B.: Revival of human hearts. Ann. Intern. Med. *10*:330, 1936.

Kouwenhoven, W. B., and Langworthy, O. R.: Cardiopulmonary resuscitation: An account of 45 years of research. Johns Hopkins Med. J. *132*:186, 1973. (This reference has been used extensively as source material.)

Kouwenhoven, W. B., et al.: Closed-chest cardiac massage. JAMA *173*:1064, 1960.

Landis, E. M., Montgomery, H., and Sparkman, D.: The effects of pressor drugs and of saline kidney extracts on blood pressure and skin temperature. J. Clin. Invest. *17*:189, 1938.

Levy, R. L., Brueen, H. G., and Russell, N. G.: The use of electrocardiographic changes caused by induced anoxemia as a test for coronary insufficiency. Am. J. Med. Sci. *197*:241, 1939.

Lillehei, C. W., and Engel, L.: Open-heart surgery. Sci. Am. *202*:77, 1960.

Lowenstein, J.: Renin assay in hypertensive disease. Ann. Rev. Med. *23*:333, 1972.

Lown, B.: Intensive heart care. Sci. Am. *219*:19, 1968.

Lown, B., Amarasingham, R., and Neuman, J.: New methods for terminating cardiac arrhythmias. JAMA *182*:548, 1962.

Mackenzie, Sir James: Diseases of the Heart, 4th ed. London, Oxford University Press, 1925.

MacLean, J.: The thromboplastic action of cephalin. Am. J. Physiol. *41*:250, 1916.

Mahomed, F. A.: Some clinical aspects of chronic Bright's disease. Guy's Hosp. Rep., 3rd Series, *24*:363, 1879.

Major, R. H.: Classic Descriptions of Disease. Springfield, Ill., Charles C Thomas, 1932.

Martin, H. N.: A New Method of Studying the Mammalian Heart. Studies from the Biology Laboratory of the Johns Hopkins University. Vol. 2. Baltimore, Johns Hopkins University Press, 1895, pp. 119–130.

Master, A. M., Friedman, R., and Dack, S.: The electrocardiogram after standard exercise as a function test of the heart. Am. Heart J. *24*:777, 1942.

McClure, R. D., and Dunn, G. R.: Transfusion of blood. History, methods, dangers, preliminary tests, present status. Report of 150 transfusions. Bull. Johns Hopkins Hosp. *28*:99, 1917.

Meek, W. J., and Eyster, J. A. E.: Experiments on the origin of propagation of the impulse in the heart. Heart *5*:227, 1914.

Merrill, J. P.: The transplantation of the kidney. Sci. Am *201*:57, 1959.

Merrill, J. P.: Present status of kidney transplantation. Disease-a-Month, November, 1974. Chicago, Year Book Medical Publishers, Inc.

Moritz, A. R., and Oldt, M. R.: Arteriolar sclerosis in hypertensive and nonhypertensive individuals. Am. J. Pathol. *13*:679, 1937.

Morris, R. E., Jr., Ransom, P. A., and Howard, J. E.: Studies on the relationship of angiotensin to hypertension in renal origin. J. Clin. Invest. *41*:1386, 1962.

Morrow, J. D., Schroeder, H. A., and Perry, H. M.: Studies on the control of hypertension by hyphex. Circulation *8*:829, 1953.

Mundth, E. D., and Austen, W. G.: Surgical measures for coronary heart disease. N. Engl. J. Med. *293*:13, 75, 124, 1975.

Oates, J., and Sjoerdsma, A.: Decarboxylase inhibition and blood pressure reduction by a-methyl-3,4-dihydroxy-DL-phenylalanine. Science *131*:1890, 1960.

Oliva, P. B., Potts, D. E., and Pluss, R. G.: Coronary arterial spasm in Prinzmetal angina. N. Engl. J. Med. *288*:745, 1973.

Osler, W.: The Lumleian lectures on angina pectoris. Delivered at the Royal College of Physicians, London, March 10–15, 1910. Lancet *1*:697, 1910.

Page, I. H.: The discovery of angiotensin. Perspect. Biol. Med. *18*:456, 1975.

Page, I. H., and Helmer, O. M.: A crystalline pressor substance (angiotonin) resulting from the reaction between renin and renin-activator. J. Exp. Med. *71*:29, 1940.

Page, I. H., and McCubbin, J. W.: Renal Hypertension. Chicago, Year Book Medical Publishers, 1968.

Paton, W. D., and Zaimis, E. J.: Clinical potentialities of certain bis-quaternary compounds causing neuromuscular and ganglionic block. Nature *162*:810, 1948.

Pickering, G. W.: High Blood Pressure. New York, Grune and Stratton, 1955.

Pickering, G. W., and Prinzmetal, M.: Some observations on renin, a pressor substance contained in normal kidney, together with a method for its biological assay. Clin. Sci. *3*:211, 1938.

Porter, W. T.: The recovery of the heart from fibrillary contractions. Am. J. Physiol. *1*:71, 1898.

Richards, D. W., Jr., et al.: Pressure in the right auricle of man, in normal subjects and in patients with congestive heart failure. Trans. Assoc. Am. Physicians *56*:218, 1941.

Richards, D. W.: The contributions of right heart catheterization to physiology and medicine, with some observations on the physiopathology of pulmonary heart disease. (Nobel Prize Lecture.) Am. Heart J. *54*:161, 1957.

Robertson, P. W., et al.: Hypertension due to a renin-secreting renal tumor. Am. J. Med. *43*:963, 1967.

Ross, R. S.: Pathophysiology of the coronary circulation. The Sir Thomas Lewis Lecture. Br. Heart J. *33*:173, 1971.

Rous, P., and Turner, J. R.: The preservation of living red blood cells in vitro. I. Methods of preservation. II. The transfusion of kept cells. J. Exp. Med. 23:219, 239, 1916.

Rowntree, L. G., and Adson, A. W.: Bilateral lumbar sympathetic neurectomy in the treatment of malignant hypertension. JAMA *85*:959, 1925.

Ruggles, H. E.: X-ray motion pictures of the thorax. Radiology *5*:444, 1925.

Rytand, D. A.: The renal factor in arterial hypertension with coarctation of the aorta. J. Clin. Invest. *17*:391, 1938.

Schroeder, H. A.: Hypertensive Disease: Causes and Control. Philadelphia, Lea and Febiger, 1953.

Seidenstricker, J. F.: Mouth to mouth resuscitation. N. Engl. J. Med. *270*:788, 1964.

Skeggs, L. T., et al.: The amino acid sequence of hypertensin II. J. Exp. Med. *104*:193, 1956.

Slaughter, F. G.: Heart surgery. Sci. Am. *182*:14, 1950.

Smithwick, R. H.: Hypertensive cardiovascular disease: Effect of thoracolumbar sympathectomy on mortality and survival rates. JAMA *147*:1611, 1951.

Sones, F. M., and Shirey, E. K.: Cine coronary arteriography. Mod. Concepts Cardiovasc. Dis. *31*:735, 1962.

Spark, R. F., and Melby, J. C.: Hypertension and low plasma renin activity: presumptive evidence for mineralocorticoid excess. Ann. Intern. Med. *75*:831, 1971.

Steele, J. M., and Cohn, A. E.: The nature of hypertension in coarctation of the aorta. J. Clin. Invest. *17*:514, 1938.

Stewart, G. N.: Researches on the circulation time and on the influences which affect it. J. Physiol. *22*:159, 1897–98.

Sturm, R. E., and Morgan, R. H.: Screen intensification systems and their limitations. Am. J. Roentgenol. Radium Ther. *62*:617, 1949.

Sweet, W. H.: Stimulation of the sino-atrial node for cardiac arrest during operation. Bull. Am. Coll. Surg. *32*:234, 1947.

Taussig, H. B.: Congenital Malformations of the Heart. New York, Commonwealth Fund, 1947.

Taussig, H. B., Kallman, C. H., Nagel, D., Baumgardner, R., Momberger, N., and Kirk, H.: Long-time observations on the Blalock-Taussig operation. VIII. 20 to 28 year follow-up on patients with a tetralogy of Fallot. Johns Hopkins Med. J. *137*:13, 1975.

Thomas, L.: The technology of medicine. N. Engl. J. Med. *284*:1366, 1971.

Veterans Administration Cooperative Study Group on Antihypertensive Agents: Effects of treatment on morbidity in hypertension: Results in patients with diastolic blood pressure averaging 115 through 129 mm Hg. JAMA *202*:1028, 1967.

Veterans Administration Cooperative Study Group on Antihypertensive Agents: Effects of treatment on morbidity in hypertension: II. Results in patients with diastolic blood pressure averaging 90 through 114 mm Hg. JAMA *213*:1143, 1970.

Weirich, W. L., Gott, V. L., and Lillehei, W.: The treatment of complete heart block by the combined use of a myocardial electrode and an artificial pacemaker. Surg. Forum *8*:360, 1957.

White, P. D.: Heart Disease, 4th ed. N.Y., Macmillan, 1951.

White, P. D.: The historical background of angina pectoris. Mod. Concepts Cardiovasc. Dis. *18*:109, 1974.

Wiggers, C. J.: The physiological basis for cardiac resuscitation from ventricular fibrillation — method for serial defibrillation. Am. Heart J. *20*:413, 1940.

Wiggers, C. J., and Wegria, R.: Ventricular fibrillation due to single, localized induction and condenser shocks applied during the vulnerable phase of ventricular systole. Am. J. Physiol. *128*:500, 1940.

Wilkins, R. W., and Judson, W. E.: The use of *Rauwolfia serpentina* in hypertensive patients. N. Engl. J. Med. *248*:48, 1953.

Willius, F. H., and Dry, T. J.: A History of the Heart and Circulation. Philadelphia, W. B. Saunders Co., 1948.

Wilson, F. N.: Report of a case showing premature beats arising in the junctional tissues. Heart *6*:17, 1915.

Wilson, F. N.: The distribution of the potential differences produced by the heart beat within the body and its surface. Am. Heart J. *5*:599, 1930.

Wilson, F. N., et al.: The electrocardiogram in myocardial infarction with particular reference to the initial deflections of the ventricular complex. Heart *16*:155, 1933.

Wolferth, C. C., and Wood, F. C.: The electrocardiographic diagnosis of coronary occlusion by the use of chest leads. Am. J. Med. Sci. *183*:30, 1932.

Wood, F. C., and Wolferth, C. C.: Angina pectoris: The clinical and electrocardiographic phenomena of the attack and their comparison with the effects of experimental temporary coronary occlusion. Arch. Intern. Med. *47*:339, 1931.

Woods, J. W., Liddle, G. W., Staut, E. G., Jr., Michelakis, A. M., and Brill, A. B.: Effect of an adrenal inhibitor in hypertensive patients with suppressed renin. Arch. Intern. Med. *123*:366, 1969.

815

Zoll, P. M.: Resuscitation of the heart in ventricular standstill by external electric stimulation. N. Engl. J. Med. *247*:768, 1952.

Zoll, P. M.: Countershock and pacemaking in cardiac arrhythmias. Hosp. Prac. February, 1975, p. 125.

Zoll, P. M., et al.: Termination of ventricular fibrillation in man by externally applied electric countershock. N. Engl. J. Med. *254*:727, 1956.

Chapter 24

Albright, F.: A page out of the history of hyperparathyroidism. J. Clin. Endocrinol. *8*:637, 1948.

Berkman, J., and Rifkin, H.: Diabetic microangiopathy. Ann. Rev. Med. *17*:83, 1966.

Browin, F. W.: The birth of insulin. Today's Health *37*:46, 66, 1959.

Clark, B. F. C., and Marcker, K. A.: How proteins start. Sci. Am. *218*:36, 1968.

Dole, V. P.: Body fat. Sci. Am. *201*:71, 1959.

Editorial: The pineal. Lancet *2*:1235, 1974.

Editorial: Somatostatin and diabetes. Lancet *1*:1323, 1975.

Feiser, L.: Steroids. Sci. Am. *192*:52, 1955.

Goldzieher, J. W., and Rudel, H. W.: How the oral contraceptives came to be developed. JAMA *230*:421, 1974.

Green, D. E.: Biological oxidation. Sci. Am. *199*:56, 1958.

Guillemin, R., and Burgus, R.: The hormones of the hypothalamus. Sci. Am. *227*:24, 1972.

Hormone treatment for immunity disorders. Medical World News, October 25, 1974, page 29.

Houssay, B. A.: Advancement of knowledge of the role of the hypophysis in carbohydrate metabolism during the last 25 years. Endocrinology *30*:884, 1942.

Howard, J. E.: Fuller Albright. Trans. Assoc. Am. Physicians *83*:110, 1970.

Jensen, E. V., and DeSombre, E. R.: Estrogen-receptor interaction. Science *182*:126, 1973.

Kolata, G. B.: Vitamin D: Investigations of a new steroid hormone. Science *187*:635, 1975.

Lehninger, A. L.: Energy transformation in the cell. Sci. Am. *202*:102, 1960.

Li, C. H.: The ACTH molecule. Sci. Am. *209*:46, 1963.

Marx, J. L.: Thymic hormones: Inducers of T cell maturation. Science *187*:1183, 1975.

Maugh, T. H., II: Diabetes: Epidemiology suggests a viral connection. Science *188*:347, 1975.

Maugh, T. H., II: Diabetes (III): New hormones promise more effective therapy. Science *188*:920, 1975.

Merrifield, R. B.: The automatic synthesis of proteins. Sci. Am. *218*:56, 1968.

Merrifield, R. B.: The synthesis of biologically active peptides and proteins. JAMA *210*:1247, 1969.

National Science Foundation: Oral Contraceptives. Interactions of science and technology in the innovative process; some case studies. Prepared for the NSF by Battelle Laboratories under contract NSF-C 667, March 19, 1973. (Extensive use has been made of this report as source material.)

Neurath, H.: Protein-digesting enzymes. Sci. Am. *211*:68, 1964.

O'Malley, B. W., Spelsberg, T. C., Schrader, W. T., Chytil, F., and Staggles, A. W.: Mechanisms of interaction of a hormone-receptor complex with the genome of a eukaryotic target cell. Nature *235*:141, 1972.

Pastan, I.: The 1971 Nobel Prize for medicine. Science *174*:392, 1971.

Pastan, I.: Cyclic AMP. Sci. Am. *227*:97, 1972.

Pfeiffer, J. E.: Enzymes. Sci. Am. *178*:29, 1948.

Phillips, D. C.: The three-dimensional structure of an enzyme molecule. Sci. Am. *215*:78, 1966.

Pike, J. E.: Prostaglandins. Sci. Am. *225*:84, 1971.

Richards, F. M.: The 1972 Nobel Prize for chemistry. Science *178*:492, 1972.

Riedman, S. R., and Gustafson, E. T.: Portraits of Nobel Laureates in Medicine and Physiology. London, New York, and Toronto, Abelard-Schuman, 1963.

Rubenstein, A. H., and Steiner, D. F.: Pro hormones. Ann. Rev. Med. *22*:1, 1971.

Salmon, W. D., Jr., and Daughaday, W. H.: A hormonally controlled serum factor which stimulates sulfate incorporation by cartilage *in vitro*. J. Lab. Clin. Med. *49*:825, 1957.

Scheinberg, M. A., Cathcart, E. S., and Goldstein, A. L.: Thymosin-induced reduction of "Null cells" in peripheral-blood lymphocytes of patients with systemic lupus erythematosus. Lancet *1*:424, 1975.

Sourkes, T. L.: Nobel Prize Winners in Medicine and Physiology, 1901–1965. (Revision of earlier work by L. G. Stevenson, M.D.) London, New York, and Toronto, Abelard-Schuman, 1966.

Stein, W. H., and Moore, S.: The chemical structure of proteins. Sci. Am. *204*:81, 1961.

Stevenson, L. G.: Nobel Prize Winners in Medicine and Physiology, 1901–1950. New York, Henry Schuman, 1953.

Sutherland, E. W.: Studies on the mechanism of hormone action. (Nobel Lecture.) Science *177*:401, 1972.

Wilkins, L.: The thyroid gland. Sci. Am. *202*:119, 1960.
Yalow, R. S., and Berson, S. A.: Immunoassay of endogenous plasma insulin in man. J. Clin. Invest. *39*:1157, 1960.
Yen, S. S. C.: Gonadotropin-releasing hormone. Ann. Rev. Med. *26*:403, 1975.
Zuckerman, S.: Hormones. Sci. Am. *196*:76, 1957.

Chapter 25

Barnes, B. A., et al.: The 12th Report of the Human Renal Transplant Registry. JAMA *233*:787, 1975.
Barr, M. L., and Bertram, E. A.: Amorphous distinction between neurones of the male and female and the behaviour of the nucleolar satellite during accelerated nucleoprotein synthesis. Nature *163*:676, 1949.
Beadle, G. W.: The genes of men and molds. Sci. Am. *179*:30, 1948.
Beadle, G. W.: Genetics and Modern Biology. Jayne Lectures for 1962. Philadelphia, American Philosophical Society, 1963.
Bearn, A. G., and German, J. L., III: Chromosomes and disease. Sci. Am. *205*:66, 1961.
Beutler, E., Yeh, M., and Fairbanks, V. F.: The normal human female as a mosaic of X-chromosome activity: Studies using the gene for G-6 PD deficiency as a marker. Proc. Natl. Acad. Sci. *48*: 9, 1962.
Carter, C. O.: The ABC of Medical Genetics. Boston, Little, Brown and Co., 1969.
Clarke, C. A.: The prevention of "Rhesus" babies. Sci. Am. *219*:46, 1968.
Coburn, A. F.: Oswald Theodore Avery and DNA. Perspect. Biol. Med. *12*:623, 1969.
Cohen, S. N.: The manipulation of genes. Sci. Am. *233*:25, 1975.
Crick, F. H. C.: The structure of the hereditary material. Sci. Am. *191*:54, 1954.
Crick, F. H. C.: The genetic code. Sci. Am. *207*:66, 1962.
Crick, F. H. C.: The genetic code, III. Sci. Am. *215*:55, 1966.
Davis, B. D.: Genetic engineering: How great is the danger. (Editorial.) Science *186*:25, 1974.
Delbruck, M.: Phage and the origins of molecular biology. Coldspring Harbor, New York, Coldspring Harbor Laboratory of Quantitative Biology, 1966.
du Vigneaud, V.: Nobel Lectures in Chemistry, 1942–62. Amsterdam, London, and New York, Elsevier Publishing Co., 1964.
Editorial: Islet-cell transplantation. Lancet *2*:909, 1975.
Franklin, E. C., Fudenberg, H., Meltzer, M., and Stanworth, D. R.: The structural basis for genetic variations of normal human gamma globulins. Proc. Natl. Acad. Sci. *48*:914, 1962.
Friedmann, T.: Prenatal diagnosis of genetic disease. Sci. Am. *225*:34, 1971.
Garrod, A.: Inborn Errors of Metabolism. London, Oxford Medical Publications, 1909.
Glass, B.: A century of biochemical genetics. Proc. Am. Philos. Soc. *109*:227, 1965.
Goodner, D. M.: Antenatal diagnosis of genetic defects. J. Reprod. Med. *10*:261, 1973.
Guillemin, R., and Burgus, R.: The hormones of the hypothalamus. Sci. Am. *227*:24, 1972.
Harboe, M., Osterland, C. K., and Kunkel, H. G.: Localization of two genetic factors to different areas of gamma globulin molecules. Science *136*:979, 1962.
Harris, H.: Garrod's Inborn Errors of Metabolism. (With supplement by H. Harris). London, Oxford University Press, 1963.
Hayes, W. (ed.): Advances in molecular genetics. Br. Med. Bull. *29*:185, 1973.
Hirschhorn, K.: Chromosome identification. Ann. Rev. Med. *24*:67, 1973.
Hoagland, M. B.: Nucleic acids and proteins. Sci. Am. *201*:55, 1959.
Holley, R. W.: The nucleotide sequence of a nucleic acid. Sci. Am. *214*:30, 1966.
Holtzman, N. A.: Dietary treatment of inborn errors of metabolism. Ann. Rev. Med. *21*:335, 1970.
Horowitz, N. H.: The gene. Sci. Am. *195*:79, 1956.
Hume, D. M.: Renal homotransplantation in man. Ann. Rev. Med. *18*:229, 1967.
Hurwitz, J., and Furth, J. J.: Messenger RNA. Sci. Am. *206*:41, 1962.
Ingram, V. M.: How do genes act? Sci. Am. *198*:68, 1958.
Ingram, V. M.: Hemoglobin and its Abnormalities. Springfield, Ill., Charles C Thomas, 1961.
Ingram, V. M.: The Hemoglobins in Genetics and Evolution. New York, Columbia University Press, 1963.
Kalckar, H. M., Anderson, E. P., and Isselbacher, K. J.: Galactosemia, a congenital defect in a nucleotide transferase: A preliminary report. Proc. Natl. Acad. Sci. *42*:49, 1956.
Keightley, R. G., Lawton, A. R., and Cooper, M. D.: Successful fetal liver transplantation in a child with severe combined immunodeficiency. Lancet *2*:850, 1975.
Kolata, G. B.: Evolution of DNA: Changes in gene regulator. Science *189*:446, 1975.
Kornberg, A.: The synthesis of DNA. Sci. Am. *219*:64, 1968.
Landsteiner, K., and Wiener, A.: Studies on an agglutinogen (Rh) in human blood reacting with anti-rhesus sera and with human isoantibodies. J. Exp. Med. *74*:309, 1941.

817

Laurence, K. M.: Fetal malformations and abnormalities. Lancet 2:939, 1974.

Levine, P., and Stetson, R. E.: An unusual case of intra-group agglutination. JAMA 113:126, 1939.

Li, C. H.: The ACTH molecule. Sci. Am. 209:46, 1963.

Luy, M. L. M.: Genetic detection—the newest use of amniocentesis. Mod. Med. 42:31, 1974.

McKusick, V. A.: The mapping of human chromosomes. Sci. Am. 224:104, 1971.

Milunsky, A., and Atkins, L.: Prenatal diagnosis of genetic disorders. JAMA 230:232, 1974.

Mirsky, A. E.: The discovery of DNA. Sci. Am. 218:78, 1968.

Motulsky, A. G.: Brave new world? Science 185:653, 1974.

Nadler, H. L.: Prenatal diagnosis of inborn defects: A status report. Hosp. Prac. 10:41, 1975.

National Science Foundation: Oral Contraceptive. Technology in Retrospect and Critical Events in Science. Vol. 2, Jan. 30, 1969. Prepared for NSF by Illinois Institute of Technology Research under Contract NSF-C535.

Nirenberg, M. W.: The genetic code, II. Sci. Am. 208:80, 1963.

Nomura, M.: Ribosomes. Sci. Am. 221:28, 1969.

Olby, R.: The Origins of Molecular Biology (The path to the Double Helix). Seattle, University of Washington Press, 1975.

Pastan, I.: Cyclic AMP. Sci. Am. 227:97, 1972.

Pike, J. E.: Prostaglandins. Sci. Am. 225:84, 1971.

Rich, A.: Polyribosomes. Sci. Am. 209:44, 1963.

Rider, A. K., et al.: The status of cardiac transplantation—1975. Circulation 52:531, 1975.

Riedman, S. R., and Gustafson, E. T.: Portraits of Nobel Laureates in Medicine and Physiology. London, New York, and Toronto: Abelard-Schuman, 1963.

Rous, P.: Karl Landsteiner, 1868–1943. Obituary notices of the Fellows of the Royal Society. Proc. R. Soc. Med. 5:295, 1947.

Scriver, G. R.: Inborn errors of metabolism: A new frontier of nutrition. Nutr. Today, 1974, p. 4.

Shaw, N. W.: Human chromosome damage by chemical agents. Ann. Rev. Med. 21:409, 1970.

Sourkes, T. L.: Nobel Prize Winners in Medicine and Physiology, 1901–1965. (Revision of earlier work by L. G. Stevenson, M.D.) London, New York, and Toronto: Abelard-Schuman, 1966.

Stein, G. S., Stein, J. S., and Kleinsmith, L. H.: Chromosomal proteins and gene regulation. Sci. Am. 232:47, 1975.

Stern, C.: The continuity of genetics in the 20th century sciences. *In* Holton, G. (ed.): Studies in the Biography of Ideas. New York, W. W. Norton and Co., 1972, p. 171.

Stevenson, L. G.: Nobel Prize Winners in Medicine and Physiology, 1901–1950. New York, Henry Schuman, 1953.

Temin, H. M.: RNA-directed DNA synthesis. Sci. Am. 226:25, 1972.

Thomas, E. D., et al.: Bone-marrow transplantation. N. Engl. J. Med. 292:832, 895, 1975.

Tjio, J. H., and Levan, A.: The chromosome number of man. Hereditas 42:1, 1956.

Woglom, W. H.: Heredity—Gregor Johann Mendel. *In* Discoverers of Medicine. New Haven, Yale University Press, 1949.

Yanofsky, C.: Gene structure and protein structure. Sci. Am. 216:80, 1967.

Chapter 26

Barrett, J. T.: Textbook of Immunology. St. Louis, The C. V. Mosby Co., 1974.

Billingham, R. E., Brent, L., and Medawar, P. B.: "Actively acquired tolerance" of foreign cells. Nature 172:603, 1953.

Bloom, B. R., and Chase, M. W.: Transfer of delayed-type hypersensitivity: A critical review and experimental study in the guinea pig. Progr. Allergy 10:151, 1967.

Bruton, O. C.: Agammaglobulinemia. Pediatrics 9:772, 1952.

Burnet, F. M.: Theories of immunity. Perspect. Biol. Med. 3:447, 1960.

Burnet, M.: The mechanism of immunity. Sci. Am. 204:58, 1961.

Burnet, M.: The thymus gland. Sci. Am. 207:50, 1962.

Chase, M. W.: The cellular transfer of cutaneous hypersensitivity to tuberculin. Proc. Soc. Exp. Biol. Med. 59:134, 1945.

Chen, K. K., and Schmidt, C. F.: The action of ephedrine, the active principle of the Chinese drug, ma huang. J. Pharmacol. Exp. Ther. 24:339, 1925.

Claude, A.: The coming of age of the cell. Science 189:433, 1975.

Cooke, R., and VanderVeer, A., Jr.: Human sensitization. J. Immunol. 1:201, 1916.

Coons, A. H., Creech, H. J., and Jones, R. N.: Immunological properties of an antibody containing a fluorescent group. Proc. Soc. Exp. Biol. Med. 47:200, 1941.

Coons, A. H., and Kaplan, M. H.: Localization of antigen in tissue cells: Improvements in method for detection of antigen by means of fluorescent antibody. J. Exp. Med. 91:1, 1950.

Cooper, M. D., Gabrielson, A. E., and Good, R. A.: Role of the thymus and other central lymphoid tissues in immunological disease. Ann. Rev. Med. *18*:113, 1967.

Cooper, M. D., and Lawton, A. R., III: The development of the immune system. Sci. Am. *231*:58, 1974.

de Duve, C.: Exploring cells with a centrifuge. Science *189*:186, 1975.

DiGeorge, A. M.: Congenital abnormalities of developing immunological apparatus. *In* Good, R. A., and Bergsma, D. (eds.): Immunologic Deficiency Diseases in Man. Birth Defects. Original article series vol. IV, no. 1. Baltimore, Williams and Wilkins Co., February, 1968.

Doherty, P. C., and Zinkernagel, R. M.: A biological role for the major histocompatibility antigens. Lancet *1*:1406, 1975.

Edelman, G. M.: The structure and function of antibodies. Sci. Am. *223*:34, 1970.

Fitz, Reginald, H.: Zabdiel Boylston, inoculator, and the epidemic of smallpox in Boston in 1721. Johns Hopkins Hosp. Bull. *22*:315, 1911.

Flexner, S., and Noguchi, H.: Snake venom in relation to haemolysis, bacteriolysis and toxicity. J. Exp. Med. *6*:277, 1902.

Glick, B., Chang, J. S., and Jaap, R. C.: The bursa of Fabricius and antibody production. Poult. Sci. *35*:224, 1956.

Good, R. A.: Progress toward a cellular engineering. JAMA *214*:1289, 1970.

Good, R. A., and Finstod, J.: The development and involution of the lymphoid system and immunologic capacity. Trans. Am. Clin. Climatol. Assoc. *79*:69, 1967.

Harris, T. N., Grimm, E., Mertens, E., and Ehrich, W. E.: The role of the lymphocyte in antibody formation. J. Exp. Med. *81*:73, 1945.

Heidelberger, M., and Avery, O. T.: The soluble specific substance of pneumococcus. J. Exp. Med. *38*:73, 1923.

Holborow, E. J.: An ABC of Modern Immunology, 2nd ed. Boston, Little, Brown and Co., 1973.

Holmes, E. C., Eilber, F., and Morton, D. L.: Immunotherapy of malignancy in humans: current status. JAMA *232*:1052, 1975.

Ishizaka, K.: Human reaginic antibodies. Ann. Rev. Med. *21*:187, 1970.

Koffler, D., Schur, P. H., and Kunkel, H. G.: Immunological studies concerning the nephritis of systemic lupus erythematosus. J. Exp. Med. *126*:607, 1967.

Lawrence, H. S.: The transfer in humans of delayed skin sensitivity to streptococcal M substance and to tuberculin with disrupted leucocytes. J. Clin. Invest. *34*:219, 1955.

Lechevalier, H. A., and Solotorovsky, M.: Three Centuries of Microbiology. New York, Dover Publications, Inc., 1974.

Lerner, R. A., and Dixon, F. J.: The human lymphocyte as an experimental animal. Sci. Am., *228*:82, 1973.

Levey, R. H.: The thymus hormone. Sci. Am. *211*:66, 1964.

Levin, A. S., Spitler, L. E., Stites, D. P., and Fudenberg, H. H.: Wiskott-Aldrich syndrome, a genetically determined cellular immunologic deficiency: Clinical and laboratory responses to therapy with transfer factor. Proc. Natl. Acad. Sci. *67*:821, 1970.

Levin, A. S., Spitler, L. E., and Fudenberg, H. H.: Transfer factor therapy in immune deficiency states. Ann. Rev. Med. *23*:175, 1973.

Levine, B. B., Stember, R. H., and Fotino, M.: Ragweed hay fever: Genetic control and linkage to HL-A haplotypes. Science *178*:1201, 1972.

Marx, J. L.: Suppressor T cells: Role in immune regulation. Science *188*:245, 1975.

Marx, J. L.: Antibody structure: Now in three dimensions. Science *189*:1075, 1975.

Maurer, P. H.: Use of synthetic polymers of amino acids to study the basis of antigenicity. Prog. Allergy *8*:1, 1964.

McDevitt, H. O.: The genetics of the immune response. Hosp. Prac., April, 1973, p. 61.

McDevitt, H. O., and Benacceraf, B.: Genetic control of specific immune responses. Adv. Immunol. *11*:31, 1969.

Medawar, P. B.: Tolerance reconsidered—a critical survey. Transplant. Proc. *5*:7, 1973.

Medawar, P. B.: The new immunology. Hosp. Prac. *9*:48, 1974.

Miller, F.: Applications of immunology to understanding mechanisms of human disease. Fed. Proc. *34*:1635, 1975.

Mills, J. A., and Cooperband, S. R.: Lymphocyte physiology. Ann. Rev. Med. *22*:185, 1971.

Nobel Laureates for 1974. MD Pacific, December, 1974, p. 9.

Nobel Prize to cell explorers. MD Pacific, December, 1974, p. 9.

Norman, P. S.: The clinical significance of IgE. Hosp. Prac., August, 1975, p. 41.

Nossal, G. J. V.: How cells make antibodies. Sci. Am. *211*:106, 1964.

Nossal, G. J. V.: Mechanisms of antibody production. Ann. Rev. Med. *18*:81, 1967.

Notkins, A. L., and Koprowski, H.: How the immune response to a virus can cause disease. Sci. Am. *228*:22, 1973.

Novikoff, A. B.: The 1974 Nobel Prize for Physiology or Medicine, Science *186*:516, 1974.

Palade, G.: Intracellular aspects of the process of protein synthesis. Science *189*:347, 1975.

Peterson, R. D. A., and Good, R. A.: Immunologic deficiency diseases in man. Natl. Found. Symp. 4th, 1968, p. 370.

819

Putnam, F. W.: Immunoglobulin structure: Variability and homology. Science *163*:633, 1969.

Rackemann, F. M.: Robert Anderson Cooke, 1880–1960. Trans. Assoc. Am. Physicians *74*:11, 1961.

Reisfeld, R. A. and Kahan, B. D.: Markers of biological individuality. Sci. Am. *226*:28, 1972.

Rich, A. R.: Inflammation in resistance to infection. Arch. Pathol. *22*:228, 1936.

Rosenau, M. J., and Anderson, J. F.: A new toxic action of horse serum. J. Med. Research *15*:179, 1906.

Ruddy, S.: The human complement system. Medical World News, October 11, 1974, p. 53.

Salmon, D. E., and Smith, T.: On a new method of producing immunity from contagious disease. Proc. Biol. Soc. Washington *3*:29, 1886.

Samter, M. (ed.): Excerpts from Classics in Allergy. Published by Ross Laboratories to commemorate the 25th Anniversary of the American Academy of Allergy, Columbus, Ohio, 1969.

Schur, P. H., and Austen, K. F.: Complement in human disease. Ann. Rev. Med. *19*:1, 1968.

Singer, C., and Underwood, E. A.: A Short History of Medicine, 2nd ed. New York and Oxford, Oxford University Press, 1962.

Singer, S. J.: The specificity of antibodies. Sci. Am. *197*:99, 1957.

Solis-Cohn, S.: The use of adrenal substance in the treatment of asthma. JAMA *34*:1164, 1900.

Speirs, R. S.: How cells attack antigens. Sci. Am., *210*:58, 1964.

Tomasi, T. B., Jr., and DeCoteau, E.: Mucosal antibodies in respiratory and gastrointestinal disease. Adv. Intern. Med. *16*:401, 1970.

Tomasi, T. B., Jr., Tan, E. M., Solomon, A., and Prendergrant, R. A.: Characteristics of an immune system common to certain external secretions. J. Exp. Med. *121*:101, 1965.

Warner, N. L., and Szeuburg, A.: Immunologic studies on normally bursectomized and surgically thymectomized chickens: Dissociation of immunologic responsiveness. *In* Good, R. A., and Gabrielson, A. E. (eds.) The Thymus in Immunobiology. New York, Hoeber-Harper, 1964, pp. 395–411.

Weissmann, G.: The meaning for medical practitioners of the work of Claude, deDuve and Palade. Medical Tribune, December 11, 1974, p. 5.

Williams, C. A., Jr.: Immunoelectrophoresis. Sci. Am. *202*:130, 1960.

Witebesky, E., Rore, W. R., Terflan, K., Paine, J. R., and Egar, R. W.: Chronic thyroidity and autoimmunization. JAMA *164*:1439, 1957.

Chapter 27

Benison, S.: The history of polio research in the United States. *In* Halton, G. (ed.): The 20th Century Sciences. Studies in the Biography of Ideas. New York, W. W. Norton Co., 1972.

Bittner, J. J.: Some possible effects of nursing on the mammary gland tumor incidence in mice. Science *84*:162, 1936.

Bodian, D.: The paralytic plague. Sci. Am. *183*:22, 1950.

Bovarnick, M. R.: Rickettsiae. Sci. Am. *192*:74, 1955.

Broad-spectrum antivirals: coming closer? Hosp. Prac., November, 1974, p. 57.

Burnet, F. M.: Viruses. Sci. Am. *184*:43, 1951.

Burnet, M.: The structure of the influenza virus. Sci. Am. *196*:37, 1957.

Caverly, C. S.: Preliminary report of an epidemic of paralytic disease, occurring in Vermont, in the summer of 1894. Yale Med. J., November, 1894.

Channock, R. M.: Control of acute mycoplasmal and viral respiratory tract disease. Science *169*:248, 1970.

Cooper, L. Z.: German Measles. Sci. Am. *215*:30, 1966.

Corner, G.: A History of the Rockefeller Institute: 1901–1953. Origins and Growth. New York, The Rockefeller Institute Press, 1964.

Dalldorf, G., and Sickles, G. M.: An unidentified filtrable agent isolated from the feces of children with paralysis. Science *108*:61, 1948.

Dalton, A. J., Maloney, J. B., Porter, G. H., Frei, E., and Mitchell, E.: Studies on murine and human leukemia. Trans. Assoc. Am. Physicians *77*:52, 1964.

Delbruck, M., and Bailey, W. T., Jr.: Induced mutations in bacterial viruses. Cold Spring Harbor Symposium Quant. Biol. *11*:33, 1946.

Dulbecco, R.: Production of plaques in monolayer tissue cultures by single particles of an animal virus. Proc. Natl. Acad. Sci. *38*:747, 1952.

Edgar, R. S., and Epstein, R. H.: The genetics of a bacterial virus. Sci. Am. *212*:71, 1965.

Editorial. Virus hepatitis updated. Lancet *1*:1365, 1975.

Eichorn, M. D.: Rubella: Will vaccination prevent birth defects? Science *173*:710, 1971.

Eisenberg, M., and Crowe, J. D.: Measles and rubella eradication in Alaska. JAMA *235*:179, 1976.

Enders, J. F., Weller, T. H., and Robbins, F. C.: Cultivation of the Lansing strain of poliomyelitis virus in cultures of various human embryonic tissues. Science *109*:85, 1949.

820

Friend, C.: The isolation of a virus causing a malignant disease of the hematopoietic system. Proc. Am. Assoc. Cancer Res. 2:106, 1956.

Gajdusek, D. C.: Slow-virus infections of the nervous system. N. Engl. J. Med. 276:392, 1967.

Gross, L.: Mouse leukemia. Ann. N.Y. Acad. Sci. 54:1184, 1952.

Gross, L.: Transmission of mouse leukemia virus through milk of virus-infected C_3H female mice. Proc. Soc. Exp. Biol. Med. 109:83, 1952.

Hahon, N.: Selected Papers on Virology. Englewood Cliffs, N.J., Prentice-Hall Inc., 1964.

Henle, G., and Henle, W.: Immunofluorescence in cells derived from Burkitt's lymphoma. J. Bacteriol. 913:1248, 1966.

Henle, G., Henle, W., and Diehl, V.: Relation of Burkitt's tumor–associated herpes-type virus to infectious mononucleosis. Proc. Natl. Acad. Sci. 59:94, 1968.

Hershey, A. D., and Chase, M.: Independent function of viral protein and nucleic acid in growth of bacteriophage. J. Gen. Physiol. 36:39, 1952.

Heubner, R. J., Rowe, W. P., and Lara, W. T.: Oncogenic effects in hamsters of human adenovirus types 12 and 18. Proc. Natl. Acad. Sci. 48:2051, 1962.

Hilleman, M. R.: Toward control of viral infections of man. Science 164:506, 1969.

Hirst, G. K.: The agglutination of red cells by allantoic fluid of chick embryos infected with influenza virus. Science 94:22, 1941.

Horne, R. W.: The structure of viruses. Sci. Am. 208:48, 1963.

Horsfall, F.: Thomas Milton Rivers. Trans. Assoc. Am. Physicians 76:16, 1963.

Hoskins, M.: A protective action of neurotropic against viscerotropic yellow fever virus in *Macacus rhesus*. Am. J. Trop. Med. 15:675, 1935.

Jacob, F., and Wollman, E. L.: Viruses and genes. Sci. Am. 204:93, 1961.

Leader, R. W., and Hurvitz, A. I.: Interspecies patterns of slow virus diseases. Ann. Rev. Med. 23:191, 1972.

Lechevalier, H. A., and Solotorovsky, M.: Three Centuries of Microbiology. New York, Dover Publications, Inc., 1974.

Maloney, J. B.: Recovery of infectious nucleic acid from a virus-induced lymphoid neoplasm. Acta Un. Int. Cancer 19:250, 1961.

Marks, G., and Beatty, W. K.: The Story of Medicine in America. New York, Charles Scribner's Sons, 1973.

Maugh, T. H.: II. Hepatitis B: A new vaccine ready for human testing. Science 188:137, 1975.

Melnick, J. L.: A new era in polio research. Sci. Am. 187:27, 1952.

Nirenberg, M. W., and Matthaei, J. H.: The dependence of cell-free protein synthesis in *E. coli* upon naturally occurring or synthetic polyribonucleotides. Proc. Natl. Acad. Sci. 47:1588, 1961.

Paul, J.: The History of Poliomyelitis. New Haven, Yale University Press, 1971.

Reed, W.: Recent researches concerning the etiology, propagation and prevention of yellow fever by the U.S. Army Commission. J. Hyg. 2:101, 1902.

Riedman, S. R., and Gustafson, E. T.: Portraits of Nobel Prize Laureates in Medicine and Physiology. New York, London, and Toronto: Abelard-Schuman, 1963.

Rivers, T. M.: Tom Rivers: Reflection on a Life in Medicine and Science. An Oral History Memoir prepared by Saul Benison. Cambridge, Mass., MIT Press, 1967.

Rivers, T. M., and Berry, G. P.: Psittacosis pneumonia experimentally induced in monkeys. Trans. Assoc. Am. Physicians 46:197, 1931.

Rivers, T. M., and Schwentker, F. F.: Vaccination of laboratory workers against psittacosis. Trans. Assoc. Am. Physicians 49:104, 1934.

Rous, P.: Transmission of a malignant new growth by means of a cell-free filtrate. JAMA 56:198, 1911.

Sabin, A. B.: Contributions of virology to human medicine during the past forty years. Isr. J. Med. Sci. 1:1090, 1965.

Salk, J. E.: Vaccines for poliomyelitis. Sci. Am. 192:42, 1955.

Schaffer, F. L., and Schwerdt, C. E.: Crystallization of purified MEF-1 poliomyelitis virus particles. Proc. Natl. Acad. Sci. 41:1020, 1955.

Sever, J., and White, L. R.: Intrauterine viral infections. Ann. Rev. Med. 19:471, 1968.

Shafer, N., and Heller, L.: Australia antigen: Update. Med. Counterpoint, Aug./Sept., 1974, p. 29.

Shope, R. E.: An intermediate host for the swine influenza virus. J. Exp. Med. 54:373, 1931.

Sinsheimer, R. L.: A single-stranded DNA from bacteriophage PHI × 174. J. Mol. Biol. 50:43, 1959.

Smith, R. T., and Bausher, J. C.: Epstein-Barr virus infection in relation to infectious mononucleosis and Burkitt's lymphoma. Ann. Rev. Med. 25:39, 1972.

Stanley, W. M.: The isolation and properties of crystalline tobacco mosaic virus. Nobel Lecture, December 12, 1946. Nobel Lectures, Chemistry, 1942–62. Amsterdam, London, and New York: Elsevier Publishing Co., 1964, p. 137.

Sternberg, G. M.: Practical results of bacteriological researches. Trans. Assoc. Am. Physicians 7:68, 1892.

821

Stewart, S. E.: Neoplasms in mice inoculated with cell-free extracts or filtrates of leukemic mouse tumors. I. Neoplasms of the parotid and adrenal glands. J. Natl. Cancer Inst. *15:* 1391, 1954.

Theiler, M.: Studies on the action of yellow fever virus in mice. Ann. Trop. Med. Parasitol. *24:*247, 1930.

Trentin, J. J., Yabe, Y., and Taylor, G.: The quest for human cancer viruses. Science *137:*835, 1962.

Witte, J. J., and Axnick, N. W.: The benefits from 10 years of measles immunization in the United States. Pub. Health Rep. *90:*205, 1975.

Wood, W. B., and Edgar, R. S.: Building a bacterial virus. Sci. Am. *217:*61, 1967.

Woodruff, A. M., and Goodpasture, E. W.: The susceptibility of the chorioallantoic membrane of chick embryos to infection with the fowl-pox virus. Am. J. Pathol. *7:*209, 1931.

Zinder, N. D., and Lederberg, J.: Genetic exchange in salmonella. J. Bacteriol. *64:*679, 1952.

Chapter 28

Ames, B. N.: Letter. Science *191:*241, 1967.

Ames, B. N., Durston, W. E., Yamasaki, E., and Lee, F. D.: Carcinogens as mutagens: A simple test system combining liver homogenates for activation and bacteria for detection. Proc. Natl. Acad. Sci. *70:*2281, 1973.

Ayres, S. M.: Cigarette smoking and lung diseases: An update. Basics of Resp. Dis. *3*(5):1, 1975.

Bertino, J. R., and Johns, D. G.: Folate antagonists. Ann. Rev. Med. *18:*27, 1967.

Bonadonna, G., et al.: Combination chemotherapy as an adjuvant treatment for operable breast cancer. N. Engl. J. Med., *294:*405, 1976.

Burchenal, J. H.: Burkitt's tumor as a stalking horse for leukemia. JAMA *222:*1165, 1972.

Burchenal, J. H., Dowling, M. D., Jr., and Tan, C. T. C.: Treatment of acute lymphoblastic leukemia. Ann. Rev. Med. *23:*77, 1972.

Cairns, J.: The cancer problem: All cancers appear to be caused by exposure to factors in the environment. Sci. Am. *233:*64, Nov., 1975.

Capizzi, R. L., Bertino, J. R., and Handschumacher, R. E.: L-Asparaginase. Ann. Rev. Med. *21:*433, 1970.

Carbone, P. P.: Non-Hodgkin's lymphoma: Recent observations on natural history and intensive treatment. Cancer *30:*1511, 1972a.

Carbone, P. P.: Combination chemotherapy for patients with malignant lymphoma. JAMA *222:*1171, 1972b.

Corner, G. W.: A History of the Rockefeller Institute: 1901–1953. Origins and Growth. New York, The Rockefeller Institute Press, 1964.

Culliton, B. J.: Cancer virus theories: Focus of research debate. Science *177:*44, 1972.

Culliton, B. J.: Breast cancer: Reports of new therapy are greatly exaggerated. Science *19:*1029, 1976.

Dao, T. L.: Ablation therapy for hormone-dependent tumors. Ann. Rev. Med. *23:*1, 1972.

DeVita, V. T., Jr., Serpick, A. A., and Carbone, P. P.: Combination chemotherapy in the treatment of advanced Hodgkin's disease. Ann. Intern. Med. *73:*881, 1970.

Djerassi, I.: Platelet transfusions and supportive care: A requirement for currently effective chemotherapy. JAMA *222:*1172, 1972.

Dodds, E. C., et al.: Synthetic oestrogenic compounds related to stilbene and diphenylethane. Part I. Proc. R. Soc. Lond., Series B, *127:*140, 1939.

Doll, R.: Pott and the prospects for prevention. Br. J. Cancer *32:*263, 1975.

Dulbecco, R.: The induction of cancer by viruses. Sci. Am. *216:*28, Apr., 1967.

Eckhart, W.: The 1975 Nobel Prize for physiology or medicine. Science *190:*650, 1975.

Editorial. Drugs for common cancers. Br. Med. J. *2:*235, 1975.

Farber, S.: Chemotherapy in the treatment of leukemia and Wilms' tumor. JAMA *198:*826, 1966.

Farber, S., Diamond, L. K., Mercer, R. D., Sylvester, R. F., Jr., and Wolfe, J. A.: Temporary remissions in acute leukemia in children produced by folic acid antagonist, 4-amino pteroylglutamic acid (aminopterin). N. Engl. J. Med. *238:*787, 1948.

Fisher, B., Carbone, P. P., Economou, S. G., et al.: L-phenylalanine mustard in the management of primary breast cancer. N. Engl. J. Med. *292:*117, 1975.

Franklin, A. L., Stokstad, E. L. R., and Jukes, T. H.: Acceleration of pteroylglutamic acid in mice and chicks by chemical antagonists. Proc. Soc. Exp. Biol. Med. *65:*368, 1947.

Frei, E., III: Combination chemotherapy of acute leukemia and Hodgkin's disease. JAMA *222:* 1168, 1972a.

Frei, E., III: Combination cancer therapy (Presidential Address). Cancer Res. *32:*2593, 1972b.

Frei, E., III: Cancer research—controversy, progress and prospects. (Editorial.) N. Engl. J. Med. *293:*146, 1975.

Freireich, E. J.: Research contributions to combination chemotherapy. JAMA *222*:1169, 1972.

Freireich, E. J., et al.: The effect of 6-mercaptopurine on the duration of steroid-induced remissions in acute leukemia: A model for evaluation of other potentially useful therapy. Blood *21*:699, 1963.

Gilman, A., and Philips, F. S.: The biological actions and therapeutic applications of the betachloroethyl amines and sulphides. Science *103*:409, 1946.

Gross, L.: Oncogenic Viruses, 2nd ed. Oxford, Pergamon Press, Ltd., 1970.

Gross, L.: The role of viruses in the etiology of cancer and leukemia. JAMA *230*:1029, 1974a.

Gross, L.: Facts and theories on viruses causing cancer and leukemia. Proc. Natl. Acad. Sci. *71*:2013, 1974b.

Gutman, A. B., and Gutman, E. B.: An "acid" phosphatase occurring in the serum of patients with metastasizing carcinoma of the prostate gland. J. Clin. Invest. *17*:473, 1938.

Henle, G., Henle, W., and Diehl, V.: Relation of Burkitt's tumor-associated herpes-type virus to infectious mononucleosis. Proc. Natl. Acad. Sci. *59*:94, 1968.

Hertz, R.: Quantitative monitoring of chemotherapy of endocrine tumors by hormone assay. JAMA *222*:1163, 1972.

Holland, J. F.: Combination therapy of acute lymphocytic leukemia of children. JAMA *222*: 1169, 1972.

Holland, J. F.: Major advances in breast-cancer therapy. (Editorial.) N. Engl. J. Med. *294*:440, 1976.

Huggins, C.: Endocrine-induced regression of cancers. Nobel Lecture, December 13, 1966. *In* Les Prix Nobel en 1966. Stockholm, The Nobel Foundation, 1967, p. 172.

Huggins, C., and Clark, P. J.: Quantitative studies of prostatic secretion. II. The effect of castration and of estrogen injection on the normal and on the hyperplastic prostate glands of dogs. J. Exp. Med. *72*:747, 1940.

Huggins, C., Stevens, R. E., and Hodges, C. V.: Studies on prostatic cancer. II. The effects of castration on advanced carcinoma of the prostate gland. Arch. Surg. *43*:209, 1941.

Jukes, T. H., Franklin, A. L., and Stokstad, E. L. R.: Pteroylglutamic acid antagonists. Ann. N.Y. Acad. Sci. *52*:1336, 1950.

Kay, H. D.: Phosphatases in growth and diseases of bone. Physiol. Rev. *12*:384, 1932.

Li, M. C.: Chemotherapeutic and immunological aspects of choriocarcinoma. JAMA *222*:1163, 1972.

Li, M. C., Hertz, R., and Spencer, D. B.: Effect of methotrexate therapy upon choriocarcinoma. Proc. Soc. Exp. Biol. Med. *93*:361, 1956.

Mashburn, L. T., and Wriston, J. C., Jr.: Tumor inhibitory effect of L-asparaginase from *Escherichia coli*. Arch. Biochem. *105*:450, 1964.

Matas, A. J., Simmons, R. L., and Jajarian, J. A.: Chronic antigenic stimulation, herpes virus infection and cancer in transplant recipients. Lancet *1*:1277, 1975.

Maugh, T. H.: II. Leukemia: A second human tumor virus. Science *187*:335, 1975.

McCann, J., Spingarn, N. E., Kobori, J., and Ames, B. N.: Detection of carcinogens as mutagens: Bacterial tester strains with R-factor plasmids. Proc. Natl. Acad. Sci. *72*:979, 1975.

Miller, J. A.: Carcinogenesis by chemicals: An overview. G. H. A. Clowes Memorial Lecture. Cancer Res. *30*:559, 1970.

Naylor, B.: The history of exfoliative cancer cytology. Univ. Mich. Med. Bull. *26*:289, 1960.

Nowell, P. C., and Hungerford, D. A.: Chromosome studies on normal and leukemic human leukocytes. J. Nat. Cancer Inst. *25*:85, 1960.

Pinkel, D.: Total therapy of acute lymphocytic leukemia. JAMA *222*:1170, 1972.

Porter, K. R., and Novikoff, A. B.: The 1974 Nobel Prize for physiology or medicine. Science *186*:516, 1974.

Rauscher, F. J., Jr.: Research and the national cancer program. Science *189*:115, 1975.

Rhoads, C. P.: Nitrogen mustards in the treatment of neoplastic disease. JAMA *131*:656, 1946.

Ross, G., Goldstein, D. P., et al.: Sequential use of methotrexate and actinomycin D in the treatment of metastatic choriocarcinoma and related trophoblastic diseases in women. Am. J. Obstet. Gynecol. *93*:223, 1965.

Rous, P.: The challenge to man of the neoplastic cell. Science *157*:24, 1967.

Rubin, H.: Carcinogenicity tests. (Letter.) Science *191*:241, 1976.

Sandberg, A. S., and Hossfeld, D. K.: Chromosomal abnormalities in human neoplasia. Ann. Rev. Med. *21*:379, 1970.

Shimkin, M. B.: Science and Cancer. Washington, D.C., U.S. DHEW Publication No. (NIH) 74-568, Second revision, 1973.

Shimkin, M. B.: Some historical landmarks in cancer epidemiology. *In* Schottenfeld, D. (ed.): Cancer Epidemiology and Prevention. Springfield, Ill., Charles C Thomas, 1975, p. 60.

Simone, J., Aur, R. J. A., Hustin, H. O., and Pinkel, D.: "Total therapy" — studies of acute lymphocytic leukemia in children. Cancer *30*:1488, 1972.

Skipper, H.: Thoughts on cancer chemotherapy and combination modality therapy. JAMA *230*:1033, 1974.

823

Spiegelman, S.: Ribonucleic acid: I. The test-tube synthesis of a viral nucleic acid. II. The development and use of molecular hybridization. JAMA *230*:1036, 1974.

Strickland, S. P.: Politics, Science and Dread Disease—A Short History of United States Research Policy. Cambridge, Mass., Harvard University Press, 1972.

Tagnon, H. J., Whitmore, W. F., Jr., and Shulman, N. R.: Fibrinolysis in metastatic cancer of the prostate. Cancer *5*:9, 1952.

Triolo, V. A., and Shimkin, M. B.: The American Cancer Society and cancer research origins and organization—1913–1943. Cancer Res. *29*:1615, 1969.

Weissmann, G.: The meaning for medical practitioners of the work of Claude, de Duve and Palade. Med. Tribune, Dec. 11, 1974, p. 5

Zubrod, C. G.: History of the cancer chemotherapy program. Cancer Chemother. Rep. *50*:349, 1966.

Zubrod, C. G.: The national program for cancer chemotherapy. JAMA 222:161, 1972.

Zubrod, C. G., Scheparts, S., Leiter, J., et al.: The chemotherapy program of the National Cancer Institute: History, analysis and plans. Cancer Chemother. Rep. *40*:349, 1960.

Chapter 29

Aserinsky, E., and Kleitman, N.: Regularly occurring periods of eye motility, and concomitant phenomena during sleep. Science *118*:273, 1953.

Axelrod, J.: Cyclic AMP in brain: Role in synaptic transmission. Science *178*:1188, 1972.

Axelrod, J.: Neurotransmitters. Sci. Am. *230*:58, 1974.

Baker, P. F.: The nerve axon. Sci. Am. *214*:74, 1966.

Barker, L. F.: The nervous system and its constituent neurons. New York, D. Appleton and Co., 1899.

Brady, J. V.: Ulcers in "executive" monkeys. Sci. Am. *199*:95, 1958.

Brady, R. O.: Cerebral lipidoses. Ann. Rev. Med. *21*:317, 1970.

Eccles, J.: The synapse. Sci. Am. *214*:74, 1966.

Eccles, J. C.: Neurosciences: Our brains and our future. *In* Kone, E. H., and Jordan, H. S. (eds.): The Greatest Adventure: Basic Research that Shapes our Lives. New York, Rockefeller University Press, 1974, p. 70.

Freidman, D. X.: The psychopharmacology of hallucinogenic agents. Ann. Rev. Med. *20*:409, 1969.

Harrison, R.: The outgrowth of the nerve fiber as a mode of protoplasmic movement. J. Exp. Zool. (Phila.) *9*:784, 1910.

Holman, R. B., Elliott, E. R., and Barcher, J. D.: Neuroregulators and sleep mechanisms. Ann. Rev. Med. *26*:499, 1975.

Howell, W. H.: Vagus inhibition of the heart and its relation to the inorganic salts of the blood. Am. J. Physiol. *15*:280, 1905.

Howell, W. H.: The effect of vagus stimulation on the output of potassium from the heart. Am. J. Physiol. *35*:131, 1906a.

Howell, W. H., and Duke, W. W.: Experiments in the isolated heart to show the relation of the inorganic salt and the action of its nerves. Am. J. Physiol. *35*:131, 1906b.

Jacobson, M., and Hunt, R. K.: The origins of nerve-cell specificity. Sci. Am. *228*:26, 1973.

Kumura, D.: The asymmetry of the human brain. Sci. Am. *228*:70, 1973.

Levi-Montalcini, R.: Growth control of nerve cells by a protein factor and its antiserum. Science *143*:105, 1964.

Marx, J. L.: Nerve growth factor: Regulatory role examined. Science 185:930, 1974.

Meek, W. J.: A brief history of American physiology. Marquette Med. Rev. *1*:51, 1937.

Miller, W. H., Ratliff, F., and Hartline, H. K.: How cells receive stimuli. Sci. Am. *205*:222, 1961.

Mountcastle, V.: Philip Bard. The Physiologist *18*:1, 1975a.

Mountcastle, V.: The view from within: Pathways to the study of perception. Johns Hopkins Med. J. *136*:109, 1975b.

Riedman, S. R., and Gustafson, E. T.: Portraits of Nobel Prize Laureates in Medicine and Physiology. New York, London, Toronto, Abelard-Schuman, 1963.

Sperry, R.: The growth of nerve circuits. Sci. Am. *201*:68, 1959.

Sperry, R.: The great cerebral commissure. Sci. Am. *210*:42, 1964.

Young, M., et al: Secretion of a nerve growth factor by primary chick fibroblast cultures. Science *187*:361, 1975.

Chapter 30

Brandt, J. L.: The National Mental Health Act of 1946. A retrospect. Bull. Hist. Med. *39*:231, 1965.

Casamajor, L.: Notes for an intimate history of neurology and psychiatry in America. J. Nerv. Ment. Dis. *98*:600, 1943.

Cowles, E.: The advancement of psychiatry in America. Am. J. Insanity 52:36, 1895.

Earle, P.: An address before the Berkshire Medical Institute, November 24, 1863: Psychologic medicine: Its importance as a part of the medical curriculum. Utica, New York, 1867.

Eisenberg, L.: Psychiatric intervention. Sci. Am. 229:116, 1973.

Freidman, D. X.: The psychopharmacology of hallucinogenic agents. Ann. Rev. Med. 20:409, 1969.

Hamilton, S. W.: The history of American mental hospitals. In Zilboorg. G. (ed.): One Hundred Years of American Psychiatry. New York, Columbia University Press, 1944, p. 167.

Howe, H. S.: Progress in neurology and psychiatry during the first half of the twentieth century. N.Y. J. Med. 51:96, 1951.

Imboden, J. B.: Psychiatry in medicine. In Harvey, A. McG., et al. (eds.): Principles and Practice of Medicine, 19th ed. New York, Appleton-Century-Crofts, 1976, p. 1605.

Mandell, A. J., and Spooner, C. E.: Psychochemical research studies in man. Science 162:1442, 1968.

Overholser, W.: The founding and the founders of the Association. In Zilboorg., G. (ed.): One Hundred Years of American Psychiatry. New York, Columbia University Press, 1944, p. 74.

Romano, J. R.: Basic contributions to medicine by research in psychiatry. JAMA 178:1147, 1961.

Romano, J. R.: The teaching of psychiatry to medical students: Past, present and future. Am. J. Psychiatry 125:90, 1970.

Romano, J.: American Psychiatry, Past, Present, and Future. Keynote Address, Southeastern Divisional Meeting, The American Psychiatric Association, The Neuropsychiatric Society of Virginia. Commemorating the Bicentennial of America's First Public Mental Hospital, Williamsburg, Va., October 8, 1973a.

Romano, J. R.: Psychiatry and medicine, 1973. Ann. Intern. Med. 79:582, 1973b.

Romano, J. R.: Psychiatric and neurologic services in the Peter Bent Brigham Hospital. Personal communication, 1975.

Shopsin, B., and Gershon, S.: The current status of lithium in psychiatry. Am. J. Med. Sci. 268:306, 1974.

Shryock, R. H.: The beginnings: From colonial days to the foundation of the American Psychiatric Association. In Zilboorg, G. (ed.): One Hundred Years of American Psychiatry. New York, Columbia University Press, 1944, p. 1.

Stallones, R. A.: Community health. (Editorial.) Science 175:839, 1972.

Whitehorn, J. C.: A century of psychiatric research in America. In Zilboorg, G. (ed.): One Hundred Years of American Psychiatry. New York, Columbia University Press, 1944, p. 167.

Chapter 31

Boldt, H. J.: The management of laparotomy patients and their modified after-treatment. N.Y. Med. J. 86:145, 1907.

Breo, D.: Hospital costs, stays vary widely across U.S. Am. Med. News March 22, 1976.

Cummings, M. M.: Your National Library of Medicine. JAMA 233:1359, 1975. [See also the 98-page brochure released in 1976 by the Department of Health, Education and Welfare, entitled *Communication in the Service of American Health: A Bicentennial Report from the National Library of Medicine* (DHEW Publication No. (NIH) 76-256).]

Dock, W.: The evil sequelae of complete bed rest. JAMA 125:1083, 1944.

Eastman, N. J.: The abuse of rest in obstetrics. JAMA 125:1077, 1944.

Firman, G. H., and Goldstein, M. S.: The future of chiropractic: A psychosocial view. N. Engl. J. Med. 293:639, 1975.

Ghormley, R. K.: The abuse of rest in bed in orthopedic surgery. JAMA 125:1085, 1944.

Gray, L. A.: Ephraim McDowell—father of abdominal surgery. Reprint of paper read before the Filson Club, Louisville, Ky., January 8, 1968.

Growth in education for family practice. JAMA 226:896, 1973.

Guerriero, W. F.: A maternal welfare program for New Orleans. Am. J. Obstet. Gynecol. 46:312, 1943.

Guerriero, W. F.: Early controlled ambulation in the puerperium. Am. J. Obstet. Gynecol. 51:210, 1946.

Halsted, W. S.: Radical cure of inguinal hernia. Johns Hopkins Hosp. Bull. 1:12, 1889.

Halsted, W. S.: The radical cure of inguinal hernia in the male. Ann. Surg. 17:542, 1893.

Harrison, T. R.: Abuse of rest as a therapeutic measure for patients with cardiovascular disease. JAMA 125:1075, 1944.

Hawley, P. R.: The American College of Surgeons. Practitioner 172:560, 1954.

Hawley, P. R.: Birth of the American College of Surgeons. Bull. Am. Coll. Surgeons 40:299, 1955.

Hellman, L. M., Kohl, S. G., and Palmer, J.: Early hospital discharge in obstetrics. Lancet 1:227, 1962.

Kaufman, M.: Homeopathy in America: The Rise and Fall of a Medical Heresy. Baltimore, Johns Hopkins University Press, 1971.

Martin, C. F.: My recollections of the period, 1925–29. *In* Morgan, W. G. (ed.): The American College of Physicians: The First Quarter Century. Philadelphia, American College of Physicians, 1940, Chap. VIII.

Menninger, K.: The abuse of rest in psychiatry. JAMA *125*:1087, 1944.

Powers, J. H.: The abuse of rest as a therapeutic measure in surgery; early postoperative activity and rehabilitation. JAMA *125*:1078, 1944.

Powers, J. H.: Evaluation of early postoperative activity. Bull. N.Y. Acad. Med. *22*:38, 1946.

Powers, J. H.: Postoperative thromboembolism: Some remarks on the influence of early ambulation. Am. J. Med. *3*:224, 1947.

Powers, J. H.: Early ambulation: Its influence on postoperative complications and return to work following hernioplasty. Ann. N.Y. Acad. Sci. *73*:524, 1958.

Powers, J. H.: Personal communication, 1976

Ries, E.: Some radical changes in the after-treatment of celiotomy cases. JAMA *33*:454, 1899.

Swanson, A. G.: Mandatory requirement versus voluntary opportunity for service in the National Health Service Corps. (Editorial.) J. Med. Educ. *50*:406, 1975.

Theobald, G. W.: Home on the second day: The Bradford experiment. Br. Med. J. *2*:1364, 1959.

Epilogue

Blendon, R. J.: The changing role of private philanthropy in health affairs. N. Engl. J. Med. *292*:946, 1975.

Bunker, J. P.: When the medical interests of society are in conflict with those of the individual, who wins? Pharos *39*:64, 1976.

Burger, E. J., Jr.: Science for medicine—time for another reappraisal. Fed. Proc. *34*:2106, 1975.

Cullen, D. J., Ferrara, L. C., Briggs, B. A., Walker, P. F., and Gilbert, J.: Survival, hospitalization charges and follow-up results in critically ill patients. N. Engl. J. Med. *294*:982, 1976.

Edwards, C. C.: The federal government in health—a personal view of current problems and future need. N. Engl. J. Med. *292*:559, 1975.

Fein, R.: Some health policy issues: One economist's view. Pub. Health Rep. *90*:387, 1975.

Hicks, N.: Doctors strong, patients weak, costs up. New York Times, Apr. 26, 1976.

McNerney, W. J.: Public and private sectors under National Health Insurance. Arch. Int. Med. *135*:910, 1975.

Morison, R. S.: Some reflections on research training and medical education. Pharos *38*:107, 1975.

Netsky, M. G.: Dying in a system of "good care"—case report and analysis. Pharos *39*:57, 1976.

Schwartz, H.: Whatever happened to the "national health care crisis." Arch. Int. Med. *135*:927, 1975a.

Schwartz, H.: Rationing medical care. New York Times, Sept. 16, 1975b.

Thomas, L.: Notes of a biology watcher: The technology of medicine. N. Engl. J. Med. *285*:1366, 1971.

Index

Numbers in *italics* refer to illustrations; numbers followed by a (t) indicate tables. See also the Chronology (p. 783) for further information.

830

837

839

843

DATE DUE